Biopsychosocial Factors in Obstetrics and Gynaecology

Biopsychosocial Factors in Obstetrics and Gynaecology

Edited by

Leroy C. Edozien
Manchester Academic Health Science Centre

P. M. Shaughn O'Brien
Keele University School of Medicine

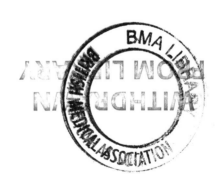

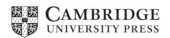

CAMBRIDGE
UNIVERSITY PRESS

CAMBRIDGE
UNIVERSITY PRESS

University Printing House, Cambridge CB2 8BS, United Kingdom

One Liberty Plaza, 20th Floor, New York, NY 10006, USA

477 Williamstown Road, Port Melbourne, VIC 3207, Australia

4843/24, 2nd Floor, Ansari Road, Daryaganj, Delhi – 110002, India

79 Anson Road, #06–04/06, Singapore 079906

Cambridge University Press is part of the University of Cambridge.

It furthers the University's mission by disseminating knowledge in the pursuit of education, learning, and research at the highest international levels of excellence.

www.cambridge.org
Information on this title: www.cambridge.org/9781107120143
DOI: 10.1017/9781316341261

First published 2017

Printed in the United Kingdom by TJ International Ltd. Padstow Cornwall

A catalogue record for this publication is available from the British Library.

Library of Congress Cataloging-in-Publication Data
Names: Edozien, Leroy C., editor. | O'Brien, P. M. Shaughn, editor.
Title: Biopsychosocial factors in obstetrics and gynaecology / edited by Leroy C. Edozien, P.M. Shaughn O'Brien.
Description: Cambridge, United Kingdom ; New York, NY : University Printing House, 2017. | Includes bibliographical references and index.
Identifiers: LCCN 2017024673 | ISBN 9781107120143
Subjects: | MESH: Genital Diseases, Female – psychology | Pregnancy Complications – psychology | Women's Health | Psychophysiology – methods
Classification: LCC RG126 | NLM WP 140 | DDC 618.1/0651–dc23
LC record available at https://lccn.loc.gov/2017024673

ISBN 978-1-107-12014-3 Hardback

....

LCE: To my daughter, Nicole

PMSO: To all the patients who have participated
in my research studies over the past 40 years

Contents

Contributors

Suzanne Abraham
Department of Obstetrics and Gynaecology, Royal North Shore Hospital, Sydney, Australia

Rachel Adams
Senior House Officer, Lewisham and Greenwich NHS Trust

Susan Ayers
Centre for Maternal and Child Health Research, City University, London, UK

Alison Barrett
Consultant Obstetrician and Gynaecologist, Waikato Hospital, Hamilton, NZ

Susan Bewley
Professor of Women's Health King's College London, and Sexual Offences Examiner The Havens Sexual Assault Referral Centre London

Olanike Bika
Consultant Obstetrician and Gynaecologist, Rotherham NHS Foundation Trust Hospital, UK

Theresa Bourne
Associate Professor, Middlesex University, London, UK

Louise D. Bryant
Associate Professor in Medical Psychology, Leeds Institute of Health Sciences, University of Leeds, UK

Gail Busby
St Mary's Hospital, Manchester, UK

Christian Cerra
Specialist Trainee in Obstetrics and Gynaecology, North Western Deanery, UK

Rebecca J. Cook
Professor Emerita, Faculty Chair in International Human Rights, University of Toronto, Canada

Jason Cooper
Consultant Gynaecologist, Royal Stoke University Hospital, UK

Zoe Darwin
School of Healthcare, University of Leeds, UK

Denise Defey
School of Midwifery
(School of Medicine), University of Uruguay. Chair, Dept. of Perinatal Psychology, Agora Institute, Uruguay

Bernard M. Dickens
Professor Emeritus of Health Law and Policy, Faculty of Law, Faculty of Medicine and Joint Centre for Bioethics, University of Toronto, Canada

Claudine Domoney
Consultant Obstetrician and Gynaecologist, Chelsea and Westminster Hospital, UK

Gail Dovey-Pearce
Consultant Clinical Psychologist, Child Health, Northumbria Healthcare NHS Foundation Trust & Associate Researcher, Newcastle University

Leroy C. Edozien
Consultant in Obstetrics and Gynaecology at the Central Manchester University Hospitals NHS Trust and Manchester Academic Health Science Centre, UK

Jane Fisher
Jean Hailes Professor of Women's Health, Monash University, Australia

Elizabeth Ford
Research Fellow in Primary Care Epidemiology, Brighton and Sussex Medical School, University of Brighton, UK

William D. Fraser
Professor, Department of Obstetrics and Gynecology, Université de Sherbrooke, Canada

Leila Frodsham
Consultant Gynaecologist and Psychosexual Medicine Lead, Guy's and St Thomas' NHS Trust, London, UK

Zeiad el Gizawy
Consultant Obstetrician and Gynaecologist, Royal Stoke University Hospital, UK

Andrea Goddard
Department of Paediatrics, St Mary's Hospital, London, UK

Helen Hall
Faculty of Medicine, Nursing and Health Sciences, Monash University, Australia

Karin Hammarberg
Jean Hailes Research Unit, School of Public Health and Preventive Medicine, Monash University, Australia

Nancy A. Haug
PGSP-Stanford University Psy.D. Consortium, Palo Alto University, Palo Alto, CA, USA

Mary Hepburn
Independent Consultant Obstetrician and Gynaecologist, Scotland, UK

Kristina Hofberg
Consultant Perinatal Psychiatrist, St George's Hospital, Stafford, UK

Caroline Hunter
Midwifery Tutor, Florence Nightingale Faculty of Nursing and Midwifery, King's College London, UK

Myra S. Hunter
Institute of Psychiatry, Psychology and Neuroscience, King's College London, UK

Tereza Indrielle-Kelly
Specialist Trainee, Royal Stoke University Hospital, Staffordshire, UK

Julie Jomeen
Professor of Midwifery, University of Hull, UK

Suman Kadian
Consultant Obstetrician and Gynaecologist, Royal Stoke University Hospital, UK

Deepthi Lavu
Specialist Trainee and Academic Clinical Fellow, Royal Stoke University Hospital, Staffordshire, UK

Lih-Mei Liao
Women's Health Division, University College London Hospitals NHS Foundation Trust, UK

Amali Lokugamage
Consultant Obstetrician and Gynaecologist, Whittington Hospital, London, UK

David McCormack
Maudsley Hospital, South London, and Maudsley NHS Foundation Trust, and Department of Psychological Medicine, King's College London, UK

Linda McGowan
Professor in Applied Health Research, School of Healthcare, University of Leeds

Elinor Milby
University of Liverpool, UK

Lamiya Mohiyiddeen
Consultant Gynaecologist, Department of Reproductive Medicine, St Mary's Hospital, Manchester, UK

Caroline E. North
Consultant Obstetrician and Gynaecologist, Royal Stoke University Hospital, UK

P. M. Shaughn O'Brien
Professor of Obstetrics and Gynaecology, Keele University School of Medicine and Consultant Obstetrician and Gynaecologist, Royal Stoke University Hospital, UK

Raquel A. Osorno
PGSP-Stanford University Psy.D. Consortium, Palo Alto University, Palo Alto, CA, USA

Amy K. Otto
Helen F. Graham Cancer Center and Research Institute, Newark, DE, USA

Hannah Rayment-Jones
Tutor in Midwifery, Florence Nightingale School of Nursing and Midwifery, King's College London, UK

Yana Richens
Consultant Midwife, University College Hospital, London, UK

Jillian S. Romm
Associate Professor, Department of Obstetrics and Gynecology, Oregon Health Sciences University, Portland, Oregon, USA

Jonathan Schaffir
Associate Professor, Department of Obstetrics and Gynecology, The Ohio State University College of Medicine, Columbus, Ohio, USA

Jean R. Séguin
Department of Psychiatry, Université de Montréal, CHU Ste-Justine Research Center, Canada

Lishiana Solano Shaffer
Assistant Professor, Department of Obstetrics and Gynecology, Oregon Health Sciences University, Portland, Oregon, USA

Gabriel D. Shapiro
Department of Epidemiology, Biostatistics and Occupational Health, McGill University, USA

Kayleigh Sheen
Postdoctoral Research Associate, University of Liverpool, UK

Laura E. Simonelli
Helen F. Graham Cancer Center and Research Institute at Newark, DE, USA

Pauline Slade
Professor of Clinical Psychology and Consultant Clinical Psychologist, University of Liverpool, UK

Melanie Smith
Manchester and Salford Pain Centre, Manchester, UK

Helen Spiby
Professor of Midwifery, University of Nottingham and Honorary Professor, University of Queensland, Australia

Mary Steen
Professor of Midwifery, University of South Australia, Adelaide, Australia

Dace S. Svikis
Professor, Department of Psychology, Virginia Commonwealth University, USA

Sibil Tschudin
Department of Obstetrics and Gynecology, University Hospital Basel, Switzerland

Judi Walsh
School of Psychology, University of East Anglia, UK

Angelika Wieck
Consultant in Perinatal Psychiatry, Manchester Mental Health and Social Care Trust, Manchester, UK

Melissa A. Yanovitch
PGSP-Stanford University Psy.D. Consortium, Palo Alto University, Palo Alto, CA, USA

Tahereh Ziaian
Senior Lecturer, Division of Health Sciences, University of South Australia, Adelaide, Australia

Editorial advisers: British Society of Biopsychosocial Obstetrics and Gynaecology (BSBOG) Executive Committee

BSBOG
BRITISH SOCIETY OF BIOPSYCHOSOCIAL
OBSTETRICS AND GYNAECOLOGY

Preface

It will be well known to anyone embarking on reading this book that the mind can influence the physiology of the body and changes in the body influence the mind – these are normal events. Internal factors can affect both the body and the mind as can external factors. If these changes occur to an excessive level, they can result in physical pathological abnormalities or psychological/psychiatric disorders. Internal factors include such things as central nervous system and bowel, hormones or blood biochemistry. External factors include weather, trauma, physical stresses, psychological or physical abuse; there are many more in both of these categories. The interplay of all of these factors impinges on all aspects of normal and abnormal life, physical and psychological health.

There has always been some confusion as to whether the term linked to these matters should be 'psychosomatic', 'psychosocial' or 'biopsychosocial', though the latter is probably the most encompassing term. Biopsychosocial factors are integral to all aspects of healthcare but perhaps more so in obstetrics, gynaecology and women's health. This is probably because so much of what occurs in the specialty involves dramatic life-changing events, from pregnancy and childbirth to malignancy and terminal cancer.

There is no suggestion that recognition of the biopsychosocial aspects of our specialty should lead to an independent specialty or subspecialty. The biopsychosocial approach should be a fundamental element in the management of the whole range of obstetric and gynaecological conditions. That said, the British Society of Biopsychosocial Obstetrics and Gynaecology (BSBOG) has become a recognized specialist society of the Royal College of Obstetricians and Gynaecologists, but its objective was not to be separate from the other subspecialties but more to engage with them in promoting the biopsychosocial elements of their function and informing their training programmes accordingly. The thought behind this textbook was initially independent of the society, but it soon became apparent that the society's aims to improve the psychological element of women's healthcare could be achieved through such a textbook. Hence, the executive committee was soon adopted as the editorial advisory board.

You will have noticed that the terms 'psychosomatic' and 'biopsychosocial' are used *almost* interchangeably. If you were to consider the titles of the various professional societies around the world – all of whom are member societies of the International Society of Psychosomatic Obstetrics and Gynaecology (ISPOG) – it will be clear that both terms are used. This is because the term 'psychosomatic' is interpreted differently in different countries. Generally speaking, in mainland Europe, the term implies the complex interaction between 'mind' and 'body', whereas in the United Kingdom and the United States, psychosomatic implies to both the medical and lay population a condition which gives rise to physical conditions which are actually psychological in origin – it is so often used pejoratively, implying that a patient's physical symptoms are imaginary or at best 'only psychological'. It is for this reason that the British Society of Psychosomatic Obstetrics, Gynaecology and Andrology (BSPOGA) changed its name to British Society of Biopsychosocial Obstetrics and Gynaecology (BSBOG) even though its umbrella body ISPOG retains 'psychosomatic' in its title.

In the development of the book the broadest content was thought to be appropriate. International contributors considered expert in the particular field were approached and the overall process was considered and approved by an editorial board comprising the members of the BSPOGA executive committee. The two editors were the outgoing (2011–2014) chairman of BSPOGA, Professor P. M. Shaughn O'Brien, and the incoming chairman (2014–2017), Mr Leroy Edozien. Whilst both of these editors are primarily obstetricians and gynaecologists in UK medical schools, both have been extensively involved in biopsychosocial aspects of the specialty over many years.

Professor O'Brien came from The Royal Free Hospital and University of London where he was a consultant and senior lecturer. He began as a professor in Keele University School of Medicine in 1989. His research and clinical care in gynaecology has centred on the menopause and the menstrual cycle, particularly on premenstrual syndrome; he is the founder and chairman of the International Society for Premenstrual Disorders (ISPMD); he devised and co-edited the textbook, *The Premenstrual Syndromes*. He initiated the textbook you are now reading and is immediate past editor in chief (joint) of the *Journal of Psychosomatic Obstetrics and Gynecology* (JPOG). In obstetrics his current research concerns pre-eclampsia and premature labour and much of his clinical practice focuses on the care of pregnant substance misuse patients.

Leroy Edozien's clinical practice and academic work focus broadly and extensively on aspects of biopsychosocial care and education in gynaecology and obstetrics. He is President-Elect of ISPOG and led the successful bid to host the 20th ISPOG International Congress in Manchester in 2022.

The principal purposes of this book are to inform clinical care and to inform both postgraduate and undergraduate education in obstetrics and gynaecology, particularly for the individual subspecialty areas. In every subspecialty area (some more than others) there is a psychological, social, biological and medical care element. All of these must be addressed if we are to provide the best care for our patients.

Biopsychosocial factors in benign gynaecology and gynaecological oncology are amply covered in this book. Each chapter ends with a list of key points. Urogynaecology has been underrepresented in the literature previously, and this is now addressed. Reproductive medicine, subfertility, psychosexual care, menopause, disorders of menstruation and premenstrual syndrome are discussed in detail as are same sex and single sex pregnancy and other gynaecological issues.

Fetal medicine has experienced great technical advances over recent years and the biopsychosocial element of this is only now catching up. For instance fetal programming has causative and consequential elements to the overall picture. Mental health and suicide are now leading causes of maternal mortality and so the editors make no apology for dealing with the topic from different angles.

The chapter authors of this textbook are highly regarded and highly qualified in this complex area of the specialty and its interrelationship with its biopsychosocial elements.

Obstetricians, gynaecologists, midwives, psychiatrists, psychologists and those in many other areas of healthcare including politicians and healthcare managers need to read this book. A distillate of its content needs to be incorporated into general and subspecialty training curricula and this will enable us to maximize the care given to our patients, partners and offspring over the coming years.

On behalf of all contributors to this book and the publisher, we express our condolences to the family of Professor Suzanne Abraham (author of Chapter 5) who passed on while the book was in production. She was a warm and highly respected colleague.

Chapter

1

Promoting and Implementing the Biopsychosocial Perspective in Obstetrics and Gynaecology
The Role of Specialist Societies

Sibil Tschudin

The Biopsychosocial Perspective in Obstetrics and Gynaecology: Nice to Have or Need to Have?

Many health problems cannot be solved and adequately treated when only the biomedical perspective, focusing on diagnostic tests and medical or surgical therapy, is taken into account. This can be assumed as well accepted in all domains of clinical medicine nowadays [1, 2]. It is particularly obvious when considering the situations and conditions of patients who turn to an obstetrician/gynaecologist: they might have experienced a pregnancy loss, be confronted with an unwanted pregnancy or with infertility, suffer from domestic violence or have to deal with a gynaecological cancer. Medically unexplained symptoms are frequent in general hospital outpatients. When comparing different specialties, Nimnuan et al. found that such symptoms were most prevalent in gynaecology and associated with being female, of younger age and of being unemployed [3]. Besides this, women also consult their obstetrician/gynaecologists for advice on

contraception, prenatal care and menopause, as well as prior to screening procedures. Nowadays, the role of the obstetrician/gynaecologist is not limited to cure but includes prevention and supportive care (see Figure 1.1). Their approach should therefore be holistic. Health professionals have to provide assistance with regard to preventive measures, decision-making and crisis intervention (see Figure 1.2).

Consequently, obstetrician/gynaecologists are confronted with many tasks requiring psychosocial competence, including patient education, counselling and management of psychosocial problems. They have also to take care of patients with pain syndromes and/or life-threatening diseases [4, 5]. If psychosocial aspects are not taken into account in these situations, the underlying cause of the problem and critical contributing factors often remain undetected and inadequately dealt with [6]. As a consequence symptoms may persist or worsen and patients' problems may develop into chronic conditions. It could be demonstrated that specific communication skills improve the ability to identify

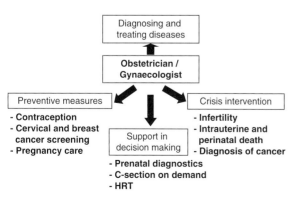

Figure 1.1 Obstetrician/gynaecologists' existing tasks

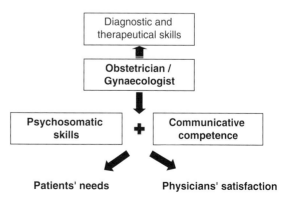

Figure 1.2 Obstetrician/gynaecologists' existing competencies profile

relevant medical and psychosocial information. Consequently, these skills have a significant impact on patient morbidity and on medical costs [2, 7–10]. Furthermore, patients' satisfaction as well as their adherence to treatment is related to physicians' communication style [5, 8, 11–16]. Lack of communication skills and psychosocial competence, however, increases physicians' stress related to patient contact and their risk of developing professional burnout syndrome [17]. In the light of these considerations, it can be argued that the psychosocial perspective is not just 'nice to have' in obstetrics and gynaecology but a perspective that we 'need to have' in our specialty.

Are Obstetrician/Gynaecologists Prepared for Their Tasks in Psychosocial Care-Giving?

Studies to date have shown that psychosomatic competence, i.e. a holistic approach based on a biopsychosocial understanding of the diagnostic as well as the therapeutic process, is an important precondition for adequate patient care. Teaching the necessary diagnostic, therapeutic and communication skills, however, is far from being an integral component of the specialty training worldwide [18, 19]. The educational committee of the International Society of Psychosomatic Obstetrics and Gynaecology (ISPOG) conducted a survey in 2012. All national member societies were approached and invited to answer the following questions:

– Which is (if existing) your currently practiced curriculum for teaching of the primary psychosomatic care in Obs/Gyn?
– Are there any teaching programmes or educational courses that involve psychosomatic topics?
– Which topics does your society consider as most important for teaching psychosomatic care in obstetrics and gynaecology?

Of a total of 19 national societies invited to take part in the survey, ten provided some information on their educational offerings. Two additional countries had provided information during a meeting of the biannual congress of the North American Society of Psychosocial Obstetrics and Gynecology (NASPOG) in 2012.

In six countries psychosocial and psychosomatic issues are covered during medical school, and in eight countries this is the case in the course of specialization. Only Germany and Switzerland have standardized compulsory curricula in psychosomatic obstetrics and gynaecology (see Table 1.1). Seven national societies indicated that they organize regular congresses or symposia on psychosomatic topics, and four countries mentioned that they have guidelines available on specific psychosomatic problems, e.g. chronic pelvic pain. Existing teaching programmes focus on general psychosomatic aspects as well as on specific pathology. A list of topics, which are addressed by most or some of the programmes, is presented in Table 1.2. From the technical perspective, the programmes focus predominantly on communication training and the establishment of

Table 1.1 Content and structure of the German and Swiss compulsory curricula in psychosomatic and psychosocial obstetrics and gynaecology

Country	Germany	Switzerland
In operation	For more than ten years	Since 2002
Target group	**Compulsory** curriculum for all residents	**Compulsory** curriculum for all residents
Extent and content	**80 lessons**: • Theory • Balint groups • Communication training • Resulting in a degree in psychosomatic basic care recognized by the German Board of Physicians	**40 lessons**: • 2 one-day courses in theory • Course in communication in ultrasound during pregnancy • Supervision groups
Provider	Eight clinical sites	Four university hospitals
Current costs	€ 1200	CHF 800

Table 1.2 Topics covered by the teaching offered by the various national societies of psychosomatic obstetrics and gynaecology

	AUS	CH	D	E	Jap	H	NL	S	UK	USA
Mood disorders	X		X			X				X
Specific psychosomatic disorders	X	X	X	X	X	X	X	X	X	X
Menopause		X	X		X	X		X	X	X
Psycho-oncology	X	X	X	X	X	X	X	X	X	X
Violence	X	X							X	X
Pregnancy	X	X	X	X	X	X	X	X		X
Childbirth and postpartum	X	X	X	X	X	X	X	X	X	
Sexuality and relationship aspects	X	X	X	X		X	X	X	X	X

AUS Austria
CH Switzerland
D Germany
E Spain
Jap Japan
H Hungary
NL Netherlands
S Sweden
UK United Kingdom
USA United States of America

a productive doctor-patient relationship, while the teaching of Balint groups, the application of role-plays, case supervision and ethics discussions were only mentioned occasionally. To conclude, there is a huge variation across countries with regard to available programmes. The array spans from established and compulsory training during medical school as well as residency to aspirational plans to install training programmes in the future.

It seems evident that not all current and future obstetricians and gynaecologists are well prepared and sufficiently trained to provide psychosomatic and psychosocial care for their patients. Even if teaching is available and provided, the question remains whether this training really improves psychosocial competence and increases communicative skills. Thus, the evaluation of educational programmes is important, even if not easy. According to Van de Wiel and Wouda the criteria used in evaluation are *effectiveness* and *efficiency* [20]. Studies investigating the effect of teaching programmes are scarce, however, especially in the domain of obstetrics and gynaecology, and generally don't go beyond the assessment of communication skills during the specialty training [21, 22]. The nationwide implementation of a compulsory psychosomatic training of all residents in

Switzerland in 2002 was an opportunity to simultaneously evaluate the teaching programme and measure the effect of its practical component consisting of supervised groups (see Figure 1.1). Participation in these groups was associated with a statistically significant increase in self-estimated psychosomatic competence [23]. Interestingly, after the completion of the teaching programme, all items assessing competence ranged on a higher level and not only those items rated lowest at the beginning of the supervised groups. Consequently, attendance at the supervision groups rather seemed to improve psychosomatic competence in general. Self-efficacy also increased significantly. Schildmann et al. present comparable results when measuring the effect of a training course on the ability to 'break bad news' at the Charité Berlin [24]. The improvement of self-rated ability to perform this task correlated with an increase in self-confidence with regard to communication skills [24]. As self-efficacy is an important protective factor against stress arising in clinical work [25], this increase may contribute to the well-being of physicians and as a non-negligible consequence to their efficiency. As perceived self-efficacy determines whether difficult topics are considered or avoided [26], the described changes are likely to result in improved patient care.

3

Thus, there seems to be growing evidence that well-shaped educational offerings may indeed improve the psychosocial competence of health professionals in the field of obstetrics and gynaecology.

The Role of ISPOG

Despite the evidence that psychosomatic competence is necessary in the practice of obstetrics and gynaecology, training in this field is, in the main, insufficient. Who else should engage in the remedy of this deficiency, and promote and implement the biopsychosocial perspective in obstetrics and gynaecology, if not the specialist society in this field, the International Society of Psychosomatic Obstetrics and Gynaecology?

Engagement of ISPOG over the Course of Time

During the 17th ISPOG Congress in Berlin in 2013, Manfred Stauber, former ISPOG president (1992–1995) and member of the ISPOG Board of Fellows, gave an overview on the history of ISPOG since its foundation in 1962. According to him the interplay between mental problems and female genital organs had already been postulated in ancient Greece, and Sigmund Freud practised psychosomatic obstetrics by treating a woman who suffered from 'psychogenic agalactia' at the end of the nineteenth century. To mention just some of the other pioneers in psychosomatics, Franz Alexander and George Groddeck conducted research into the interrelation of mind and body and the treatment of physical disorders through psychological processes. Further important milestones in the introduction of the biopsychosocial perspective in medicine were set by the US-American psychiatrist George L. Engel and the German internist Thure von Uexküll [27].

The first steps in promoting an understanding of psychosomatic and psychosocial aspects in obstetrics and gynaecology were taken by the founding members of ISPOG, i.e. Leon Chertok (France), Norman Morris (Great Britain), Niles and Michael Newton (USA), Hans J. Prill (Germany), Myriam de Senarclens (Switzerland), Pierre Vellay (France), Lucio Zichella (Italy), Alberto Cardenas Escovar (Spain), Elliot Philip (Great Britain), Murray Enkin (Canada), Hugo Husslein (Austria), Herrmann Hirsch (Israel) and Ferrucio Miraglia (Italy). The founding of the society took place at the first International ISPOG Congress

in 1962 in Paris. After a decade of rather informal exchange, the society became more organized and structured and from 1972 onwards ISPOG congresses were held regularly on a triennial basis. Over the subsequent years the spheres of interest were infertility/reproductive medicine, sexual disorders, family planning, abortion/pregnancy conflicts, pregnancy loss/miscarriage, antenatal care, psychosomatic obstetrics, menopausal disorders, chronic pelvic pain and psycho-oncology. Besides organizing congresses, ISPOG was visible in the media through regular ISPOG newsletters and the *Journal of Psychosomatic Obstetrics and Gynecology* (JPOG). The journal was founded in 1982 in order to provide a scientific forum for obstetricians, gynaecologists, psychiatrists and psychologists, academic health professionals and all others who share an interest in the psychosocial and psychosomatic aspects of women's health. All these efforts were, and still are, important in stimulating obstetricians and gynaecologists to pay more attention to this important facet of their profession. Even if the majority of ISPOG members are obstetrician-gynaecologists, the society always supported and propagated a multidisciplinary strategy by targeting and including other health professionals, such as psychiatrists, psychologists and midwives.

While the above-mentioned efforts and activities helped to promote awareness of psychosomatic and psychosocial issues, it was necessary to develop other strategies for implementing the biopsychosocial perspective in everyday clinical practice. This became more and more obvious in the last decade and led to a sharper focus on educational activities.

ISPOG Educational Committee

All national societies were invited to an informal and exploratory meeting held during the NASPOG congress in Providence, USA, in 2012. A few months later, at the International Federation of Gynecology and Obstetrics (FIGO) congress in Rome, Italy, an educational committee was established within ISPOG.

Goals of the ISPOG Educational Committee

The committee, chaired by the author of this chapter, defined its goals and formulated strategies to achieve these goals as follows:

The principal goal of ISPOG with regard to education is 'to promote access to a psychosomatic approach for all health care providers in the field of obstetrics and gynaecology in order to fulfil the needs of the patients they treat and/or care for'.

The educational goals of ISPOG are the following:

1. To develop an e-learning academy that aims at serving as a platform for exchange of knowledge considering cultural differences and local characteristics providing a theoretical basis as well as teaching materials and specific tools that may serve as a reference for all national societies and that may be incorporated into
    i. Teaching of residents
    ii. Continuous medical education (CME) for all obstetricians/gynaecologists and other health professionals in obstetrics and gynaecology
    iii. Clinical discussions within the activity of the national societies
2. To provide access to the talks of psychosomatic symposia/congresses by means of webcasts
3. To offer and encourage workshops to give members the opportunity to experience the psychosomatic approach personally.

To reach these goals the following strategies are envisaged:

1. Installation and maintenance of a server
2. Development and maintenance of a knowledge database on the ISPOG website
3. Formation of an 'editorial board' that is responsible for the quality control of the files available for download from the ISPOG website
4. Development of quality criteria, which will be discussed and installed by the ISPOG Executive Committee and afterwards published on the ISPOG website
5. Development of the theoretical framework for e-learning as well as e-learning teaching material in a step-by-step process
6. Constant identification of congresses – e.g. FIGO, European Board and College of Obstetrics and Gynaecology (EBCOG), International Association for Women's Mental Health (IAWMH) and World Association for Infant Mental Health (WAIMH) – that qualify as platforms for psychosomatic contributions.

Current Achievements of the Educational Committee

With regard to the aims set in 2012, ISPOG has to date successfully achieved some, though certainly not all of them. The server and the ISPOG website are well prepared to develop and expand the knowledge database. The editorial board has been constituted and quality criteria for educational resources will be discussed periodically by the ISPOG Executive Committee. A promising strategy for sensitizing young colleagues to psychosocial aspects and teaching communication skills on a practical level is to hold workshops during congresses organized by ISPOG or affiliated societies. 'Hands-on' training is in fact not limited to surgical and interventional skills training. The positive feedback of participants at workshops offered at the EBCOG congress in Glasgow in 2013 and the European Network of Trainees in Obstetrics and Gynaecology (ENTOG) scientific meeting in 2015 in Utrecht as well as the positive evaluation of partly interactive symposia with case discussions offered at the European Society of Contraception (ESC) congress in Lisbon in 2014 and the IAWMH congress in Tokyo in 2015 speak for an even more widespread offer of such training modules. Even if electronic media are very helpful in facilitating communication and exchange, personal contacts still carry great significance, especially in a field where communication is the basic and predominant skill.

The Role of Other Specialist Societies

ISPOG has a central role in promoting and implementing the biopsychosocial perspective in obstetrics and gynaecology. It is, however, of utmost importance to gain the support of other societies with similar and somehow overlapping interests. To profit not only from professional but also from economical synergies is crucial in a world of economic dependence and financial restriction. Thanks to the constant engagement of the former ISPOG presidents, Marieke Paarlberg and Carlos Damonte Khoury, contacts and collaboration with several societies have been initiated and established. Mutual invitations to hold symposia at the congresses of the mentioned associations are just one of the achievements. Even more important are joint declarations and the collaborative development of guidelines. EBCOG invited ISPOG to contribute to the EBCOG Standards of Care for Women's Health in Europe released in 2014 in order to guarantee that psychosocial aspects are sufficiently considered in the document [28].

The national psychosomatic obstetric and gynaecology societies each relate differently to their respective national societies or colleges of obstetrics and gynaecology. Some are independent; others are so-called working or special interest groups of their 'mother' society/college. As the psychosocial perspective should be considered in any condition and every obstetrician/gynaecologist should possess basic knowledge and skills, a close collaboration is essential and should be pursued.

The best way to guarantee the incorporation of psychosocial issues into professional training is to have a compulsory basic curriculum, as has been established in Germany and Switzerland. Although ISPOG encourages and supports the idea that more (if not all) countries should integrate a mandatory basic training in psychosocial issues into their programme for specialization in obstetrics and gynaecology, it also acknowledges that the prerequisite resources and underlying framework are currently not available in many nations. Pending the development of these prerequisites, we should concentrate on identifying options to at least partly fill this gap in professional training and education. To enhance the attractiveness of these options the national societies/colleges of obstetrics and gynaecology should develop Continuing Professional Development (CPD) accreditation of such offers.

Conclusions, Practical Implications and Future Strategies

Health professionals will be better positioned to promote and implement the biopsychosocial perspective in obstetrics and gynaecology if they are equipped with the pertinent skills and acquire psychosocial competence through formal training. Specialist societies in general and ISPOG in particular have an indispensable role not only in devising such training but also in promoting awareness through the mass media, through advocacy and through contacts with governmental and regulatory authorities. It is also their role to promote fruitful and sustainable developments with regard to clinical protocols and research into psychosocial issues in obstetrics and gynaecology. Professionals in countries where there is currently no national specialist society for psychosocial obstetrics and gynaecology are welcome to liaise with ISPOG with a view to setting up one in their country.

Key Points

- The psychosocial perspective is not just 'nice to have' in obstetrics and gynaecology but a perspective that we 'need to have' in the specialty.
- Not all current and future obstetricians and gynaecologists are well prepared and sufficiently trained to provide psychosomatic and psychosocial care for their patients.
- Worldwide, the teaching of diagnostic, therapeutic and communication skills necessary for psychosocial competence is far from being an integral component of specialty training in obstetrics and gynaecology.
- Well-shaped educational offerings may improve the psychosocial competence of health professionals.
- In the last decade, the International Society of Psychosomatic Obstetrics and Gynaecology (ISPOG) has focused more sharply on educational activities.
- A promising way to guarantee the incorporation of psychosocial issues into professional training is to have a compulsory basic curriculum, as has been established in Germany and Switzerland.

Acknowledgement

It would not have been possible to write this chapter without the support and contribution of a number of colleagues. Special thanks go to Vivian Pramataroff Hamburger, who conducted the survey about educational activities of the national member societies of ISPOG, and all other members of the educational committee; Brigitte Leeners, who co-authored the evaluation of the compulsory teaching programme in Switzerland; Manfred Stauber, who provided an excellent overview on the history of ISPOG; Levente Lázar, who initiated the development of a web-based knowledge database; all members of the current ISPOG board and especially the former ISPOG presidents, Marieke Paarlberg and Carlos Damonte Khoury, who untiringly and efficiently engage in ambassadorial activities.

References

1. Borrell-Carrio, F., A.L. Suchman, and R.M. Epstein, The biopsychosocial model 25 years later: principles, practice, and scientific inquiry. *Annals of Family Medicine*, 2004. **2**(6): pp. 576–82.

2. Stewart, M.A., Effective physician-patient communication and health outcomes: a review. *CMAJ*, 1995. **152**(9): pp. 1423–33.

3. Nimnuan, C., M. Hotopf, and S. Wessely, Medically unexplained symptoms: an epidemiological study in seven specialities. *Journal of Psychosomatic Research*, 2001. **51**(1): pp. 361–7.

4. Bitzer, J. et al., [Psychosocial and psychosomatic basic competence of the gynecologist – from intrinsic conviction to a learnable curriculum]. *Gynakol Geburtshilfliche Rundsch*, 2001. **41**(3): pp. 158–65.

5. Leeners, B. et al., Satisfaction with medical information in women with hypertensive disorders in pregnancy. *J Psychosom Res*, 2006. **60**(1): pp. 39–44.

6. Barsky, A.J., E.J. Orav, and D.W. Bates, Somatization increases medical utilization and costs independent of psychiatric and medical comorbidity. *Arch Gen Psychiatry*, 2005. **62**(8): pp. 903–10.

7. Jünger, J. and V. Köllner, Integration of a doctor/patient-communication-training into clinical teaching: examples from the reform-curricula of Heidelberg and Dresden Universities. *Psychother Psych Med*, 2003. **53**: pp. 56–64.

8. Langewitz, W.A. et al., Improving communication skills – a randomized controlled behaviorally oriented intervention study for residents in internal medicine. *Psychosom Med*, 1998. **60**(3): pp. 268–76.

9. Levinson, W., Doctor-patient communication and medical malpractice: implications for pediatricians. *Pediatr Ann*, 1997. **26**(3): pp. 186–93.

10. Mead, N., P. Bower, and M. Hann, The impact of general practitioners' patient-centredness on patients' post-consultation satisfaction and enablement. *Soc Sci Med*, 2002. **55**(2): pp. 283–99.

11. Bertakis, K.D. et al., The influence of gender on physician practice style. *Med Care*, 1995. **33**(4): pp. 407–16.

12. Christen, R.N., J. Alder, and J. Bitzer, Gender differences in physicians' communicative skills and their influence on patient satisfaction in gynaecological outpatient consultations. *Soc Sci Med*, 2008. **66**(7): pp. 1474–83.

13. Hall, J.A. and D.L. Roter, Do patients talk differently to male and female physicians? A meta-analytic review. *Patient Educ Couns*, 2002. **48**(3): pp. 217–24.

14. Krupat, E. et al., The practice orientations of physicians and patients: the effect of doctor-patient congruence on satisfaction. *Patient Educ Couns*, 2000. **39**(1): pp. 49–59.

15. Topacoglu, H. et al., Analysis of factors affecting satisfaction in the emergency department: a survey of 1019 patients. *Adv Ther*, 2004. **21**(6): pp. 380–8.

16. Trummer, U.F. et al., Does physician-patient communication that aims at empowering patients improve clinical outcome? A case study. *Patient Educ Couns*, 2006. **61**(2): pp. 299–306.

17. Whippen, D.A. and G.P. Canellos, Burnout syndrome in the practice of oncology: results of a random survey of 1,000 oncologists. *J Clin Oncol*, 1991. **9**(10): pp. 1916–20.

18. Herzler, M. et al., Dealing with the issue 'care of the dying' in medical education – results of a survey of 592 European physicians. *Med Educ*, 2000. **34**(2): pp. 146–7.

19. Whitehouse, C.R., The teaching of communication skills in United Kingdom medical schools. *Med Educ*, 1991. **25**(4): pp. 311–8.

20. van de Wiel, H.B. and J.C. Wouda, Evaluative studies in (medical) education. *J Psychosom Obstet Gynecol*, 2008. **29**(1): pp. 1–2.

21. Alder, J. et al., Communication skills training in obstetrics and gynaecology: whom should we train? A randomized controlled trial. *Arch Gynecol Obstet*, 2007. **276**(6): pp. 605–12.

22. van Dulmen, A.M. and J.C. van Weert, Effects of gynaecological education on interpersonal communication skills. *BJOG*, 2001. **108**(5): pp. 485–91.

23. Tschudin, S. et al., Psychosomatics in obstetrics and gynecology – evaluation of a compulsory standardized teaching program. *Journal of Psychosomatic Obstetrics and Gynecology*, 2013. **34**(3): pp. 108–15.

24. Schildmann, J. et al., Evaluation of a 'breaking bad news' course at the Charite, Berlin. *Med Educ*, 2001. **35**(8): pp. 806–7.

25. Buddeberg-Fischer, B. et al., Chronic stress experience in young physicians: impact of person- and workplace-related factors. *Int Arch Occup Environ Health*, 2010. **83**(4): pp. 373–9.

26. Hulsman, R.L. et al., Teaching clinically experienced physicians communication skills. A review of evaluation studies. *Med Educ*, 1999. **33**(9): pp. 655–68.

27. Edozien, L.C., Beyond biology: the biopsychosocial model and its application in obstetrics and gynaecology. *BJOG: An International Journal of Obstetrics and Gynaecology*, 2015. **122**(7): pp. 900–3.

28. EBCOG. Standards of Care for Women's Health in Europe. 2014; Available from: www.ebcog.eu.

Psychosocial Context of Illness and Well-Being in Women's Health

Susan Ayers and Elizabeth Ford

Introduction

Women's reproductive health encompasses a wide range of topics, including menstruation, conception, abortion, pregnancy, miscarriage, childbirth and menopause. Although mainly focussed on women, these events involve issues that affect both men and women and include sexual dysfunction, infertility and becoming a parent. Reproduction also encompasses a range of illnesses, such as endometriosis, sexually transmitted diseases, pelvic pain, premenstrual syndrome and testicular cancer. These disorders and their treatments can have implications for fertility and reproduction. For example, endometriosis is associated with reduced fertility in women. Common procedures and treatments associated with reproduction include contraception, cervical smears and hormone replacement therapy. Reproductive issues raise unique ethical dilemmas, such as the point at which terminating a pregnancy is morally defensible; the rights of donor parents and children of donors; whether a subsequent pregnancy should be used by parents to provide a child with the right genetic make-up to be an organ or tissue donor for a sick older sibling.

All these events can be viewed from different perspectives: biomedical, psychological, social and cultural. Which perspective we take affects both our understanding and treatment of disorders [1]. For example, a biomedical perspective would see premenstrual syndrome as caused by fluctuations and imbalances in hormones associated with the menstrual cycle. Treatment would therefore involve pharmacological methods to counteract hormonal imbalances or influence mood. A psychological perspective of premenstrual syndrome might examine how women's patterns of stress and behaviour contribute to worsening mood around menstruation, such as noticing particular triggers and maladaptive responses. Treatment might involve identifying and changing maladaptive thinking or behaviour, and

finding coping strategies to help women respond in a more adaptive way. A social perspective of premenstrual syndrome might examine women's sociodemographic circumstances and levels of support, or cultural beliefs and narratives about premenstrual syndrome. This might lead to treatment providing practical or emotional support to women during critical times, or public health campaigns to change cultural beliefs and narratives.

It is clear that none of these perspectives on their own offer adequate explanation or treatment of premenstrual syndrome. Therefore a **biopsychosocial approach**, which considers all the perspectives outlined previously, will lead to more informed and holistic approaches to treatment.

Psychosocial Views of Health

Concepts of well-being, health and illness are not easy to define, and there is large variation between cultures and individuals. For example, research shows that people with terminal illnesses generally report reduced quality of life. Yet quality of life is not a single entity and, even if people report more physical symptoms, pain and disability, they may also report increased appreciation of life and family and other positive benefits. Reproductive health issues are therefore complex and we need to recognize that, for individuals, health and illness are subjective states of well-being. In other words, a person may *think* he or she is healthy or ill regardless of the underlying pathology. For example, with chronic pelvic pain many women have no identifiable underlying abnormality; or the pain can persist after an abnormality is treated [2] – see Chapter 16.

Health also can be thought of in terms of physical, psychological and social health. A survey of 9,000 people [3] found that we generally think of health in six different ways:

1. not having symptoms of illness
2. having physical or social reserves

3. having healthy lifestyles
4. being physically fit or vital
5. psychological well-being
6. being able to function

The World Health Organization (WHO) broadly defined health as 'a state of complete physical, mental, and social well-being and not merely the absence of disease or infirmity' [4]. The value of this definition is that it is inclusive and the emphasis on well-being accounts for individual differences in subjective perception of health. However, this definition has been criticized for referring to a utopian 'perfect' state that few of us reach, even when we feel healthy.

As with the biopsychosocial perspective, how we define health has implications for which treatments we provide. If we aim for health as defined by the WHO it could put unrealistic pressure on countries to provide social circumstances and medical systems that mean everyone lives in a state of complete well-being. Others have pointed out that the concept of complete well-being confuses happiness with health [5]. This potentially validates the pursuit of happiness as a legitimate medical goal. The rapid increase in cosmetic surgery in order for people to feel happier with their appearance is an example of this. Definitions of health are also intertwined with cultural norms and have implications for social policy and laws. In western countries the dominant view is that individuals have responsibility for their health through lifestyle choices. Policies have therefore been implemented that attempt to improve our lifestyles and health, such as banning smoking in public places.

Psychosocial Issues in Women's Reproductive Health

Thus, how we examine reproductive health depends on the perspective we take and how we define health. Health can be considered in biomedical, psychological and social terms and may also impact on these areas of women's lives. In this section we illustrate this by examining psychosocial factors in menstruation and menopause, pregnancy and childbirth.

Menstruation and Menopause

The age at which girls start menstruating – menarche – has fallen markedly through the twentieth century. This change is thought to be due to not only better health and basic nutrition but also increased weight and obesity in young girls. The correlates of the menstrual cycle have been examined in relation to a range of behaviours such as sexual behaviour, sleep and diet. The follicular phase prior to and during ovulation has been associated with increased libido [6]. From an evolutionary perspective, increased sexual behaviour at this time increases a woman's chances of conception. The menstrual cycle might also influence our choices of mate: there is some evidence that women in the fertile phase of the menstrual cycle have a greater preference for men with more typically masculine characteristics, e.g. taller, more masculine faces and bodies, more social presence and sexual competitiveness [7]. However, this is only the case when women are asked to rate or choose men for short-term relationships and not when they are instructed to choose men for long-term relationships.

The menstrual cycle does not appear to affect sleep and diet as much as is commonly believed. One study in which women kept detailed daily sleep records found that although women rated their quality of sleep as worse in the days before and during menstruation, there was no actual difference in amount of sleep or waking during the night [8]. Similarly, research suggests that changes in food preferences are more strongly influenced by cultural norms than biological changes. For example, chocolate cravings during the menstrual cycle differ strongly between cultures [9], suggesting that any effect of the menstrual cycle on food preferences is culturally defined.

Premenstrual Syndrome (PMS)

Physical and psychological symptoms often occur in the luteal phase just before menstruation. These symptoms are commonly referred to as premenstrual tension (PMT) or premenstrual syndrome (PMS) – see Chapter 12. PMS includes a range of psychological and physical symptoms such as irritability, sleep problems, depression, labile mood and abdominal bloating. PMS is reported by up to 30% of women, and is most common among those aged 25–35. Around 1–2% of these women experience a severe form of PMS referred to as premenstrual dysphoric disorder (PMDD). PMDD is diagnosed when there are marked disturbances in home life, social life and work due to significant changes in sleep, appetite, energy, concentration, mood and anxiety which appear during most of the last week of the luteal phase and abate in the week after menses [10]. PMDD is not simply the exacerbation of an existing mood disorder during the premenstrual period: it is supposed to be 'switched on' during days of the menstrual cycle, and 'switched off' for the remainder of the cycle. However, women with a past history of depression are more likely to suffer from PMDD, and PMDD is associated with poor overall health.

The relative contribution of physical and psychological factors to PMS and PMDD is unclear and the diagnosis therefore remains controversial. Timing of symptoms suggests that fluctuations in hormone levels play some causal role in psychological symptoms [11]. The increased vulnerability of women with a history of depression suggests that predisposing factors can be exacerbated by the menstrual cycle. However, cultural differences in PMS suggest that the interpretation of symptoms is influenced by cultural norms. Interventions should therefore take into account biological, psychosocial and cultural factors.

Proper diagnosis of PMS entails monitoring a woman's symptoms over the course of at least one menstrual cycle. Various aids have been developed to help with this, such as the PMT-Cator [12] which is a simple wheel on which women record experiences of five common symptoms every day for six weeks. The recommended treatment of PMS in the UK and the USA focusses on anti-depressants. Meta-analyses have shown that progesterone or progestogen treatment is not clinically effective [13]. Other hormonal approaches appear more effective, particularly those which suppress ovulation (Chapter 12). Despite this, practices vary between countries, illustrating cultural influences on treatment. A study of PMS and PMDD treatment in different countries found that doctors in the USA, the UK, and Canada favoured anti-depressants, French doctors favoured hormone and analgesic treatment, and German doctors favoured complementary medicine [14].

Psychological treatment for PMS may be effective. Meta-analyses show that, although education and monitoring are of limited use, cognitive behavioural therapy (CBT) and CBT-based interventions result in reduced depression and anxiety, less interference of symptoms on daily functioning and more positive behaviour changes [15]. Standard intervention packages are therefore now available. One trial found an eight-session intervention was as effective as anti-depressants over six months and more effective over the first year [16].

Menopause

Menopause is a good illustration of cultural influences on reproductive issues as it is associated with a range of symptoms that vary between cultures. Symptoms include hot flushes, night sweats, poor memory, loss of libido, irritability, problems with skin or hair, vaginal dryness, anxiety and headaches. In western cultures between 50 and 70% of women report symptoms, such as hot flushes and night sweats, but a much lower incidence of symptoms is reported in cultures where menopause is viewed positively and increases the prestige of the women [17]. Reporting of hot flushes in cultures such as Japan has also increased as cultural awareness of the menopause, or *kônenki*, has increased [18]. Thus, cultural discourses influence interpretation of menopause symptoms.

There is mixed evidence on the psychological impact of menopause such as whether women are more vulnerable to depression during this time. A review concluded that fluctuations and declines in ovarian hormones may influence the onset and progression of depression [19]. Ovarian hormones are known to have specific modulatory effects on the serotonergic and noradrenergic systems, both of which are involved in depression. In western cultures, however, it has been found that concurrent stressful events are important predictors of women's well-being during menopause. For example, one study found that depressed mood in menopausal women is strongly influenced by a history of depression, history of premenstrual complaints, negative attitudes towards aging or menopause and poor current health [20]. Menopause also often coincides with significant life role changes, such as children leaving home. There are therefore likely to be multiple physical, psychological and cultural causes of depressed mood during menopause.

Pregnancy and Childbirth

Pregnancy and childbirth are times of huge physical and psychosocial transition. It is undoubtedly a positive time for many women, but can be associated with impaired physical functioning, health and wellbeing [21].

In early pregnancy most women experience nausea and vomiting. This is commonly referred to as 'morning sickness', but only 2% of women have symptoms restricted to the morning and 80% experience nausea and vomiting all day. Although postnatal depression is most well known, mental health problems are almost as frequent in pregnancy as they are after birth. Severe depression occurs in up to 12% of women during pregnancy and 19% of women after birth [22]. Anxiety disorders affect a similar proportion of women during pregnancy and after birth [23], although research has typically examined anxiety symptoms rather than disorders, so more research is needed to establish the prevalence of diagnostic anxiety disorders.

Anxiety symptoms, stress and distress are important in pregnancy when they have the potential to influence birth outcomes, fetal development and infant characteristics. There is now substantial evidence that severe or chronic stress in pregnancy is associated with preterm birth and low birth weight. For example, women who are victims of domestic abuse are 1.4 times more likely to have a low birth weight baby [24]. Job stress can also result in adverse outcomes. Women who work in physically demanding jobs, do shift work or report work fatigue are more likely to have a preterm birth, hypertension and birth complications [25]. Emotional distress in pregnancy has a similar effect. Depression and anxiety are associated with obstetric complications, pregnancy symptoms, preterm labour, more requests for delivery by caesarean section and increased use of pain relief during labour [26].

Antenatal stress can also affect fetal and infant development. Ultrasound studies have shown various effects of maternal anxiety on fetal behaviour, such as reduced fetal movement [27]. Longitudinal research has shown that stress and anxiety in pregnancy are associated with poor cognitive, behavioural and emotional development in children, and that these effects remain even after controlling for prenatal, obstetric and other psychosocial factors [28]. Further evidence comes from animal research, where the offspring of pregnant rats or monkeys exposed to stressors are significantly more likely to be stillborn or have low birth weight, and are more likely to have impaired neuromotor functioning, impaired learning, greater behavioural disturbance and hypothalamic-pituitary-adrenal axis dysfunction in response to stress [29, 30].

The effects of stress and distress on infant characteristics could be due to a range of factors. First, it may be that the mother and child have genes that increase the likelihood of anxiety and emotional problems. Second, women exposed to stress during pregnancy may live in adverse circumstances.

If adversity continues after birth it can also influence the development of the baby. Related to this, adversity may be associated with lifestyle factors that affect the developing fetus and baby (e.g. poor nutrition). A third explanation is that there are critical periods during pregnancy during which fetal stress responses are programmed or 'hard wired'. The *fetal programming hypothesis* proposes that the fetus is particularly sensitive to maternal stress during mid-pregnancy and at the end of pregnancy. The effect of stress on fetal development is thought to occur through reduced utero-placental blood supply, reduced nutrients and increased transmission of stress hormones. However, it is important to note that research shows that if infants have a nurturing early environment and positive attachment with their main caregivers then the impact of antenatal stress is reversible [31].

In terms of medical care this has several implications – the main one being that if we reduce stress and anxiety in pregnancy it may have the potential to reduce caesarean sections and improve maternal and infant outcomes. An example of where this is an issue is the impact of stress on female healthcare professionals who are pregnant. Research on women healthcare professionals shows they are at increased risk of pregnancy complications, especially in late pregnancy. One study found that during pregnancy female doctors working in hospitals report that the physical demands of the job (e.g. night shifts, standing for long periods) are stressful and there is poor support from colleagues. Institutional support for healthcare professionals during pregnancy is therefore lacking and needs to be properly examined [32].

In childbirth, the greatest social change over time has been the context and type of birth. Births have moved from home to hospital and caesarean births in the UK have risen from under 5% in the 1950s to almost 30% today. The reasons for this rise are not clear. One suggestion is that more women are requesting caesarean section in preference to vaginal birth. However, an Australian study found that only 6% of pregnant women wanted caesarean births – and most of these had obstetric complications or a previous complicated delivery [33]. In the UK most caesareans are performed as emergency births after labour has started, suggesting that the rise in caesarean sections is due to increased complications during labour and/or increased tendency for doctors to carry out caesareans rather than continue with non-operative births.

Discourses and ideologies around birth and maternity care are culturally determined but also vary within cultures. For example, within society, individuals may have contrasting views that birth is risky and care should be highly medicalized, or that birth is a natural process where interference is harmful [34]. Maternity services and practitioners usually have internalized or embraced a set of ideologies around birth and, for hospital birth, this is likely to driven by a biomedical approach. Differences in beliefs and notions of risk between healthcare professionals and a woman's own perception may result in conflict and misunderstandings. Giving birth in a hospital may be reassuring, informed, technologically advanced and 'safe' to women with a biomedical view of birth, but it may feel cold, stressful and perilous to women with different assumptions [35]. For example, a study from Australia, where hospital birth is highly medicalized, found that women who chose homebirth against medical advice or without trained health professionals were well educated about the risks of birth. However, they perceived hospital care to be riskier than staying at home, with 17 out of 20 having had a previous birth experience and four women being midwives themselves [36]. Women in this study had therefore intensely scrutinized, or personally experienced, the risks inherent in giving birth in a hospital, and decided that the harmful activities of healthcare providers and organisations were riskier than the birth process itself. Other studies show that around 10% of women would prefer a home delivery – most of them because they think they will have more control [37]. However, research in the Netherlands, where approximately 30% of women give birth at home, suggests place of birth makes no difference to the proportion of women who find birth traumatic [38].

The events of birth can impact significantly on women's transition to motherhood and her mental health. For example, research shows between 20 and 30% of women find giving birth traumatic and around 3% develop postnatal post-traumatic stress disorder (PTSD) [39]. Women who have assisted or caesarean births are more likely to develop PTSD, but it is not a straightforward relationship: individual risk factors interact with what happens during birth to determine whether women find it traumatic [40]. Risk factors include depression in pregnancy or previous PTSD, negative birth experiences, assisted or caesarean birth and lack of support during labour [41]. The symptoms of women who develop PTSD include flashbacks to the birth, intrusive thoughts about what happened, avoidance of reminders of the birth and hyperarousal including increased anger and irritability [10]. The majority of women with PTSD also develop depression. Women who miscarry or who suffer perinatal loss are particularly at risk of PTSD and other psychological disorders, and this risk increases with greater gestational age at which the loss occurs [42].

Psychosocial factors such as support from others during labour also have a critical influence on birth outcomes and psychological well-being. Women are more likely to be traumatized by birth if they feel poorly informed, not listened to, inadequately cared for, or have little support from staff or their partner [40]. The provision of support for women during labour is not standard in many poorly resourced countries. This means experimental studies have been possible, where women are randomly allocated a person to support them or not. A meta-analysis of these studies shows that simply providing a lay person ('Doula') to support a woman during labour results in better physical outcomes for both mother and baby, including shorter labours, less analgesia, fewer assisted or operative deliveries and higher maternal satisfaction with the birth experience [43].

Summary and Conclusion

In this chapter we have looked at how reproductive health can be defined and viewed from biomedical, psychological and social perspectives; and how the perspective we take influences our understanding of the causes and treatment of reproductive health issues. We have also shown how reproductive events, such as menstruation, pregnancy and birth, are influenced by psychological and social factors, and conversely how they can impact on women's psychological health, as illustrated by PMDD, or PTSD following childbirth. Cultural factors, such as views of individual responsibility for health and discourses around events, such as menopause and birth, will influence how women view and respond to these events and can differ both between and within a particular culture.

The interplay between psychosocial and biomedical factors in how women experience and respond to reproductive events is therefore critical. Reproductive events and health are naturally embedded in the wider social context of women's lives, and therefore, these events, adjustment to these events and the impact on women's psychological and social functioning must all be considered in this wider sociocultural setting.

Key Points

- Concepts of well-being, health and illness are not easy to define, and there is a large variation between cultures and individuals.
- How we define health has implications for which treatments we provide.
- Psychosocial factors are integral to the holistic management of menstruation, premenstrual syndrome, menopause, pregnancy and childbirth.
- Discourses and ideologies around birth and maternity care are culturally determined but also vary within cultures. Maternity services and practitioners usually have internalized or embraced a set of ideologies around birth and, for hospital birth, this is likely to driven by a biomedical approach.
- The events of birth can impact significantly on women's transition to motherhood and mental health.
- Women are more likely to be traumatized by birth if they feel poorly informed, not listened to, inadequately cared for, or have little support from staff or their partner.

References

1. Ayers, S., & de Visser, R. (2011). *Psychology for Medicine*. London: Sage.
2. Brawn, J., Morotti, M., Zondervan, K.T., Becker, C.M., & Vincent, K. (2014). Central changes associated with chronic pelvic pain and endometriosis. *Human Reproduction Update*, 20(5), 737–747.
3. Blaxter, M. (1990). *Health and Lifestyles*. London: Routledge.
4. World Health Organization (1992). *Basic Documents* (39th *Edition*). Geneva: WHO.
5. Saracci, R. (1997). The World Health Organisation needs to reconsider its definition of health. *British Medical Journal*, 314, 1409.
6. Gangestad, S.W., & Cousins, A.J. (2001). Adaptive design, female mate preferences, and shifts across the menstrual cycle. *Annual Review of Sex Research*, 12, 145–185.
7. Little, A.C., Jones, B.C., & Burriss, R.P. (2007). Preferences for masculinity in male bodies change across the menstrual cycle. *Hormones and Behavior*, 51, 633–639.
8. Baker, F.C., & Driver, H.S. (2004). Self-reported sleep across the menstrual cycle in young, healthy women. *Journal of Psychosomatic Research*, 56, 239–243.
9. Zellner, D.A., Garriga-Trillo, A., Centeno, S., & Wadsworth, E. (2004). Chocolate craving and the menstrual cycle. *Appetite*, 42, 119–121.
10. American Psychiatric Association (2000). *Diagnostic and statistical manual of mental disorders* (4th ed., Text Revision). Washington, DC: American Psychiatric Publishing.
11. Rapkin, A. (2003). A review of treatment of premenstrual syndrome & premenstrual dysphoric disorder. *Psychoneuroendocrinology*, 28, 39–53.
12. Magos, A.L., & Studd, J.W.W. (1988). A simple method for the diagnosis of the premenstrual syndrome by use of a self-assessment disk. *American Journal of Obstetrics and Gynecology*, 158, 1024–1028.
13. Wyatt, K., Dimmock, P., Jones, P., Obhrai, M., & O'Brien, S. (2001). Efficacy of progesterone and progestogens in management of premenstrual syndrome: Systematic review. *British Medical Journal*, 323, 776–780.
14. Weisz, G., & Knaapen, L. (2009). Diagnosing and treating premenstrual syndrome in five western nations. *Social Science and Medicine*, 68, 1498–1505.
15. Busse, J.W., Montori, V.M., Krasnik, C., Patelis-Siotis, I., & Guyatt, G.H. (2008). Psychological intervention for premenstrual syndrome: A meta-analysis of randomized controlled trials. *Psychotherapy and Psychosomatics*, 78, 6–15.
16. Hunter, M., Ussher, J., Cariss, M., Browne, S., & Jelly, R. (2002). A randomised comparison of psychological (cognitive behaviour therapy, CBT), medical (fluoxetine) and combined treatment for women with Premenstrual Dysphoric Disorder. *Journal of Psychosomatic Obstetrics and Gynecology*, 23, 193–199.
17. Freeman, E.W., & Sherif, K. (2007). Prevalence of hot flushes and night sweats around the world: A systematic review. *Climacteric*, 10, 197–214.
18. Melby, M.K., Lock, M., & Kaufert, P. (2005). Culture and symptom reporting at menopause. *Human Reproduction Update*, 11, 495–512.
19. Deecher, D., Andree, T.H., Sloan, D., & Schechter, L.E. (2008). From menarche to menopause: Exploring the underlying biology of depression in women experiencing hormonal changes. *Psychoneuroendocrinology*, 33, 3–17.
20. Dennerstein, L., Guthrie, J.R., Clark, M., Lehert, P., & Henderson, V.W. (2004). A population-based study of

negative mood in middle-aged, Australian-born women. *Menopause, 11*, 563–568.

21. Haas, J.S., et al. (2004). Changes in the health status of women during and after pregnancy. *Journal of General Internal Medicine, 20*, 45–51.

22. Gavin, N.I., Gaynes, B.N., Lohr, K.N., Meltzer-Brody, S., Gartlehner, G., & Swinson, T. (2005). Perinatal depression: A systematic review of prevalence and incidence. *Obstetrics & Gynecology, 106*(5), 1071–83.

23. Ross, L.E., & McLean, L.M. (2006). Anxiety disorders during pregnancy and the postpartum period: A systematic review. *Journal of Clinical Psychiatry, 67*, 1285–1298.

24. Murphy, C.C., Schei, B., Myhr, T.L., & Du Mont, J. (2001). Abuse: A risk factor for low birth weight? A systematic review and meta-analysis. *Canadian Medical Association Journal, 164*, 1567–1572.

25. Mozurkewich, E.L., Luke, B., Avni, M., & Wolf, F.M. (2000). Working conditions and adverse pregnancy outcome: A meta-analysis. *Obstetrics and Gynecology, 95*, 623–635.

26. Alder, J., Fink, N., Bitzer, J., Hösli, I., & Holzgreve, W. (2007). Depression and anxiety during pregnancy: A risk factor for obstetric, fetal and neonatal outcome? A critical review of the literature. *Journal of Maternal-Fetal and Neonatal Medicine, 20*(3), 189–209.

27. Van den Bergh, B.R.H., Mulder, E.J.H., Mennes, M., & Glover, V. (2005). Antenatal maternal anxiety and stress and neurobehavioural development of the fetus and child: Links and possible mechanisms: A review. *Neuroscience and Biobehavioral Reviews, 29*, 237–258.

28. Talge, N.M., Neal, C., & Glover, V. (2007). Antenatal maternal stress and long-term effects on child neurodevelopment: How and why? *Journal of Child Psychology and Psychiatry, 48*, 245–261.

29. Chapillon, P., Patin, V., Roy, V., Vincent, A., & Caston, J. (2002). Effects of pre- and postnatal stimulation on developmental, emotional, and cognitive aspects in rodents: A review. *Developmental Psychobiology, 41*, 373–387.

30. Schneider, M.L., Moore, C.F., Roberts, A.D., & Dejesus, O. (2001). Prenatal stress alters early neurobehavior, stress reactivity and learning in non-human primates: A brief review. *Stress, 4*, 183–193.

31. Rice, F., Jones, I., & Thapar, A. (2007) The impact of gestational stress and prenatal growth on emotional problems in offspring: A review. *Acta Psychiatrica Scandinavica, 115*, 171–183.

32. Finch, S.J. (2003). Pregnancy during residency: A literature review. *Academic Medicine, 78*, 418–428.

33. Gamble, J., & Creedy, D. (2001). Women's preference for a caesarean section: Incidence and associated factors. *Birth, 28*, 101–110.

34. Malacrida, C., & Boulton, T. (2012) Women's perceptions of Childbirth 'Choices'. Competing discourses of motherhood, sexuality and selflessness. *Gender & Society, 26*(5), 748–772.

35. Miller, A.C., & Schriver, T. (2012) Women's childbirth preferences and practices in the United States. *Social Science and Medicine, 75*, 709–716.

36. Jackson, M., Dahlen, H., & Schmied, V. (2012) Birthing outside the system: perceptions of risk amongst Australian women who have freebirths and high risk homebirths. *Midwifery, 28*, 561–567.

37. Davies, J., Hey, E., Reid, W., & Young, G. (1996). Prospective regional study of planned home births. *BMJ, 313*, 1302–1306.

38. Stramrood, C., Paarlberg, K.M., Huis In 't Veld, E.M., Berger, L.W., Vingerhoets, A.J., Schultz, W.C., & van Pampus, M.G. (2011). Post-traumatic stress disorder following childbirth in home-like and hospital settings. *Journal of Psychosomatic Obstetrics & Gynecology, 32*(2), 88–97.

39. Grekin, R., & O'Hara, M. W. (2014). Prevalence and risk factors of postpartum posttraumatic stress disorder: A meta-analysis. *Clinical Psychology Review, 34*(5), 389–401.

40. Ayers, S., & Ford, E. (2015). Post-traumatic stress during pregnancy and the postpartum period. In A. Wenzel & S. Stuart (Eds.) *Oxford Handbook of Perinatal Psychology*. Oxford: Oxford University Press, 182–200.

41. Ayers, S., Bond, R., Bertullies, S., & Wijma, K. (2016). The aetiology of post-traumatic stress following childbirth: A meta-analysis and theoretical framework. *Psychological Medicine, 46*(6), 1121–1134.

42. Munk-Olsen, T., Hammer Bech, B., Vestergaard, M., Li, J., Olsen J., & Munk Larsen, T. (2014). Psychiatric disorders following fetal death: A population-based cohort study. *BMJ Open, 4*, doi:10.1136/bmjopen-2014–005187.

43. Hodnett, E., Gates, S., Hofmeyr, G.J., & Sakala, C. (2007). Continuous support for women during childbirth. *Cochrane Database of Systematic Reviews, 3*, art. no. CD003766.

Epigenetics
The Bridge between Biology and Psychosocial Health

Leroy C. Edozien

Introduction

In delivering and researching women's health care, the traditional approach has focussed on biological mechanisms and biomedical interventions. This approach has taken women's health care to great heights, facilitated by advances in science and technology; however, it is increasingly recognized in clinical practice that biopsychosocial factors are critical to the promotion, maintenance and enhancement of women's health. Health and illness are closely associated with behaviour, emotions and thoughts and, in the sphere of women's health, the UK Confidential Enquiries into Maternal Deaths and similar programmes elsewhere have drawn attention to the major role played by maladaptive health behaviour, psychosocial stress and emotional problems in maternal mortality and morbidity. There is increasing recognition of the importance of social and behavioural factors – such as inactivity, stress, poor nutrition, smoking, drug and alcohol abuse, exposure to risk and risk taking. Furthermore, there is increasing awareness that health and behaviour in pregnancy have significant implications not only for fetal health in utero but also for the immediate and long-term well-being of the child. These developments call for a biopsychosocial approach to the delivery of women's health services and to research in this field. The biopsychosocial approach aims to obtain a comprehensive picture of health conditions and events by using biological, behavioural, psychological and social measures. It adopts the life course approach to health (which emphasizes the connection between the individual and the socioeconomic and historical context in which the individual lives) [1], and integrates 'nature' with 'nurture'.

Despite its potential strengths, the biopsychosocial model is yet to become firmly entrenched in health care. The 'bio' (biology) has not been integrated with the 'psychosocial', largely because of health professionals' bias for 'hard science', with the psychological and social domains being regarded as 'fluffy stuff'.

Although the association between psychosocial factors and health outcomes is recognized, the underlying biological mechanisms have hitherto been poorly understood. It is arguable that until health professionals and scientists, who are usually brought up in the positivist tradition, have a better understanding of these mechanisms insufficient attention will be paid to the biopsychosocial approach.

There is, however, a development on the horizon that portends a climate change: epigenetics, reportedly the fastest growing branch of medicine, is bridging the gap between biology and psychosocial health.

Psychosocial Health

The World Health Organization defines health as a state of complete physical, mental and social well-being and not just the absence of disease. It is, however, still common in biomedical discourse for 'health' to be construed narrowly as physical health. The term 'well-being' has emerged as a holistic alternative, aimed particularly at capturing the emotional dimension of health. In this chapter, psychosocial health is taken to mean a state of mental, emotional, social and spiritual wellness.

Physical ill-health could induce psychological problems or lead to social isolation and economic losses. On the other hand, psychosocial ill-health (or the state of suffering adverse psychosocial conditions) may precipitate physical ill-health. For example, African American women with upward economic mobility from early life impoverishment tend to have lower rates of preterm birth and infant mortality compared with African American women with lifelong residence in impoverished neighbourhoods [2]. Lifestyle factors such as tobacco, alcohol, exercise and diet strongly influence the incidence rates of cancer, obesity, metabolic disease and cardiovascular disease. Social isolation has been found to have a deleterious effect on the immune system.

Adverse psychosocial conditions affect not only the index woman but also her offspring and subsequent generations. The Dutch Famine Birth Cohort Study showed that women who were exposed to famine (caused by a German blockade of supplies during World War II) gave birth to children with adverse metabolic and mental phenotypes (i.e. were more susceptible to conditions such as diabetes, obesity and schizophrenia) [3, 4].

The social environment has also been shown to have a neurobiological impact: early life experience of abuse, neglect and challenging parenting style have been shown to affect cognition and behaviour [5].

While epidemiological studies have established that psychosocial health and physical health are closely associated, the underlying biological mechanisms have been uncertain, and sometimes controversial. A relatively new field of investigation – epigenetics – promises to yield some answers to age-old questions.

Genome, Genes and DNA

To understand the basics of epigenetics, a knowledge of some basic terminology is essential. Biological information essential for human development is stored in the molecule deoxyribonucleic acid (DNA). The complete set of DNA in an organism is known as a *genome*, and all nucleated cells in a human contain a copy of the entire genome. A *gene* is a piece of the genome, and different genes determine different traits. The DNA wraps around proteins called *histones*, forming a compact unit.

The set of genes (i.e. the particular DNA sequence) that accounts for a specific trait (e.g. hair colour) is the *genotype*. The appearance of that trait is known as the *phenotype*. A variety of phenotypes (the outward manifestation of the genetic code) can occur among cells with identical DNA. In other words, identical genotypes can manifest as different phenotypes. It is known, for example, that monozygotic twins may share identical genotype but manifest different phenotype (differences in physical and psychological characteristics and vulnerability to disease) [6].

This variation in phenotype is partly due to mutation (a change in the DNA sequence) but mostly due to changes in the production of gene products ('gene expression').

What Is Epigenetics?

Some biochemical changes alter gene expression without altering the DNA sequence. These changes are known as 'epigenetic' changes. The term 'epigenetics' was first used by the developmental biologist Conrad H Waddington to describe the processes by which the genotype brings about the associated phenotype [7]. He observed that environmental factors can cause the phenotype to be different from to the one expected from a particular genotype and that the new phenotype could be inherited by offspring even in the absence of the original environmental stimulus. At the time, the structure of the DNA had not been unravelled. Today, 'epigenetics' refers to changes in gene expression that do not entail a change in the DNA sequence itself. The underlying biochemical processes ('epigenetic modifications') include DNA methylation and histone modification (such as acetylation, methylation and phosphorylation). There are other mechanisms of epigenetic change, but DNA methylation and histone modification are the most studied. Methylation of the DNA involves the coupling of a methyl group to a cytosine (one of the four main bases found in the DNA). The source of the methyl group is *S*-adenosyl-L-methionine (SAM). This addition of chemical compounds to the DNA and histone modifies the activity of the genes within the genome, and the modifications can be inherited by offspring. Usually, methylation switches off the gene.

When compounds attach to the DNA and modify its function, they are said to have 'marked' the genome. All the chemical compounds attached to the DNA in the organism as part of epigenetic modification constitute the *epigenome*.

The methylation of the DNA is catalysed by the enzymes DNA methyltransferases (DNMTs). Histone modification, which affects how tightly the DNA is wound around the histone, is catalysed by histone methyltransferase and other enzymes. Any condition that alters the tissue levels of these enzymes can affect methylation or histone modification and thus affect gene expression.

The chromosomes that we inherit from our parents contain not only DNA but also proteins. The DNA carries genetic information, while the proteins carry epigenetic information.

It is thought that, through epigenetic mechanisms, nutrition, stress, sleep and other environmental factors induce changes in gene expression and thereby influence health and well-being. Significantly, epigenetic changes can be passed on from one generation to the next. Given the huge attention that DNA has commanded in scientific research, it is remarkable that the psychosocial context of the parent can affect the gene expression of the offspring without any change in the DNA sequence, and it is now clear that science has to look beyond the genome for answers to key questions in epidemiology, human development and medical sociology.

Developmental and Clinical Implications of Epigenetics

Epigenetic changes have been implicated in both normal and disease states. They have been found to influence human reproduction, behaviour, susceptibility to disease and fetal programming. Adverse outcomes could result from either inhibition of methylation (through deficiency of methyl donors or altered enzyme activity) or errors in methylation (e.g. methylation occurring at the wrong site). Abnormal or altered methylation has been found in many cancers, vascular diseases, immune disorders and even in poorly nurtured, but otherwise healthy, offspring. It has been suggested that epigenetics may play a role in the pathogenesis of leiomyomas [8] and endometriosis [9].

We can't change our genome but we can change our epigenome. The epigenome can be changed during intrauterine life but also at any time during the lifetime of the person. As discussed next, lifestyle has a strong potential to induce changes in the epigenome.

Unlike genetic mutations, epigenetic changes are potentially reversible, and a number of epigenetic drugs are in development for treating specific diseases. Various fields of investigation have developed in response to the growing interest in epigenetics. These include behavioural epigenetics (which studies the role of epigenetics in shaping behaviour), epigenetic epidemiology, nutritional epigenetics, developmental epigenetics (investigating how factors in the early life environment determine an individual's phenotype) and medical epigenetics.

Ageing

In the Belfast Elderly Longitudinal Free-Living Ageing STudy (BELFAST study), hundreds of nonagenarians who were 'very good' for their age were recruited and subjected to a range of assessments which included anthropometric measurements, diet and lifestyle history, lipid profile and immune status. It has been suggested that the findings of this study emphasize the need to look after the epigenome [10]. Ageing is associated with alterations in histone and DNA methylation [11]. This may be due to changes with exposure to factors (such as diet) that inhibit DNA methylation or to decreases in the activity of methyltransferase (DNMT).

Adults may have a biological age that is older or younger than their chronological age, and this may reflect epigenetic changes. Hannum and colleagues have developed a measure of biological age based on the degree of methylation associated with 71 sites in the human genome that are strongly associated with chronological age [12]. This measure can be used to compare a person's biological age with their chronological age. It is not yet in clinical use but marks a further milestone in the coming together of biological and psychosocial aspects of health and well-being.

Diet

One of the most striking manifestations of epigenetic change and the heritability of such change was an experiment which showed that the coat colour and disease susceptibility of newborn agouti mice could be changed by feeding their mothers extra vitamins during pregnancy [13]. Agouti mice have the agouti gene which makes them fat and yellow and prone to cancer and diabetes. When agouti mice were fed a diet rich in methyl donors, their offspring were slender, brown and not prone to cancer and diabetes. Significantly, this change was achieved without altering the DNA sequence of the agouti mice. Rather, the diet led to a change in gene expression.

The potential influence of diet on epigenetic change is huge. Dietary deficiencies could alter SAM metabolism, thereby altering methylation of DNA and influencing gene expression. Deficiency of micronutrients in pregnancy is associated with increased risk of neural tube defects, preeclampsia and small-for-gestational age baby, and this may have to do with DNA methylation.

The micronutrients folate, vitamin B12, vitamin B6, choline, betaine and methionine are involved in the production of SAM, the methyl donor for methylation (Figure 3.1). Folate is involved in the re-methylation of homocysteine to methionine which is adenosylated to form SAM. Betaine, present in wheat and spinach, breaks down the toxic by-products of SAM synthesis.

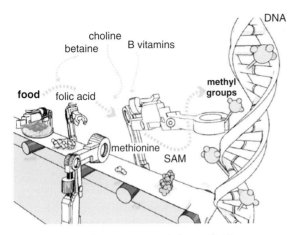

Figure 3.1 Role of B-Vitamins in methylation of DNA
Source: Reprinted with kind permission from http://learn.genetics
.utah.edu.

'Folate' is a general term for a group of water-soluble B-vitamins found in foods, predominantly in the form of 5-methyl-tetrahydrofolate (THF). Folic acid, the oxidized synthetic compound commonly prescribed to pregnant women, needs to be reduced and methylated to THF in the liver before it can be useful in metabolism. High levels of unreduced folic acid could have adverse effects and for this reason dietary sources of folate are preferable for non-pregnant women. Dietary deficiency of folate is a cause of hyperhomocysteinaemia, a risk factor for vascular disease, recurrent miscarriage, placental abruption, pre-eclampsia, congenital disorders such as cleft lip and other pregnancy complications.

Epigenetic processes are also affected by polyphenols; these alter the activities of methylation enzymes such as such as 5-cytosine DNMT. Polyphenols (also known as phenolics) are antioxidants found in bran, purple potatoes, wine, seeds, green tea, food supplements and some complementary medicines; their contribution to epigenetic change could be exploited for disease prevention and treatment [11].

Maternal Smoking

Smoking in pregnancy is associated with increased risk of miscarriage, preterm labour and fetal growth restriction. The adverse effects of smoking extend beyond birth: maternal smoking is associated with neurodevelopmental delay, impaired general cognitive ability and conduct disorder. These consequences of maternal smoking have been attributed to aberrant DNA methylation and gene expression. DNA methylation was found to be altered in the placenta and in cord blood of newborns whose mothers smoked during pregnancy [15].

Sleep

Epigenetic mechanisms are thought to be involved in the development and maintenance of insomnia [16]. Also, stress induced by sleep deprivation could affect gene expression.

The circadian rhythm, the 24-hour cycle referred to as the 'body clock', regulates physiological processes and tells the body when to sleep. It plays an important role in health and well-being, and disruptions to this rhythm have been associated with shortened life span, cancer and degenerative diseases. There is evidence that epigenetic changes are involved in the link between circadian rhythm and these abnormalities [17, 18]. Persons doing long-term shift work were found to have alterations in the levels of DNA methylation associated with the pertinent genes.

Exercise

It is well recognized that exercise improves motor and cognitive function and reduces the risk of cardiovascular, metabolic and degenerative disease. While the impact of exercise is partly due to the genetic constitution of the individual, epigenetic mechanisms are also thought to play a role. Both acute and chronic exercises significantly influence the methylation of genes involved in metabolism, muscle growth and inflammation in humans [19]. The impact of acute exercise on DNA methylation appears to depend on the intensity of the exercise, but it is not known whether aerobic exercise and anaerobic exercise influence DNA methylation in a similar way. It has also been shown that exercise causes other epigenetic changes such as histone modification.

The Social Environment

Social experiences may induce epigenetic change at any stage in the life of an individual – from infancy through adolescence to adulthood – and the social environment can have long-term physiological and behavioural effects [20]. This was demonstrated in a study of mothering style and methylation in rats [21]. The mothers frequently lick and groom their offspring. The study found that, through epigenetic mechanisms, the amount of such nurturing received by the offspring affects their brain development and their stress response. Richly nurtured rats grew up to be relaxed and sociable, and neglected rats grew up to be nervous and more sensitive to stress

Similarly, childhood neglect has been shown to have persistent effects in the human brain [22].

As epigenetics may underlie the impact of improved social circumstances on health, it could be that this is a mechanism by which psychological therapies exert their effects. Mindfulness has been found to cause epigenetic changes, thus influencing genetic expression [23].

Fetal Programming

During embryogenesis there is a high rate of DNA synthesis and there is extensive epigenomic marking as cell differentiation takes place, so the risk of aberrant epigenetic change is higher than at any other time.

The Barker hypothesis, that adult diseases have their origins in fetal life, stemmed from the observation that growth-restricted babies were at increased risk of developing cardiovascular disease, diabetes mellitus, obesity and metabolic syndrome as adults. These effects of early life environment on susceptibility to adult disease are now thought to be explained, at least in part, by epigenetics. Direct evidence in support of epigenetics as the mechanism underlying the developmental origins of health and disease in adult humans is, however, far from robust, and many more years of research are required [24].

Conclusion

One of the benefits of the emergence of epigenetics is that the scientific credentials of the biopsychosocial approach to health care delivery are greatly enhanced. The biomedical model of care has not yet paid sufficient attention to the role of the physical and social environment and of psychological factors in the aetiology, prevention and management of ill-health, but that is beginning to change.

It may well be that, in the future, a person's susceptibility to diseases will be identified early by genetic markers and receive effective preventative intervention. The ability to reverse epigenetic marks

may open up new treatments for cancer. Above all there may be greater impetus for people of all ages to adopt healthier lifestyles.

Key Points

- Health is a state of complete physical, mental and social well-being and not just the absence of disease. Psychosocial health is a state of mental, emotional, social and spiritual wellness.
- Adverse psychosocial conditions affect not only the index woman but also her offspring and subsequent generations.
- 'Epigenetics' refers to changes in gene expression that do not entail a change in the DNA sequence itself. The underlying biochemical processes include DNA methylation and histone modification.
- Through epigenetic mechanisms diet, exercise, stress, sleep and other environmental factors induce changes in gene expression and thereby influence health and well-being.
- The effects of epigenetics could be harnessed for disease prevention and treatment, including the development of pharmacological and non-pharmacological therapies.

References

1. Royal College of Obstetricians and Gynaecologists. Why should we consider a life course approach to women's health care? Scientific Impact Paper No. 27. London; RCOG August 2011.
2. Collins J, Rankin K, David R. African American Women's lifetime upward economic mobility and preterm birth: The effect of fetal programming. *American Journal of Public Health.* 2011;**101**(4):714–9.
3. Heijmans BT, Tobi EW, Stein AD, Putter H, Blauw GJ, Susser ES, Slagboom PE, Lumey LH. Persistent epigenetic differences associated with prenatal exposure to famine in humans. *Proc Natl Acad Sci U S A.* 2008;**105**(44):17046–9. doi: 10.1073/pnas.0806560105.
4. Painter RC, de Rooij SR, Bossuyt PM, Simmers TA, Osmond C, Barker DJ, Bleker OP, Roseboom TJ. Early onset of coronary artery disease after prenatal exposure to the Dutch famine. *Am J Clin Nutr.* 2006;**84**:322–7.

5. Spratt EG, Friedenberg SL, Swenson CC, Larosa A, De Bellis MD, Macias MM, Summer AP, Hulsey TC, Runyan DK, Brady KT. The effects of early neglect on cognitive, language, and behavioral functioning in childhood. *Psychology (Irvine).* 2012;**3**(2):175–82.

6. Haque FN, Gottesman II, Wong AH. Not really identical: Epigenetic differences in monozygotic twins and implications for twin studies in psychiatry. *Am J Med Genet C Semin Med Genet.* 2009;**151C**(2): 136–41. doi: 10.1002/ajmg.c.30206.

7. Waddington CH. The epigenotype. *Endeavour.* 1942; 18–20 Reprinted in *Int. J. Epidemiol.* 2012;**41**:10–13. doi: 10.1093/ije/dyr184.

8. Yang Q, Mas A, Diamond MP, Al-Hendy A. The mechanism and function of epigenetics in uterine leiomyoma development. *Reprod Sci.* 2016;**23**(2): 163–75. doi: 10.1177/1933719115584449.

9. Guo SW. Epigenetics of endometriosis. *Mol Hum Reprod.* 2009;**15**(10):587–607. doi: 10.1093/molehr/gap064.

10. Rea IM, Dellet M, Mills KI. ACUME2 Project. Living long and ageing well: Is epigenomics the missing link between nature and nurture? *Biogerontology.* 2016;**17** (1):33–54. doi: 10.1007/s10522-015-9589-5.

11. Weidner CI, Wagner W. The epigenetic tracks of aging. *Biol Chem.* **395**(11):1307–14. doi: 10.1515/hsz-2014-0180.

12. Hannum G, Guinney J, Zhao L, Zhang L, Hughes G, Sadda S, Klotzle B, Bibikova M, Fan JB, Gao Y, Deconde R, Chen M, Rajapakse I, Friend S, Ideker T, Zhang K. Genome-wide methylation profiles reveal quantitative views of human aging rates. *Mol Cell.* 2013;**49**(2):359–67. doi: 10.1016/j.molcel.2012.10.016.

13. Waterland RA, Jirtle JL. Transposable elements: Targets for early nutritional effects on epigenetic gene regulation. *Molecular and Cell Biology.* 2003;**23**: 5293–300.

14. Pan MH, Lai CS, Wu JC, Ho CT. Epigenetic and disease targets by polyphenols. *Curr Pharm Des.* 2013;**19**(34):6156–85.

15. Knopik VS, Maccani MA, Francazio S, McGeary JE. The epigenetics of maternal cigarette smoking during pregnancy and effects on child development. *Dev Psychopathol.* 2012;**24**(4):1377–90. doi: 10.1017/S0954579412000776.

16. Palagini L, Biber K, Riemann D. The genetics of insomnia – evidence for epigenetic mechanisms? *Sleep Med Rev.* 2014;**18**(3):225–35. doi: 10.1016/j.smrv.2013.05.00.

17. Qureshi IA, Mehler MF. Epigenetics of sleep and chronobiology. *Curr Neurol Neurosci Rep.* 2014;**14** (3):432. doi: 10.1007/s11910-013-0432-6.

18. Masri S, Kinouchi K, Sassone-Corsi P. Circadian clocks, epigenetics, and cancer. *Curr Opin Oncol.* 2015;**27**(1):50–6. doi: 10.1097/CCO.0000000000000153.

19. Voisin S, Eynon N, Yan X, Bishop DJ. Exercise training and DNA methylation in humans. *Acta Physiol (Oxf).* 2015;**213**(1):39–59. doi: 10.1111/apha.12414.

20. Champagne A, Curley JP. Epigenetic Influence of the Social Environment. In: Petronis A and Mill J (eds.), *Brain, Behavior and Epigenetics, Epigenetics and Human Health,* doi 10.1007/978-3-642-17426-1_10, Springer-Verlag Berlin Heidelberg, 2011.

21. Weaver IC, Cervoni N, Champagne FA, D'Alessio AC, Sharma S, Seckl JR, Dymov S, Szyf M, Meaney MJ. Epigenetic programming by maternal behavior. *Nat Neurosci.* 2004;**7**(8):847–54.

22. McGowan PO, Sasaki A, D'Alessio AC, Dymov S, Labonté B, Szyf M, Turecki G, Meaney MJ. Epigenetic regulation of the glucocorticoid receptor in human brain associates with childhood abuse. *Nat Neurosci.* 2009;**12**(3):342–8. doi: 10.1038/nn.2270.

23. Kaliman P, Alvarez-López MJ, Cosín-Tomás M, Rosenkranz MA, Lutz A, Davidson RJ. Rapid changes in histone deacetylases and inflammatory gene expression in expert meditators. *Psychoneuroendocrinology.* 2014;**40**:96–107. doi: 10.1016/j.psyneuen.2013.11.004.

24. Saffery R, Novakovic B. Epigenetics as the mediator of fetal programming of adult onset disease: What is the evidence? *Acta Obstet Gynecol Scand.* 2014;**93**(11): 1090–8. doi: 10.1111/aogs.12431.

Communicating Effectively

The Patient–Clinician Relationship in Women's Healthcare

Jillian S. Romm and Lishiana Solano Shaffer

At the center of medicine there is always a human relationship between a patient and a doctor.
—*Michael Balint* [1]

Skillful communication is a critical element in developing the patient–clinician relationship and serves as a potential strength in the healing process for patients. 'Communication between patients and clinicians is the bedrock of the patient-clinician relationship' [2]. Studies are finding significant connection between functional clinician–patient relationships and patient and clinician satisfaction[3, 4].

Due to the nature of women's healthcare specialties and the intimacy and trust embedded in the clinician–patient relationship, we believe that there are essential communication competencies which build upon basic communication techniques, and they are necessary skills for the women's healthcare clinician. Many clinicians care for women throughout their patients' life cycles and are involved in multiple significant life events. The clinician–patient relationship is of critical importance in women's healthcare.

Developing and maintaining communication skills allows for productive and empathetic healthcare relationships. In addition to patient and clinician satisfaction, empathetic communication is associated with increased adherence to treatment and fewer malpractice complaints. More importantly, patients cared for by clinicians who they perceive as empathetic have more favorable health outcomes and are more satisfied with their care [5, 6].

There is ample evidence of the power of empathy in clinical relationships. For example, diabetic patients who scored their physicians with higher empathy scores had significantly better diabetes control [5, 7]. In this case, empathy resulted in physicians better understanding their patients' circumstances and allowing for recommendation and treatment options catered to unique lifestyles. This patient-centered care fostered

better adherence to treatment, with significantly improved health outcomes. Research also indicates that patient-centeredness and empathic communication lead to better immune function, shorter post-surgery hospital stays and fewer complications [8], decreased migraine disability and symptoms [9] and shorter duration of colds[10].

Patients report that their relationships with their clinicians are important and highly valued.

Patients who perceive a lack of caring or collaboration are more likely to litigate and cite feeling devalued, being given information poorly and sensing that the physician was not understanding them or their wishes [11]. Indeed, patients have indicated that what is most important to them is their relationship with their clinician and that relationship is more important to them than their treatment. Baile et al. reported that patients identify their physicians as one of their most important sources of psychological support [12]. The Physician's Foundation also surveyed patients and identified how critically important their relationships are with their doctors and clinical specialists [13].

The Schwartz Center's focus group research in 2013–2014 identified that patients cited compassionate care as being the most important aspect of their healthcare. They described the compassionate relationship as one in which they receive understandable information, are involved in decisions, are listened to attentively, and are shown respect. These behaviors are indicators of productive communication and are essential aspects of a healthy clinical relationship [14].

There is also evidence that clinicians with productive and functional relationships who deliver quality care are more satisfied, less burned out, and likely to remain in their careers.

Research by the Rand Corporation for the American Medical Association found that a primary driver of job satisfaction among physicians was the ability to provide high-quality patient care [15].

To date, most information regarding patient preferences about healthcare relationships has been acquired from research in primary care medicine. These preferences are likely to be similar to those for obstetrical and gynecological patients. The very nature of women's health specialties, which includes caring for patients during significant milestones in their lives, many of which are quite intimate, provides opportunities for skillful utilization of the clinician–patient relationship.

Empathic Communication

'The state of empathy, or being empathic, is to perceive the internal frame of reference of another with accuracy and with the emotional components and meanings which pertain thereto as if one were the person' [16]. Empathy is the human quality that recognizes and sustains human connection and understanding. In patient–clinician relationships, as patients experience empathy, they also feel understood, accepted and respected.

Historically in medical training, recommendations about clinical relationships included development of 'detached concern' and caution against affective empathy was urged. A more clinical, or 'cognitive empathy,' was encouraged. There is little support in the literature for such caution and for the recommended emotional avoidance [17].

Currently, there is a greater appreciation for the value of skilled communication in service of the clinician–patient relationship, and empathy is encouraged and normalized. Empathy is a natural socio-emotional competency that has evolved with the mammalian brain to form and maintain social bonds [18] and is the metaphorical cornerstone of human relationships. In clinical relationships, this social bonding creates and sustains the clinician–patient relationship.

Communication and Healthcare Relationships

The clinician–patient relationship is essentially a moral enterprise that is grounded in trust. Such relationships require skilled communication. In healthy and functional clinical relationships, empathy develops as the relationship develops. The clinician's empathy for the patient, as well as for themselves, naturally develops and deepens, and serves as a positive feedback loop, enhancing relationships with patients,

which results in both increased patient and clinician satisfaction.

The capacity for empathy naturally exists in humans. Studies have shown that it is possible to increase or decrease empathy in response to the environment and context[19]. Indeed, one's mindset and beliefs about empathy determine how much effort they will exert to experience empathy[20]. There appears to be a naturally self-protective process for healthcare professionals who have demonstrated a down-regulation in their pain empathy responses after exposure to patients in pain and suffering, allowing them to be objective and thoughtful as they care for their patients[21].

There is agreement that empathy commonly decreases during training [22, 23] due to numerous factors, including the focus on professional distance and clinical neutrality, paucity of role models, and harsh/non-compassionate treatment of trainees. Other factors are objectification of the patient [24], increased workload, mistreatment by supervisors, lack of emotional support, and interpersonal conflict [25].

Among the many skills in which medical providers must be proficient, the human and primitive abilities to understand and connect with and have empathy for their patients are critical components of effective communication and clinical care. These essential skills require training and ongoing support to maintain them over a professional career.

Basic Communication Skills

Communication is verbal and non-verbal, and becoming proficient in communication skills ensures adequate data collection during the medical interview, sharing of information, and recognizing concerns and priorities of the patient and provider. These basic skills establish the groundwork for building a strong patient–clinician relationship [26].

Healthcare relationships are complex, and the thoughts and feelings of both parties are influenced by the social and medical context and setting, as well as the perceptual skills of the clinician [27]. Attentive listening skills, empathy, and use of open-ended questions are examples of skillful communication.

Collaborative communication involves the two-way exchange of information. It requires that clinicians provide opportunities to suggest and discuss treatment options and to share the decision-making process with the patient and family. In discussing available treatments, the skilled clinician elicits and recognizes the patient's expectations, hopes and level of risk acceptance [28].

Communication Strategies

There is a developing worldwide consensus of the importance of teaching and training medical professionals in basic communication skills as well as in challenging conversations, such as giving bad news, acknowledging medical errors, and cultural communication and competencies. The European Consensus on Learning Objectives for Core Communication Curriculum has outlined three levels of communication training [29]. These include key communication tasks and recommended skills, including empathy and reflective skills and special and difficult discussions. In the United States, the Accreditation Council for Graduate Medical Education competencies include interpersonal and communication skills and evaluation of the effectiveness of communication with both patients and families, as well as other healthcare professionals and team members as an aspect of professionalism [30].

In 2003, the Institute of Medicine in the United States called upon educators and licensing organizations to strengthen health professional training requirements in the delivery of patient-centered care. They specified communication skills, such as open-ended inquiry, reflective listening and empathy. In addition, the report recommended training healthcare professionals to respond to the unique needs, values, and preferences of individual patients. This 'patient-centered model' relies on effective and skillful healthcare communication and clinician–patient/family relationships [31].

Teaching Communication and Empathy Skills

As hospital, educational, and healthcare organizations are increasingly committed to trainee and employee education and continuous quality improvement in the area of communication, they are offering programs to refine healthcare communication and relationship skills. These programs include didactic and lecture formats, group work, self-reflection and self-awareness activities, and web-based courses and programs. Training ranges from basic communication skills to more complex, self-reflection-based interpersonal and self-management skills.

Courses and programs should be aimed at offering information about the importance of communication and the patient–clinician relationship. Training should build upon learners' native empathetic abilities such as recognizing paralanguage, reflection and self-awareness, as well as increased knowledge of others' cultures and religions. These skills are in support of clinical relationships and enhance communication and understanding.

In reviewing the communication trainings options, we find a wide array of programs, from those providing basic communication information and strategies, to programs that promote self-reflection and empathy for the patient and for oneself in the clinical encounter.

Several programs offer basic communication skills training. For example, AIDET [32] and BATHE [33] offer information to enhance the clinician's cognitive understanding of the importance and basic components of communication. Beckman et al. [34] recommended core communication skills, including active listening and soliciting attribution, as a model of co-participation between the patient and clinician. Empathetic training expands upon basic communication understanding, and presents a neurobiological and physiological frame for appreciating the value of interpersonal communication[35]. This training offers additional coursework for complex patient interactions, such as delivering bad news. Web-based training and utilizing simulation/patient-actors to recreate medical encounters may provide new and additional options for clinical education about interpersonal skills. Several researchers are evaluating the efficacy of such novel forums [36].

We acknowledge that there are basic communication skills that are necessary in healthcare, such as engaged listening, conveying acceptance, developing rapport and encouraging dialogue. These skills enhance the medical interview, which leads to more efficient care, and are important foundation skills that are required in all healthcare professionals.

There are more complex and nuanced skills that are necessary in women's healthcare specialties. These skills support clinical practice and are based on competencies beyond basic communication skills. These competencies provide the framework for productive clinician–patient relationships. The essential communication competencies include effective communication, self-awareness, and relationship development and refinement. Each competency builds upon the

BOX 4.1 Communication Strategies and Education/Training Programs

Communication with Patients

AIDET: A simple communication training technique, identifying aspects of communication as Acknowledge, Introduce, Duration, Explain, Thank you. Focuses exclusively on verbal communication skills.

Balint Groups: Group members and the leader sit round in a circle; a case is presented and then discussed, with emphasis on the doctor–patient relationship. Named after Michael Balint who, with his wife Enid, held psychological training seminars for GPs in London.

RESPECT: Intercultural communication, with training in cultural awareness, knowledge, skill, and encounters leading to the provider becoming 'culturally desiring' of cultural knowledge, skillful, and familiar with cultural encounters.

BATHE Technique: Recommended for eliciting information about a new patient – or a new problem, this model utilizes mnemonic device: Background, Affect, Trouble, Handling, Empathy. Clinicians are encouraged to inquire about the patient's response to the problem, how troubled they are, and empathic responses are recommended. The experience of feeling empathy for the patient is presumed.

Empathetic Training: Web-based, self-paced didactic instruction includes basic neuroscience of interpersonal connections, detection and management of patients' emotional states, and offers recommendations for provider responses and self-management skills.

Mindfulness: Based on an eight-week behavioral program and educational course that offers first hand experience of meditation techniques, including mindful awareness of daily activities and communication. Evidence suggests that mindfulness-based stress reduction (MBSR) can improve empathy skills in clinicians. MBSR reduces burnout and develops self-awareness and self-compassion, and assists in development of empathy with others, as well as with oneself.

Narrative Med: Taught in small groups and workshops, narrative medicine training teaches one to recognize, absorb, interpret, and honor the stories of patients' illnesses. Clinicians are encouraged to imagine and enter patients' worlds, to better understand, and reflect on their own experiences in patient care.

REDE: Provides peer training in basics of healthcare communication training, with additional options for such concerns as managing conflict and difficult conversations.

Schwartz Reflection Rounds: Multidisciplinary forum where staff reflect on psychosocial issues that arise in caring for patients. These interactive discussions are anchored in a case presentation and focus on clinicians' experiences, thoughts, and feelings and encourage staff to share insights, vulnerabilities and support.

Sharing Bad News

SPIKES: Developed for oncology originally, recommends a six-step process in delivering bad news, with the goal of fulfilling the objectives of the discussion, gathering information from the patient, transmitting the medical information, providing support, and eliciting the patient's collaboration in developing a plan.

Oncotalk/VitalTalk: Communication programs designed for oncology, end-of-life and palliative care conversations. This training may include four-day residential training, small group discussions, role-playing, standardized patient experiences, and self-evaluation.

Cultural Communication

RESPECT: Model using action-oriented communication and behaviors to build trust across race ethnicity, culture, and power differences. Utilizes mnemonic device including respect, explanatory model, social context, power, empathy, concerns and trust/therapeutic alliance. Specific responses to patients are suggested within the model.

Communication with Colleagues

PEEER: Training recommends critical elements in intra-professional communication, including Plain Language, Engagement, Empathy, Empowerment, Respect. Specific examples of communication skills are offered.

rapprochement resulting from basic communication strategies and techniques.

Effective communication in service of clinical relationships requires flexibility, the ability to engage in the clinical encounter and develop the relationship to benefit the patient. As rapport is established, there is increase in the clinician's awareness of the patient's and of their own feelings. The clinician can then interpret these feelings as reflecting those of the patient. Gleichgerrcht suggested that the ability to engage in self-other awareness and regulate one's emotions, along with the tendency to help others, contributes to the sense of compassion that comes from clinical practice [37]. Informed by both verbal and non-verbal communication, the skilled clinician can then refine and further develop the trusting and shared relationship.

To do this effectively the clinician must feel comfortable within the interpersonal relationship, be aware of one's own biases, concerns, and context, and use the knowledge of their own internal experience as a reflection of the patient's internal experience. This process is the clinical application of empathy, where the clinician is aware that they are sensing the patient's feelings within themselves. In addition, the efficacious use of self in the medical encounter expands the capacity for communication and connection and deepens the clinician–patient relationship.

The essential communication competencies require that the clinician use one's self as an instrument in medical care. Philip Hopkins, as he reflected on the power of the healthcare relationship, stated, "The most frequently used drug in medicine is the doctor himself" [38].

The ability to skillfully use oneself in the healthcare relationship requires competence in communication, interpersonal skills, insight, self-awareness and empathy. As clinicians gain experience and confidence in their basic interpersonal skills, providing opportunities for reflective practices will support and sustain clinician–patient relationship development, as well as increase both patient and clinician provider satisfaction.

Programs such as Balint Groups [39], reflection rounds [40], and self-reflective processes, such as mindfulness practices [41], provide opportunities for deeper understanding of both patients and clinicians. Such programs provide interventions that enhance

communication and develop empathy, utilizing inductive-based strategies.

The most innovative programs are grounded in the clinical encounter while providing reflection and self-awareness skills development. Balint Groups are an example of a strategy that enhances reflection and increases understanding of both the patient and the clinician's experiences. In this case-based group process, the discussion focuses on the clinicians' relationships with their patients. Participants report feeling more expansive, creative, and compassionate and less isolated as the result of Balint Group work. Although historically embedded in primary care medicine, several programs offer Balint Group work in women's healthcare training [42, 43], and currently additional specialties are piloting Balint Groups to support professionalism, communication skills development, and as a buffer for professional burnout [44, 45, 46].

Reflection rounds are multidisciplinary forums for staff reflection on emotional and psychosocial issues that arise in caring for patients. These interactive discussions are anchored in a case presentation and focus on clinicians' experiences, thoughts and feelings. Attendees are encouraged to share insights, vulnerabilities and support. Preliminary research indicates that reflection rounds enhance team and provider communication and support [47].

Mindfulness training has many benefits for clinicians. Well established as practices to decrease anxiety, depression and pain [48], mindfulness training is being piloted among healthcare clinicians. Medical students demonstrated increased empathy as well as decreased anxiety and depression, after mindfulness training [49]. Mindfulness-trained primary care physicians reported enhanced attentive listening skills and the ability to more effectively respond to patients, and had developed greater self-awareness [50]. Mindfulness training has also been shown to reduce psychological distress and burnout and to increase empathy [51].

Difficult Conversations and Specific Communications

Complex communication skills are also required in clinical practice, such as when sharing concerning news or prognoses, dealing with angry and difficult patient encounters, and caring for patients from different cultures and languages.

Sharing difficult news and prognoses is challenging, and clinicians report inadequate training and modeling for such encounters. Unfortunately, these are not rare encounters for the women's healthcare clinician [52]. Many of the techniques used for communicating bad news can also be used for other difficult encounters.

The SPIKES Protocol provides a template for disclosing unfavorable information. This protocol consists of six steps, with the goal being to enable the clinician to fulfill the four primary objectives of disclosing bad news, including gathering information from the patient, transmitting the medical information, providing support to the patient, and eliciting the patient's collaboration in developing a strategy or treatment plan for the future. Originally piloted with oncologists, SPIKES is currently utilized by other specialties. SPIKES users report increased confidence in their ability to disclose unfavorable medical information to their patients [53]. Oncotalk was also targeted at oncologists, and was piloted as a four-day residential training program, offering reflective practices and communication skills training. Skills include basic communication and difficult conversations, such as giving bad news, palliative care discussions and family conferences.

As modeled by Kubler-Ross, inviting patients to serve as educators delivering bad news may be an effective teaching strategy [54]. Specific advice and recommendations shared by patient-educators included setting the scene and pacing the discussion, non-verbal messages of caring, and allowing patients to maintain hopefulness.

Skilled and effective inter-colleague communication is essential in healthcare. Medical care lends itself to teams and systems and, when well functioning, patients and the clinicians benefit. Designed for all health professionals, the PEEER model represents Plain Language, Engagement, Empathy, Empowerment, Respect, and these goals are met with training about specific communication skills [55]. The skills of patient-centered communication transfer to inter-colleague communication, increasing self-efficacy in communication in general [56].

Electronic Medical Records (EMR) and Healthcare Communication

In addition to difficult patient encounters, the challenges and demands of modern healthcare systems must be noted as impacting clinicians' practices. Electronic medical records (EMR) are being utilized to enhance patient charting and communication between colleagues and between patients and their clinicians. Research indicates that patients view EMR communication with their clinicians positively [57]. However, feedback from medical professionals suggests that the computer has negative effects on communication between clinicians and patients, distracting and preventing them from having meaningful personal interactions with their patients [58]. Discussing a patient's care via electronic communication presents challenges for clinicians who benefit from face-to-face discussions with colleagues.

Attending to verbal and non-verbal messages is critical when incorporating computer and keyboard work into the clinical encounter. After establishing the relationship, purposeful and transparent charting may be done in the patient's presence. Prior to coming in the exam room, the clinician should review relevant medical records. When a clinician takes time to review the EMR, even if briefly, and then reflects this review back to the patient, the patient is likely to perceive that the EMR is of value and an integral aspect of their care. Shared decision making and a recap of the plan can be done with the patient and, with the assistance of the EMR, relevant educational materials may be reviewed on the screen and printed for the patient's use. We recommend a discussion about electronic email follow-up, which can save significant time for the clinician, and feel personal to patients.

In addition, some medical practices are piloting the use of medical scribes, who are individuals trained in transcription of the pertinent medical details of the clinical interaction. Scribes allow clinicians to devote 100% of their verbal and non-verbal attention to the patient, and evidence suggests they may improve clinician satisfaction, productivity, time-related efficiencies, revenue, and patient–clinician interactions [59]. As the use of EMR expands, developing and sustaining relationships and utilizing effective communication strategies in conjunction with electronic tools will be more critical than ever.

Cultural Communication Competencies

Culture and ethnicity have often been cited as barriers in establishing effective and satisfying clinician–patient relationships. Schouten and Meeuwesen's review of cultural communication literature found major differences in doctor–patient communication as a consequence of patients' ethnic backgrounds. They noted that physicians behaved less effectively when interacting with ethnic minority patients, as compared to patients of the dominant culture. Ethnic minority patients themselves are also less verbally expressive, less assertive, and less effective during medical encounters than patients of dominant culture [60].

It is helpful to develop strategies to enhance awareness of patients' attitudes, beliefs, biases, and behaviors that may influence patient care and adherence to treatment. Understanding the role of culture will allow clinicians to explore the meaning of illness, understand patient's social and family context, and provide patient-centered and culturally competent care [61].

Summary

Women's healthcare specialties provide opportunities for long and productive relationships with patients and families. Specialists in obstetrics and gynecology may follow patients through puberty, childbearing and the years of aging, and form trusting and healthy relationships that serve the patients during routine care and significant life events. Using the patient–clinician relationship skillfully leads to significant health benefits, as well as patient and clinician satisfaction.

In that empathetic communication is the cornerstone of caring relationships, ensuring adequate training and support to maintain empathetic skills is critical during training years and beyond. Incorporating the essential communication competencies of skilled communication – rapport development, self-awareness, and relationship refinement – will elevate the clinician from basic communication skills to excellence and provide enhanced patient and provider satisfaction. Many tools and trainings are available to aid in this process. We favor a method that actively incorporates reflection and self-awareness such as Balint Groups, reflection rounds, and mindfulness-based training.

In this fast-paced, high-tech era of medicine, where knowledge and information are ever expanding, it is imperative that we stay focused on what is truly at the center: the clinician–patient relationship.

Imagination is not only the uniquely human capacity to envision that which is not, and, therefore, the foundation of all invention and innovation. In its arguably most transformative and revelatory capacity, it is the power that enables us to empathize with humans whose experiences we have never shared [62].

Key Points

- Developing and maintaining communication skills allows for productive and empathetic healthcare relationships. Being empathic is to perceive the internal frame of reference of another with accuracy and with the emotional components and meanings which pertain thereto as if one were the person.
- In addition to patient and clinician satisfaction, empathetic communication is associated with increased adherence to treatment and fewer malpractice complaints. Empathy serves as a positive feedback loop, enhancing relationships with patients, which results in both increased patient and clinician satisfaction.
- Due to the nature of women's healthcare specialties and the intimacy and trust embedded in the clinician–patient relationship, more complex and nuanced communication skills are required of women's healthcare clinicians.
- These include rapport development, self-awareness, and relationship refinement, and could be acquired through training initiatives such as Balint Groups, reflection rounds, and mindfulness-based training. Templates such as the SPIKES protocol and the PEEER model enhance empathy and communication.
- As the use of EMR expands, developing and sustaining relationships and utilizing effective communication strategies in conjunction with electronic tools will be more critical than ever.
- Patients can be engaged as educators, for example, in teaching how to communicate challenging news.

References

1. Balint M. *The doctor, his patient and the illness*. London: Tavistock Publications; 1957.

2. Medical Oncology Communication Skills Training Modules; 2002. Available at: www.vitaltalk.org/sites/default/files/Oncotalk_Fundamental_Skills.pdf. Accessed 22 March 2017.

3. Esposito CL, Macciaroli JM, Witter J, DeGoias E, Morote ES. Patients tell the story: Interrelationships among patient satisfaction, communications with providers, and emergency department care. *JNY State Nures Assoc*. 2014;**44**(1):4–10.

4. Moreno-Jimenez B, Galvez-Herrer M, Rodriquez-Carvajal R, Sanz Vergel AI. A Study of physician's intention to quit: The role of burnout, commitment, and difficult doctor-patient interactions. *Psicothema*. 2012 May;**24**(2):263–70.

5. Hojat M, Louis DZ, Markham FW, Wender R, Rabinowitz C, Gonnella JS. Physician's empathy and clinical outcomes for diabetic patients. *Acad Med.* 2011 March;**86**(3):359–64.

6. Rakel DP, Hoeft TJ, Barrett, BP, Chewning BA, Craig BM, Niu M. Empathy and the duration of the common cold. *Fam Med.* 2009 July–August;**41**(7):494–501.

7. Del Canale S, Louis DZ, Maio V, Wang X, Rossi G, Hojat M, Connella JS. The relationship between physician empathy and disease complications: An empirical study of primary care physicians and their diabetic patients in Parma, Italy. *Acad Med.* 2012 September;**87**(9):1243–9.

8. Steinhausen S, Ommen O, Antoine SL, Koehler T, Pfaff H, Neugebauer E. Short- and long-term subjective medical treatment outcome of trauma surgery patients: The importance of physician empathy. *Patient Prefer Adherence.* 2014 September;**18**(8):1239–53.

9. Attar HS, Chandramani S. Impact of physician empathy on migraine disability and migraineur compliance. *Ann Indian Acad Neurol.* 2012 August;**15**(Suppl 1):S89–94.

10. Rakel D. Perception of empathy in the therapeutic encounter: Effects on the common cold. *Patient Educ Couns,* 2011 December;**85**(3):390–7.

11. Beckman HB, Markakis KM, Suchman AL, Frankel RM. The doctor-patient relationship and malpractice: Lessons from plaintiff depositions. *Arch Intern Med.* 1994 June 27;**154**(12):1365–70.

12. Baile WF, Buckman R, Lenzi R, Glober G, Beale EA, Kudelka AP. SPIKES – a six-step protocol for delivering bad news: Application to the patient with cancer. *Oncologist.* 2000; **5**(4):302–11.

13. The Physician's Foundation, Consumer Survey, October 2012. Available at: www.physiciansfoundation .org/healthcare-research/consumer-survey. Accessed 22 March 2017.

14. The Schwartz Center: Focus Group Report 2012–2013. Available at: www.theschwartzcenter.org/partnering-with-patients/understanding-what-patients-want/. Accessed 22 March 2017.

15. Friedberg MW, Chen, PG, Van Busum KR, Aunon FM, Pham C, Caloyeras JP, Mattke S, Pitchforth E, Quigley DD, Brook RH, Crosson FJ, Tutty M. Rand Corporation Report Study: Factors affecting physician professional satisfaction and their implications for patient care, health systems, and health policy. Available at: www.rand.org/content/dam/rand/pubs/research_reports/RR400/RR439/RAND_RR439.pdf. Accessed 22 March 2017.

16. Rogers CR. Empathetic: An unappreciated way of being. *Couns Psych.* 1975; **5**(2).

17. Decety J, Jackson PL. The functional architecture of human empathy. *Behav Cogn Neurosci Rev.* 2004 June;**3**(2):71–100.

18. Decety J, Norman GJ, Berntson GG, Cacioppo JT. A neurobehavioral evolutionary perspective on the mechanisms underlying empathy. *Prog Neurobiol.* 2012 July;**98**(1):38–48.

19. Decety J, Yang CY, Cheng Y. Physicians down-regulate their pain empathy response: An event-related brain potential study. *Neurimage.* 2010 May 1;**50**(4):1676–82.

20. Schumann K, Zaki J, Dweck CS. Addressing the empathy deficit: beliefs about the malleability of empathy predict effortful responses when empathy is challenging. *J Pers Soc Psychol.* 2014 September;**107**(3):475–93.

21. Decety J, Michalska KJ. Neurodevelopmental changes in the circuits underlying empathy and sympathy from childhood to adulthood. *Dev Sci.* 2010 November;**13**(6):886–99.

22. Hojat M, Connella JS. Eleven years of data on the Jefferson scale of empathy-medical student version (JSE-S): Proxy norm data and tentative cutoff scores. *Med Princ Pract.* 2015; **24**:344–50.

23. Williams B, Boyle M, Fielder C. Empathetic attitudes of undergraduate paramedic and nursing students towards four medical conditions: A three-year longitudinal study. *Nurse Educ Today.* 2015 February;**35**(2):e14–8.

24. Haque OS, Waytz A. Dehumanization in medicine: Causes, solutions and functions. *Perspect Psychol Sci.* 2012 March;**7**(2):176–86.

25. Riess H. Empathy in medicine – a neurobiological perspective. *JAMA.* 2010 October 13;**304**(14):1604–5.

26. Chio A, Montuschi A, Cammarosano S, DeMercanti S, Cavallo E, Ilardi A, Ghiglione P, Mutani R, Calvo A. ALS patients and caregivers communication preferences and information seeking behavior. *Eur J Neurol.* 2008 January;**15**(1):55–60.

27. Ghaffarifar S, Ghofranipour F, Ahmadi F, Khoshbaten M. Barriers to effective doctor-patient relationship based on PRECEDE model. *Glob J Health Sci.* 2015 March 25;**7**(6):43280.

28. Feudtner C. Collaborative communication in pediatric palliative care: A foundation for problem-solving and decision-making. *Pediatr Clin North Am.* 2007;**54**(5):583–607.

29. Bachmann C, Abramovitch H, Barbu CG, Cavaco AM, Elorza RD, Haak R, Loureiro E, Ratajska A, Silverman, J, Winterburn S, Rosenbaum M.

A European consensus on learning objectives for core communication curriculum in health care professions. *Patient Ed Couns.* 2003; (93): 18–26.

30. ACGME Program Requirements for Graduate Medical Education in Obstetrics and Gynecology. Accreditation Council for Graduate Medical Education. 2014. Available at: www.acgme.org/acgmeweb/Portals/0/PFAssets/ProgramRequirements/220_obstetrics_and_gynecology_07012014.pdf.

31. Greiner AC, Knebel E, editors. *Health professions education: A bridge to quality.* The National Academies Press; 2008.

32. AIDET: Five Fundamentals of Patient Communication DVD. Available at: www.firestarterpublishing.com/videos/sample-category/aidet-reg;-five-fundamentals-of-patient-commun-(1)#.Va7QkMZVhHw.

33. Stuart MR, Lieberman J. *The fifteen minute hour: Therapeutic talk in primary care* 5th Edition. Radcliffe Publishing Ltd. 2015.

34. Beckman H, Markakis K, Suchman A, Frankel R. Getting the most from a 20-minute visit. *Am J Gastroenterol.* 1994 May;**89**(5):662–4.

35. Empathetics Website. Available at: http://empathetics.com/products/.

36. Kleinsmith A, Rivera-Gutierrez D, Finney G, Cendan J, Lok B. Understanding empathy training with virtual patients. *Comput Human Behav.* 2015 November 1;**52**:151–8.

37. Gleichgerrcht E, Decety J. Empathy in clinical practice: How individual dispositions, gender, and experience moderate empathic concern, burnout, and emotional distress in physicians. *LoS One.* 2013 Apr 19;**8**(4).

38. Maxwell H, editor. *Integrated medicine: The human approach.* Available at: www.goodreads.com/book/show/3500352-integrated-medicine.

39. Balint E. The possibilities of patient-centered medicine. *J R Coll Gen Pract.* 1969 May; **17**(82): 269–76.

40. Penson RT, Schapira L, Mack S, Stanzler M, Lynch TJ Jr. Connection: Schwartz center rounds at Massachusetts general hospital cancer center. *Oncologist* 2010;**15**(7):760–4.

41. Kabat-Zinn J. An outpatient program in behavioral medicine for chronic pain patients based on the practice of mindfulness meditation: Theoretical considerations and preliminary results. *Gen Hosp Psychiatry.* 1982 April;**4**(1):33–47.

42. Ghetti C, Chang J, Gosman G. Burnout, psychological skills, and empathy: Balint training in obstetrics and gynecology residents. *J Grad Med Educ.* 2009 December;**1**(2):231–5.

43. Adams KE, O'Reilly M, Romm J, James K. Effect of Balint training on resident professionalism. *Am J Obstet Gynecol.* 2006 November; **195**(5):1431–7.

44. Koloroutis M. The therapeutic use of self: Developing three capacities for a more mindful practice. *Creat Nurs.* 2014;**20**(2):77–85.

45. Epner DE, Baile WF. Difficult conversations: Teaching medical oncology trainees communication skills one hour at a time. *Acad Med.* 2014 April;**89**(4):578–84.

46. Lelorain S, Sultan S, Zenasni F, Catu-Pinault A, Jaury P, Boujut E, Rigal L. Empathic concern and professional characteristics associated with clinical empathy in French general practitioners. *Euro J Gen Prac.* 2013;**19**:23–28.

47. Lown BA, Manning CF. The Schwartz Center Rounds: Evaluation of an interdisciplinary approach to enhancing patient-centered communication, teamwork, and provider support. *Acad Med.* 2010 June;**86**(6):1073–81.

48. Ludwig DS, Kabat-Zinn J. Mindfulness in medicine. *JAMA.* 2008 September 17;**300**(11):1350–2.

49. Shapiro SL, Schwartz GE, Bonner G. Effects of mindfulness-based stress reduction on medical and premedical students. *J Behav Med.* 1998 December;**21**(6):581–99.

50. Beckman HB, Wendland M, Mooney C, Krasner MS, Quill TE, Suchman AL, Epstein RM. The impact of a program in mindful communication on primary care physicians. *Acad Med.* 2012 June;**87**(6):815–9.

51. Krasner MS, Epstein RM, Beckman H, Suchman AL, Chapman B, Mooney CJ, Quill TE. Association of an educational program in mindful communication with burnout, empathy, and attitudes among primary care physicians. *JAMA.* 2009 September 23;**302**(12):1284–93.

JAMA. 2009 September 23;**302**(12):1284–93. doi: 10.1001/jama.2009.1384.

52. Guerra FA, Mirlesse V, Baiao AE. Breaking bad news during prenatal care: A challenge to be tackled. *Cien Saude Colet.* 2011 May;**16**(5):2361–7.

53. Baile WF, Buckman R, Lenzi R, Glober G, Beale EA, Kudelka AP. SPIKES-A six-step protocol for delivering bad news: Application to the patient with cancer. *Oncologist.* 2000;**5**(4):302–11.

54. Romm J. Breaking bad news in obstetrics and gynecology: Educational conference for resident physicians. *Arch Womens Ment Health.* 2002 November;**5**(4):177–9.

55. Conigliaro R, Kupersteing J, Dupuis J, Welsh D, Taylor S, Weber D, Jones M. *The PEEER model: Effective healthcare team-patient communications.* MedEdPORTAL Publications. 2013. Available at: http://dx.doi.org/10.15766/mep_2374-8265.9360#sthash.lmi62wvi.dpuf.

56. Norgaard B. Communication with patients and colleagues. *Dan Med Bull.* 2011 December;**58**(12): B4359.

57. Zarcadoolas C, Vaughon WL, Czaja SJ, Levy J, Rockoff ML. Consumers' perceptions of patient-accessible electronic medical records. *J Med Internet Res.* 2013 August 26;**15**(8):e168.

58. O'Malley AS, Grossman JM, Cohen GR, Kemper NM, Pham HH. Are electronic medical records helpful for care coordination? Experiences of physician practices. *J Gen Intern Med.* 2010 March; **25**(3):177–85.

59. Schultz CG, Holmstrom HL. The use of medical scribes in health care settings: A systematic review and future directions. *J Am Board Fam Med.* 2015 May–June;**28** (3):371–81.

60. Schouten BC, Meeuwesen L. Cultural difference in medical communication: A review of the literature. *Patient Educ Couns.* 2006 December;**64**(1–3):21–34.

61. Markova T, Broome B. Effective communication and delivery of culturally competent health care. *Urol Nurs.* 2007 June;**27**(3):239–42.

62. Rowlings, JK. *The fringe benefits of failure, and the importance of imagination.* Harvard Gazette. 2008 June 5. Available at: http://news.harvard.edu/gazette/story/2008/06/text-of-j-k-rowling-speech/. Accessed 22 March 2017.

Biopsychosocial Aspects of Eating Disorders in Obstetrics and Gynaecology

Suzanne Abraham

Presentation of Eating Disorders

The prevalence of eating disorders (EDs) depends on the diagnostic criteria employed, the population studied, their age and gender. It is believed at least 20% of cases do not present for help; these people may have the resilience and support from family, friends and community to make changes and maintain a good quality of life without professional help. There may be even more who present for help with fertility and gastrointestinal problems, rather than their ED. Unfortunately, women tend not to report the presence of an ED to obstetricians and gynaecologists, or physicians, perhaps because they may be labelled as having a 'mental health problem', and many doctors do not ask [1,2]. Physicians consider their training in diagnosing and treating EDs is poor [2].

A few women may choose their ED as a lifestyle. Websites encouraging and perpetuating disordered eating also negatively affect individuals who have never suffered from an ED [3].

Asking about disordered eating and weight control should be included during assessment of menstrual irregularities and infertility.

Asking about exercise should be included during assessment of menstrual irregularities and infertility.

Asking about disordered eating and weight control should be included during assessment of gastrointestinal disorders.

Have a list of reliable local websites for people with eating disorders.

What Is an Eating Disorder?

In simple terms, ED is when eating- and/or energy-controlling behaviours significantly affect a person's quality of life. These behaviours are commonly food restriction, binge eating, overeating, excessive exercise, self-induced vomiting and laxative use. A range of other medications, including prescribed, online and illegal drugs, can be included.

The behaviours cover up or provide an escape or short term relief from dysphoric moods and stressful anxious feelings and symptoms.

EDs are considered addictive disorders by some professional bodies. Anxiety, particularly social anxiety, and depressive moods are common. Although most ED patients do not have a personality disorder, they may have some of the features, the most common being anxious/avoidant, followed by borderline and dependent [4]. There may be other comorbid medical and psychiatric problems, such as diabetes mellitus or coeliac disease, present, but these should not explain the disordered eating.

Body Image

This chapter includes discussion of anorexia nervosa with and without body image problems, bulimia nervosa and bulimia nervosa–like disorders, including purging disorder, and binge eating and overeating disorders. Although obesity, BMI above 30 kg/m^2, is not necessarily associated with an ED, it is when the disordered eating leads to obesity and continuing weight gain. For a few obese people the ED does not become apparent until after bariatric surgery.

An ED does not have to include major issues with body image (see functional gastrointestinal disorders). What constitutes a disturbed body image can be hard to assess in some people. Most women want to be lighter than they are and the heavier they are, the more weight they wish to lose; this is normal. Women without an ED are happy at a BMI of 18–19 kg/m^2 (actual BMI equals desired BMI); an ED woman who does not purge is content at a BMI of 17–18, and below this wants to be heavier. This degree of disturbance overall appears small.

The characteristics of the EDs are given in Table 5.1. Criteria for the EDs are available online DSM-5 (2013) and ICD 10 (2010).

Table 5.1 Eating disorder types

Types of eating disorders
Anorexia nervosa–like: preoccupation with control of food, eating and weight-losing behaviours with sustained low body weight.
Bulimia nervosa–like: episodic binge eating with use of dangerous weight control measures
Purging disorder: self-induced vomiting or other purging behaviour for control of weight
Exercise disorder: preoccupation with control of excessive exercise
Binge eating disorder: binge eating without compensatory weight control methods
Overeating disorders: unwanted out-of-control overeating leading to chronic obesity

These disorders may overlap or occur at different times in a person's life; purging may continue after binge eating has ceased or vice versa, binge eating and purging may occur at very low body weight.

Binge Eating and Other Eating Behaviours

Binge eating is considered to be discrete episodes of the overeating of a large amount of food; persons feel outside their own control. Out-of-control overeating may not have the urgency of a binge, does not occur in episodes or not a lot of food is necessarily eaten in an episode.

One-fifth to one-third of obese women experience disordered eating. Overeating behaviours leading to obesity are 'grazing', eating small amounts of food throughout the day, experiencing a constant drive to eat, waking up at night and eating, 'comfort eating' and 'emotional eating'.

Other patterns also occur: chewing and spitting, regurgitating and re-swallowing or spitting out; following bariatric surgery other variations can be seen.

The type, frequency and duration of the behaviours, intensity of body image problems and poor self-esteem are important to ascertain during assessment.

EDs also occur in men with onset a few years later than women. Adolescent men continue to grow and lay down muscle rather than fat after their growth spurt. In younger males excessive exercise usually plays a major role and there is a greater incidence of psychopathology. Problems with binge eating appear to be more common especially among older men.

Excessive Exercise

It is hard to define excessive exercise as many people, for example athletes and dancers, do a lot of exercise which is considered healthy. When does exercise become unhealthy?: when the reproductive system is switched off, when it is compulsive, when there are

withdrawal symptoms if it is stopped, when exercising interferes with the person's quality of life? Excessive exercise may occur before or after the onset of disordered eating.

Exercise helps control moods and feelings.
Exercise can replace eating and body image as the main focus of the disorder.
Many sports and some careers support disordered eating and exercise.

Eating Disorders and Functional Gastrointestinal Disorders (FGID)

Gastrointestinal symptoms that occur without evidence of structural gastrointestinal disease are a well-recognized feature of patients with EDs. Disordered eating can be associated with gastrointestinal disorders among women with no or little body image problem. Women may restrict the amount or types of foods they eat, induce vomiting or take laxatives to relieve their gastrointestinal discomfort and bloating.

Discomfort from slow gastric emptying can exacerbate undereating in starving patients with anorexia nervosa by enhancing satiety [5].

Reassure low weight women their discomfort following eating meals will cease as they continue eating a normal amount of food.
A history of physical and sexual abuse is common to FGID and EDs [6,7].
Enquiry about sexual, physical and emotional abuse is important in women with eating disorders and FGIDs.

Among anorexia and bulimia-like ED patients, over 90% report at least one FGID and 33% report three or more [8,9,10]. The most prevalent FGIDs using ROME III questionnaire were postprandial distress syndrome (an unpleasant sense of fullness in the abdomen after a meal), irritable bowel syndrome (IBS), followed by unspecified functional bowel disorders, and functional heartburn (symptoms of heartburn not related to gastro-oesophageal reflux). The most significant predictor of postprandial distress syndrome was starvation; depression was a very weak predictor. The predictor of functional heartburn and unspecified functional bowel disorders was somatisation, and of IBS laxative use [9]. A recent study also found obese patients with a binge eating behaviour showed a significantly higher prevalence of postprandial distress syndrome [11].

A greater understanding of postprandial distress syndrome may help in the management of ED patients.

Bloating among ED patients leads to fears of weight gain, food avoidance, greater weight-losing methods and general self-loathing. Bloating is reported more frequently than distension (78% versus 58%). After controlling for BMI, IBS was the most significant predictor of bloating [12].

What Causes an Eating Disorder?

The onset of disordered eating most commonly occurs in women in the years after menarche.

When a young woman gains weight before her first menstrual period, her self-esteem may decrease and she may become aware of psychological feelings of anxiety and depression. The changes in body image are thought to challenge her self-esteem and initiate dieting and disordered eating.

Earlier signs of disordered eating, prior to menarche, may reflect other psychiatric disorders such as autism, bullying and childhood emotional sexual or physical abuse.

Other adolescent triggers among women with a genetic/epigenetic propensity to develop EDs can be academic challenges, change in the amount of exercise, boyfriend or family issues, media, viral illness, depression and anxiety.

Many young women have a phase of disordered eating and experiment with changing their eating and body weight and experience binge eating without developing a chronic ED.

Onset after 25 years is usually associated with other medical or psychiatric problems or life crises such as, chemotherapy, bipolar depression.

Risk and Perpetuating Factors

The risk factors for the development of an ED are impaired learning of 'normal' eating and exercise; a daily family meal is protective. Childhood emotional deprivation and abuse are risk factors.

The perpetuating factors involve the reward of the behaviours themselves, self-induced vomiting being one of the most addictive behaviours and one of the most difficult to extinguish. Self-induced vomiting is associated with a quick relief from anxious and depressive feelings. Stressful life events, personality characteristics, psychiatric or medical problems and lack of support exacerbate these behaviours and allow them to continue. There are many advantages to having an ED such as avoiding making decisions, being looked after and to feel in control of life.

The perceived advantages of having an eating disorder are explored during treatment.
The risk and perpetuating factors are addressed during treatment.

Explaining Why Eating Disorders Happen

There are many theories put forward to explain the occurrence of EDs. These include theories relating to genetic and epigenetic factors, childhood and adolescent development, sexual and physical abuse, social, personality, physiological factors and recently the gut microflora [13,14,15].

The healthy immune system of an adult is dependent on the microflora acquired at birth and early life, and these microflorae are thought to play a role in control of body weight [16]. Whether changes in the gut bacteria that produce large quantities of epigenetically active metabolites result in turning on an ED has not been explored. The gut microbiota may be responsible for increased intestinal permeability, resulting in the development of a chronic low-grade inflammatory state that contributes to obesity and associated chronic metabolic diseases [17].

Have you ever been told you have any autoimmune problems, e.g. diabetes, coeliac?

Menarche and Menstruation

When did you have your first menstrual period?

Menarche occurs earlier in overweight and obese girls. Earlier menarche is associated with a greater likelihood of binge eating behaviour developing [18]. Late or delayed menarche can reflect excessive exercise associated with training, failure to gain weight or the onset of weight loss before menarche.

> *Have you ever lost your periods?*
>
> *Has there been a time when your periods were reasonably regular and you were not taking 'the pill'?*
>
> *Women with underlying menstrual irregularity may believe they are having normal menstrual cycles when they are taking oral contraception.*
>
> *Women will not know if they have amenorrhoea when taking oral contraception except at very low weight – the pill may mask an underlying amenorrhoea.*
>
> *When the body is under stress the first system to switch off is the reproductive one.*

Women with normal BMI can also become amenorrhoeic, as frequently happens with athletes, dancers and women with bulimia nervosa, purging or exercise disorders [19]. This may reflect lack of available energy or stress from the behaviours. Cortisol is involved in energy regulation and reported to be associated with both increases and decreases in eating and body weight. Cortisol levels are high in anorexia nervosa, women who eat in response to stress and those who are obese. Relapses in binge eating occur following emotional stress. Although we queried the usefulness of amenorrhoea in the diagnosis of anorexia nervosa, it remains a good indicator of insufficient energy and a body under stress [20].

> *Asking about the type, intensity and duration of activity is important.*

Although BMI is a useful tool to assess body weight, including low weight, it is not an accurate measure of body composition in people who exercise, particularly those involving weight requirements for competition [21,22]. In a study of female athletes, both 'under-' and 'overfat' athletes self-reported menstrual dysfunction, stress fractures, history of weight fluctuation and use of weight control methods, and were diagnosed with clinical EDs and/or low bone density [22].

Recommendations have been suggested to help prevent and detect ED behaviour among male and female athletes before they become chronic, including education and treatment. Like non-athletic people with EDs they recover from their ED 10–20 years later [23].

Bone Mineral Density (BMD)

Weight loss and amenorrhoea are associated with loss of BMD, particularly neck of femur and lumbar vertebrae. Bone loss occurs within 12 months of amenorrhoea and over 50% of women with long-standing amenorrhoea will be osteopenic within two years. Patients can be reassured their menstrual periods will return when they are above and remain above a BMI of 19 kg/m^2 and if they are not employing other weight-controlling behaviours, particularly exercise.

Treatment for Low Bone Density

*Optimal treatment to prevent osteopenia and osteoporosis is restoration of body weight **and** return of menses as soon as possible.*

Both are necessary; weight gain alone will not result in recovery of bone. In the case of excessive exercise, ceasing exercise completely may be necessary for return of menses. Recovery of BMD to age-related levels can take many years; up to six years has been reported [24].

Doctors frequently prescribe oral contraception for young women for low BMD. This can allow the patient to believe she is no longer losing bone and delay recovery from her ED [25].

> *There is debate about hormone replacement in women with eating and exercise disorders in their teens, 20's and 30's.*

There is no evidence from studies that 'the pill' improves bone density, even if body weight is gained [24]. In adolescents 'the pill' may prevent peak bone density being reached [25]. In older women it may slow down the recovery of bone. One recent study, using physiological levels of oestrogen, has shown improvement with the transdermal oestrogen patch (and cyclic progesterone) in both spine and hip [26].

Supplementation with calcium and vitamin D does not improve bone outcome, although low-weight ED patients are more likely to have low vitamin D levels [27].

Polycystic Ovarian Syndrome (PCOS)

Have you ever been told you have PCOS?

Great care must be taken in the diagnosis of polycystic ovarian syndrome (PCOS) in women with irregular cycles, particularly in women 25 years and less. Androgenisation (free testosterone) must be measured. Follicle count is greater in many young women than that needed for diagnosis, and the ultrasound may look 'polycystic' in appearance in amenorrhoeic women. An eating, weight-controlling and exercise history may help to clarify the diagnosis, particularly in normal or low-weight women. Obese women who have oligomenorrhoea or amenorrhoea and hirsutism may have PCOS.

Care must be taken before diagnosing PCOS in young women with disordered eating.

Premenstrual Syndrome (PMS) and Menopause

There is little known about premenstrual syndrome (PMS) and EDs. One of the accepted PMS symptoms is a premenstrual increased appetite. Patients report greater overeating or binge eating in the luteal phase.

Late-onset EDs have been reported. Whether this is an exacerbation of a dormant ED in response to the events around menopause is unknown [28]. The predominant ED among middle-age women is binge eating disorder [28].

Recovery from an Eating Disorder

The outcome studies involve patients who have been treated at major institutions. Among those studied, recovery from an ED can take many years and relapses occur. After 10–15 years approximately 80% of patients have recovered and have a good quality of life, with about half still 'watching their weight' similar to other women in the community. Of the 20% who have a chronic condition, most improve and a few die (suicide or ED-related).

The predictors of a good outcome are treatment is sought early, never been at very low or very high weight, no self-induced vomiting, no medical or psychiatric comorbidity and no sexual or physical abuse [13].

In the two years following bariatric surgery there is marked weight loss and improvements in medical comorbidities and psychological functioning. Unfortunately, a minority also experience problems, such as reoccurring or new psychiatric disorders including EDs [29].

Sexuality

Are you using any type of contraception?

If a woman is or likely to be sexually active it is important to discuss her need for contraception.

Fertility can return unexpectedly, particularly during treatment and so amenorrhoea cannot be relied upon for pregnancy prevention.

Amenorrhoea is not a form of contraception.

Women with ED show a wide range of sexual knowledge, attitudes and practices. A decrease in sexual interest is reported with both weight loss and weight gain. Anorexia nervosa patients who binge eat and purge are likely to be less inhibited, have more than one sexual partner and have experienced oral-genital sex. Sexual matters, usually associated with boyfriends, are often associated with onset or exacerbation of their ED [29].

Bulimia nervosa women are more likely to describe their libido as 'above average' and to have had an abortion. Marital breakdown is also more common [30].

In the first two years following bariatric surgery, body contouring to remove the excess folds of skin improves sexual intimacy, body image and psychological variables and decreases weight regain [31].

Gynaecological Examination of a Woman with a Current or Past History of an Eating Disorder

A careful and sensitive history, including sexuality and abuse, can help your approach.

Conducting a gynaecological examination with sensitivity is important. Women, particularly those who have been at low weight, may have had little sexual experience when they present with amenorrhoea or infertility. Care approaching and explaining why you would like to conduct the examination and how it is done are important [32,33].

Getting Pregnant

Both underweight and obese women, and women with eating and exercise disorders, may have difficulties falling pregnant.

Small changes in behaviour can help conception.

Commencing appropriate changes in body weight and decreasing the frequency or ceasing extreme methods of weight control improve the chances of conception. Learning to eat regular meals and snacks during the day and exercising sensibly may be sufficient for normal-weight women who are recovering from their ED (see 'normal eating', Table 5.2).

Table 5.2 What is 'normal' eating?

Normal eating for people with disordered eating is establishing regular structured eating that is flexible and appropriate in different situations [13].

Eating three meals and two or three snacks each day

Eating at approximately the same time each day (usually)

Eating in discrete intervals of time (not grazing)

Being able to eat spontaneously on social occasions with others

Eating a wide range of foods

Knowing what proportions of food and size of meals are appropriate

Being able to eat more or less on occasions

Learning to eat or not eat when you are happy, sad or anxious

Treatment of disordered eating and exercise can prevent the need for assisted conception.

Induction of ovulation or other assisted conception will usually result in pregnancy. Unfortunately, these methods of assisted conception are more likely to result in miscarriage and several attempts may be needed. Changing eating and exercise patterns will help.

It is usually suggested induction of ovulation is deferred until the ED is no longer active because of the relapse rate and possible complications associated with pregnancy, childbirth and postpartum [34,35].

Infertility clinic doctors should inquire about exercise and EDs before inducing ovulation.

Eating Disorders and Management during Pregnancy

The pregnancy and postnatal complications associated with ED are shown in Table 5.3.

Relapse prevention is a major aim of antenatal and postnatal care.

Women with active symptoms of an ED at the time of conception can continue with their disordered eating or relapse at any time during pregnancy and the following year. Relapse among recovered women is much less frequent [36, 37]. Follow-up of bulimia nervosa patients for 10–15 years found recovered patients had no perinatal problems [30].

Table 5.3 Complications of pregnancy in women with eating disorder

Women with disordered eating are more likely to experience complications during their pregnancy and after the birth [13].

Complications during pregnancy include:

increased risk of miscarriage

hyperemesis gravidarum

pregnancy-induced hypertension

gestational diabetes

delivery of a growth-restricted baby

delivery of a small-for-gestational-age baby

delivery of a premature baby

delivery of a large-for-gestational-age baby

need a caesarean section

anxiety and depression

Complications after birth include:

postpartum haemorrhage

postnatal depression

feelings of distress

Women delivering growth-restricted babies (small for gestational age [SGA]) are more likely to have ED pathology before and after the birth, to be at low body weight before pregnancy, have low maternal weight gain during pregnancy and be more likely to smoke compared with women who had small babies who were born early. Women with a past history of an ED were at no greater risk of delivering a low-birth-weight infant [38].

A large multicentre study confirmed obesity is an independent risk factor for adverse obstetric outcome and is significantly associated with an increased caesarean delivery rate. Obese women may also have small or large babies who may grow up and become obese adults with the metabolic syndrome [39]. Women who have had bariatric surgery also need to be monitored carefully as they have an increased risk of SGA infants, and possibly an increase in stillbirth and neonatal death, although other obesity-related risks are decreased [40]. Adjustable band surgery may be preferable for women in their reproductive years as the band can be released during pregnancy.

Women with disordered eating at conception must be assessed and monitored more frequently during pregnancy.

Body Image and Pregnancy

The following information can help to reassure women and help prevent relapse:

Deposition of fat in the breasts, hips and thighs is essential for the growth and development of the fetus and is a normal part of pregnancy.

Most of the weight gain during pregnancy is fluid, baby and placenta.

It is normal for a woman to be less active as pregnancy proceeds, to increase the energy available for the baby.

Decreased activity can be a challenge for women with EDs who exercise for control of body weight and their emotions. Constipation of pregnancy can also be a trigger for some women.

Weight Gain during Pregnancy

Underweight women need to gain an amount of weight to reach a BMI of over 19, in addition to the normal weight gain expected during pregnancy. Overweight and obese women do not need to put on as much weight during pregnancy, probably because they already have energy reserves for the development of their baby. Knowing her body weight can trigger relapse for some women.

Do you want to be told your weight at antenatal visits?

Eating during Pregnancy

Many women, including women with EDs, report that their eating and nutrition improves during pregnancy [41]. Food cravings are common and vary from woman to woman.

'Picking' (eating small amounts of food more often) is reported as the most common unwanted behaviour.

Binge eating can be experienced by women, but less than 10% report it to be a 'severe' problem. This may explain the increase in binge eating disorder found in some studies.

It is thought binge eating occurs at times of rapid fetal growth when there is inadequate maternal food intake.

Binge eating may also follow the nausea and vomiting of early pregnancy, because insufficient energy may have been available for storage in the mother's body.

Binge eating is more common in the second half of pregnancy.

Binge eating, fear of weight gain, vomiting, exercise, constipation coupled with changes in mood may be associated with relapses in women who have not recovered.

Eating Disorders and the Postnatal Period

Body Weight

A comparison of women with and without EDs suggest most women adjust positively to changes in body weight during pregnancy. In the year following childbirth women with EDs lose weight rapidly (some to below pre-pregnancy levels) leading to an improvement in their body weight satisfaction, while women without an ED remained dissatisfied with their weight for most of the postpartum year [42].

Knowing that it takes most of the year after childbirth for weight to return to pre-pregnancy levels can be reassuring and may help to prevent relapse.

Mental State

Postnatal distress is associated with body weight and shape concerns, with disordered eating before and during pregnancy and with vomiting during pregnancy. Women with EDs are at risk for peri- and postnatal depressive and anxiety problems in addition to other women with a history of depression [43,44].

Assessment of mood and exploring her worries during and after childbirth is necessary.

Breastfeeding

Women with an eating disorder do breastfeed but are more likely to stop breastfeeding earlier than other women [45]. Whether this reflects the rapid loss of weight in the first months after the birth or is associated with anxiety and depression is not known [46].

Early intervention to prevent infant feeding difficulties is needed.

Children of Parents with Eating Disorders

There is good evidence that children of parents with EDs disorders are at increased risk of disturbances in their development. Five possible ways this may occur are suggested: genetic influences, mothers overfeeding or underfeeding their infants, impaired parental availability or attachment, poor eating role models and the presence of dysfunctional parental and family relationships [47]. The psychopathologies are different in boys and girls [48].

Treatment of Eating Disorders

The most important part of treatment is ongoing biopsychosocial assessment and support.

Most treatment is supportive psychotherapy, dietetic counselling and cognitive behavioural therapies as indicated. Family and partners are included as appropriate. The dietitian is an important part of the treatment team and may play a major role in less severe cases [49,50]. Family doctors and a dietitian see and treat people with EDs and may refer them to a physician, psychiatrist, psychologist or other health professional for assessment and/or treatment. In more severe cases referral to a multidiscipline eating disorder specialist team is suggested.

As each person is an individual with a unique range of problems continuing assessment and examination is crucial.

Treatment in an outpatient setting is usually adequate but for others lenient inpatient treatment may be needed for physical or psychological/psychiatric reasons. Cognitive behavioural therapy (CBT) delivered online, by a therapist or self-help group, is useful. Help with sexual and physical abuse issues may be needed and different versions of CBT employed [51,52].

Treatment involves learning to cope with uncomfortable feelings associated with every day matters and the bigger life events as they occur without resorting to ED or inappropriate behaviours.

In general medications have little effect on the eating disorder. Antidepressants prescribed for comorbid depression have little effect on the eating disorder or the time to relapse. For other medications adverse side effects limit their use [53]. Atypical antipsychotics in low doses show some positive effects on depression and anxiety, but there is insufficient evidence to say they aid weight gain in anorexia nervosa [54].

Follow-up women with eating disorders for 2 years after entering the recovery phase.

Key Points

- Eating disorders (EDs) include food restriction, binge eating, overeating, excessive exercise, self-induced vomiting and laxative use.
- The type, frequency and duration of the eating behaviours, the intensity of body image problems and the degree of self-esteem should be assessed.
- Onset of ED prior to menarche may reflect other psychiatric disorders such as autism, bullying and childhood emotional, sexual or physical abuse. Onset after the age of 25 years is usually associated with other medical or psychiatric problems or life crises such as chemotherapy and bipolar depression.
- Risk factors for ED include childhood emotional deprivation and abuse. Stressful life events, personality characteristics, psychiatric or medical problems and lack of support exacerbate disordered eating behaviours.
- The complications of ED include low bone mineral density, subfertility, miscarriage, fetal growth restriction, perinatal depression and anxiety.
- Gastrointestinal symptoms that occur without evidence of structural gastrointestinal disease are a well-recognized feature of EDs.
- Women who present with menstrual irregularities and infertility should be asked about exercise, disordered eating and weight control.
- Issues of sexuality and contraceptive needs should be explored.
- The most important part of treatment is ongoing biopsychosocial assessment and support. Cognitive behavioural therapy (CBT) is helpful. Antidepressants prescribed for comorbid depression have little effect on eating behaviour, weight gain or the time to relapse.

References

1. Abraham S. Obstetricians and maternal body weight and eating disorders during pregnancy. *J Psychosom Obstet Gynecol.* 2001; **22**: 159–163.
2. Leddy MA, Hal H, Schulkin J. Obstetrician-gynaecologist and women's mental health: Findings of the collaborative ambulatory

research network. *Obstet Gynaecol Surv.* 2011; **66**: 316–323.

3. Bardone-Cone A, Cass K. What does viewing a pro-anorexia website do? An experimental examination of website exposure and moderating effects. *Int J Eat Disorder.* 2007; **40**: 537–548.

4. von Lojewski A, Fisher A, Abraham S. Have personality disorders been overdiagnosed among eating disorder patients? *Psychopathology.* 2013; **46**: 421–426.

5. Robinson OH, Clarke M, Barrett J. Determinants of delayed gastric emptying in anorexia nervosa and bulimia nervosa. *Gut.* 1988; **29**: 458–464.

6. Leserman J, Drossman DA. Relationship of abuse history to functional gastrointestinal disorders and symptoms. *Trauma Violence Abuse.* 2007; **8**: 331–343.

7. Alander T, Heimer G, Svardsudd K, et al. Abuse in women and men with and without functional gastrointestinal disorders. *Dig Dis Sci.* 2008; **53**: 1856–1864.

8. Boyd C, Abraham S, Kellow J. Psychological features are important predictors of functional gastrointestinal disorders in patients with eating disorders. *Scand J Gastroenterol.* 2005; **40**: 929–935.

9. Wang X, Luscombe GM, Boyd C, et al. Functional gastrointestinal disorders in eating disorder patients: Altered distribution and predictors using ROME III compared to ROME II criteria. *World J Gastroenterol.* 2014; **20**: 16293–16299.

10. Boyd C, Abraham S, Kellow J. Appearance and disappearance of functional gastrointestinal disorders in patients with eating disorders. *Neurogastoentrol Motil.* 2010; **22**: 1279–1283.

11. Santonicola A, Angrisani L, Ciacci C, et al. Prevalence of functional gastrointestinal disorders according to Rome III criteria in Italian morbidly obese patients. 2013 *The Scientific World Journal.* http://dx.doi.org/10.1155/2013/532503.

12. Abraham S, Luscombe GM, Kellow J. Pelvic floor dysfunction predicts abdominal bloating and distension in eating disorder patients. *Scand J Gastroenterol.* 2012; **47**: 625–631.

13. Abraham S. *Eating disorders, the facts.* 7th ed. Oxford, Oxford University Press, 2015.

14. Bulik CM, Sullivan PF, Wade TD, et al. Twin studies of eating disorders: A Review. *Int J Eat Disord.* 2000; **27**: 1–20.

15. Campbell IC, Mill J, Uher R, Schmidt U. Eating disorders, gene – environment interactions and epigenetics. *Neurosc Biobehav Rev.* 2011; **35**: 784–793.

16. Kleiman SC, Carroll IM, Tarantino LM, et al. Gut feelings: A role for the intestinal microbiota in anorexia nervosa? *Int J Eat Disord.* 2015; **48**: 449–451.

17. Tsukumo DM, Carvalho BM, Carvalho Filho MA, et al. Translational research into gut microbiota: New horizons on obesity treatment: Updated 2014. *Arch. Endocrinol. Metab.* 2015; 59. http://dx.doi.org/10.1590/2359-3997000000029.

18. Day J, Schmidt U, Collier D, et al. Risk factors, correlates, and markers in early onset bulimia nervosa and EDNOS. *Int J Eat Disord.* 2011; **44**: 287–294.

19. Abraham S, Pettigrew B, Boyd C, Russell J. Predictors of functional and exercise amenorrhoea among eating disorder and exercise disordered patients. *Hum Reprod.* 2006; **21**: 257–261.

20. Abraham S, Pettigrew B, Russell J, Taylor A. Usefulness of amenorrhoea in the diagnosis of eating disorder patients. *J Psychosom Obstet Gynecol.* 2005; **26**: 211–215.

21. Abraham S, Luscombe G, Boyd C, Olesen I. Predictors of the accuracy of self-reported height and weight in adolescent female school students. *Int J Eat Disord.* 2004; **36**: 76–82.

22. Torstveit MK, Sundgot-Borgen J. Are under- and overweight female elite athletes thin and fat? A controlled study. *Med Sci Sports Exerc.* 2012; **44**: 949–957.

23. Sundgot-Borgen J, Meyer NL, Ackland TR, et al. How to minimise the health risks to athletes who compete in weight-sensitive sports review and position statement on behalf of the Ad Hoc Research Working Group on Body Composition, Health and Performance, under the auspices of the IOC Medical Commission. *Br J Sports Med.* 2013; **47**: 1012–1022.

24. Howgate DJ, Graham SM, Leonidou A, et al. Bone metabolism in anorexia nervosa: Molecular pathways and current treatment modalities. *Osteoporosis Int.* 2013; **24**: 407–421.

25. Bergstrom I, Crisby M, Engstrom A, et al. Women with anorexia nervosa should not be treated with estrogen or birth control pills in a bone sparing effect. *Acta Obstet et Gynecol Scand.* 2013; **92**: 877–880.

Zigler S, Hunter TS. The effect of hormonal contraception on acquisition of peak bone density of adolescents and young women. *J Pharmac Pract.* 2012; **25**: 331–340.

26. Misra M. Physiologic estrogen replacement increases bone density in adolescent girls with anorexia nervosa. *J Bone Miner Res.* 2011; **26**: 2430–2438.

27. Velickovic KMC, Makovey J, Abraham SF. Vitamin D. Bone mineral density and body mass

index in eating disorder patients. *Eating Behav.* 2013; **14**: 124–127.

28. Mangweth-Matzek B, Hoek HW, Rupp CI, et al. Prevalence of eating disorders in middle aged women. *Int J Eat Disord.* 2014; **47**: 320–324.

29. Green DD, Engel SG, Mitchell JE. Psychological aspects of bariatric surgery. *Curr Opin Psychiat.* 2014; **27**: 448–452.

29. Beumont PJV, Abraham S, Simson KG. The psychosexual histories of adolescent girls and young women with anorexia nervosa. *Psychol Med* 1981; **11**: 131–140.

30. Abraham S. Sexuality and reproduction in bulimia nervosa patients over 10 years. *J Psychosom Res.* 1998; **44**: 491–502.

31. Ramalho S, Bastos AP, Silva C, et al. Excessive skin and sexual function: Relationship with psychological variables and weight regain in women after bariatric surgery. *Obes. Surg.* 2015; **25**: 1149–1154.

32. Abraham S. Gynaecological examination: a teaching package integrating assessment with learning. *Med Educat.* 1998; **32**: 76–81.

33. Sanfilippo JS, Lara-Torre E. Adolescent gynaecology. *Obstet Gynecol.* 2009; **113**: 935–947.

34. Abraham S, Mira M, Llewellyn-Jones D. Should ovulation be induced in women recovering from an eating disorder or who are compulsive exercisers? *Fertil Steril.* 1990; **53**: 566–568.

35. Stewart DE. Reproductive functions in eating disorders. *Ann Med.* 1992; **24**: 287–291.

36. Micali N, Treasure J, Simonoff E. Eating disorders symptoms in pregnancy: A longitudinal study of women with recent and past eating disorders and obesity. *J Psychosom Res.* 2007; **63**: 297–303.

37. Coker EL, Mitchell-Wong LA, Abraham SF. Is pregnancy a trigger for recovery from an eating disorder? *Acta Obstet Gynecol Scand.* 2013; **92**: 1407–1413.

38. Conti J, Abraham S, Taylor A. Eating behavior and pregnancy outcome. *J Psychosom Res.* 1998; **44**: 465–477.

39. Weiss JL, Malone FD, Emig D, et al. Obesity, obstetric complications and Cesarean delivery rate–a population-based screening study. *Am J Obstet Gynecol.* 2004; **190**: 1091–1097.

40. Johansson K, Cnattingius S, Näslund I, Roos N, et al. Outcomes of Pregnancy after Bariatric Surgery. *N Engl J Med.* 2015; **372**: 814–824.

41. Abraham S, King W, Llewellyn-Jones D. Attitudes to body weight, weight gain and eating behavior in pregnancy. *J Psychosom Obstet Gynecol.* 1994; **15**: 189–195.

42. Coker E, Abraham S. Body weight dissatisfaction: A comparison of women with and without eating disorders. *Eat Behav.* 2014; **15**: 453–459.

43. Abraham S, Taylor A, Conti J. Postnatal depression, eating, exercise, and vomiting before and during pregnancy. *Int J Eat Disord.* 2001; **29**: 482–487.

44. Micali N, Simonoff E, Treasure J. Pregnancy and post-partum depression and anxiety in a longitudinal general population cohort: The effect of eating disorders and past depression. *J Affect Disord.* 2011; **131**: 150–157.

45. Torgersen L, Ystrom E, Haugen M, Meltzer HM, et al. Breastfeeding practice in mothers with eating disorders. *Maternal Child Nutr.* 2010; **6**: 243–252.

46. Micali N, Simonoff E, Stahl D, Treasure J. Maternal eating disorders and infant feeding difficulties: Maternal and child mediators in a longitudinal general population study. *J Child Psychol Psychiat.* 2011; **52**: 800–807.

47. Patel P, Wheatcroft R, Park RJ, Stein A. The children of mothers with eating disorders. *Clin Child Famil Psychol Rev.* 2002; **5**: 426–230.

48. Micali N, Stahl D, Treasure J, Simonoff E. Childhood psychopathology in children of women with eating disorders: Understanding risk mechanisms. *J Child Psychol Psychiat.* 2014; **55**: 124–134.

49. Hart S, Russell J, Abraham S. Nutrition and dietetic practice in eating disorder management. *J. Hum Nutr.* 2011; **24**: 144–153.

50. American Dietetic Association. Position of the American dietetic association: Nutrition intervention in the treatment of anorexia nervosa, bulimia nervosa, and other eating disorders. *J Am Diet Assoc.* 2006; **106**: 2073–2082.

51. National Institute for Health and Care (NICE) Guidelines. Eating disorder: core interventions in the treatment and management of anorexia nervosa, bulimia nervosa, and related disorders. 2004.

52. Hay P, Chinn D, Forbes D, et al. Royal Australian and New Zealand college of psychiatrists clinical practice guidelines for the treatment of eating disorders. *ANZ J Psychiat.* 2014; **48**: 977–1008.

53. Hay PJ, Claudino AM. Clinical psychopharmacology of eating disorders: A research update. *The Int J Neuropsychopharmacol* 2012; **15**: 209–222.

54. McKnight RF, Park RJ. Atypical antipsychotics and anorexia nervosa: A review. *Eur Eat Disord Rev.* 2010; **18**: 10–21.

6

The Brain, Heart and Human Behaviour

Leroy C. Edozien

Introduction

The mind is not easy to define but comprises a person's consciousness, feeling, thinking, judgement and experience. The biomedical model of clinical practice separates the mind from the body and focusses on the latter. Attempts to bridge this divide led to the emergence of 'psychosomatic' medicine. One problem with the term 'psychosomatic' is that it does not quite succeed in eliminating the dualism of the biomedical model: while it conjoins *psyche* (mind) and *soma* (body), it fails to capture and reflect the web of interconnectedness between them. Physically, the mind and the body cannot be one because the mind is not a physical entity; functionally, they may also not be in unison – for example, the body may be relaxed while the mind is agitated. Nevertheless a rigid distinction between the mind and body, as historically advocated by dualist philosophers and scientists, cannot be supported given current knowledge in neurosciences, sociobiology and psychobiology. Functionally, it can be said of the mind and the body that they are not one but not two either – and the interactions between the brain, the heart and behaviour illustrate this. The brain and the heart have a complex but close relationship to each other. They strongly influence, and are influenced by, behaviour (exercise, diet, smoking, sleep, relaxation, risk taking) and behaviour-related factors (anxiety, depression, anger, aggression, risk aversion, social support, psychological and social stress).

Basic Anatomy of the Brain

The brain is composed of the cerebrum, cerebellum and brainstem. The cerebrum comprises two hemispheres, each of which has four lobes – frontal, parietal, temporal and occipital – each of which is predominantly responsible for particular functions. The frontal lobe is concerned with decision-making and problem-solving; the occipital lobe is concerned

with vision and the temporal lobe is involved in hearing, memory and emotion. The parietal lobe integrates sensory information emanating from various receptors. The neocortex, made up of grey matter, is the outermost, most developed and largest part of the cerebrum. The cerebellum is responsible for coordination and balance. The brain stem comprises the medulla oblongata, pons and midbrain. Neural connections from the cortex pass through the brainstem to connect with the peripheral nervous system. The brain stem also serves as a regulatory centre for cardiac, respiratory and various other functions. The midbrain includes the thalami (collections of nuclei) and inferiorly adjacent to these is the hypothalamus.

The brain is most commonly associated with cognition, which is the function of the neocortex, but an equally important role of the brain pertains to emotion, and this is the function of the limbic system.

The Limbic System

The limbic system is a group of structures in the brain that are involved in emotion, motivation, behaviour and memory. It includes the hippocampus, hypothalamus, amygdala, the basal ganglia, mammillary body, cingulate gyrus and parahippocampal gyrus (Figure 6.1). These structures have very complex neural connections with each other, with other parts of the brain and with the autonomic nervous system.

The amygdala is the emotion centre of the brain, while the hippocampus plays an essential role in the formation of new memories about past experiences. The cingulate gyrus is involved in the coordination and regulation of a range of activities and experiences including aggressive behaviour, reaction to pain and memories of smells and sights. The basal ganglia comprise nuclei lying deep in the subcortical white matter of the frontal lobes. The functions of this group of nuclei include organizing motor behaviour and coordinating habit learning.

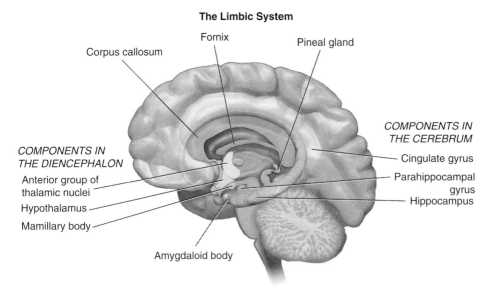

The Limbic System

Fornix

Corpus callosum

Pineal gland

COMPONENTS IN
THE CEREBRUM

Cingulate gyrus

Parahippocampal
gyrus

Hippocampus

COMPONENTS IN
THE DIENCEPHALON

Anterior group of
thalamic nuclei

Hypothalamus

Mamillary body

Amygdaloid body

Figure 6.1 The limbic system

Source: Image courtesy of Bruce Blausen; Blausen.com staff. 'Blausen gallery 2014'. Wikiversity Journal of Medicine. DOI:10.15347/wjm/ 2014.010. ISSN 20018762. (Own work) [CC BY 3.0 (http://creativecommons.org/licenses/by/3.0)], via Wikimedia Commons.

The hypothalamus, which could be described as the Polaris of the limbic constellation, receives a multiplicity of inputs from the hippocampus, amygdala, vagus nerve, olfactory nerves, optic nerve and other structures in the limbic and central nervous systems. It has osmoreceptors, thermoreceptors, steroid receptors and other receptors that mediate regulatory functions. Activities and perceptions regulated through the hypothalamus include temperature, appetite, hunger, thirst, pain, pleasure, sexual satisfaction, anger, aggression and other forms of arousal. The hypothalamus also regulates blood pressure, heart rate, breathing, digestion and sweating. It is neurally and chemically connected to the pituitary gland, which in turn releases into the bloodstream hormones that are important in the regulation of the endocrine system, growth and metabolism.

The Cognitive Brain and the Emotional Brain

The limbic system is described as the 'emotional brain' and the higher centres as the 'cognitive brain'.

The emotional brain modulates not only emotions but also the physical activities of the cardiovascular, digestive, immune and other systems. In a similar vein, the cognitive brain controls emotions as well as cognition. Without this control, life is ruled by raw emotions, untamed by rational consideration. Emotion must be moderated by reason. Cognitive control of behaviour entails the selection of behaviours aimed at achieving specific goals. The cognitive processes involved in this control – termed 'executive functions' – include attentional control, inhibitory control and working memory [1].

When this control by the cognitive brain is switched off as happens in a panic attack, the limbic system is in overdrive. This manifests as sweating, trembling, vomiting and spasms. A similar switching off of cognitive control could account for symptoms of posttraumatic stress disorder (PTSD) (see Chapter 39).

On the other hand, excessive control by the cognitive brain stifles emotions to the extent that one may disconnect from warning signals coming from the emotional brain or lose the ability to relate to other persons in a sensitive manner. Complete well-being (physical and psychological) requires a balance between emotion and reason. The extent to which this is achieved is determined by Emotional Intelligence – the ability to recognize, manage and respond appropriately to one's emotion and the emotion of others.

Hormones and the Brain

The brain regulates metabolism, growth, reproduction, emotions and other physiological and social functions through not only the nervous system via neurotransmitters but also the endocrine system. Hormones (the chemical messengers released from endocrine glands) can influence behaviour, for example, sexual inclinations, lifestyle and parenting style.

The brain has receptors for a range of hormones, including metabolic hormones (such as insulin and leptin), thyroid hormones, steroid hormones and others that are produced in response to stress, the circadian rhythm and emotional states. In response to incoming signals, neurones in the brain induce the pituitary gland to secrete factors into the blood that increase or decrease hormone production by the target endocrine gland. The neurones in the hypothalamus produce gonadotropin-releasing hormone which stimulates the pituitary gland to release follicle-stimulating hormone (FSH) and luteinizing hormone (LH) into the bloodstream. These act on the ovary to induce follicular development, production of oestrogen, ovulation, luteinisation and production of progesterone. In males, they promote spermatogenesis and release of testosterone.

A feedback loop transmits signals back to the brain to maintain hormone levels as required. Through such feedback loops the brain acts as a control centre for a range of human behavioural responses to environmental and social challenges. These responses include eating, drinking, learning, coping with stress and formation of social bonds. Thus, for example, oestradiol influences sex motivation and behaviour, vasopressin affects memory and learning, testosterone mediates aggression and oxytocin controls social bonding. Maternal care-giving (see Chapter 25) is influenced by not only social conditions but also oxytocin and dopamine [2].

Just as hormones could affect behaviour, so could behaviour affect hormone levels. For example, the anticipation of sexual intercourse has been shown to increase testosterone levels in women [3]. Breastfeeding induces a surge of oxytocin. More frequent partner hugs result in higher oxytocin levels which in turn are associated with lower blood pressure and heart rate in premenopausal women [4].

Interruptions and aberrations in the hormone–brain interaction result in anxiety disorders, psychopathology, maternal neglect and other morbidities. For example, fluctuations in sex steroid hormones are associated with the premenstrual syndrome which manifests not only as physical

---

BOX 6.1 Behaviours, Roles and Effects Attributed to Oxytocin

Prosocial behaviours

Trust

Attachment

Empathy

Social recognition (memory for faces)

Sexual behaviour ('love hormone')

Arousal

Orgasm

Feeding behaviour

Regulation of hunger states (suppresses food intake)

Cognitive regulation of food craving in women

Parturition and lactation

Uterine contraction

Milk ejection ('let down') reflex

Initiation of maternal behaviour

Anxiolytic and anti-stress effects

Modulation of the immune system and inflammation; promotion of wound healing

Modulation of peripheral hormones

Insulin

Cholecystokinin

Release of Atrial natriuretic peptide (ANP)

Modulation of autonomous functions

Aetiology of autism, schizophrenia

---

symptoms but also as changes in emotions and thought processes (see Chapter 12). Premature menopause is associated with reduced cognitive performance later in life [5].

The hormone oxytocin, which has a key (physical) role in pregnancy, labour and lactation, is also a particularly important determinant of behaviour [6, 7]. The specialized cells in the adenohypophysis (anterior lobe of the pituitary gland) secrete adrenocorticotropic hormone, thyroid-stimulating hormone, prolactin, growth hormone, LH and FSH. This secretory activity is modulated by oxytocin. By this and other mechanisms oxytocin influences a wide range of behaviours and physiological processes – see Box 6.1. Epigenetic changes (see Chapter 3) may account for some of the effects of oxytocin [8].

The Brain-Hormone-Heart Nexus

The emotional brain has a two-way connection with the heart through the autonomic nervous system. This system consists of parasympathetic and sympathetic divisions. These divisions release different neurotransmitters and function in opposite but complementary fashion. The sympathetic division releases epinephrine and norepinephrine (adrenaline and noradrenaline) which speed up the heart. The parasympathetic division, with the vagus nerves as its primary nerves, releases acetylcholine which slows down the heart. The heart rate reflects the relative activity of the sympathetic and parasympathetic systems. Ideally a balance should prevail. In some conditions excessive sympathetic activity (or parasympathetic underactivity) may persist, with associated physical and psychological distress and behavioural problems [9].

The interval between beats is not regular – 'a healthy heart is not a metronome' [10]. The change in the time intervals between adjacent heartbeats is known as heart rate variability (HRV). Excessive variability, as occurs in arrhythmia, is detrimental to health but so too is decreased variability. Decreased parasympathetic or increased sympathetic activity reduces HRV. HRV is a marker of resilience. Functional magnetic resonance studies show that specific areas of the brain (amygdala and prefrontal cortex) that are involved in perceptions of threat are also associated with variable cardiac rhythm[11].

There is a positive relationship between emotion regulation ability and level of resting HRV. Negative emotions (such as anger, anxiety and everyday worries) reduce cardiac variability, while positive emotions (such as joy, love and satisfaction) optimize cardiac variability. Adverse psychosocial work conditions are associated with reduced HRV [12]. Compared to people who are sedentary, those who engage in regular exercise have higher HRV [13]. HRV is reduced in people who are distressed and in those with PTSD. Those with low HRV tend to be less stress tolerant (as assessed by cortisol responses) and more impaired cognitively (as assessed by tests of executive function and working memory) [14, 15].

The autonomic imbalance underlying these findings is the putative 'final common pathway linking psychosomatics and psychopathology' [14]. Thayer and colleagues suggest that 'HRV may be more than just an index of healthy heart function, and may in fact provide an index of the degree to which the brain's "integrative" system for adaptive regulation provides flexible control over the periphery' [11].

The term 'cardiac coherence' has been applied to the state of optimal HRV [16]. Cardiac coherence theory holds that persons can be trained (by self or others) to optimize their HRV.

Growing recognition of the links between the brain, heart and behaviour has led to the emergence of neurocardiology and behavioural cardiology, fields which incorporate knowledge from psychology and psychiatry [17, 18].

Nutrition, Brain and Behaviour

Deficiencies of micronutrients and polyunsaturated fats are associated with behavioural problems. A study conducted in Egypt, Kenya and Mexico found positive associations between meat intake and cognitive function, school performance and social behaviours, and a cause-and-effect relationship was subsequently confirmed in a random allocation trial [19]. While the consumption of too much meat is associated with cancer, too little results in cognitive impairment [20]. In another study, supplementation with omega-3 fatty acids was found to be associated with reduced behaviour problems in children and teenagers [21]. A systematic review published in 2013 showed that 'broad-spectrum micronutrients' were effective in the treatment of antisocial behaviour and some psychiatric symptoms [22]. More recently, a UK study has added to the evidence that nutrition supplement may be protective against disruptive behaviour [23].

Neurobiological factors underlie these findings. Two-thirds of the brain is made up of fatty acids. Fatty acids consist of a chain of carbon atoms, with a methyl group at one end and an acid group at the other. Unsaturated fatty acids have at least one missing hydrogen atom which has been replaced by a double bond between carbon atoms. A fatty acid is described as polyunsaturated if it has two or more double bonds. Omega-3 and omega-6 are polyunsaturated fatty acids in which the first double bond occurs at the third and sixth carbon atoms respectively, counting from the methyl end ('omega'). Omega-6 fatty acids are essential nutrients but they are pro-inflammatory and they compete with omega-3 fatty acids for use in the body. For these reasons an excess of omega-6 should be avoided (the ratio of omega-6 to omega-3 should be between 1:1 and 4:1). Omega-3 fatty acids are essential for the development of brain cells and, by enhancing cell membrane permeability, they facilitate neurotransmission. The enzymatic reactions involved in the production of neurotransmitters require vitamins and minerals as cofactors. Low omega-3 levels are associated with reduced HRV [24].

There are three common types of omega-3 fatty acids: EPA (eicosapentaenoic acid), DHA (docosahexaenoic acid) and ALA (alpha-linolenic acid). These are 'essential polyunsaturated fatty acids' because while they are important for body functions the body does not produce them *de novo*, and they must be obtained through the dietary ALA (the body synthesizes DHA and EPA from ALA). Dietary sources of omega-3 include salmon, mackerel, grassfed beef, brussels sprouts, cauliflower and walnuts.

Other nutrients required for brain development and function include vitamins and iron. The fetus requires iron for the development of brain cells and synthesis of neurotransmitters. There is evidence that iron deficiency in newborns and infants affects brain and behavioural function through alterations in dopamine metabolism, myelination and hippocampal structure and function [25, 26]. Sleep quality is also affected [27].

Practical Implications

Knowledge of the interactions between the brain, heart and behaviour mediated by hormones and neurotransmitters underscores the biopsychosocial model of care. It should be an essential part of the undergraduate and postgraduate training in women's health based on the life course approach advocated by the Royal College of Obstetricians and Gynaecologists [28]. This would equip specialists to counsel and manage women in a more holistic manner and promote the adoption of multidisciplinary approaches to diagnosis and treatment. Women presenting to obstetricians and gynaecologists commonly have problems that are rooted in wider public health concerns and which require behavioural and psychosocial interventions. A better understanding of brain-heart-behaviour interactions could facilitate the management and treatment of the various conditions discussed elsewhere in this book. For example, studies of oxytocin and the brain could be 'the first step in developing novel, pharmacological treatments in support of behavioral and psychosocial interventions' for maternal neglect [2].

Conclusion

The brain is more than a computer and the heart is more than a pump. The heart is commonly regarded as the seat of emotions and the brain as the seat of cognition, but the key modulators of emotion are in the brain, not in the heart. In everyday discourse the brain and the heart are often pitched against each other ('Don't allow your heart to rule your head') but in reality they work in harmony. The dynamics of the brain-heart-behaviour interactions are highly complex, and what has been presented in this chapter is a simplified account. An understanding of these interactions, even if rudimentary, should facilitate the practice of a biopsychosocial approach to women's health care.

Key Points

- Functionally, the brain comprises a cognitive brain and an emotional brain.
- The autonomic nervous system is the main channel of communication between the brain and the heart. For maintenance of health there should be vagal balance. In conditions of chronic stress or anxiety there is relative overactivity of the sympathetic system and concomitant pathology.
- Variable cardiac rhythm is a marker of health and well-being.
- Negative emotions (such as anger, anxiety and everyday worries) reduce cardiac variability, while positive emotions (such as joy, love and satisfaction) optimize cardiac variability.
- Hormones such as oxytocin produced under the control of the brain modulate behaviour.
- Deficiencies of micronutrients and polyunsaturated fats are associated with behavioural problems.

References

1. Diamond A. Executive functions. *Annu Rev Psychol.* 2013;**64**:135–68. doi:10.1146/annurev-psych-113011–143750.

2. Strathearn L. Maternal neglect: Oxytocin, dopamine and the neurobiology of attachment. *J Neuroendocrinol.* 2011;**23**(11):1054–65. doi: 10.1111/j.1365–2826.2011.02228.x.

3. van Anders SM, Hamilton LD, Schmidt N, Watson NV. Associations between testosterone secretion and sexual activity in women. *Horm Behav* 2007;**51**(4):477–82.

4. Light KC, Grewen KM, Amico JA. More frequent partner hugs and higher oxytocin levels are linked to lower blood pressure and heart rate in premenopausal women. *Biol Psychol.* 2005;**69**(1):5–21.

5. Ryan J, Scali J, Carrière I, Amieva H, Rouaud O, Berr C, Ritchie K, Ancelin ML. Impact of a premature menopause on cognitive function in later life. *BJOG.* 2014;**121**(13):1729–39.

6. Lee HJ, Macbeth AH, Pagani JH, Young WS. Oxytocin: The great facilitator of life. *Progress in Neurobiology.* 2009;**88**(2):127–51. doi:10.1016/j. pneurobio.2009.04.001.

7. Yang HP, Wang L, Han L, Wang SC. Nonsocial functions of hypothalamic oxytocin. *ISRN Neurosci.* 2013;**2013**:179272. doi: 10.1155/2013/179272.

8. Haas BW, Filkowski MM, Cochran RN, Denison L, Ishak A, Nishitani S, Smith AK. Epigenetic modification of OXT and human sociability. *Proc Natl Acad Sci U S A.* 2016;**113**(27):E3816–23. doi: 10.1073/pnas.1602809113.

9. Grassi G, Quarti-Trevano F, Seravalle G, Dell'Oro R. Cardiovascular risk and adrenergic overdrive in the metabolic syndrome. *Nutr Metab Cardiovasc Dis.* 2007;**17**(6):473–81.

10. Shaffer F, McCraty R, Zerr CL. A healthy heart is not a metronome: an integrative review of the heart's anatomy and heart rate variability. *Front Psychol.* 2014;**5**:1040. doi: 10.3389/fpsyg.2014.01040.

11. Thayer JF, Ahs F, Fredrikson M, Sollers JJ 3rd, Wager TD. A meta-analysis of heart rate variability and neuroimaging studies: Implications for heart rate variability as a marker of stress and health. *Neurosci Biobehav Rev.* 2012;**36**(2):747–56. doi: 10.1016/j. neubiorev.2011.11.009.

12. Jarczok MN, Jarczok M, Mauss D, Koenig J, Li J, Herr RM, Thayer JF. Autonomic nervous system activity and workplace stressors – a systematic review. *Neurosci Biobehav Rev.* 2013;**37**(8):1810–23. doi: 10.1016/j.neubiorev.2013.07.004.

13. Routledge FS, Campbell TS, McFetridge-Durdle JA, Bacon SL. Improvements in heart rate variability with exercise therapy. *Can J Cardiol.* 2010;**26**(6): 303–12.

14. Thayer JF, Brosschot JF. Psychosomatics and psychopathology: Looking up and down from the brain. *Psychoneuroendocrinology* 2005;**30**: 1050–58.

15. Thayer JF, Lane RD. Claude Bernard and the heart-brain connection: Further elaboration of a model of neurovisceral integration. *Neurosci Biobehav Rev.* 2009;**33**(2):81–88. doi: 10.1016/j. neubiorev.2008.08.004.

16. Servan-Schreiber D. *Healing without Freud or Prozac.* London: Rodale International 2005.

17. Pereira VH, Cerqueira JJ, Palha JA, Sousa N. Stressed brain, diseased heart: A review on the pathophysiologic mechanisms of neurocardiology. *Int J Cardiol.* 2013;**166**(1):30–37. doi: 10.1016/j.ijcard.2012.03.165.

18. Rozanski A. Behavioral cardiology: Current advances and future directions. *J Am Coll Cardiol.* 2014;**64**(1): 100–10. doi:10.1016/j.jacc.2014.03.047.

19. Neumann CG, Murphy SP, Gewa C, Grillenberger M, Bwibo NO. Meat supplementation improves growth, cognitive, and behavioral outcomes in Kenyan children. *J Nutr.* 2007;**137**(4):1119–23.

20. Gupta S. Brain food: Clever eating. *Nature.* 2016;**531** (7592):S12–3. doi: 10.1038/531S12a.

21. Raine A, Portnoy J, Liu J, Mahoomed T, Hibbeln JR. Reduction in behavior problems with omega-3 supplementation in children aged 8–16 years: A randomized, double-blind, placebo-controlled, stratified, parallel-group trial. *J Child Psychol Psychiatry.* 2015;**56**(5):509–20. doi: 10.1111/jcpp.12314.

22. Rucklidge JJ, Kaplan BJ. Broad-spectrum micronutrient formulas for the treatment of psychiatric symptoms: A systematic review. *Expert Rev Neurother.* 2013;**13**(1):49–73. doi: 10.1586/ern.12.143.

23. Tammam JD, Steinsaltz D, Bester DW, Semb-Andenaes T, Stein JF. A randomised double-blind placebo-controlled trial investigating the behavioural effects of vitamin, mineral and n-3 fatty acid supplementation in typically developing adolescent schoolchildren. *Br J Nutr.* 2016;**115**(2):361–73. doi: 10.1017/S0007114515004390.

24. Carney RM, Freedland KE, Stein PK, Steinmeyer BC, Harris WS, Rubin EH, Krone RJ, Rich MW. Effect of omega-3 fatty acids on heart rate variability in depressed patients with coronary heart disease. *Psychosom Med.* 2010;**72**(8):748–54. doi: 10.1097/PSY.0b013e3181eff148.

25. Lozoff B, Georgieff MK. Iron deficiency and brain development. *Semin Pediatr Neurol.*2006;**13**:158–65.

26. Georgieff MK. Long-term brain and behavioral consequences of early iron deficiency. *Nutr Rev.* 2011;**69**(Suppl 1):S43–8. doi: 10.1111/j. 1753–4887.2011.00432.x.

27. Peirano PD, Algarín CR, Chamorro RA, Reyes SC, Durán SA, Garrido MI, Lozoff B. Sleep alterations and iron deficiency anemia in infancy. *Sleep Med.* 2010;**11** (7):637–42. doi: 10.1016/j.sleep.2010.03.014.

28. Royal College of Obstetricians and Gynaecologists. Why should we consider a life course approach to women's health care? Scientific Impact Paper No. 27. August 2011.

Complementary Medicine for Women's Healthcare

Helen Hall

Complementary Medicine

Complementary medicine (CM) describes a variety of healthcare practices with a history of use or origins, outside of conventional Western medicine. While the variety of therapies included under the CM rubric is extensive, most sit within one of two major categories: natural products (herbal medicine, dietary supplements, etc.), and mind and body practices (acupuncture, chiropractic, massage, meditation, yoga, etc.) [1]. In contrast to the conventional approach taken in biomedicine, CM is underpinned by a holistic perspective, which promotes the body's natural healing ability and the individual as an active participant in their healthcare [2]. CM therapies may be used as single modalities, or incorporated in whole medical systems. An example is seen with acupuncture which may be employed as a stand-alone intervention, or integrated with other therapies (such as herbal medicines) within a Traditional Chinese Medicine (TCM) approach.

Integrative medicine (IM) refers to the use of evidence-based CM therapies in combination with conventional biomedical treatments. This healthcare approach takes a holistic perspective and aims to optimize well-being at all stages of life [3, 4]. Hence, IM broadens the range of therapeutic options and allows for more individualized healthcare.

Prevalence and Motivation of CM Use by Women

Surveys undertaken in numerous countries, including the USA [5], the UK [6] and Australia [7] indicate that many women use CM. Indeed a systematic review of the literature found that CM users tend to be middle age (in the broadest sense), well-educated females with more than one medical condition; although they do not necessarily consider their health to be poorer than non-users [8]. While some women turn to CM because they are disillusioned with biomedical treatments, most use the therapies as an adjunct to, rather than a replacement for, conventional medicine. Women utilize CM not only to manage illness but also to promote general well-being. Various therapies are utilized by women to manage a variety of their health problems, including dysmenorrhoea [9], infertility [10], breast cancer [11] and conditions associated with menopause [12] and pregnancy [13].

CM Use during Pregnancy

The discourses of holistic, 'natural' treatments appeal to pregnant women, and many integrate CM therapies into their maternity care [14]. With the increasing medicalisation of normal pregnancy and birth, women may turn to CM in an attempt to retain control and reduce unwanted medical intervention [15]. Furthermore, midwives are often supportive of women's use of these therapies [16, 17]. Many women report that CM helps them to manage conditions associated with normal healthy pregnancy and to assist them during labour and birth [18]. CM modalities are often used to manage symptoms such as back pain, fatigue, urinary tract infection, nausea and vomiting and in preparation for labour [18–20]. Popular therapies utilized during pregnancy include nutritional supplements, herbal medicine, relaxation therapies and aromatherapy [14].

CM and Patient Safety

CM and Evidence-Based Medicine

Evidence-based medicine (EBM) integrates clinical expertise, the best available evidence and the patient's preference. However, the research component has gained prominence with the randomized control trial (RCT) considered the gold standard. In this context, concerns have been raised regarding the lack of robust scientific evidence for many CM therapies. Yet there is ongoing debate about the appropriateness of applying the EBM approach, particularly the use of RCTs, to CM. Indeed there are fundamental ideological differences which need to be considered; while biomedicine values an objective and reductionist approach, many CM therapies have emerged from a holistic paradigm which emphasizes complex systems and individual differences. Further to these ideological challenges, additional barriers to CM research include lack of available funding, infrastructure, professional expertise and suitable validated research instruments [21].

Currently, much of CM expertise is based on traditional knowledge and empirical wisdom, rather than scientific verification. However, a growing number of therapies are now being subjected to rigorous scientific enquiry. For example, acupuncture has a long history of being used to stimulate labour, and the effectiveness of this intervention has recently been supported with findings from clinical trials [22]. Yet it should be noted that while traditional use may provide some level of confidence, it does not ensure either safety or efficacy. A case in point is seen with blue cohosh (*Caulophyllum thalictroides*), which was traditionally used for birth preparation but is now contraindicated due to evidence associating it with an increase in the risk of congenital problems [21].

Regardless of the current debate, healthcare providers should remember that while EBM has become entrenched in the modern biomedical approach, women are likely to continue to use CM regardless of the lack of scientific evidence. For instance, a study exploring menopausal women's views towards CM found women were not deterred by a lack of scientific validation and they expected their conventional health provider to respect their decision to use it [23]. Furthermore, it is worth reflecting upon the fact that many medical procedures have not been assessed according to the principles of EBM [21]. Nonetheless, it is widely accepted that there needs to be more quality scientific research into effects of CM therapies and a significant amount of work is now being undertaken [21].

Communication and Information

The exchange of appropriate information and open dialogue between patients and healthcare professionals is fundamental to good care. Yet women often base their decisions to use CM therapies on non-professional sources of information (such as family and friends), without their healthcare providers' knowledge or input. Research indicates that women may not disclose their CM use because they are concerned that they will encounter a negative response or they recognize that mainstream health providers have a poor understanding of the therapies [24]. In fact many conventional health professionals do have limited understanding of CM, and this problem is further exacerbated by lack of collaboration with qualified CM practitioners.

Given the popularity of CM, all health professionals should have the basic understanding to engage in open dialogue regarding use of the therapies and, when appropriate, refer to CM practitioners [25]. Improved CM education and communication would help address the current disconnect between the acceptance of CM in the community and its marginalisation in modern biomedicine.

Useful information can be accessed via the web sites outlined below.

The National Center for Complementary and Integrative Health (NCCIH) is a leading agency for scientific research on complementary and integrative health approaches – https://nccih.nih.gov

CM on PubMed® was developed jointly by the National Library of Medicine (NLM) and NCCIH and contains citations to journal articles related to CM – https://nccih.nih.gov/research/camonpubmed.

Medline plus is produced by the NLM and has reliable, up-to-date health information, for the free consumers about drugs and over-the-counter medicines, including herbal and dietary supplements – https://medlineplus.gov/druginformation.html

CM Modalities and Women's Health

The use of specific CM therapies for women's health conditions varies significantly according to context (e.g. country) and acceptability by women and their health providers. An extensive search of the evidence is beyond the scope of this chapter, however common therapies are highlighted here to provide examples.

Natural Products

Natural products are therapeutic substances derived from nature such as herbs and dietary supplements. While they generally have less serious adverse effects than conventional drugs, the underlying assumption that natural products are safe is largely unsubstantiated [17]. As well as the intrinsic toxicity of some plants, CM supplements are generally not subject to the same level of regulation or formal assessment of safety and efficacy as pharmaceuticals. Moreover, inconsistencies in harvesting and manufacturing process and problems with adulteration can all lead to adverse events. Added to this risk is the potential for some natural products to interact with pharmaceutical drugs. Indeed, both adverse and beneficial interactions have been reported with a number of products [26].

In addition, a number of behaviours increase a person's risks when they consume natural products. These actions include individuals using CM supplements and pharmaceuticals concurrently, self-prescribing without advice from a qualified practitioner and failure to inform their biomedical doctor of their use.

Herbal Medicines and Women's Health

Herbal medicine refers to the use of a plant, or plant part, for its medicinal properties. Herbs are incorporated into numerous approaches, including the Western herbal tradition, Ayurveda, TCM and many local indigenous medicinal systems. One of the challenges with investigating the efficacy of herbal medicines for women's health conditions lies in the very nature of plants themselves. While modern pharmaceuticals are usually based on a highly regulated dose of an active ingredient, herbal medicines have been derived from plants containing multiple constituents with a synergistic effect. In addition to this, herbal medicines are often a compound mix of a variety of plants. Therefore the therapeutic activity of herbal medicine is due to its complex interaction of different constituents, rather than one specific active ingredient that can be isolated and tested.

Nevertheless, an evidence base for the use of herbal medicines to various women's health conditions is beginning to emerge. For instance a Cochrane review found promising evidence for the use of Chinese herbal medicine for primary dysmenorrhoea [7]. There is also evidence that soy extracts are effective against vasomotor complaints in some menopausal women [27] and ginger reduces pregnancy-induced nausea [28]. Alternatively, there are now concerns that some commonly used herbal medicines may not be safe. For example black cohosh (*Actaea racemosa*), that is commonly used to manage menopausal symptoms, may cause liver problems [27].

Nutritional Medicine and Women's Health

There has been increasing appreciation of the impact of diet on well-being and nutritional assessment is now considered an important aspect of a health history. In addition, surveys reveal that many women consume nutritional supplements [29]. This surge in interest may be in part due to the decreasing nutritional value of the modern Western diet. It is clear that, despite the availability of food, malnutrition is prevalent. In contrast to undernutrition where there is insufficient food to sustain healthy life, malnutrition relates to poor-quality diet. Evidence from the USA, Australia and the UK indicates declining levels of nutritional value in our food [3]. Furthermore, research confirms that most people do not consume a balanced diet. More adults are becoming overweight or obese, and vitamin and mineral deficiencies are common in these people [30]. In fact the majority of patients seen by doctors in today's society are at a high risk of having or developing a nutritional deficiency [3]. In addition to the problems of a poor diet, some drugs may cause nutrient deficiency. For example medications containing oestrogen have been associated with a decrease in the serum zinc and magnesium levels [26]. Research indicates that as well as correcting dietary insufficiencies, nutritional supplementation may prevent or improve a wide variety of women's health conditions, including dysmenorrhoea, cervical cancer, miscarriage, pregnancy-induced nausea and vomiting, premature birth, osteoporosis and more [3, 4].

Mind-Body Therapies

The NCCIH states 'mind-body medicine focusses on the interactions among the brain, mind, body, and behaviour, and the powerful ways in which emotional, mental, social, spiritual and behavioural factors can directly affect health' [1]. Hence, mind-body therapies are based on the premise that supporting the well-being of the mind will promote physical health and vice versa. In addition, most diseases have a psychological component as a trigger and/or as an outcome and therefore stress management can improve well-being generally. Women often use mind-body therapies to support their health [31]. Common examples of therapies categorized as 'mind-body medicine' include massage, yoga, meditation, hypnosis, tai chi, acupuncture, chiropractic and osteopathy.

Massage and Women's Health

Massage involves the systematic manipulation of the body tissue for a curative effect. While the exact mechanism is not fully understood, massage can reduce muscle tension and promote circulation as well as improve psychological well-being. As such it is a popular therapy for a wide range of conditions from sports injuries to stress relief. Although caution must be taken, massage has few risks and can be provided in multiple settings, from a person's home to a hospital ward. There has been extensive assessment of the effectiveness of massage for a variety of medical problems and patient populations. The findings of studies exploring its use for women's health problems indicate that it is safe and acceptable treatment for many conditions. For example prenatally depressed women who received massage twice weekly from their partners reported less pain, depression, anxiety and improvements in their relationship [32]. Likewise, women with breast cancer who received a 35-minute massage three times a week for a month had improved quality-of-life scores compared to a control group [33].

Yoga and Women's Health

Yoga aims to achieve balance of body, mind and spirit using three basic components: posture (asana), breathing (pranayama) and meditation (dhyana). Advocates of yoga assert that practising the postures improves flexibility and strength, learning to control breathing supports relaxation while undertaking meditation focusses the mind. There are a number of different approaches, with hatha yoga being the most widely practised in the West. Although yoga is a holistic system, the common approach tends to focus on various postures as a stress-reducing practice. The use of yoga for various women's health issues has received considerable attention from researchers. For example a review of the studies investigating the effectiveness of yoga to manage menopause found moderate evidence for short-term effectiveness on psychological symptoms but no evidence for somatic, vasomotor or urogenital symptoms [34]. Other studies have reported that the practice of yoga is associated with reductions in severity of dysmenorrhea [35] and positive effects on pain, balance and general health in postmenopausal osteoporotic women [36].

Meditation and Women's Health

Meditation involves undertaking a set of intentional practices which lead to increased awareness, greater presence and a more integrated sense of self. Typically, the practice involves a combination of repeating a mantra, listening to the breath, self-directed mental practices or detaching from the thought process. Common types of meditation include concentrative and mindfulness. *Concentrative* meditation comprises focussing attention on an object (sound, light, idea) and sustaining attention until the mind achieves stillness. Transcendental Meditation (TM) is a form of concentrative meditation that is based on Hindu teachings. Another approach is *mindfulness* meditation which involves a person focussing on the present and being aware of their current actions, emotions and thoughts without judging them. While not its primary purpose, relaxation may also occur as a result of mindfulness meditation. There is a growing repertoire of research investigating the effectiveness of these practices for a wide range of health conditions, including those specific to women. For example, there is now good evidence that meditation is an effective intervention to support women's mental health when they are dealing with a range of conditions, including pregnancy [37], infertility [38], breast cancer [39] and menopause [40].

Hypnosis and Women's Health

Hypnosis uses suggestions that are aimed at enabling a person to focus narrowly and intensify their concentration. During hypnosis the conscious mind is placed 'on hold' and beneficial suggestions made by a therapist can be accepted more readily into the subconscious mind. Commonly used to help people stop smoking or reduce food intake, hypnosis is now being used for some women's health conditions. A systematic review of the literature found promising evidence for the effectiveness of hypnosis in breast cancer care; in particular, it was found to be useful in the management of pain distress, fatigue, nausea and hot flashes [41]. Hypnosis has also been shown to significantly improve hot flashes in postmenopausal women [42].

Tai chi and Women's Health

Tai chi is a type of mindfulness-based exercise that has its origins in China as a martial art. The practice of tai chi involves slow, gentle movements and elements of meditation (such as imagery and deep breathing), with the aim of rebalancing the body's healing capacity. Due to the gentle nature of tai chi, it is an appropriate therapy for many people, including the elderly and those with physical limitations. In light of its practicality for an aging population, it is interesting to note that there is evidence that tai chi may be an effective and safe intervention for maintaining bone mineral density, reducing fall frequency and increasing musculoskeletal strength in postmenopausal women [43]. Tai chi also shows promise for other health concerns, including the management of anxiety and depression in women with a range of medical conditions [44].

Acupuncture and Women's Health

According to TCM, the body has a network of invisible channels through which life energy (qi) flows, known as *meridians*. Blockage of the meridians can result in an inadequate life energy leading to imbalance and ultimately illness. This obstruction may result from stress, poor diet, pathogens, environmental conditions and lifestyle factors. Acupuncture involves the stimulation of specific points along the meridians to remove blockages of the energy and restore balance. Acupressure is similar to acupuncture; however, it employs gentle, firm pressure to stimulate energy rather than penetrating the skin with fine needles. There is an increasing volume of research investigating the use of acupuncture for women's health conditions. For example an RCT found that acupuncture can reduce the duration of the third stage of labour [22], while a pilot study found a reduction in the fatigue experienced by breast cancer survivors who received acupuncture [45].

Spinal Manipulation/Mobilization and Women's Health

Spinal manipulation/mobilization aims to re-establish a healthy balance within the body by restoring normal alignment. Treatment is usually characterized by the application of biomechanical force (high- or low-velocity thrust) to a localized joint. In addition to its impact on pain via spinal 'gating' mechanism, spinal manipulation may also improve mobility. Although the safety of spinal manipulation remains contentious, most of the adverse events are benign and transitory, with only rare reports of serious complications [46]. Women commonly seek out chiropractors and osteopaths to support their health; however, a review of the scientific evidence regarding the effectiveness of manual therapies reported mixed results; spinal manipulation was useful for back pain and migraine, but the evidence for its role in premenstrual syndrome was not conclusive and lacking for dysmenorrhea [47].

Conclusion

In summary, there is a growing interest in the integration of evidence-based CM therapies into women's healthcare. IM has the potential to support women to manage a wide range of their health conditions. Although many CM therapies are recommended on the basis of traditional practices, a scientific evidence base is beginning to develop. The increasing popularity of these therapies places an onus on the healthcare professions to develop the relevant knowledge and referral systems. Healthcare providers need to acquire the information and confidence to communicate openly so women who are interested in CM have the appropriate support to make informed and safe decisions.

Key Points

- Most CM therapies can be classified into one of two categories: natural products (herbal medicine, dietary supplements, etc.) and mind and body practices (acupuncture, chiropractic, massage, meditation, yoga, etc.).
- Integrative medicine (IM) refers to the use of evidence-based CM therapies in combination with conventional biomedical treatments.
- While some women turn to CM because they are disillusioned with biomedical treatments, most use the therapies as an adjunct to, rather than a replacement for, conventional medicine.
- Women may not disclose their CM use because they are concerned that they will encounter a negative response or they recognize that mainstream health providers have a poor understanding of the therapies.
- Biomedicine values an objective and reductionist approach; however, CM adopts a holistic view which emphasizes complex systems and individual differences.
- There needs to be more quality research into CM therapies and a significant amount of work is now being undertaken.
- Randomized controlled trials have demonstrated the benefits of various CM modalities for a range of obstetric and gynaecological conditions.
- Health professionals should have the basic understanding of CM in order to support women to make well informed therapeutic decisions.

References

1. National Center for Complementary and Integrative Health. Complementary, alternative, or integrative health: What's in a name? 2015 [1/7/15]; Available from: https://nccih.nih.gov/health/integrative-health [accessed 11 March 2017].

2. Hall, H., Complementary therapies., in *Fundamentals of nursing and midwifery; a person centred approach*, R. Hill, H. Hall and P. Glew, Editors. 2017, Wolters Kluwer: Australia. pp. 718–34.

3. Kotsirilos, V., L. Vitetta, and A. Sali *A guide to evidence based Integrative and complementary medicine.* 2011, Sydney: Churchill Livingstone Elsevier.

4. Leach, M., *Clinical decision making in complementary and alternative medicine.* 2010, Sydney: Churchill Livingstone Elsevier.

5. Upchurch, D., et al., Demographic, behavioral, and health correlates of complementary and alternative medicine and prayer use among midlife women: 2002. *Journal of Womens Health*, 2010. **19**(1): pp. 23–30.

6. Coulson, C. and J. Jenkins, Complementary and alternative medicine utilisation in NHS and private clinic settings: A United Kingdom survey of 400 infertility patients. *J Exp Clin Assist Reprod*, 2005. **2**(5): doi:10.1186/1743-1050-2-5

7. Zhu, X., et al., Chinese herbal medicine for primary dysmenorrhoea. *Cochrane Database Syst Rev*, 2008. **4** (6): pp. 389–91.

8. Bishop, F. and G. Lewith, Who uses CAM? A narrative review of demographic characteristics and health factors associated with CAM use. *Evidence-based Complementary and Alternative Medicine*, 2010. **7**(1): pp. 11–28.

9. Cho, S. and E. Hwang, Acupuncture for primary dysmenorrhoea: A systematic review. *BJOG an international journal of obstetrics and gynaecology*, 2010. **117**(5): p. 509.

10. Perry, T. and J. Hirshfeld-Cytron, Role of complementary and alternative medicine to achieve fertility in uninsured patients. *Obstet Gynecol Surv*, 2013. **68**: pp. 305–11.

11. Greenlee, H., et al., Complementary and alternative therapy use before and after breast cancer diagnosis: The pathways study. *Breast Cancer Res Treat*, 2009. **117**(3): pp. 653–65.

12. Posadzki, P., et al., Prevalence of complementary and alternative medicine (CAM) use by menopausal women: A systematic review of surveys. *Maturitas*, 2013. **75**: pp. 34–43.

13. Pallivalappila, A., et al., Complementary and alternative medicines use during pregnancy: A systematic review of pregnant women and healthcare professional views and experiences. *Evidence-Based Complementary and Alternative Medicine*, 2013. doi: 10.1155/2013/205639.

14. Hall, H., D. Griffiths, and L. McKenna, The use of complementary and alternative medicine by pregnant women: A literature review. *Midwifery*, 2011. **27**(6): pp. 817–24.

15. Mitchell, M. and S. McClean, Pregnancy, risk perception and use of complementary and alternative medicine. *Health Risk Soc*, 2014. **16**(1): pp. 101–16.

16. Adams, J., et al., Attitudes and referral practices of maternity care professionals with regard to complementary and alternative medicine: An integrative review. *Journal of Advanced Nursing*, 2011. **67**(3): pp. 472–83.

17. Hall, H., L. McKenna, and D. Griffiths, Midwives' support for complementary and alternative medicine: A literature review. *Women and Birth*, 2012. **25**(1): pp. 4–12.

18. Skouteris, H., et al., Use of complementary and alternative medicines by a sample of Australian women during pregnancy. *Australian and New Zealand Journal of Obstetrics and Gynaecology*, 2008. **48**(4): pp. 384–90.

19. Frawley, J., et al., Prevalence and determinants of complementary and alternative medicine use during pregnancy: Results from a nationally representative sample of Australian pregnant women. *Aust NZ J Obstet Gynaecol*, 2013. **4**: pp. 347–52.

20. Adams, J., D. Sibbritt, and C. Lui, The use of complementary and alternative medicine during pregnancy: A longitudinal study of Australian women. *Birth*, 2011. **38**: pp. 200–6.

21. Hall, H., L. McKenna, and D. Griffiths, Complementary and alternative medicine: Where's the evidence? *British Journal of Midwifery*, 2010. **18**(7): pp. 436–40.

22. López-Garrido, B., et al., Influence of acupuncture on the third stage of labor: A randomized controlled trial. *Journal of Midwifery & Women's Health*, 2015. **60**(2): pp. 199–205.

23. Gollschewski, S., et al., Women's perceptions and beliefs about the use of complementary and alternative medicines during menopause. *Complement Ther Med*, 2008. **16**(3): pp. 163–8.

24. Hall, H., D. Griffiths, and L. McKenna, Complementary and alternative medicine: Interaction and communication between midwives and women. Women and Birth, 2015.

25. Hall, H., L. McKenna, and D. Griffiths, From alternative, to complementary to integrative medicine: Supporting Australian midwives in an increasingly

pluralistic maternity environment. *Women and Birth*, 2013. **26**: pp. e90–e3.

26. Stargrove, M., J. Treasure, and D. McKee, *Herb, nutrient ad drug interactions: Clinical implications and therapeutic strategies*. 2008, Missouri: Mosby Elsevier.

27. Depypere, H. and F. Comhaire, Herbal preparations for the menopause: Beyond isoflavones and black cohosh. *Maturitas*, 2014. **77**(2): p. 191.

28. Matthews, A., et al., Interventions for nausea and vomiting in early pregnancy. *The Cochrane Database of Systematic Reviews*, 2010. **8**(9) doi: 10.1002/14651858. CD007575.pub4

29. Xue, C., et al., Complementary and alternative medicine use in Australia: A national population-based survey. *The Journal of Alternative and Complementary Medicine*, 2007. **13**(6): pp. 643–50.

30. Marovic, T. and S. Natoli, Paradoxical nutrient deficiency in overweight and obesity: The importance of nutrient density. *Medical Journal of Australia*, 2009. **190**: pp. 149–51.

31. Sibbritt, D., J. Adams, and P. van der Riet, The prevalence and characteristics of young and mid-age women who use yoga and meditation: Results of a nationally representative survey of 19,209 Australian women. *Complementary therapies in medicine*, 2011. **19**(2): p. 71.

32. Field, T., et al., Massage therapy reduces pain in pregnant women, alleviates prenatal depression in both parents and improves their relationships. *Journal of Bodywork and Movement Therapies*, 2008. **12**: pp. 146–50.

33. Ovayolu, Ö., et al., The effect of aromatherapy and massage administered in different ways to women with breast cancer on their symptoms and quality of life. *International Journal of Nursing practice*, 2014. **20**(4): pp. 408–17.

34. Cramer, H., et al., Effectiveness of yoga for menopausal symptoms: A systematic review and meta-analysis of randomized controlled trials. *Evidence-Based Complementary and Alternative Medicine*, 2012 doi: 10.1155/2012/863905.

35. Chien, L.-W., H.-C. Chang, and C.-F. Liu, Effect of yoga on serum homocysteine and nitric oxide levels in adolescent women with and without dysmenorrhea. *The Journal of Alternative and Complementary Medicine*, 2013. **19**(1): pp. 20–23.

36. Tüzün, S., et al., Yoga might be an alternative training for the quality of life and balance in postmenopausal osteoporosis. *European Journal of Physical and Rehabilitation Medicine*, 2010. **46**(1): pp. 69–72.

37. Woolhouse, H., et al., Antenatal mindfulness intervention to reduce depression, anxiety and stress: A pilot randomised controlled trial of the MindBabyBody program in an Australian tertiary maternity hospital. *BMC Pregnancy and Childbirth*, 2014. **14**(369): doi: 10.1186/s12884-014-0369-z

38. Sherratt, K. and S. Lunn, Evaluation of a group programme of mindfulness-based cognitive therapy for women with fertility problems. *Journal of Obstetrics and Gynaecology*, 2013. **33**(5): p. 499.

39. Zainal, N., S. Booth, and F. Huppert, The efficacy of mindfulness-based stress reduction on mental health of breast cancer patients: A meta-analysis. *Psycho-oncology*, 2013. **22**(7): p. 1457.

40. Carmody, J., et al., Mindfulness training for coping with hot flashes: Results of a randomized trial Menopause. *Menopause*, 2011. **18**(6): pp. 611–20.

41. Cramer, H., et al., Hypnosis in breast cancer care: A systematic review of randomized controlled trials. *Integr Cancer Ther*, 2015. **14**(1): pp. 5–15.

42. Elkins, G., et al., Clinical hypnosis in the treatment of postmenopausal hot flashes: A randomized controlled trial. *Menopause*, 2013. **20**(3): pp. 291–8.

43. Wayne, P., et al., The effects of Tai Chi on bone mineral density in postmenopausal women: A systematic review. *Arch Phys Med Rehabil*, 2007. **88**(5): pp. 673–80.

44. Sharma, M. and T. Haider, Tai Chi as an alternative and complimentary therapy for anxiety: A systematic review. *Journal of Evidence-Based Complementary & Alternative Medicine*, 2015. **20**(2): pp. 143–53.

45. Smith, C., et al., The effect of acupuncture on post-cancer fatigue and well-being for women recovering from breast cancer: A pilot randomised controlled trial. *Acupuncture in Medicine: Journal of the British Medical Acupuncture Society*, 2013. **31**(1): p. 9.

46. Gouveia, L., P. Castanho, and J. Ferreira, Safety of chiropractic interventions: A systematic review. *Spine*, 2009. **34**(11): pp. E405–13.

47. Bronfort, G., et al., Effectiveness of manual therapies: The UK evidence report. *Chiropractic & Osteopathy*, 2010. **18**(3): doi: 10.1186/1746-1340-18-3

Domestic Violence and Abuse

Rachel Adams and Susan Bewley

Introduction

Once per clinic, once per night shift, a clinician is likely to meet a patient who is currently experiencing domestic violence and abuse (DVA) [1]. Although it can impact upon every aspect of health and well-being, DVA is misunderstood, often undisclosed, and when survivors of DVA present in healthcare contexts, professionals feel ill-equipped to respond.

Domestic violence and abuse can be defined as:

Any incident or pattern of incidents of controlling, coercive or threatening behaviour, violence or abuse between those aged 16 or over who are or have been intimate partners or family members, regardless of gender or sexuality. This can encompass, but is not limited to, the following types of abuse:

Psychological
Physical
Sexual
Financial
Emotional [2]

Those experiencing violence have described their needs and expectations when they become patients. Survivors want their experiences heard, and responses to be respectful and empathic. They need safe and confidential spaces for disclosure, and for health professionals to signpost them towards multidisciplinary support [3].

At face value these seem simple, and within the central remit of healthcare. However, significant barriers to health professional enquiry, and survivor disclosure, have been described. This chapter takes the literature on barriers as its starting point and focusses on the example of doctors as front-line healthcare professionals. It examines the context of doctors' work, their questions and the underlying assumptions that may challenge engagement with DVA. In so doing, important comparisons between survivor and clinician experiences are found, which may offer a new approach to clinician engagement.

Barriers in Context

Barriers occur at different levels. By its nature, DVA demands an understanding of power, gender, class and culture dynamics [4]; this language may be unfamiliar to many clinicians. For example, while this chapter focusses on violence experienced by women and perpetrated by men as the most common, most chronic, and most severe form of DVA [5], it is not meant to exclude other patterns. It is intended as a starting point for learning, specifically for obstetrician/gynaecologists.

The medical context poses further challenges. For example, the literature focusses on barriers from senior healthcare perspectives [6], but in practice the front-line doctors (and nurses and midwives) engaging with survivors of DVA are junior and non-specialist [7]. Doctors at all levels lack training in DVA, but juniors also lack experience of their professional and structural context [4]. The pressurized setting of a labour ward or emergency department may be a challenging [8], or even hostile, environment to the 'problem' of women with DVA.

The global context is one of recognition of the harms of violence against women and girls, and newly trained doctors have grown up with WHO gender mainstreaming and resurgent feminism [9]. However, after a decade of austerity, the local context of healthcare is changing. Preventative, community-based work is being lost and crises of violence are presenting in healthcare settings more regularly [10]. Concurrently, more legalistic and punitive approaches are taken; healthcare training on DVA often appears solely as an adjunct to child safeguarding, whilst 'target-driven' pushes for female genital mutilation convictions enter the health arena [11]. Doctors will see more violence, and it may be framed in a legalistic (rather than therapeutic) way.

At the individual doctor–patient level, barriers can be re-imagined as a series of questions that may arise

Table 8.1 Barriers to Domestic Violence and Abuse disclosure and enquiry

	Barriers	Facilitators
Survivors	Fear of perpetrator	Confidentiality
	Fear of losing children	Multidisciplinary response
	Shame	Acknowledgement
	Stage of change/ awareness	Non-judgmental listening
	Powerlessness	
Professionals	Desribed as "External"	Exposure
	Time	Support
	Resources	Training
	Job definition	
	'Obstructive patients'	
	Lack of training	
	Described as "Internal"	
	Frustration	
	Powerlessness	
	Prejudicial attitudes	
	Exposure (professional / personal)	

as the front-line doctor is confronted with DVA. As shown in Table 8.1, this chapter asks:

- Is it my job to address DVA?
- What effect will it have on patient management?
- How will I change my clinical practice to incorporate DVA enquiry?

Against the backdrop of barriers and questions, there are examples of junior doctors as champions and innovators [12,13]. This chapter aims to empower like-minded 'front-line doctors' and supportive seniors to explore why colleagues may have doubts.

Working through Barriers

A history of DVA is an important social determinant of health. Figure 8.1 maps this onto a typical Obstetrics & Gynaecology doctor's clerking structure and demonstrates how DVA awareness is an essential part of this process

Making links with an individual patient's presentation during the initial enquiry forms part of a front-line response, which is further described in Tables 8.2–8.4 and Figure 8.2.

Despite this, neither screening nor case-based enquiry about DVA has become routine in practice [17]. What prevents DVA enquiry becoming an essential part of history and formulation?

'Is It My Job?'

It is not uncommon to hear clinicians say 'dealing with domestic violence is not part of my job'. They might argue that DVA is not a disease, and that it is not the job of medicine to address social phenomena but merely its downstream ill-effects. However, as Figure 8.1 demonstrates, the connections between physical, psychological and social manifestations of DVA are thoroughly enmeshed. For example, survivors of violence are over-represented in cases of chronic abdominal/pelvic pain and subsequent diagnostic laparoscopies, as their doctors search for physical causes for unexplained symptoms [18,19]. The 'reason' will never simply be 'violence', but acknowledging its association with pain will influence the clinical workup – and thus associated risks and harms [20].

A clinician may respond negatively to DVA as a 'taboo', associated with sex, mental illness, addiction and the 'private sphere' [15,21]. Nevertheless, there is evidence that women find enquiry about DVA acceptable, even welcome. Patients test whether it's safe (psychologically and practically) to reveal DVA, often dropping hints within their minor physical complaints and repeat visits [22], but are unlikely to disclose unless actually asked directly [23]. Even if this were not hidden, doctors in their special societal position must often confront taboos that affect health and

Demographics
- Domestic violence and abuse (DVA) affect all ages, genders, sexualities, cultures and classes.
- Risk factors include young age, poverty, and presence of a male partner.
- **The most prevalent, severe and repeated violence is experienced by women in heterosexual relationships [5].**

Presenting complaint
- Abuse is often chronic, types of violence overlap, and there is complex interplay of biological-psychological-social factors by the time of presentation.
- The history often does not point to a clear diagnosis and there is a **high rate of medically unexplained symptoms [17].**
- This is considered a pattern of help-seeking behaviour [18].

Past history
- Increased rate of chronic abdominal and pelvic pain, and an increased number of diagnostic laparoscopies [19].
- **Dose-response relationship** between common physiological symptoms of pregnancy and the severity of sexual abuse [20].
- Risk of DVA increases with common mental disorders e.g. depression (lifetime OR 2.7), and PTSD (lifetime OR 7.3) [21].

Gynaecology history
- **Reduced reproductive control:** Increased rate of sexually transmitted infections and symptoms. Increased rates of termination of pregnancy (TOP), repeat and concealed TOP [22].
- **Shame, fear and re-traumatizing:** Less likely to participate in cervical screening [23].
- More likely to experience increased pain, fear and embarrassment with intimate examination [24**].**

Obstetric history
- **Chronic effect on maternal-fetal health** – associations with small-for-gestational age, intrauterine growth restriction, stillbirth and premature labour.
- **Traumatic effect on maternal-fetal health-** association between violent abdominal trauma and abruption [17,25].

Social History
- Relationship breakdown is time of high risk [26].
- Smoking, alcohol, and substance abuse high [27].
- Successive Confidential Enquiries into Maternal Death document the patterns of late booking, frequent non attendance and chaotic social situations among the lives of women who died of all causes with DVA in their history [28].

Figure 8.1 The clinical history of a DVA survivor: Mapping onto a doctor's clerking

Table 8.2 Front-line response: Asking the question

Ask the question:
Open questions and /questions that link with clinical presentation (see Figure 8.1)

The HARK questions are an evidence-based tool designed to identify DVA in clinical context[29] See also Figure 8.2:
Have you been humiliated, or emotionally abused by your partner/ex?
Are you afraid of your partner/ex?
Have you been forced to have sexual contact, have you been raped?
Have you been kicked, punched or physically threatened?

Power and control:
Power and control are central to a woman's experience of DVA – consider specific questions.
Be aware that survivors may decline help or even react negatively.
A sensitive enquiry is still valuable.

Table 8.3 Front-line response: Initial response to a disclosure

Vocalize reassurance and acknowledgement:
'no-one has the right to harm you'. Assume there is more she is not telling you but don't push for information that is not necessary.

Adapt examination and environment as needed [13,35].

Avoid breaches of confidentiality: open waiting rooms, computer 'reminders' and entries in patient-held maternity notes. Keep DVA history strictly separate from material that the partner, family or public may see.

Safe and confidential written documentation is vital to validate, record and provide legal evidence for victims. It may be needed for criminal or civil actions years later. Do not avoid documentation altogether [38].

Formal risk assessment requires training, but all frontline doctors must be alert to high-risk presentations. Knowledge of formal risk assessment tools such as CAADA-DASH and Department of Health advice can inform clinical practice [39,40].

Except where you suspect significant and imminent harm, your patient is the best judge of her safety.

Power and control:
A safe disclosure and secure documentation can empower a survivor to take the next steps on her own terms.

Table 8.4 Front-line response: Next Steps

All doctors can perform a limited advocacy role. For example, believe your patient, share decisions, find and provide a 24hr helpline number: UK **0808 2000 247** [43].

Independent domestic violence advocates (IDVAs) are specially trained patient advocates who stand by survivors and navigate routes to safety and self-efficacy.
IDVA referral improves mother and child well-being and helps reduce violence [4].

Involving IDVAs is a way that doctors can facilitate their patient's safety and well-being whilst acknowledging the limits of their role. This is especially true when there are concerns about child safeguarding:
'What you tell me is confidential unless I think there is a serious risk to you or your children. But I want to help, and have found services who can support you'.

Power and control:
Child safeguarding is the clinician's priority, but there may be conflicting responsibilities that disempower patients.
Work alongside your patient; discuss decisions wherever possible [42].

that require otherwise intrusive questioning (e.g. harmful alcohol use, suicidality, rectal bleeding). DVA should be considered in a similar light.

A rebuttal may be that doctors are not the best professionals to deal with DVA, suggesting it is up to social workers, the police or violence/safeguarding specialists instead [14]. DVA certainly demands a multidisciplinary response, but there is evidence that survivors present more often, and more quickly, to health professionals [3]. As such, it is worth reiterating that these will be junior, unsupported doctors in frontline roles such as emergency departments and

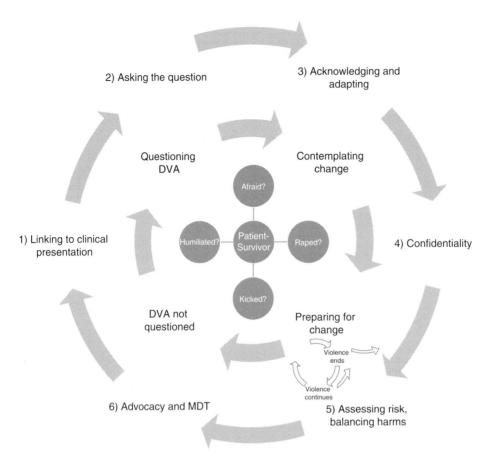

Figure 8.2 A patient's journey through DVA; a front-line doctor's response.
Adapted from [20,29]

general practices. Pregnancy in particular is a heightened time for DVA onset and escalation, but also a rare period of close contact with survivors [24]. These clinical encounters are a 'window of opportunity' for women to seek help on their own terms, which is more difficult once criminal justice, social services or education systems are involved [25]. This aspect changes the imperative to act:

> To ignore the offered 'calling card' is to collude with the continuing concealment of domestic violence behind closed doors [26].

The harm caused by DVA cannot be measured and explained in terms of an epidemic. Instead, the active vector is human behaviour, fraught with injustice and inequality [27]. Doctors, perhaps especially in Obstetrics & Gynaecology, are actors in these issues of social justice, and responding to DVA should be a priority [28].

'I Don't Have Enough Time'

This is the most prominent barrier in the literature, and taps into ever-present, complex concerns for medical professionals [16,30,31].

> We're overwhelmed ... [by] physical ... and mental problems ... and now social problems ... its probably easier not to ask [about DVA] ... to open that can of worms [32].

Suggesting you create more time or give more resources might seem a reasonable solution. Yet it is not actually quantities of *time* that women want [33] and delays and wrong turns can occur if the issue is not addressed. 'Time' may not really be the barrier at hand. 'Not enough time' is perhaps better understood under a theme of 'external barriers' (see Table 8.1) where doctors seem to reject the job of engaging with DVA. This is in contrast to 'internal barriers' which reflect feelings, attitudes and behaviours [16,30,31].

Furthermore, when external barriers are expressed, doctors often simultaneously use powerful imagery: 'opening a Pandora's Box' [21] or the 'can of worms' [15,32] This hints at hidden aspects of their reluctance to engage:

> Focusing on lack of time may mask other barriers that are more challenging for practitioners to address, such as feelings of frustration, a sense of futility or helplessness about how best to respond. [16]

'Will It Change Management?'

Doctors are usually action-oriented and motivated by observing demonstrable change. This may act as a barrier to addressing DVA in contrasting ways:

'Will I Cause Harm?'

The fear of confronting taboos has been addressed previously, but there is also a fear of causing psychological harm. Professionals fear re-traumatizing the patient through enquiry or examination [14,31], and pain and distress during intimate examination certainly have been found to be higher in survivors of sexual violence [34]. However, this barrier may be short-sighted. If examination proceeds without the doctor acknowledging violence, it seems likely that for some women distress would be greatly compounded. Minor adaptations can be easily overlooked, e.g. offering a choice of position, or allowing women to guide the speculum during examination, but these can greatly increase a patient's sense of control over a frightening situation [13,35] and might enhance all consultations where women do not disclose previous bad experiences.

There are also concerns of causing a dramatic negative outcome such as increased violence resulting from disclosure, and disengagement with care for fear of safeguarding intervention [16]. These barriers are paramount to women and are addressed next.

'Will It Change Outcomes?'

Some doctors report that their attempted intervention failed. This is often accompanied by a sense of futility or even resentment towards their patient:

> I have been repeatedly frustrated by women who, after I have taken the trouble to provide alternatives for them, have 'backed down' and returned to their abusive partners [16].

It appears the desired outcome here was dramatic and public – the cessation of an abusive relationship and change of life this would trigger. These expectations may stem from an inaccurate characterization of DVA.

Doctors tend to focus on 'physical and visible' harms and feel competent identifying cases on this basis [31].This leads to vast under-detection of DVA [6], but also contributes to an overly 'physical and visible' definition of an intervention. If the problem is always imagined as an acute, violent, physical crisis, then the corresponding intervention may naturally aim to match this urgency and visibility.

What Is the Evidence?

Mechanisms for Harm

There *is* a potential risk of harm when doctors enquire about DVA. Women are most at risk of being murdered in the aftermath of leaving a violent relationship, and violence often escalates if the perpetrator discovers a disclosure [36]. Therefore pressurizing a woman to leave, or making an unsafe breach of confidentiality, are mechanisms by which doctors can cause harm, and there are case studies which demonstrate this [37].

Likewise, child protection interventions, intended to avoid catastrophic harms, are also capable of causing suffering to parent and child. More than three quarters of women endure the erosion of their own personal safety and agency for long periods, and make a change specifically and solely to protect their children [36]. However, many women feel portrayed as 'part of the problem' for failing to leave an abusive partner immediately, and fear their children will be 'taken away' [41]. Although little researched, there are potential mechanisms by which doctors could compound these fears.

A doctor may feel that because social services involvement is protocol-driven (and in some situations mandated), triggering this is a straightforward way to pass responsibility. At this point, the doctor might disengage from the reality of DVA ('not my job'), which may be perceived by the woman as shaming or uncompassionate. Furthermore, under time pressure and lacking experience, they may not even explain that a referral has taken place. This undermines basic principles of shared decision-making – even when safeguarding concerns might override consent – and for the patient it profoundly compromises trust in healthcare professionals [42].

In such a fraught situation there are multiple competing interests, one of which is the vital responsibility to safeguard children. Even in overview, it is clear that a front-line clinician cannot represent all parties. Referral to specialists such as an independent domestic violence advocate is essential (see Table 8.4).

Benefits and Outcomes

Having focussed on crisis points, the risks need to be put back in context. The experience of DVA (and the process of change to escape it) is not usually a linear or explosive event. It is best described as a cycle, with multiple steps and changes of direction [20,44]. Doctors meet survivors for a few short moments on this journey, and the interactions will not always coincide with crisis, visible injury or turning points for change. This is illustrated in Figure 8.2.

Taking this more balanced view, at meta-analysis level, no study chose 'leaving the partner' as an endpoint and there is no evidence that clinician enquiry about DVA causes harm. There is limited evidence of any benefit either, and it may be that the endpoints of 'intervention' need more careful definition. For example, 'case identification' may be too conservative an endpoint and only a proxy for any action. Making a compassionate and humane enquiry of itself is likely to have an impact because it opens a 'broader discussion opportunity' with the patient and resets social norms over time [45].

Acknowledging this changes the locus of the intervention, situating the important moral and clinical work in the initial conversations. It demands attention, due to the serious potential harm to avoid, but it may also have a positive effect on barriers: you can avoid doing harm and you can make a difference by listening, acknowledging and providing a safe environment. **This alternative intervention for frontline clinicians is outlined in** Figure 8.2.

'How Will I Change My practice?'

Despite addressing many barriers and outlining a different intervention, unless health professionals are conscious of this shift, they may continue to feel they have failed:

> Help-seeking and self-empowerment behaviours may be subtle and are sometimes not recognized by health providers who want to see major changes [44].

Health professionals engage daily with enquiries and management plans which may fail, e.g. smoking cessation or diabetes management, yet would rarely characterize the encounters as failures that didn't deserve raising in a medical consultation. Nor would 'poor outcomes' be suggested as a reason to avoid

enquiry altogether. Yet, with DVA, this appears to be a major barrier [46].

Looking into the 'Pandora's box' may help explain the difference. With DVA, it is not just the condition or situation that is characterized as difficult or 'bad', but the patient herself. Survivors of DVA have been characterized as 'non-compliant', misusers of services and liars [14,21]. Survivor testimony records incidents such as this:

> The GP wrote 'raped' in inverted commas in my notes … When my case went to court, it got thrown out on the basis that the GP didn't believe me [47].

Women are also sometimes blamed for the situation [31], for example male doctors theorizing that abuse was a result of women withholding sex in relationships [48]. It is likely that negative attitudes will have a negative downstream effect on clinician behaviours [6]:

> Domestic violence is a big morass which we will never escape. I get a headache thinking about it. And that attitude translates into the type of care we give those patients [21].

There are many other ways in which confronting DVA is difficult or challenging. Many clinicians themselves will have experienced, witnessed or even perpetrated violence. Bringing the issue 'close to home' raises difficult emotions, especially for women clinicians who tend to identify with and be affected by the patient's experience [21,48]. However, a sense of personal connection to the problem, unlike negative emotions of frustration or blame, has also been seen to act as a facilitator for engagement in certain circumstances [15].

Doctors often cite lack of training as a barrier for avoiding enquiry and non-intervention [15,16], but we argue that to change practice, the 'negative patient' characterization and its potential rationalization of 'problematic' medical behaviour also need to be addressed: 'There is no such thing as a difficult patient, just a patient with difficult problems'.

Reframing DVA

Similarities between Patient and Provider

Exploring doctors' barriers has illuminated a link between negative clinician attitudes and potentially avoidant behaviours. Similarities between patient and provider voices may help to overcome this, for example acknowledging that there is a shared dissatisfaction with the 'fix and solve approach'[14] of the biomedical model [15,21,31].

There is also a shared experience of 'powerlessness', although experienced very differently and for different reasons. A web of 'power and control' is exerted by perpetrators over every part of survivors' lives, best illustrated by the Duluth Wheel which in turn has informed simple clinical tools for enquiry such as the HARK questions, shown in Table 8.2 [29, 49].

Doctors' responses similarly mention a sense of powerlessness [26]:

> Many physicians were frustrated by their inability to control the patient's behaviour, and the patient's inability to control the circumstances of their lives. This . . . was one of the major obstacles to physicians' willingness to address domestic violence[21].

Powerlessness in Clinical Encounters

These challenges can collide during a clinical encounter but can also offer a solution. A common example is a DVA survivor who appears to reject help or refuses to leave her partner:

> A senior emergency department doctor was distressed when a patient reacted to a DVA enquiry by . . . storming out and complaining loudly to her partner and the entire waiting room 'How dare anyone think [I am a victim of violence]', and threatening legal action[50].

Here the doctor's distress could easily turn into a 'bad' patient characterization. However, by bringing powerlessness to the surface, it can remind the clinician to ask *why* the patient may have reacted in this way. DVA victims are often under constant surveillance and restriction by their oppressors and changing the situation is a high-stakes decision:

> She [the doctor] realized her patient had acted to protect herself . . . She had made the abuse public, and her partner now knew that people were aware of it. She had also demonstrated her complete loyalty to him[50].

In this example, focussing on the two experiences of powerlessness helps explain and potentially overcome a negative reaction.

Likewise, a social services referral can be profoundly disempowering for a woman, especially if the referral and its implications are not explained, (as would routinely be done for the dangers of emergency surgery). The alternative approach is more

a shift of viewpoint than a great change in clinical practice. Open and inclusive communication can address power imbalances and allow doctor and patient to work together. One survivor describes:

> When I told my [children's social work] nurse she **listened to me** carefully and **believed me.** She **told me what she was going to do** and **let me hear** her on the phone talking to the police [47].

It may not take much more time than cannulation or writing a drug chart and can transform the healthcare professional from opponent to advocate.

Conclusion

A Front-Line Doctor's Response

Doctors are duty bound to help their patients, and a fair starting point assumes that they earnestly strive to achieve this [51]. When the type of problem a patient presents is not easily amenable to help, doctors may feel that their identity is challenged [52]:

> The difficult patient is one that makes me feel ineffective[53].

This is hard to acknowledge and has rarely been linked to the characterization of DVA survivors by health professionals. However, facing up to this may actually help to transform interactions [16, 54].

Figure 8.2 sets out a model for front-line doctors' engagement in DVA which has elsewhere been called a 'first-responder' role[20]. It is patient-centred but also holds clinical attention on the dynamics of power and control, as illustrated by the HARK clinical questions.

It demonstrates the cycle of change a woman goes through, sometimes over years, whereas a doctor's role is peripheral and must adapt to the stage of the cycle. The clinical signposts and clerking map within the text come together to form this front-line intervention: identification, initial response and referral for next steps.

Perhaps the most empowering aspect of this approach, for a clinician, is that it puts emphasis on the everyday skills of communication and the central professional tenets of confidentiality and shared decision-making. This intervention is short, allows the doctor to avoid doing harm and aims to overcome negative patient characterization. In so doing it aims to address the main barriers to enquiry outlined previously. Even if the brief encounter stays at the level of an unanswered empathic enquiry about violence, it can 'lessen feelings of shame and apprehension' [44], 'interrupt and prevent recurrence of violence' [28,31], and improve clinician confidence and competence [46].

Next Steps

Doctors do not routinely discuss power dynamics and hierarchies, yet these are certainly key issues for DVA work and more broadly [4]. The effect of poor staff morale and bullying on patient outcomes is a political headline [55]. Proportionally more staff in Obstetrics & Gynaecology experience bullying than in any other specialty, and responses appear problematic and 'victim-blaming' [56]. A specialty that advocates for women patients must enable its doctors to look into the 'Pandora's box' and engage with power-and-control dynamics, both for their patients and the profession.

Other unintended benefits from this approach may be that it sheds light on urgent topical issues of bullying, whistle-blowing, obstetric violence and other issues of social justice within medicine [57]. Furthermore, a relatively 'universal' approach may have applications for other topics where patients themselves are characterized in problematic ways: mental health and addiction for example.

Often these topics are kept within the remit of academic discussion, but much could be gained from helping doctors see 'power-and-control' dynamics in their everyday work: in emergency departments, during night shifts and busy clinics, and be equipped with the front-line skills to respond.

Key Points

- Domestic violence and abuse (DVA) can encompass, but are not limited to, the following types of abuse: psychological, physical, sexual, financial, emotional.
- A history of DVA is an important social determinant of health but doctors at all levels lack training in DVA.
- Barriers and facilitators associated with DVA enquiry and disclosure should be explored in DVA training – both groups experience powerlessness.
- Patients experiencing DVA are subject to a web of 'power and control' exerted by perpetrators. Considering presentation in light of these factors may facilitate the clinical encounter.

- Women find enquiry about DVA acceptable, even welcome. Patients test whether it's safe (psychologically and practically) to reveal DVA, but are unlikely to disclose unless actually asked directly.
- Doctors often feel powerless to help women with a history of DVA, maybe particularly if they expect to see dramatic change, thus leading to negative characterization of their patients.
- The experience of DVA (and the process of change to escape it) is cyclical rather than a one-off event. Doctors should consider their supportive enquiry and communication as interventions in their own right, even if not leading to cessation of violence.
- Open and inclusive communication, especially around safeguarding and support, can address power imbalances and allow doctor and patient to work together.
- The HARK questions are an evidence-based tool designed to identify DVA in a clinical context.

References

1. Office of National Statistics. Intimate Personal Violence and Partner Abuse. chapter 4 in Crime Survey for England and Wales (CSEW). 2014. www.ons.gov.uk/ons/dcp171776_352362.pdf. (Accessed 11 March 2017).

2. Home Office. Guidance: Domestic Violence and Abuse. 2013. https://www.gov.uk/guidance/domestic-violence-and-abuse (Accessed 11 March 2017).

3. Feder GS, Hutson M, Ramsay J, Taket AR. Women exposed to intimate partner violence: expectations and experiences when they encounter health care professionals: A meta-analysis of qualitative studies. *Arch Intern Med* 2006;**166**:22–37.

4. NICE. PH50: Domestic violence and abuse: How health services, social care and the organisations they work with can respond effectively. 2014. www.nice.org.uk/guidance/ph50 (Accessed 17 March 2017).

5. Smith K, Osborne S, Lau I, Britton A. *Homicides, firearm offences and intimate violence 2010/11: Supplementary volume 2 to Crime in England and Wales 2010/11.* London. Home Office. 2012.

6. Roelens K, Verstraelen H, Van Egmond K, Temmerman M. A knowledge, attitudes, and practice survey among obstetrician-gynaecologists on intimate

partner violence in Flanders, Belgium. *BMC Public Health* 2006;**6**:238.

7. RCOG. Future Workforce in Obstetrics and Gynaecology – England and Wales. Overview and Summary. 2009. www.rcog.org.uk/globalassets/documents/guidelines/rcogfutureworkforcesummary.pdf (Accessed 11 March 2017).

8. O'Campo P, Kirst M, Tsamis C, Chambers C, Ahmad F. Implementing successful intimate partner violence screening programs in health care settings: Evidence generated from a realist-informed systematic review. *Soc Sci Med* 2011;**72**(6):855–66.

9. World Health Organization. Global plan of action to strengthen role of health systems in addressing interpersonal violence, in particular against women and girls, and against children 2014. www.who.int/reproductivehealth/topics/violence/en. (Accessed 11 March 2017).

10. Woman's Aid. Press Release: Doctors increasingly relied on to support survivors of domestic violence. 2013.

11. Avalos L. This FGM trial should never have happened. In Opinion, Guardian Online. 2015. www.theguardian.com/commentisfree/2015/feb/05/fgm-is-better-tackled-by-grassroots-work-than-prosecution. (Accessed 11 March 2017).

12. Halsted S. Junior doctors stand up against domestic violence in BMJ Policy Debate Blog. 2014. https://communities.bma.org.uk/policy_debate/b/weblog/archive/2014/12/24/junior-doctors-stand-up-against-domestic-violence (Accessed 11 March 2017).

13. MyBodyBackProject. *About- My body back*. 2015. www.mybodybackproject.com/services-for-women/mbb-clinics/. (Accessed 11 March 2017).

14. Rose D, Trevillion K, Woodall A, Morgan C, Feder G, Howard L. Barriers and facilitators of disclosures of domestic violence by mental health service users: Qualitative study. *Br J Psychiatry* 2011;**198**:189–94.

15. Gutmanis I, Beynon C, Tutty L, Nadine Wathen C, Macillan HL. Factors influencing identification of and response to intimate partner violence: A survey of physicians and nurses *BMC Public Health* 2007;**7**:12.

16. Beynon C, Gutmanis I, Tutty L, Nadine Wathen C, Macillan HL. Why physicians and nurses ask (or don't) about partner violence: A qualitative analysis. *BMC Public Health* 2012;**12**:473.

17. Stöckl H, Hertlein L, Himsl I et al. Acceptance of routine or case-based inquiry for intimate partner violence: a mixed method study *BMC Pregnancy and Childbirth* 2013;**13**:77.

18. Drossman DA, Leserman J, Nachman G et al. Sexual and physical abuse in women with functional or organic gastrointestinal disorders. *Ann Int Med* 1990;**113**(11):828–33.

19. Latthe P, Mignini L, Gray R, Hills R, Khan K. Factors predisposing women to chronic pelvic pain: Systematic review. *BMJ* 2006;**332**:749.

20. García-Moreno C, Hegarty K, Lucas d'Oliveira AF, Koziol-McLain J, Colombini M, Feder G. The health-systems response to violence against women. Lancet violence against women and girls series. *Lancet* 2014;**385**(9977):1567–79.

21. Sugg NK, Inui T. Primary care physicians' response to domestic violence. opening pandora's box. *JAMA* 1992;**267**(23):3157–60.

22. Eide H, Frankel R, Haaversen AC, Vaupel KA, Graugaard PK, Finset A. Listening for feelings: Identifying and coding empathic and potential empathic opportunities in medical dialogues. *Patient Educ Couns* 2004;**54**:291–7.

23. Ramsden C, Bonner M. A realistic view of domestic violence screening in an emergency department. *Accid Emerg Nursing* 2002;**10**:31–39.

24. Bowen E, Heron J, Waylen A, Wolke D. ALSPAC Study Team. Domestic violence risk during and after pregnancy: Findings from a British longitudinal study. *BJOG* 2005;**112**:1083–9.

25. Devries KM, Kishor S, Johnson H. Intimate partner violence during pregnancy: Analysis of prevalence data from 19 countries. *Reprod Health Matters* 2010;**18**: 158–70.

26. Heath, I. Domestic violence: the general practitioner's role. In Policy Areas, Royal College of General Practitioners. 1998. www.rcgp.org.uk/clinical-and-research/a-to-z-clinical-resources/domestic-violence.aspx (Accessed 11 March 2017).

27. Carter J. Patriarchy and violence against women and girls. *Lancet* 2015;**385**(9978):e40–41.

28. Van Parys A, Verhamme A, Temmerman M, Verstraelen H. Intimate partner violence and pregnancy: A systematic review of interventions. *PLoS ONE* 2014; **9**(1):e85084.

29. Sohal H, Eldridge S, Geder G. The sensitivity and specificity of four questions (HARK) to identify intimate partner violence: A diagnostic accuracy study in general practice. *BMC Fam Pract* 2007;**8**:49.

30. Roelens K. Intimate partner violence: The gynaecologist's perspective. *Verh K Acad Geneeskd Belg* 2010;**72**(1–2):17–40.

31. Virrkl T, Husso M, Notko M, Holma J, Laitila A, Mantysaari M. Possibilities for intervention in domestic violence: Frame analysis of health care professionals' attitude. *Journal of Social Service Research* 2015; **41**(1):6–24.

32. Mildorf, J. *Setting the scene in Storying Domestic Violence: Constructions and Stereotypes of Abuse in the Discourse of General Practitioners.* Lincoln: University of Nebraska Press. 2007; 91.

33. Peckover S. Supporting and policing mothers: An analysis of the disciplinary practices of health visiting. *J Adv Nurs* 2002;**38**(4):369–77.

34. Weitlauf JC, Finney JW, Ruzek JI et al. Distress and pain during pelvic examinations: Effect of sexual violence. *Obstet Gynecol* 2008;**112**(6):1343–50.

35. Bewley S. A doctor who changed my practice: Putting women in control. *Br Med J.* 2000;**321**:1454.

36. Humphreys C, Thiara R. *Routes to Safety: Protection Issues Facing Abused Women and Children and the Role of Outreach Services.* Bristol: Woman's Aid Publications. 2002.

37. Bacchus LJ, Bewley S, Vitolas CT, Aston G, Jordan P, Murray SF. Evaluation of a domestic violence intervention in the maternity and sexual health services of a UK hospital. *Reproductive Health Matters* 2010;**18**(36):147–57.

38. Rhodes KV, Frankel RM, Levinthal N, Prenoveau E, Bailey J, Levinson W. 'You're not a victim of domestic violence, are you?' Provider– Patient Communication about Domestic Violence. *Ann Intern Med.* 2007;**17**(9): 620–7.

39. Safelives. CAADA-DASH checklist with quick start guide. In: Resources for identifying the risk victims face. www.safelives.org.uk/practice-support/resour ces-identifying-risk-victims-face (Accessed 11 March 2017).

40. Department of Health (2013) Health Visiting and School Nursing Programmes: supporting implementation of the new service model No.5: Domestic Violence and Abuse – Professional Guidance.www.gov.uk/government/uploads/system/u ploads/attachment_data/file/211018/9576-TSO-Health_Visiting_Domestic_Violence_A3_Posters_ WEB.pdf (Accessed 11 March 2017).

41. London Child Protection Services. Chapter 27. Safeguarding children affected by domestic abuse and violence. London Safeguarding Children Board. 5th edition. www.londoncp.co.uk/chapters/sg_ ch_dom_abuse.html#barriers (Accessed 11 March 2017).

42. Shakespeare J. Domestic Violence in families with children. Guidance for primary health care professionals in Policy Areas. Royal College of General Practitioners. 2002.www.rcgp.org.uk/policy/rcgp-policy-areas/domestic-violence.aspx (Accessed 29 August 2015).

43. National Domestic Violence Helpline. 24 hr telephone number. 11 March 2017).

44. Chang JC, Dado D, Hawker L et al. Understanding turning points in intimate partner violence: Factors and circumstances leading women victims toward change. *J Womens Health (Larchmt)* 2010; **19**(2): 251–59.

45. Taft A, O'Doherty L, Hegarty K, Ramsay J, Davidson L, Feder G. Screening women for intimate partner violence in healthcare settings. *Cochrane Database Syst Rev* 2013;**30**(4):CD007007.

46. Gerbert B, Gansky SA, Tang JW et al. Domestic violence compared to other health risks: A survey of physicians' beliefs and behaviors. *Am J Prev Med* 2002;**23**(2):82–90.

47. Taskforce on the Health Aspects of Violence against Women and Children. Responding to violence against women and children – the role of the NHS. 2010. htt p://www.health.org.uk/sites/health/files/Respondingto ViolenceAgainstWomenAndChildrenTheRoleofTheN HS_guide.pdf (Accessed 11 March 2017).

48. Lo Fo Wong SH, De Jonge A, Wester F, Mol SS, Römkens RR, Lagro-Janssen T. Discussing partner abuse: Does doctor's gender really matter?. *Fam Pract* 2006;**23**:578–86.

49. Domestic Violence Intervention Project. Power and Control Wheel http://www.theduluthmodel.org/train ing/wheels.html (Accessed 11 March 2017).

50. Stephens, L. Box 12.8 Chapter 12: Emergency Medicine and Surgical Specialties in: Bewley S, Welch J (eds). *ABC of Domestic and Sexual Violence.* Oxford: Wiley, 2015; 56.

51. GMC. Duties of A Doctor in Good Medical Practice. 2013. www.gmc-uk.org/guidance/good_medical_prac tice/duties_of_a_doctor.asp (Accessed11 March 2017).

52. Lorenzetti R, Jacques M, Donovan C, Cottrell S, Buck J. Managing difficult encounters: Understanding physician, patient, and situational factors. *Am Fam Physician* 2013;**87**(6):419–25.

53. Schwartz D. Uncooperative patients. *Am J Nurs* 1958 Jan;**58**(1):75–7.

54. Hill T. How clinicians make (or avoid) moral judgments of patients: Implications of the evidence for relationships and research. *Philosophy, Ethics, and Humanities in Medicine* 2010;**5**:11.

55. Francis R. Independent Inquiry into care provided by Mid Staffordshire NHS Foundation Trust. Jan 2005–2009;2010. www.gov.uk/government/publi cations/independent-inquiry-into-care-provided-by-mid-staffordshire-nhs-foundation-trust-january-2001 -to-march-2009. (Accessed 11 March 2017).

56. RCOG. Improving resilience in Workplace and Workforce Issues. 2015. www.rcog.org.uk/en/careers-training/workplace-workforce-issues/improving-workplace-behaviours-dealing-with-undermining/un

dermining-toolkit/unit-trust-and-local-education-provider-interventions/improving-resilience/ (Accessed 11 March 2017).

57. Bohren MA, Vogel JP, Hunter EC et al. The mistreatment of women during childbirth in health facilities globally: A mixed-methods systematic review. *PLoS Med* 2015;**12**(6): e1001847.

Further Reading

58. Campbell JC. Health consequences of intimate partner violence. *The Lancet* 2002;**359**:1331–6.

59. Lukasse M, Henriksen L, Vangen S, Schei B. Sexual violence and pregnancy-related physical symptoms. *BMC Pregnancy and Childbirth* 2012;**12**:83.

60. Trevillion K, Oram S, Feder G, Howard LM. Experiences of domestic violence and mental disorders: A systematic review and meta-analysis. *PLoS ONE* 2012;**7**(12):e51740.

61. Hall M, Chappell L, Parnell B, Seed P, Bewley S. Associations between intimate partner violence and

termination of pregnancy: A systematic review and meta-analysis. *PLOS Medicine* 2014;**11**(1): e1001581.

62. Cadman L, Waller J, Ashdown-Barr L, Szarewski A. Barriers to cervical screening in women who have experienced sexual abuse: An exploratory study. *J Fam Plann Reprod Health Care* 2012;**38**:214–20.

63. Campbell JC, Webster D, Koziol-McLain J et al. Risk factors for femicide in abusive relationships: Results from a multisite case control study. *Am J Public Health* 2003;**93**(7):1089–1097.

64. Humphreys C, Regan L, River D, Thiara RK. Domestic violence and substance Use: Tackling complexity. *Br J Soc Work* 2005;**35**:1303–20.

65. Lewis G. Chapter 12.1 Domestic abuse in Saving Mothers' Lives Reviewing maternal deaths to make motherhood safer: 2006–2008. The Eighth Report of the Confidential Enquiries into Maternal Deaths in the United Kingdom. 2011. http://onlinelibrary.wiley.com /doi/10.1111/j.1471–0528.2010.02847.x/epdf (Accessed19 September 2015).

Female Genital Cutting

Leroy C. Edozien

Introduction

Female genital cutting (FGC), also called female genital mutilation (FGM), is defined by the World Health Organization as 'all procedures involving partial or total removal of the external female genitalia or other injuries to the female genital organs for non-medical reasons' [1]. It is performed routinely in many communities, particularly Africa, the Middle East and Asia. It was estimated in 2016 that 200 million women had undergone the procedures in Africa, Asia and elsewhere. One of the Sustainable Development Goals (SDGs) set by the global community under the auspices of the United Nations Organisation is the elimination of FGC by the year 2030. The UN reported in 2016 that while there has been a reduction in the prevalence of FGC, the rate of progress is insufficient to keep up with population growth, and that if trends continue the number girls and women undergoing FGC will continue to rise in the next 15 years [2].

Clitoridectomy was used in nineteenth-century Britain to suppress female masturbation, but FGC is alien to contemporary western norms and values and is referred to as mutilation. The affected women do not wish to be described as having mutilated bodies, and they sometimes feel that they have been treated with disrespect by health professionals [3], or that their 'mutilation' has taken precedence over the health problem that they presented with [4]. The term 'female genital mutilation' is pejorative, and the more neutral term 'female genital cutting' is preferable in culturally sensitive discourse [4].

Health Professionals' Knowledge about FGC

With global trends in immigration and multiculturalism, doctors, nurses and midwives in the western world are increasingly likely to encounter in their clinical practice girls or women who have had, or are at risk of having, FGC. There is evidence, however, that health professionals worldwide do not know enough about FGC [5, 6]. Studies on healthcare providers' awareness, knowledge and attitudes regarding FGC have shown a lack of awareness of the prevalence, diagnosis and management of FGC, but there are no robust studies showing whether the training to improve the knowledge and attitude of healthcare providers has an impact on the quality of the care offered [6].

Girls born to immigrants from communities that practise FGC are at risk, and health professionals in both community and hospital practice should have both the knowledge and the cultural competence to offer appropriate and sensitive care to the women [4–6]. Health professionals should know what action to take when they encounter a child or woman who has had or is at risk of FGC. They should also know the law in their country pertaining to FGC. The Royal College of Obstetricians and Gynaecologists recommends that all gynaecologists, obstetricians and midwives should receive mandatory training on FGC [7]. Each health board should have a designated obstetrician and/or gynaecologist responsible for FGC care. These lead clinicians should be aware of local and/or regional specialist multidisciplinary FGC services and should be competent in all aspects of FGC (including child safeguarding protocols).

Reasons for FGC

There are no health benefits to FGC and the reasons for doing it are sociocultural. A fundamental reason is the belief in patriarchal societies that FGC would preserve the chastity of the woman, preserve her virginity and prevent extramarital sexual activity [8].

FGC is often deemed to be a rite of passage and in some communities an uncircumcised vulva is seen as dirty [9]. The practice is often perpetuated by women who believe that their daughters or granddaughters will not find a husband or will not bear a male child if there is no genital cutting. Girls may submit to the ritual in order to belong to the community and for fear of social isolation if they are different from their peers.

Types of FGC

The WHO [10] classifies FGC as follows:

Type 1: Clitoridectomy – removal of the clitoral hood and/or removal of all or part of the clitoris.

Type 2: Excision – partial or total removal of the clitoris and labia minora, with or without removal of the labia majora.

Type 3: Infibulation – narrowing of the introitus by creating a seal, formed by cutting and repositioning the labia. On examination, the vulva is flat, without labia and with only a small opening allowing egress of urine and menstrual flow.

Type 4   Other (piercing, scraping, pricking, labial elongation and cauterizing).

The operation is usually performed by non-medical persons, using knives, scissors, scalpels, broken glass or razor blades, and without anaesthesia or sepsis precautions. In some countries it is performed by doctors.

Complications of FGC

The complications vary with the type of FGC and the environment (sepsis, equipment, medical/non-medical operator) in which it was performed. They include haemorrhage (with potentially massive bleeding from laceration of the internal pudendal artery or the clitoral artery), infection, vulval cysts, keloids, chronic pelvic or vulval pain, menstrual and urinary flow problems, subfertility and problems during labour and childbirth. A study of 28,393 women at 28 obstetric centres in six countries found that women with type 3 FGC have on average 30% more caesarean sections and 70% increase in incidence of postpartum haemorrhage compared with those who have not had any FGC [10]. A meta-analysis of obstetric consequences showed that women who have undergone FGC were over three times more likely to have a difficult labour and twice as likely to suffer obstetric haemorrhage [11]. FGC is associated with an increased need for neonatal resuscitation and increased risk of perinatal mortality.

Psychological and psychosexual complications include loss of libido, lack of pleasurable sensation, dyspareunia, flashbacks, loss of self-esteem and risk of self-harm [12]. Women who have undergone FGC have a significantly lower Sexual Quality of Life-Female score than control women [13].

The Law

FGC is illegal in various countries of the world [14, 15] but enforcement of the laws has been difficult and not been prioritized. In the United States federal law (18 US Code § 116) makes it illegal to perform FGC in the United States or knowingly transport a girl out of the United States for purpose of inflicting FGC. Also, at least 23 states in the United States have laws against FGC, with sentencing provisions ranging from 5 to 30 years. In Germany, the 47th Criminal Law Amendment Act introduced new provisions in 2013 making FGC a separate criminal offence in section 226a of the German Criminal Code. All states and territories in Australia have laws that ban FGC. In England, Wales and Northern Ireland FGC is illegal under the Female Genital Mutilation Act 2003. In Scotland and in the Republic of Ireland it is illegal under the Prohibition of Female Genital Mutilation (Scotland) Act 2005 and the Criminal Justice (Female Genital Mutilation) Act 2012 respectively. Under US, Irish and UK laws, a person is guilty of an offence if they excise, infibulate or otherwise mutilate the whole or any part of a girl's or woman's labia majora, labia minora or clitoris. Necessary operations performed by a registered medical practitioner on physical and mental health grounds and any operation performed by a registered medical practitioner or midwife on a woman who is in labour or has just given birth, for purposes connected with the labour or birth, do not count as infringement of the law on FGC. Operations performed as part of gender reassignment, for example, do not count as FGC as defined by the law.

Under these laws anyone who performs FGC could face up to 14 years in prison. In Germany, offenders can be sentenced to 15 years' imprisonment. In 2016 a former midwife, a mother of two girls and a community leader were each sentenced to a maximum of 15 months in prison after Australia's first criminal prosecution for FGC.

Despite existing legislation the practice of FGC continues, and this necessitated strengthening of the UK law and there are proposals to strengthen the legal framework in Australia [16]. In the United Kingdom, the Serious Crime Act 2015 extends the extraterritorial reach of FGC offences, provides anonymity to victims, creates a new offence of failing to protect a girl under 16 from the risk of FGC and makes provision for FGC Prevention Orders to protect victims and likely victims. It imposes a new duty on professionals to notify the police of acts of FGC. Anyone found guilty of failing to protect a girl from FGC can face up to seven years in prison.

Reporting Requirements and Referrals in the United Kingdom

In the United Kingdom a health professional who identifies FGC in a child under the age of 18 years has a legal duty to report this information to the police. For the purposes of this duty, the relevant age is the girl's age at the time of the disclosure/identification of FGC (i.e. it does not apply where a woman aged 18 or over discloses she had FGC when she was under 18).

There is no requirement to report a non-pregnant adult woman aged 18 or over to the police or social services unless a related child is at risk. It is not mandatory to report every pregnant woman identified as having had FGC to social services or the police unless the unborn child, or any related child, is considered to be at risk of FGC. Indicators that a girl is at risk include the following:

- Her family or community is known to practise FGC.
- There are indications that she is to be taken out of country for a prolonged period.
- She expresses concern about a planned overseas travel.
- Her mother or siblings have undergone FGC.

Risk assessment can be facilitated by use of an FGC safeguarding risk assessment tool [17].

Any suspicion that a child under the age of 18 years has undergone or is at risk of undergoing FGC should be referred to the Children's Social Care and multi-agency FGC safeguarding guidelines should be followed. The doctor or midwife making the referral should consult the local safeguarding specialist midwife if such a position exists within the unit.

The psychological health needs of any child under 18 years who has been subjected to FGC should be assessed, and she should be referred to the appropriate specialist services.

Recording Information

Healthcare professionals must amply record any identified or suspected FGC and related safeguarding concerns in the health records, and information should be shared with the GP and other professionals. When a patient with FGC is identified, this must be documented in the medical records regardless of whether FGC is the reason for presentation. An FGC Risk Indication System was introduced in the United Kingdom to help safeguard girls up to 18 years who are at risk of FGC. An indicator is added to a girl's electronic healthcare record, thus alerting other healthcare professionals.

A mandatory requirement to accurately record information about FGC was introduced in the United Kingdom in March 2014. In April 2015, an enhanced dataset was introduced, requiring health organizations to record FGC data and return patient-identifiable data to the Health and Social Care Information Centre (HSCIC, now NHS Digital). Data should be submitted every time the woman or girl has treatment related to her FGC and every time FGC is identified, not just the first time. Formal consent is not required but the woman should be advised that information about her FGC will be submitted to the FGC Enhanced Dataset. She should be informed that her personal data will be submitted without anonymization to NHS Digital, in order to prevent duplication of data, but reassured that all personal data are anonymized at the point of statistical analysis and publication.

Care of Women with FGC

Health professionals caring for women with FGC should ensure that their approach is sensitive and non-judgemental. Skilled communication (see Chapter 4) is essential. Discussions, examination and treatment could trigger flashbacks, and this should be anticipated. Counselling should be offered as appropriate to the partner/husband as well as to the woman.

The law on FGC should be explained. Where it is necessary to use an interpreter, efforts should be made to obtain a female interpreter and preferably one who does not support the practice of FGC. A family member should not be used as an interpreter.

Written information should be provided. The 'Statement Opposing Female Genital Mutilation' leaflet [18], also known as the FGC Health Passport, is a written declaration by the UK government which stresses that FGC is a serious criminal offence. It is designed for girls and their families to keep in their passport, purse or bag and show to families when there is a threat of FGC.

Antenatal Care

When booked for antenatal care, every woman should be asked directly if she has undergone FGC (e.g. 'Have you been cut ...') and their response should be documented. Women who disclose FGC should be referred to the lead clinician for FGC and a safeguarding risk assessment should be done. A birth plan should be documented. If the woman has type 3 FGC she should be offered deinfibulation (see discussion). Deinfibulation is performed between 20 and 32 weeks' gestation, early enough for the scar to heal before birth.

Intrapartum Care

Some women will require deinfibulation in labour – because either they have chosen to have it at this time or the FGC was identified for the first time in labour. Deinfibulation can be performed in the first stage of labour to facilitate catheterization and vaginal examinations.

An episiotomy will usually (but not invariably) be required. When repairing episiotomies and perineal tears the operator should take care to avoid reinfibulation. Declining a request from the woman or her husband to reinfibulate is relatively straightforward; avoiding a spontaneous reinfibulation (due to apposition of raw edges), which could leave the surgeon vulnerable to allegations of intentional reinfibulation, is more challenging. All findings, repair details and advice given to the woman should be fully documented.

Postnatal Care

The type of FGC and its current status, child protection concerns and advice given to the woman should be documented, and this information should be shared with the community midwife, health visitor and GP. It should be documented in the neonatal examination charts that the baby has normal genitalia (unless there are any recognized congenital anomalies). Where applicable an indicator should be added to a baby girl's electronic healthcare record, per the FGC Risk Indication System, with consent

from the parent and/or guardian. The mother's history of FGC should also be documented in the child's Red Book.

Gynaecological Interventions

Women presenting with dyspareunia and some with urinary problems will require deinfibulation (see discussion). Those with urethral strictures may benefit from cystoscopy and urethral dilation. Where there is doubt, the woman should be referred to a urologist or urogynaecologist. A multidisciplinary approach should be taken, so that the associated psychological and psychosexual issues are also addressed.

Deinfibulation

Deinfibulation (also known as defibulation) is the division of scar tissue formed by the apposition of cut labia. The scar tissue may be thin or thick and is divided by means of a longitudinal midline incision starting at the narrowed vaginal opening and proceeding upwards until the urethral meatus becomes visible. This operation is usually done under a local anaesthetic, but the woman may prefer a general or regional anaesthetic for psychological reasons. Postoperatively woman should be advised to keep the area dry and clean and to periodically part the labia so that they don't spontaneously fuse again. Suturing is not usually required if the divided scar tissue is thin.

Educational Resources for Health Professionals

The Royal College of Obstetricians and Gynaecologists [7], Royal College of Midwives [19], Royal College of Nursing [20], Society of Obstetricians and Gynaecologists of Canada [21], Royal Australia and New Zealand College of Obstetricians and Gynaecologists [22], American College of Obstetricians and Gynecologists [23] and the UK Department of Health [17, 24, 25] have produced guidelines and educational materials on FGC for health professionals.

Conclusion

In the United Kingdom and other countries there is a push for greater enforcement of existing and new laws against FGC. Health professionals have a major role to play in implementing the law while also offering culturally competent care. This role requires an understanding of the sociocultural issues, the legal framework and the safeguarding protocols that apply.

Key Points

- Female genital cutting is illegal in various countries. In the United Kingdom it is illegal not only to perform FGC but also to take a child outside the United Kingdom for FGC and to fail to protect a child from FGC.
- Health professionals in the United Kingdom have a legal duty to report to the police if a child reports that she has had or is found on examination to have had FGC.
- Doctors, nurses, midwives and other professionals should be aware of the legal and safeguarding frameworks pertaining to FGC that are applicable in their place of work.
- Complications of FGC include loss of libido, lack of pleasurable sensation, dyspareunia, flashbacks, loss of self-esteem and risk of self-harm. Long-term physical complications include urinary problems, vulval cysts, subfertility and difficulties in labour and childbirth.
- Deinfibulation, the division of scar tissue formed by the apposition of cut labia, may be required, to facilitate sexual intercourse, micturition or childbirth. Reinfibulation after childbirth is illegal.
- Health professionals caring for women with FGC should ensure that their approach is sensitive and non-judgemental.

References

1. World Health Organization. Eliminating Female Genital Mutilation: An Interagency Statement – UNAIDS, UNDP, UNECA, UNESCO, UNFPA, UNHCHR, UNHCR, UNICEF, UNIFEM, WHO. Geneva: WHO, 2008.

2. UNICEF Data: Monitoring the Situation of Children and Women. Female genital mutilation and cutting. https://data.unicef.org/topic/child-protection/female-genital-mutilation-and-cutting/. Accessed 11 March 2017.

3. Chalmers B, Omer-Hashi K. What Somali women say about giving birth in Canada. *Journal of Reproductive and Infant Psychology.* 2002;**20**:267–328.

4. Upvall MJ, Mohammed K, Dodge PD. Perspectives of Somali Bantu refugee women living with circumcision in the United States: A focus group approach. *J Nurs Stud.* 2009;**46**:360–368. doi: 10.1016/j.ijnurstu.2008.04.009.

5. Zurynski Y, Sureshkumar P, Phu A, Elliott E. Female genital mutilation and cutting: A systematic literature review of health professionals' knowledge, attitudes and clinical practice. *BMC Int Health Hum Rights.* 2015;**15**:32. doi: 10.1186/s12914-015–0070-y.

6. Balfour J, Abdulcadir J, Say L, Hindin MJ. Interventions for healthcare providers to improve treatment and prevention of female genital mutilation: A systematic review. *BMC Health Serv Res.* 2016 August 19;**16**(1):409. doi: 10.1186/s12913-016–1674-1.

7. The Royal College of Obstetricians and Gynaecologists. Female Genital Mutilation and its Management. Green-top Guideline No. 53. London: RCOG, July 2015.

8. Ekwueme OC, Ezegwui HU, Ezeoke U. Dispelling the myths and beliefs toward female genital cutting of woman: Assessing general outpatient services at a tertiary health institution in Enugu state, Nigeria. *East Afr J Public Health.* 2010;**7**:64–67.

9. Alo OA, Gbadebo B. Intergenerational attitude changes regarding female genital cutting in Nigeria. *J Womens Health (Larchmt).* 2011;**20**:1655–1661.

10. WHO study group on female genital mutilation and obstetric outcome, Banks E, Meirik O, Farley T, Akande O, Bathija H, Ali M. Female genital mutilation and obstetric outcome: WHO collaborative prospective study in six African countries. *Lancet* 2006;**367**:1835–1841.

11. Berg RC, Underland V. The obstetric consequences of female genital mutilation/cutting: A systematic review and meta-analysis. *Obstet Gynecol Int.* 2013;**2013**:496564. doi: 10.1155/2013/496564.

12. Utz-Billing I, Kentenich H. Female genital mutilation: An injury, physical and mental harm. *J Psychosom Obstet Gynecol.* 2008;**29**:225–229. doi: 0.1080/01674820802547087.

13. Andersson SH, Rymer J, Joyce DW, et al. Sexual quality of life in women who have undergone female genital mutilation: A case-control study. *BJOG.* 2012;**119**:1606–1611. doi: 10.1111/1471–0528.12004.

14. https://cyber.harvard.edu/population/fgm/fgm.htm. Accessed 11 September 2016.

15. Mathews BP. Female genital mutilation : Australian law, policy and practical challenges for doctors. *Medical Journal of Australia.* 2011;**194**:139–141.

16. Attorney-General's Department. Review of Australia's Female Genital Mutilation Legal Framework. Final Report. March 2013. Available at www.ag.gov.au/publications/documents/reviewofaustraliasfemalegenitalmutilationlegalframework/review%20of%20australias%20female%20genital%20mutilation%20legal%20framework.pdf. Accessed 11 March 2017.

17. Department of Health. Female Genital Mutilation Risk and Safeguarding; Guidance for Professionals. London: DH, May 2016. Available at www.gov.uk/government/uploads/system/uploads/attachment_data/file/525390/FGM_safeguarding_report_A.pdf. Accessed 11 March 2017.

18. HM Government. A Statement Opposing Female Genital Mutilation www.gov.uk/government/uploads/system/uploads/attachment_data/file/451478/FGM_June_2015_v10.pdf. Accessed 11 March 2017.

19. Royal College of Midwives. Tackling FGM in the UK: Intercollegiate Recommendations for Identifying, Recording and Reporting. London: RCM, 2013.

20. Royal College of Nursing. Female Genital Mutilation. An RCN Educational Resource for Nursing and Midwifery Staff. London: RCN, 2006.

21. Society of Obstetricians and Gynaecologists of Canada. Female Genital Cutting. Clinical Practice Guidelines No. 299, November 2013.

22. The Royal Australia and New Zealand College of Obstetricians and Gynaecologists. Female Genital Mutilation. Information for Australian Health Professionals. RANZCOG, 1997. See also RANZCOG, Genital Mutilation (FGM) www.ranzcog.edu.au/component/docman/doc_view/1078-female-genital-mutilation-c-gyn-01.html. Accessed 11 March 2017.

23. American College of Obstetricians and Gynecologists. Female Genital Mutilation. ACOG Committee Opinion No. 151. ACOG Comm Opin. 1995; No. 151:1.

24. Department of Health Guideline. Multi-Agency Statutory Guidance on Female Genital Mutilation. 2016; London: DH.

25. Health Education England. E-Learning for Healthcare. Available at www.e-lfh.org.uk/programmes/female-genital-mutilation/. Accessed 11 September 2016.

Chapter

10 Diverse Sex Development
Critical Biopsychosocial Perspectives

Lih-Mei Liao

Diverse Sex Development

The dimorphic sex categories obscure the important fact that the embryonic tissues that develop into testes, penis and scrotum are initially the same as those that develop into ovaries, womb, vagina, clitoris and labia. Sex differentiation typically begins at about six weeks of embryonic life, and a sex-undifferentiated fetus soon assumes the anatomical structures and appearance of what we think of as female or male. Certain genetic conditions may lead to some changes in the developmental pathway so that the usual markers of sex – gonads, genitalia and karyotype are not female- or male-typical.

Historically, the term 'hermaphroditism' was used in Anglophone societies to refer more specifically to genitals deemed not clearly differentiated. The hermaphroditic myth of a dual set of functioning male and female reproductive organs in one individual is impossible in humans. Nevertheless, the term was adopted in medicine from the 1870s, before the science of anatomy revealed internal structures/functionality [1]. The term 'intersex' was introduced in 1917 to represent a number of heterogeneous conditions, not all of which are associated with ambiguous external genitalia and some are associated with physical health problems requiring medical treatment. Prevalence depends on inclusion criteria. Using a very broad definition, prevalence of intersex live births has been estimated to be as high as one in two hundred [2], although each of the numerous named condition is very much rarer.

The past two decades have witnessed rapid advances in molecular biotechnology that have resulted in the identification of more variants of intersex conditions so that a different categorization scheme was needed to facilitate the burgeoning basic science research. In 2006, the intersex nomenclature underwent major revision and development in the (first international) 'Consensus Statement on the Management of Intersex Disorders' [3]. The term 'disorders of sex development' was invented to encompass all 'congenital conditions in which the development of chromosomal, gonadal or anatomical sex is atypical'. Genetic diagnosis has begun to replace clinical diagnosis as the gold standard. Unsurprisingly, 'disorders of sex development' has been greeted with mixed reactions [4]. 'Diverse sex development' (DSD) is adopted in this chapter to reflect the fact that many affected individuals consider their bodies different rather than disordered. The gynaecological subspecialty most likely to work with women diagnosed with DSD is Paediatric and Adolescent Gynaecology (PAG) [5].

Until relatively recently, psychologists in the field have been preoccupied with brain gender research [6, 7] rather than contributions to health care. Professional interests have more recently shifted to care provision, and any psychologically attuned clinician can make useful contributions. It is, however, argued that a strong conceptual framework underpinned by transparent social values is foundational [8].

Traditional Medical Management

DSD may present in childhood or adulthood, sometimes alongside other bodily differences and/or medical problems. Detection in childhood is usually triggered by visible genital differences, which do not apply to all conditions. Normalising genital surgery on atypical genitalia of children who cannot give consent continues to be controversial. Another major criticism is the concealment of diagnosis and treatment information, especially for girls and women with initial presentations in adolescence and adulthood.

Phallocentric Gender Assignment in Infancy

Erectile and penetrative potential of the phallus has been an overriding consideration in male assignment, and fertility potential the overriding factor in female assignment. Children presenting ambiguous genitalia at birth were assigned female in the ratio of approximately 9:1 [9].

In the past, paediatricians stated that the decision to raise a child as a boy should be 'dictated entirely by the size of the phallus' [10] and that phallus size was 'of paramount importance' in gender assignment [11]. Newborn penile size charts were first used in the 1960s, and any child with a penis of stretched length of less than 2.5 cm was likely to be assigned female regardless of the underlying diagnosis [10]. For a child with a 46,XY karyotype, the phallus and testes would typically be removed and the child would undergo feminizing genital surgery and female gender of rearing. The leaning towards female assignment may also have been influenced by the technical difficulties in penile reconstructive surgery. Multiple procedures may create a penile structure, but the capacity for erection and penetration is often limited.

A larger group that presents ambiguous external genitalia at birth comprises 46,XX children with congenital adrenal hyperplasia (CAH). These children, who have a female-typical karyotype, have been exposed to male-typical amounts of androgens in utero. The metabolic consequences relating to salt loss and dehydration require endocrine management [12]. The child may present externally with a larger clitoris and/or fused labia and/or absence of a vaginal opening and internally with both ovaries, a uterus and an internal (upper) vagina. Because of their fertility potential, these children tend to be assigned female.

Childhood Feminizing Genital Surgery

In contrast to the justifiably cautious tone around penile construction, paediatric urologists have been much more confident in their ability to construct female-typical genital anatomies that meet cultural expectations of appearance and function. Cosmetic surgery to reduce the size of the clitoris has evolved from clitoridectomy (amputation of the clitoris) to clitoral recession (pleating together the erectile tissue to shorten the clitoris) and clitoral reduction (removal of the erectile tissue and attempted preservation of the nerve and blood vessels) [13]. The highly popular 'one stage genitoplasty' means refashioning the scrotal appearance of the labia where applicable and creating a vagina at the same time. The vagina has no anatomical purpose for the child. Postoperatively, she has

to perform daily dilation to keep the cosmetic vagina open and, controversially, if too young to manage this, her adult caretakers would have to perform dilation on her.

Ambiguous genitalia have been known to many premodern cultures in different parts of the world, and community responses have been highly variable across temporal and geographical loci. Surgery to erase genital ambiguity began in Europe and North America in the mid-nineteenth century, though the rationale is often wholly attributed to the protocol developed much later in Johns Hopkins in the late 1950s. The protocol was based on the psychological theory that all infants are gender neutral at birth until about two years old. From then on, the child's appearance, including genital appearance, was thought to be pivotal for unambiguous gender development. Parents and child must be left in no doubt of the assigned gender. Parents were advised to withhold information about the diagnosis and treatments from the child. This particular gender theory has been abandoned, and today's surgeons cannot agree on ethics and techniques [14]. However, surgery appears to be continuing [15].

Sexual outcomes of feminizing genital surgery by definition can only be examined longitudinally, when the children who have been operated on reach puberty and adulthood, i.e. many years after the procedures are initially performed. The widespread practice of childhood surgery has meant that there are very few children available for comparative research. Nuanced longitudinal follow-up of the children may have been possible, but there has been a collective neglect to investigate potential multiple outcomes.

Persistent concerns expressed by recipients of childhood surgery have prompted some clinicians to recall adults who have been lost to paediatric follow-up. In a landmark study, 44 adolescent girls with CAH who had undergone feminizing genitoplasty in childhood were reviewed by a team of gynaecologists [16]. Despite multiple childhood operations, nearly all of the study participants had required further surgery for either menstrual flow or vaginal intercourse, or both, in adolescence and adulthood. Case notes enabled the authors to conclude that the initial surgery had been positioned as 'one-off' for the majority of the participants. These findings raise issues about how accurately informed were the consenting parents. Subsequent research has identified more difficulties with orgasm for women who had undergone clitoral surgery [17] and diminished sensitivity specific to the site of surgery [18]. The quality of the flurry of more recent reports is variable, but it is undeniable that there is a groundswell of provider and recipient opinions that interrogate the practice of childhood feminizing surgery.

Adolescent and Adult Presentations

Some DSD conditions are more typically diagnosed in adolescence and adulthood. For example, women and girls with Mayer-Rokitansky-Küster-Hauser (MRKH) syndrome may present to gynaecological services in adolescence and adulthood for absence of menarche. Sometimes the process is triggered by difficulties during attempts at a smear test or vaginal sex. These women and girls are usually physically healthy with a 46,XX karyotype and functioning ovaries and therefore do not require estrogen replacement. They do not have a womb or a cervix and have a smaller vagina which the majority elect to have treated (see discussion). Rare subtypes of MRKH may be associated with certain medical complications.

Women with complete androgen insensitivity syndrome (CAIS) also tend to present in adolescence and adulthood. They have a 46,XY karyotype female-typical external genitalia and a smaller vagina. Internally, they have testes that produce male-typical quantities of androgens but lack receptors to decode them, and they do not have a womb or cervix. Because of the absence of visible signs at birth, almost all of the children are reared as female. They may present for medical investigations in adolescence because periods have not started – as for MRKH, although in CAIS some girls may have been presented to paediatricians prompted by the identification of protruding testes in the pelvic area. Reports consistently suggest that women and girls with CAIS identify unambiguously as female [19].

Secrecy has been central to traditional medical management of intersex but especially for women with XY conditions such as CAIS. One would think that, given the nature of the investigations and treatments, continued dialogue between doctor, patient and family would be unavoidable. However, difficulties in getting full diagnostic and treatment information have been corroborated by personal [20, 21, 22] and professional accounts [23, 24, 25]. Complaints range from inadequate information and non-discussion to outright deception (e.g. being told that the procedure was a hysterectomy when testes were being removed).

Some people have taken decades to piece together their medical history; catalysts in the process might have been a television programme or magazine article on intersex, a smear test that could not take place or fertility investigations that did not identify a womb. Medical secrecy had hindered for some decades the development of peer support and psychological care as well as quality evaluative research.

Gynaecological management is focussed upon hormonal management in the case of CAIS, and vagina construction in both CAIS and MRKH. A number of surgical techniques exist. The type of surgery would depend on the genital anatomy and whether or not the woman has already had surgery [13, 26]. All vaginoplasties are major operations and complications are not uncommon. Quality scientific evaluation of morphological, cosmetic and psycho-sexual impact is sparse.

In the light of the uncertainties surrounding surgical vagina construction which in most circumstances would require a dilation regime to be maintained by the patient afterwards, non-surgical dilation has become the first line approach for vaginal agenesis in some countries. Dilation involves daily insertion into the vaginal space cylindrical shapes that graduate in width and length, not unlike those prescribed for women presenting at psychosexual clinics for 'vaginismus'. Generally women are advised to dilate daily for some months and thereafter less frequently to keep the vagina open unless they engage in regular vaginal penetrative sex.

Multidisciplinary Team and Psychological Care

The 1990s saw the emergence of intersex patient advocacy/support groups campaigning for a number of changes to clinical management. Some argued that parental distress should not be treated by surgery on the child, and that all children should be assigned as boy or girl without surgery. New and non-medical narratives of intersex sparked a proliferation of media reports, psychosocial analyses and ethical debates in the 1990s and 2000s. Since then, formal acknowledgment of the need for care from a multidisciplinary team (MDT) including access to psychological input can be identified in almost all clinical recommendations, including the consensus statement a decade ago [3]. The role of care user groups is also formally acknowledged in recent care documents [27]. The level of implementation is unknown. By far the most verifiable impact of the consensus statement is the widespread use of the term disorders of sex development and exponential genetic research output.

In terms of access to psychological support, the consensus statement recommends thus: 'Psychosocial care provided by mental health staff with expertise in DSD should be an integral part of management to promote positive adaptation. This expertise can facilitate team decisions about gender assignment/reassignment, timing of surgery and sex-hormone replacement' [3]. Whilst the importance of psychological care is frequently alluded to, its remit, scope, theories, methods and accountability have not yet been coherently articulated [28]. Therefore the range, depth and quality of psychological work can be expected to be highly variable between services [29]. It is, however, self-evident that an individualistic approach based on the diagnosis and treatment of psychopathology is not appropriate. In recognition of the need for methodical development of psychosocial research, practice and education in DSD, psychologists and care users have recently founded the European Network for Psychosocial Studies of Intersex/Diverse Sex Development (www.europsi.org). Following are example situations that justify the need for advance psychological skills and conceptualizations including a norm-critical approach to body differences [30].

Emotional Safety

Qualitative analysis by psychosocial professionals [23] and narratives published by affected adults [20, 21] and parents [31] point to a risk of significant psychological harm in case of poor emotion care [32]. Uncontained emotional distress may render it difficult for parents to prioritize the child's future in their appraisal of the risks of irrevocable surgical interventions for their child; as such it compromises the principles of informed consent [33].

Atypical sex anatomies fascinate clinicians and researchers so that intimate examination and medical photography may not always be optimally managed [see 20]. Professional eagerness to correct what is deemed an aberration could set off a negative chain reaction in affected people and their families, making open communication within families a near impossibility. An important role for psychosocial professionals is to facilitate team reflections, to prioritize emotional containment for affected persons [32] and

to help to overcome the significant communication barriers imposed by the binary language on sex and gender [29].

Gender Assignment

As a result of the emergent evidence from adolescents and adults, it is now generally accepted that phallus size alone should not dictate gender assignment. Some XY adolescents and adults who had been female assigned and subjected to feminizing surgery have reported latent gender dysphoria leading to reassignment to the male gender [34]. It had been assumed that all XY babies with ambiguous genitals were infertile but, with the advent of intracytoplasmic sperm injection, there are reports of pregnancies even in the presence of oligospermia or even azoospermia for people with a number of 46,XY diagnoses [35, 36]. Furthermore, recent reports suggest that a stable gender identity is possible in male assigned adolescents with 46,XX CAH [37].

Gender assignment of infants with DSD is currently understood as a collaborative process between team and family, taking into account the results of a range of investigations as well as parental preferences that may be influenced by family, culture and religion. Given the negative reports on feminizing surgery from XX and XY individuals however assigned, and some possibility of reassignment in adolescence and adulthood, a more conservative approach to childhood genital surgery is needed.

The process of gender assignment and decision-making about normalizing surgery is characterized by uncertainties and dilemmas and can be expected to be highly stressful for parents [31]. Psychological support from professionals and user groups is pivotal. It is a team responsibility to protect the time and space for parents and support staff to manage emotional distress so that the future of the child can be at the forefront of clinical decisions. An alternative psychosocial care pathway should be developed for families who opt to delay surgery [38].

Managing Stigma

Stigma is defined as a negative sense of social difference from others or as an adverse reaction to the perception of a negatively evaluated difference [39]. This 'difference' is outside of the socially defined norm and therefore deeply discrediting [40]. Fear of devaluation can be part of the psychological landscape of many XY women [23]. Research participants have also spoken of feeling like outsiders un-entitled to relationships [24]. Supported exploration of feelings of stigmatization is perhaps the most important focus in psychosocial interventions for the adult woman. Stigma, shame and avoidance often surface in dilemmatic decisions on self-disclosure about DSD in social situations [25]. Openness is generally felt to be high risk (e.g. 'people would flip if they find out'), whilst withholding information may be experienced as a moral lack of integrity (e.g. 'what kind of person does my secrecy make me?').

Whereas a person can choose not to disclose in many situations, given the presence of physical signs including those left behind by surgery, choosing not to disclose to sexual partners is more difficult. Some individuals may withdraw from intimate relations in order to avoid having to explain. Avoidance and safety seeking despite a desire for relationships and intimacy can persist for years. Distress may be expressed in seeking (further) surgery to afford 'normality' in identity, relationships and sexual practices. However, expressions of happiness and joy appear to be far more identifiable in the narratives of people who embrace their differences and engage with likeminded people [32].

Parents may require assistance to talk to their child about DSD in developmentally appropriate ways and to encourage the children to ask questions. Fear of shaming and stigmatizing the child may make this task challenging even for the most committed parents [32]. Talking to the child may mean also talking to siblings and perhaps the extended family and wider communities. This is easier said than done. Paediatric psychological interventions to support parental tasks should receive adequate resource allocation to translate this recommendation into reality.

Reconsidering Sex

The belief that all genitals look discretely male or female and that they are not only capable of but are naturally inclined towards blissful union with each other seldom comes into question in society. The normalization/naturalization of genital intercourse frames a wide range of pleasurable and meaningful sexual experiences as 'other' and vastly limits the construction of these experiences as satisfying and affirming. It is unsurprising that many women with DSD who have already accessed pleasurable sexual experiences seek vagina construction in order to 'have sex', reflecting a strong linguistic and conceptual conflation of 'sex' and coitus in society [24]. In other words [41], *'Full genital performance during heterosexual intercourse is the essence of sexual functioning, which excludes and demotes nongenital possibilities for pleasure and expression'* (p. 53, emphasis original)

Research has identified a higher prevalence of anticipatory and experienced sexual difficulties regardless of diagnosis and whether or not women have undergone genital surgery [24, 41, 17, 42, 43]. In psychosexual education and support, a move away from 'normal sex' and a greater emphasis in sensuality rather than gender performance can offer greater scope for pleasure as people become more open to opportunities for good-enough sexual relating [28]. Therapeutic exploration might focus on the developmental trajectories of the following: (1) gender positioning of self; (2) gender(s) of preferred partners; (3) body perceptions; (4) sexual concerns and experiences – actual and fantasized; (5) sexual and relationship aspirations and (6) knowledge and attitude relating to a range of sexual activities.

Some of these ideas were taken up in the development of a vagina dilation protocol as a less invasive alternative to surgery for women seeking vagina construction [44, 45]. The development was in response to some of the difficulties aptly expressed by a research participant: 'I felt … like [] I hadn't learned all the social sort of skills that were needed to [] you know to-to establish a relationship and that maybe that was the main problem, and having a vagina wouldn't really help … there's more going on than just vaginal length'.[24, p.579] Unlike surgery, self-managed dilation takes several months which affords time and space to rethink sexuality [44]. Engaging materials have been developed by a user advocacy group (www.dsdteens.org) to enable more services to access the multidisciplinary approach.

Facilitating Informed Choice

DSD does not preclude people from living well. However, the diagnosis could propel individuals into dilemmatic decisions. Although psychological support is more clearly indicated at the point of the initial diagnosis, there are subsequent time points where such help may also be beneficial. A few brief examples are as follows.

In infancy and early childhood, parents may be presented with the option of feminizing surgery. As it does not affect the child's health, DSD teams should ensure that it is presented as a choice, and give weight to non-intervention also as a choice [33]. Parents should be allowed plenty of time to recover from the shock of the diagnosis, digest all of the information, consult with support groups if they wish and, most importantly, bond with their child [31]. When parents decide on normalizing surgery, they are likely to be seeking 'normality' for their children in future identity, sexuality and relationships. Psychosocial professionals can gently guide parents to question what is normal in identity, sexuality and relationships. They can help parents to weigh up the reality of the surgical trajectory, which may involve repeat operations and examinations, and uncertainties about the anatomical and psychological impact. For the currently small proportion of parents who decide to defer surgery until their child can give consent, psychological input may need to be intensified, to co-create the best approach to educate and support the affected child, the siblings, the extended family and perhaps the wider community.

In the past, prophylactic gonadectomy was routine for XY girls and women to reduce cancer risks and for gender compatibility. The patient would require hormone replacement therapy for long-term health [46]. In recent years, more women with functioning testes are choosing to retain their testes to avoid taking exogenous hormones. Ongoing research suggests that the cancer risk is relatively small for some conditions but high for others [47]. Decision counselling regarding the gonadectomy trade-off can support women to make an informed choice.

Choice is important not just for surgery. Studies with other populations suggest that genetic testing could pose significant dilemmas for family members who may struggle to discuss certain conditions and carrier status [48]. The Androgen Insensitivity Syndrome Support Group in the United Kingdom (www.aissg.org) has documented how genetic testing could fill people with dread about having to discuss DSD within the family. A collaborative approach means plenty of time and opportunities to help people explore the potential implications of genetic testing for family relationships, as well as education and support for potential carriers to consider the implications (including the communication challenges with the next generation) [29].

This leads to the issue of supporting individuals and couples in their parenthood considerations. Choosing to be childfree is entirely valid for all individuals and couples with or without a DSD diagnosis. For those who wish to be parents, adoption is a viable

option across all diagnostic groups. In terms of fertility potential, women with CAH have a uterus and ovaries and the potential for natural conception and pregnancy subject to optimal steroidal replacement [12]. Regarding assisted reproduction, women with MRKH have ovaries but no uterus and therefore the potential to have genetic children via surrogacy. Fertility considerations for XY women can be complex. Women with gonadal dysgenesis have an intact Müllerian system and can carry a pregnancy conceived via ovum donation and in vitro fertilization. There are reports of pregnancies successfully carried to term for this group of women [11]. For women with CAIS, sperm could potentially be aspirated from a testis and used to fertilize an ovum which could then be carried by a surrogate. The ethical and psychosocial considerations are complex and there are no reported cases in the literature.

Consumption of assisted reproductive technology is characterized by overwhelming uncertainties and dilemmas. Complex treatment with uncertain timing and outcome should not be presented as a straightforward solution for a desire or longing, however understandable. Rather, many individuals and couples need psychological input to manage expectations and emotions and to maintain a healthy engagement with the broadest possible range of life goals [49].

Public Engagement and Education

Medicine has helped to preserve the sex and gender dichotomy by erasing anatomical characteristics that speak of the continuity between maleness and femaleness. The secrecy and taboo has resulted in an impoverished linguistic framework with which to address diverse sex characteristics. Normalizing interventions can be physically and psychologically costly for some individuals. Medicalization can furthermore marginalize systemic solutions, perhaps especially public engagement with DSD.

Social tolerance that fosters self-acceptance in individuals born different reflects a healthier society than social intolerance that fosters shame and stigma that underpins normalization. Public understanding is a possible goal. Bodily characteristics deemed insufficiently gendered do not only affect people with DSD but the general population. For example, healthy men may also have breasts and healthy women may not, and healthy men may have sparse facial or body hair and healthy women may have a lot. The burden of social pressure to do gender in particular ways is widely shared in society.

Summary

DSD encompasses numerous congenital conditions associated with atypical development of chromosomal, gonadal or anatomical sex. Traditional medical management has been dominated by a surgical focus. Phallus size was the main consideration in gender assignment of babies with ambiguous genitalia, and there has been a leaning towards female assignment. Longitudinal evaluation has been sparse. Strong reservations from adults so treated as children and recent research have prompted a re-examination of the approach.

A shift from a surgical focus to multidisciplinary team working is evident in clinical recommendations. Integral psychological care is now emphasized. Perhaps most importantly, the role of care user groups in service development and peer support is now acknowledged. The change in ethos has not eliminated normalizing interventions, but it has opened up more possibilities for psychosocial professionals and care users to explore a wider range of narratives and educational strategies relating to diversity in sex and gender.

Key Points

- Terms such as 'hermaphroditism', 'intersex' and 'disorder of sex development' have been used to describe atypical development of the lower genital tract, but these terms have limitations. 'Diverse sex development' (DSD) is adopted by some workers to reflect the fact that many affected individuals consider their bodies different rather than disordered.
- DSD conditions may be diagnosed at birth or later, when an adolescent girl presents to gynaecological services with primary amenorrhoea.
- For children diagnosed at birth, the process of gender assignment and decision-making regarding surgery to normalize the genitalia is characterized by uncertainties and dilemmas and can be highly stressful for parents.
- A more conservative approach is currently advocated for medically non-essential surgery in childhood. Issues of informed choice and consent to treatment should be addressed through a transparent process.

- The management of DSD across the life span requires a multidisciplinary team approach including access to psychological input and involvement of care user groups.
- Although the importance of psychological care is frequently alluded to, its remit, scope, resource allocation, methods and accountability have not yet been coherently articulated.

References

1. Dreger, A.D., Chase, C., Sousa, A., Gruppusso P.A., & Frader J. (2005). Changing the nomenclature/taxonomy of intersex: A scientific and clinical rationale. *Journal of Pediatric Endocrinology & Metabolism*, **18**, 735–738.

2. Blackless, M., Charuvastra, A., Derryck, A., & Fausto-Sterling, A. (2000). How sexually dimorphic are we? Review and synthesis. *American Journal of Human Biology*, **12**, 151–166.

3. Lee, P.A., Houk, C.P., Ahmed, S.F., & Hughes, I.A. (2006). Consensus statement on management of intersex disorders. International Consensus Conference on Intersex. *Pediatrics*, **118**(2), e488–500.

4. Davis G. (2013). The power in a name: Diagnostic terminology and diverse experiences. *Psychology & Sexuality*, doi:10.1080/19419899.2013.831212.

5. Balen, A., Breech, L., Creighton, S., & Liao, L. An Introduction to Pediatric & Adolescent Gynaecology. In S. Creighton, A. Balen, L. Breech & L. Liao (eds.) *Pediatric & Adolescent Gynecology: A Problem-Based Approach*. Cambridge University Press, in press.

6. Jordan-Young R.M. (2011). Hormones, context and 'Brain Gender': A review of evidence from congenital adrenal hyperplasia. *Social Science & Medicine*, doi:10.1016/jsocscimed.2011.08.026.

7. Stout, S.A., Litvak, M., Robbins, N.M., & Sandberg, D.E. (2010). Congenital adrenal hyperplasia: Classification of studies employing psychological endpoints. *International Journal of Pediatric Endocrinology*, doi:10.1155/2010/191520.

8. Liao, L.M. & Simmonds, M. (2013). A values-driven and evidence-based health care psychology for diverse sex development. *Psychology & Sexuality*, doi:10.1080/19419899.2013.831217.

9. Newman, K., Randolph, J., & Anderson, K. (1992). The surgical management of infants and children with ambiguous genitalia: Lessons learned from 25 years. *Annals of Surgery*, **215**, 644–653.

10. Donaghoe, P.K. (1991). Clinical management of intersex abnormalities. *Current Problems in Surgery*, **28**, 519–579.

11. American Academy of Pediatrics (2000). Evaluation of the newborn with developmental anomalies of the external genitalia. *Pediatrics*, **106**, 138–142.

12. Han T.S., Walker B.R., Arlt W., & Ross R.J. (2015). Treatment and health outcome in adults with congenital adrenal hyperplasia. *Nature Reviews Endocrinology*, **10** (2), 115–124.

13. Creighton S., Chernausek S., Romao R., Ransley P., & Pippi Salle J. (2012). Timing and nature of reconstructive surgery for disorders of sex development – Introduction. *Journal of Pediatric Urology*, **8**, 602–610.

14. Lee P.A., Nordenström A., & Houk C.P. (2016). Global Disorders of Sex Development Update since 2006: Perceptions, Approach and Care. *Hormone Research in Paediatrics*, doi: 10.1159/000442975.

15. Michala L., Liao L.M., Wood D., Conway G.S., & Creighton S.M. (2014). Practice changes in childhood surgery on ambiguous genitalia? *Journal of Pediatric Urology*, **10**(5), 934–939.

16. Creighton, S., Minto, C., & Steele S.J. (2001). Feminising childhood surgery in ambiguous genitalia: Objective cosmetic and anatomical outcomes in adolescence. *Lancet*, **358**, 124–125.

17. Minto, C.L., Liao, L.M., Woodhouse, C.R.J., Ransley, P.G., & Creighton, S.M. (2003). Adult outcomes of childhood clitoral surgery for ambiguous genitalia. *Lancet*, **361**, 1252–1257.

18. Crouch N.S., Liao, L.M., Woodhouse, C.R., Conway, G.S., & Creighton, S.M. (2008) Sexual function and genital sensation following feminising genitoplasty for congenital adrenal hyperplasia. *J Urol*, **179**(2), 634–638.

19. Wisniewski A.B., Migeon C.J., Meyer-Bahlburg, H.F.L., Gearhart, J.P., Berkovitz, G.D., Brown, T.R., & Money, J. (2000). Complete androgen insensitivity syndrome: Long-term medical, surgical, and psychosexual outcome. *Journal of Clinical Endocrinology and Metabolism*, doi: 10.1210/jcem.85.8.6742.

20. Anonymous, 1994. Once a dark secret. *BMJ*, **308**, 542.

21. Davis, G. & Feder, E.K. (eds.) (2015) Narrative Symposium: Intersex. *Narrative Inquiry in Bioethics*, **5**(2), 87–125.

22. Simmonds, M. Patients and parents in decision making and management. In AH Balen (ed.) *Paediatric and adolescent gynaecology – A multidisciplinary approach.* Cambridge, UK: Cambridge University Press, 2004, 205–228.

23. Alderson, J., Madill, A., & Balen, A. (2004). Fear of devaluation: Understanding the experience of intersexed women with androgen insensitivity syndrome. *British Journal of Health Psychology*, **9**(1), 81–100.

24. Boyle, M., Smith, S., & Liao L.M. (2005). Adult genital surgery for intersex: A solution to what problem? *Journal of Health Psychology*, **10**, 573–584.

25. Liao L.M. (2003). Learning to assist women born with atypical genitalia: Journey through ignorance, taboo and dilemmas. *Journal of Reproductive & Infant Psychology*, **2**, 229–238.

26. Rokhal R.S. & Creighton S.M. (2012). Management of Vaginal Agenesis. *Journal of Pediatric & Adolescent Gynecology*, doi: 10.1016/j.jpag.2011.06.003.

27. Baratz A.B., Sharp M.K., & Sandberg D.E. Disorders of sex development peer support. In O. Hiort & S. Ahmed (eds.) *Understanding differences and disorders of sex development (dsd)*. Basel: Karger, 2014, pp 99–112.

28. Liao L.M. Towards a clinical-psychological approach for addressing the hetero sexual concerns of intersexed women. In V. Clarke & E. Peel (eds.) *Out in psychology: lesbian gay bisexual transgender and queer perspectives.* Wiley 2007, pp 391–408.

29. Liao L.M. & Simmonds M. Communicating about diverse sex development. In J. Wiggens & A. Middleton (eds.) *Getting the message across: practical advice for genetics health care professionals.* Oxford University Press, 2013, pp 42–60.

30. Alderson, J., Roen, K., & Muscarella, M. Psychological Care: Addressing the Effects of Sexual and Gender Norms. In S. Creighton, A. Balen, L. Breech & L. Liao (eds.) *Pediatric & Adolescent Gynecology: A Problem-Based Approach*. Cambridge University Press, in press.

31. Magritte E. (2012). Working together in placing the long term interests of the child at the heart of the DSD evaluation. *Journal of Pediatric Urology*, doi:10.1016/j.jpurol.2012.07.011.

32. Liao L.M. Stonewalling emotion. In G. Davis & E. Feder (eds.) *Narrative Symposium: Intersex.* Narrative Inquiry in Bioethics, 2015, **5**(2), 143–150.

33. Tamar-Mattis A., Baratz A., Baratz Dalke K., & Karkazis K. (2013). Emotionally and cognitively informed consent for clinical care for differences of sex development. *Psychology & Sexuality*, doi: 10.1080/19419899.2013.831215

34. Reiner W.G. & Gearhart J.P. (2004). Discordant sexual identity in some genetic males with cloacal exstrophy assigned to female sex at birth. *N Engl J Med*, **350**, 333–341, doi: 10.1056/NEJMoa022236.

35. Palermo G., Joris H., Devroey P., & Van Stertegham A. C. (1992). Pregnancies after intracytoplasmic injection of a single spermatozoon into an oocyte. *Lancet*, **340**, 12–18.

36. Katz M.D., Kligman I., Li-Qun C., Yuan-Shan Z., Fratianni C. et al. (1997). Paternity by intrauterine insemination with sperm from a man with 5-alpha reductase 2 deficiency. *NEJM*, **336**, 994–998.

37. Houk C.P. & Lee P.A. (2013). Approach to assigning gender in 46,XX congenital adrenal hyperplasia with male external Genitalia: Replacing Dogmatism with Pragmatism. *JCEM*, doi: 10.1210/jc.2010-0714.

38. Liao L.M., Wood D., & Creighton S.M. (2015). Between a rock and a hard place: Parents choosing normalising cosmetic genital surgery for their children. *BMJ*, **351**:h5124.

39. Susman J. (1994). Disability, stigma and deviance. *Social Science & Medicine*, **38**(1), 15–22.

40. Goffman E. *Stigma: Notes on the Management of Spoiled Identity*. New York: Prentice-Hall, 1963.

41. Tiefer L. *Sex is not a Natural Act and Other Essays*. Oxford: Westview Press, 1995.

42. May, B., Boyle, M., & Grant, D. (1996). A comparative study of sexual experiences: Women with diabetes and women with congenital adrenal hyperplasia due to 21-hydroxylase deficiency. *Journal of Health Psychology*, **1**, 479–492.

43. Minto, C.L., Liao, K.L.M., Conway, G.S., & Creighton, S.M. (2003). Sexual function and complete androgen insensitivity syndrome. *Fertility and Sterility*, **80**, 157–164.

44. Liao, L.M., Doyle, J., Crouch, N.S., & Creighton, S.M. (2006). Dilation as treatment for vaginal agenesis and hypoplasia: A pilot exploration of benefits and barriers as perceived by patients. *Journal of Obstetrics & Gynecology*, **26**, 144–148.

45. Ismail-Pratt, I.S., Bikoo, M., Liao, L.M., Conway, G.S., & Creighton, S.M. A prospective outcome study of vaginal dilation therapy as first line treatment for vaginal agenesis. Manuscript submitted for publication.

46. Berra M., Liao L-M., Creighton S.M., & Conway G.S. (2010). Long-term health issues of women with XY karyotype. *Maturitas*, **65**, 172–178.

47. Deans R., Creighton S.M., Liao L-M., & Conway G.S. (2012). Timing of gonadectomy in adult women with complete androgen insensitivity syndrome: Patient preferences and clinical evidence. *Clinical Endocrinology*, doi: 10.1111/j.1365–2265.2012.04330.x.

48. Shaw, A., & Hurst, J.A. (2009). 'I don't see any point in telling them': Attitudes to sharing genetic information in the family and carrier testing of relatives among British Pakistani adults referred to a genetics clinic. *Ethnicity and Health*, **14**(2), 205–224.

49. Slade, P., O'Neil, C., Simpson, A.J., & Lashen, H. (2007). The relationship between perceived stigma, disclosure patterns, support and distress in new attendees at an infertility clinic. *Human Reproduction*, **22**, 2309–2317.

Biopsychosocial Factors in Paediatric and Adolescent Gynaecology

Gail Busby, Gail Dovey-Pearce and Andrea Goddard

Introduction

A wide range of gynaecological conditions is managed within paediatric and adolescent gynaecology (PAG). Broadly speaking the conditions can be subdivided into general PAG, disorders of puberty and adolescence and developmental abnormalities. (Developmental abnormalities are not discussed in this chapter and are covered in Chapter 10.)

The aim is to explore the interaction between gynaecological health and the changes occurring in childhood and through adolescence. Suggestions for clinical practice (in both paediatric and adult settings) will be discussed. There is a distinct lack of empirical study in this area, so clinical case law and extrapolations from other areas of paediatric and adolescent health will be the basis for this discussion. Adolescent health as a specialist area and the needs of young people are increasingly being discussed and addressed [1], but no specific guidelines exist for children and young people presenting in gynaecology, and few studies examine the views of those accessing gynaecological services [2]. Training tools are being developed but clinicians often have to navigate consultations using the skills they have developed as either a paediatrician or adult clinician. The need for further research and professional training will be outlined, and the importance of the integrated, multidisciplinary approach will be emphasized.

The term 'young people' will be used to refer to those aged 11–25, to reflect the developmental changes occurring during these years. Physically, they are experiencing pubertal changes and, cognitively, they are moving from concrete to more abstract thinking. In terms of social and self-development, young people are acquiring autonomy and beginning to broaden their focus from salient tasks of childhood (e.g. friendships and academic goals) to include emerging tasks of adulthood, such as work, partnership and family [3]. Neurologically, the brain undergoes a period of significant remodelling from early adolescence into the third decade of life. The structural, connective and neurochemical changes allow young people to be primed for salient developmental tasks (e.g. the primacy of social reward systems, to prompt relationship building outside of the immediate family). Predominant neural circuits become more efficient and the integration of brain functions increases [4].

Communicating with Children, Young People and Parents

Clinicians need to build rapport and sustain discussion in order to know what children and young people understand about their condition and treatment and the fears they may have. Having an interest in the individual patient will enable rapport and lead to more effective history-taking, information giving and health education [5]. Key communication skills enable dialectical, rather than didactic, discussion with children and young people presenting in gynaecology: avoiding problem-saturated talk; asking questions in an easy-to-answer way; acknowledging that you expect them to have different perspectives and shaping discussion by using analogies that fit with their interests. It should be said that these skills are equally important when working with adults.

Children and young people can be reluctant to offer up information early on in the clinical relationship, especially considering their stage of self-identity and body image development and the likely embarrassment of discussing gynaecological issues. Assessment and treatment planning might need to happen at a slower pace to facilitate trust. Young people describe the importance of staff consistency and civility, accessible services, age-appropriate information and education, and support around their emotional, social and developmental needs being impacted upon by their health [6].

Managing the patient-parent-clinician triad of communication is key, and the child or young person has to remain central to the consultation. Asking questions directly to them and giving the young person the opportunity to be seen alone are vital. This might constitute just two minutes of the consultation with an 11-year-old and the entire time with a 25-year-old. Equally, some pre-teens will feel confident to have more time alone, and some 20-somethings will want their parent or partner in the room for most of the time. It will work best if clinicians and departments offer the opportunity to be seen alone as standard practice, thus being able to normalize and explain the reasons for it. Parents of 11–16s could usefully be given information about confidentiality and being seen alone, prior to the appointment, either in the post or when booking in upon arrival.

Parents will have their own needs in relation to their child's health and they are an important source of support for them, so their questions and concerns must be elicited and addressed, yet not at the expense of supporting the child's ownership of their health issues or the development of the young person's autonomy within the consultation.

Examining Children

Approaches to examining the genital area in childhood depend on age and developmental stage. At all ages it is important to establish a good rapport with the child and carer first. The examination setting should be child-friendly and contain pictures and activities to reassure and distract the child. A normal examination couch is sufficient for examination in the 'frog leg' position. A couch that children can 'help' to raise and lower is a useful distraction tool. Younger children can be examined on their mother's knees or lap.

Babies and toddlers up to about 2 years or 3 years are accustomed to having their nappy changed, and there is usually no difficulty examining the genital area. Examining older children with developmental difficulties varies from child to child. In both cases the presence of a familiar, reassuring parent or carer is essential and it may be that the parent is needed to help with the examination – for example by separating the labia to allow the examining doctor or nurse to inspect the vestibule and peri-urethral area. At about 4 years of age children become aware of the 'private' nature of the genital area. Before starting any examination, a discussion should be held with the child and

the parent explaining the reasons for examining the genital area, an explanation given to the child outlining what is going to happen and reassurance provided that the examination will be halted if requested. It is good practice to explain to the child that the genital area is 'private' so that normally only a parent/carer and in certain cases a doctor or nurse should be looking or touching that area. Throughout the procedure, age-appropriate explanations should be provided to describe exactly what is happening. Note that the hymen and vestibule are extremely sensitive before puberty and that even taking a swab will be painful for the child. Digital or instrumental vaginal examination is very rarely indicated in prepubertal girls. If so, this should be conducted under a general anaesthetic. Once the examination is complete, the child should be told how helpful she was and thanked for agreeing to be examined [7].

Examination of a child when there is a disclosure or concern about sexual abuse is a specialized area and the local Sexual Assault Referral Centre (SARC) or specialist service should be contacted.

Although it is impossible to cover every condition seen in PAG within the confines of this chapter, several conditions have been chosen to highlight the significant biopsychosocial aspects which need to be considered in order to manage these conditions in a holistic manner. This list is by no means exhaustive, and many other conditions may also have overt or more difficult to elicit biopsychosocial implications.

Vulvovaginitis

Redness, irritation and discomfort of the external genitalia and dysuria are the common symptoms of what is called vulvovaginitis (VV) in prepubertal girls. Vaginal discharge is sometimes present. VV is ascribed to the low oestrogenic environment of the prepubertal genital area once the influence of intrauterine maternal oestrogens has worn off in infancy resulting in thin, sensitive external genitalia. Aggravating factors for VV are thought related to hygiene, though the evidence for this is not robust. Some young girls have considerable difficulties which include missing school. Infection, especially with streptococcus, needs to be excluded, as does identifying a vaginal foreign body. Swabbing the genital area is painful for young girls. Girls presenting with problematic vulvovaginitis need a sensitive enquiry into all aspects of their physical and emotional health. The possibility of sexual abuse, or other psychological issues, e.g. bullying at school, needs to be looked into. A multidisciplinary approach with a paediatrician, specialist in vulval disorders and psychologist can be very helpful in severe or persistent cases [8].

Lichen Sclerosus

Lichen sclerosus (LS) is an uncommon inflammatory skin disorder with a predilection for the anogenital area. The cause is unknown but there are genetic and autoimmune associations. The disease is mostly seen in prepubertal and postmenopausal females. The lesions present as sharply demarcated white plaques encircling the vagina and anus. Pruritus, dysuria, bleeding and constipation are the dominant complaints, although patients may be asymptomatic. Delay in diagnosis and/or misdiagnosis are reported and cause significant problems and frustration for both the patient and her family. Lesions may mimic the findings of sexual abuse. An experienced clinician can usually make the diagnosis of lichen sclerosus by examination alone, but skin biopsy is recommended if the diagnosis is not certain, or if another vulvar skin disease might be present. Potent corticosteroids are very effective in symptomatic treatment [9].

Traumatic Gynaecologic Injuries (Including Straddle Injuries and Puncture Injuries)

Accidental trauma is commonly seen in the prepubertal girls, with straddle injuries the most prevalent. Sexual abuse must always be a consideration in the evaluation. Genital injuries in girls often cause great anxiety because of the location and concern for future gynaecological and sexual development. The non-oestrogenized prepubertal genital tissues are friable (with excellent blood flow) and lack distensibility and, therefore, even minor trauma can cause injury and bleeding which may appear extensive. Though urogenital trauma frequently raises the question of sexual abuse, it is uncommonly associated with it. It is important to be able to correlate the history of the injury with physical findings on examination. Thorough documentation and appropriate referral of cases suspicious for abuse is a priority of care. The majority of cases require no surgical intervention; however, penetrating injuries or hemodynamic instability may require immediate laparotomy or laparoscopy [10].

Delayed and Precocious Puberty in Girls

Normal, true or central GnRH-driven puberty in girls usually begins with thelarche (the onset of breast buds) which can start anywhere between age 8 and 14 but typically start about age 11 years. Pubarche (the onset of pubic hair) is usually caused by secretion of adrenal androgens, the initiation of which is termed adrenarche. Pubarche usually follows thelarche by a few months, with menarche (the onset of periods) usually starting about 2 years after breast buds are first noticed. Girls have their growth spurt fairly early in puberty and by the time they start their periods, a lot of their growing will have been done. Most girls will have started their periods by the time they are 13 and finish growing by about the age of 15. It is normal for there to be some variation in the age at which puberty starts and most girls will start theirs 2 years before or after the average. Thus 95% of girls start their periods between the ages of 11 and 15. Problems most commonly arise through 'mistiming' of puberty which is either early ('precocious') or delayed.

In the last 20 to 30 years there has been a great deal of controversy over the issue of timing of puberty in girls with concerns about vulnerability and sexualization of a generation of girls reaching puberty earlier than previous generations and before they are emotionally ready. Longitudinal studies from the 1990s show that while thelarche, especially in black girls, may be earlier than studies done in the 1950s suggested, the age of menarche is only minimally earlier, with most current studies documenting an average age between 12 and 12.5 years, only four months younger than documented in the mid-twentieth century.

Precocious Puberty

Causes of abnormally early pubertal maturation may be separated into GnRH-dependent and GnRH-independent processes.

Central precocious puberty is GnRH-dependent, resulting from activation of the hypothalamic-pituitary-gonadal axis by a variety of central nervous system abnormalities, including malignancies, trauma, infection, malformation, neurocutaneous syndromes. However, by far the most common is idiopathic.

Two common variants of GnRH-independent precocious puberty exist. Premature thelarche refers to the isolated development of breast tissue. Typically, there are no other pubertal findings, such as accelerated linear growth, rapid progression of breast development or advanced skeletal maturation. Classical premature thelarche does not progress and usually regresses over several months. It often occurs in toddlers but may also be seen in older girls.

Premature adrenarche is a variant in which mildly elevated concentrations of adrenal-derived androgens cause gradually progressive pubic and/or axillary hair growth. Breast development is absent, and skeletal maturation may be mildly advanced [11].

Psychosocial effects of early normal and precocious puberty

Psychosocially, early puberty raises concerns about being different from peers and, for example, having to cope with periods while still in primary school. Significant concerns arise in relation to physical and sexual maturity not being accompanied by emotional maturity and the vulnerability that can arise as a result. The long-term behavioural and emotional outcomes of girls with puberty occurring in the normal time frame but earlier than average suggest that adverse outcomes are limited to adolescence with more risk-taking behaviours, including being delinquent and advanced sexual experiences. By adult age, there were no differences in psychosocial adjustment between the early- and late-developed women [12].

The relevance of these studies to those with true precocious puberty is unclear, and there is little current literature addressing this subject.

Delayed Puberty in Girls

A girl who has not reached thelarche by the age of 13 is considered to be delayed.

Causes include:

- constitutional delayed puberty, more likely to occur if the mother started her periods after age 14.
- decreased body fat seen in girls who are very athletic, particularly in gymnasts, ballet dancers and competitive swimmers.
- decreased body fat seen in girls with anorexia nervosa – see 'Eating Disorders'.
- chronic illnesses in which body fat is often decreased, e.g. inflammatory bowel disease where it can be a presenting feature.
- primary ovarian insufficiency with Turner syndrome being a major cause.

- damage to the ovaries due to radiation, usually to treat leukaemia or certain other kinds of cancer.
- pituitary insufficiency, which may be accompanied by evidence of other pituitary disorders.

Menstrual Disorders in Adolescence

In the United Kingdom, the onset of puberty occurs at approximately 10 years of age, with a median age of menarche of 12.9 years. The establishment of regular menstrual cycles can take several more years. Variations in menstrual patterns (frequency, volume, duration, irregularity) can create anxieties regarding ill health or serious underlying disorders.

Normal Menstrual Cycle

The hypothalamic-pituitary-ovarian axis is active during fetal life and quiescent during childhood. It is reactivated at puberty due to removal of the inhibitory mechanisms that are responsible for the release of gonadotrophin-releasing hormone from the hypothalamus. This results in increased pulsatility of follicle-stimulating hormone and luteinizing hormone. Menarche occurs towards the end of puberty when the complex cascade of hormonal events results in sufficient oestrogens to promote endometrial proliferation [13].

Early menstrual life is associated with anovulatory cycles. The frequency of ovulation is related both to the time since menarche and age at menarche. Early menarche is associated with early onset of ovulatory cycles. When the age at menarche is <12 years, 50% of cycles are ovulatory in the first year. In contrast, it may take 8–12 years after menarche until females with later-onset menarche become fully ovulatory [14].

The menstrual problems experienced by young people include dysmenorrhoea, oligo/amenorrhoea, heavy menstrual bleeding and premenstrual syndrome. There is currently a limited exploration of health-related quality of life and menstrual problems in the younger age range, but studies suggest lower quality-of-life scores across physical health and psychosocial health domains. Comparing these scores with those from other studies of chronic diseases demonstrates statistically lower scores than adolescents with cystic fibrosis and a lower score in psychosocial health compared with adolescents with juvenile arthritis [15].

Dysmenorrhoea may impact more upon physical functioning and school attendance and amenorrhoea more upon psychosocial functioning [16], but very little has been studied about psychosocial functioning in young people with menstrual-related problems and much more research is needed.

A young person's experience of these difficulties will be influenced by their understanding and beliefs about what is happening to their body and developmentally appropriate information and education will be needed, with an awareness of the person's cultural context, and further assessment and support for young people showing the lowest mood and/or social functioning should be considered.

Menstrual Suppression in Adolescents

Physicians who treat adolescents commonly use extended cycles of combined hormonal contraception to treat menstrual symptoms. This is in keeping with the preference of many adolescents to experience fewer menses (also of reproductive health professionals).

Some of the conditions for which extended cycles have been specifically studied are premenstrual syndrome, dysmenorrhoea and menorrhagia, headaches, haematology and oncology disorders, and menstrual hygiene.

Menstrual Problems in Adolescents with Physical or Developmental Disabilities

For adolescents with physical or developmental disabilities, the onset of menstrual cycles, the expression of sexuality and the possibility of abuse can provide many challenges for patients and their caregivers [17]. Patients and caregivers will often present for help and direction, from anticipatory guidance before menarche to assistance with menstrual suppression, hygiene and menstrual symptoms [18].

Concerns regarding the onset of menarche can include behaviour deterioration, vulnerability to pregnancy or difficulty managing the actual bleeding. Although it is important to acknowledge the concerns these often-overwhelmed parents/carers feel, for general health and optimal growth, the adolescent should usually be allowed to go through puberty at their pace and timing. Once the menses have started, the effects on the teenager can be addressed [17].

The menstrual flow, whether normal or abnormal, may affect daily living for these young women by causing difficulties in maintaining hygiene or the

resulting behaviours. For some teenagers with developmental delay, blood may be associated with pain or injury and the concept of 'normal' blood may be difficult to understand. Thus the sight of menstrual blood can be extremely distressing to the patient. Cyclical mood or behaviour changes can be a manifestation of dysmenorrhoea in non-verbal patients. The patient's behaviour can be significantly affected, especially in teenagers with autism.

The available modalities of treatment for menstrual suppression include depot medroxyprogesterone acetate (DMPA) injections, continuous oral progestogens, continuous combined hormonal contraceptives and gonadotrophin-releasing hormone (GnRH) analogues. Surgical options include insertion of a levonorgestrel-releasing intrauterine system and, rarely endometrial ablation or hysterectomy [19]. Complete amenorrhoea is difficult to obtain with any hormonal treatment, and scheduled withdrawal bleeds may be better tolerated than erratic unpredictable bleeding. The choice of treatment can only be made in partnership with the parents/carers and the young woman herself. If after full explanation therapy is warranted, an assessment of bone mineral density (BMD) status should be made and other factors such as acceptability of injections, oral medications or patches, anticonvulsant use, thromboembolic risk factors, family history of malignancy, patient weight and need for contraception should be assessed. Surgical options should be considered a last resort when symptoms are severe and other treatment options have failed. The ethical and legal situations are also difficult in a patient who is unable to understand the issues surrounding surgery and likely sterility which would be a consequence of endometrial ablation or hysterectomy.

Eating Disorders

Eating disorders begin mostly in adolescence and may hinder or delay adolescent development. They have long-standing physical and psychosocial effects in adulthood. Although the rates of eating disorders continue to increase, the age of onset remains unchanged. The peak age of onset is 15 years of age, which corresponds with the time of greatest adolescent challenges [20,21].

The onset of puberty starts the process during which adolescents have to adapt to a changing body and new demands of maturing sexuality. Very early puberty in girls has been associated with depressive disorders, eating disorders, disruptive behaviour disorders and comorbid depression and substance disorders [22].

The presenting symptom of eating disorders may be menstrual irregularity and therefore may present to the gynaecologist.

There are three major groups of eating disorders: anorexia nervosa (AN), bulimia nervosa (BN) and those who have features of an eating disorder but do not fit the criteria for either AN or BN, referred to as eating disorders not otherwise specified (EDNOS), which accounts for the majority of adolescents presenting for treatment.

The features of AN are self-imposed weight loss leading to a weight less than 85% of that expected for age and height, a distorted body image in which patients see themselves as being too fat, an intense fear of gaining weight and amenorrhoea for at least three months.

The main feature of BN is the binge episode in which a large amount of food is consumed over a short period of time. The binge is associated with a feeling of lack of control and is followed by behaviours such as self-induced vomiting, excessive exercise, periods of prolonged starvation or the use of laxatives.

The EDNOS group comprises those who have not yet lost enough weight to meet the criteria, who have been amenorrhoeic for less than three months, who purge but do not binge and who binge but do not purge. The female athlete triad also falls under this category [23].

The Female Athlete Triad

The athlete triad refers to the combination of low energy availability, menstrual dysfunction and low BMD.

Energy restriction in female athletes: This ranges from an inadvertent decrease in energy intake or failure to increase caloric consumption for exercise to pathologic restrictive behaviours in the context of eating disorders. The prevalence of disordered eating ranges from 1% to 62% in female athletes with higher rates in sports reliant on weight categories or lean build (e.g. gymnastics, running, dancing) [24].

Menstrual dysfunction: From delaying the onset of menarche, oligomenorrhoea and amenorrhoea, exercise can impact menstrual function in several ways. These disorders occur in 12% to 79% of female athletes and are more prevalent in lean sports [25].

Low BMD: This ranges from optimal bone health to osteoporosis. The International Society for Clinical Densitometry recommends that BMD in children and premenopausal women be expressed as Z-scores. A Z-score below -2.0 is termed low bone density for chronological age. Osteoporosis in children refers to the presence of both a fracture history and low BMD.

Low energy availability and hypo-oestrogenism have independent and cumulative effects on bone health. It was previously thought that low BMD was solely a function of hypo-oestrogenism, but weight gain has been reported to have favourable effects of BMD, whereas lack of complete recovery of BMD with oral contraceptive pills in patients with AN or exercise-induced amenorrhoea suggests that oestrogen levels are not the only factor involved in the maintenance of BMD [26].

Management of eating disorders and the female athlete triad is multidisciplinary and should involve a physician, dietician and, if an eating disorder is present, a mental health professional. Treatment should aim for nutritional recovery, which offers the best response in terms of BMD and the metabolic abnormalities seen in these patients [27]. Nutritional rehabilitation is associated with restoration of menses at weights approximately 90% of the median for age and height [28].

The mainstays of treatment are nutritional therapy, psychological therapy including psychotherapy, cognitive behavioural therapy and family therapy which have been shown to be of benefit [29].

Pharmacological therapy may include antidepressants and anxiolytics [29]. Calcium and vitamin D supplements may be necessary [30]. The oral contraceptive pill, in the absence of nutritional recovery, has not had consistent efficacy in reversing low BMD and may provide false reassurance while the underlying problem of energy deficit continues to undermine skeletal health. Exogenous hormone-induced monthly bleeding will also obscure resumption of spontaneous menses, an objective indicator of return to biological health.

Due to a lack of safety data in women of reproductive age, bisphosphonates should be avoided [27].

Premature Ovarian Insufficiency

Premature ovarian insufficiency (POI) arises from a predetermined reduced number of ovarian follicles at birth, accelerated follicular atresia or follicular dysfunction [14]. The majority of cases are idiopathic

(90%) but known causes include ovarian injury due to chemotherapy, radiotherapy or surgery, and genetic factors involving the X chromosome. It has also been associated with autoimmune diseases, infections and smoking. In adolescents with POI, a karyotype should be performed to rule out sex chromosome translocation, short arm deletion, X chromosome excess or deficiency or the presence of an occult Y chromosome, which is associated with an increased risk of gonadal tumours. About 16–20% of women who are carriers of the permutation of Fragile X syndrome (FMR1 gene) experience POI and must undergo testing for this permutation [31]. Up to 40% of women with POI have autoimmune abnormalities, usually autoimmune thyroiditis. Approximately 20% have an autoimmune disease such as diabetes, thyroid disease or adrenal disease.

Adolescents with POI have a 5–10% chance of spontaneous conception at some time after diagnosis [32]. Appropriate contraceptive advice must therefore be given to avoid unwanted pregnancy. Referral to a reproductive medicine clinic for counselling regarding fertility options is also appropriate. This would usually involve donor egg in vitro fertilization and embryo transfer.

Oestrogen deficiency should be corrected to avoid symptoms including vasomotor symptoms, atrophic vaginitis and dyspareunia. These women are also at risk of osteoporosis and cardiovascular disease. Adolescents with POI should be given appropriate counselling prior to starting oestrogen replacement therapy.

The three management issues in adolescents with this condition are the effect of the diagnosis on the psychological health of the patient, the consequent fertility issues and the short- and long-term effects of oestrogen deficiency. Adolescents and their parents may experience a sense of helplessness, anger, sadness and guilt which may also give rise to a negative impact on body image and perception of femininity. Evaluation by a psychologist is important to evaluate levels of depression, anxiety and coping mechanisms.

Contraception in Adolescents

Hormonal contraceptives are prescribed to adolescents for a range of indications including contraception, dysmenorrhoea, endometriosis, ovarian cyst suppression, polycystic ovarian syndrome, dysfunctional uterine bleeding and hormone replacement therapy for POI.

A working knowledge of contraception is therefore essential in dealing with adolescents in gynaecology. Best practice in adolescent anticipatory guidance and screening include a sexual health history, screening for pregnancy and sexually transmitted infections, counselling and, if indicated, providing access to contraceptives [33].

The 2008 WHO Consensus statement on Sexual health in Young People noted that 'responsible adolescent intimate relationships' should be 'consensual, non-exploitative, honest, pleasurable and protected against unintended pregnancy and STDs if any type of intercourse occurs' [34].

The decision to embark upon sexual activity is a positive choice for most adolescents, but may for some be associated with issues of regret, particularly with the co-use of alcohol.

Sexual Competence and the Law Relating to Adolescent Sexual Activity:

The age for consent for sexual activity in the United Kingdom is 16 years. Research indicates that the median age for coitarche is 16 years – so quite a few adolescents are sexually active before the age of 16. The Sexual Offences Act 2003, England and Wales, brought together all laws designed to protect persons under 16 years of age from sexual abuse. This law is not intended to prosecute mutually agreed sexual activity between two adolescents of a similar age, unless it involves abuse or exploitation [35].

In England, Wales and Northern Ireland, young people can access contraception at any age if they are deemed to be 'Fraser Competent' according to Fraser Guidelines.

Fraser Guidelines

These are guidelines set out by Lord Fraser (House of Lords 1985). They relate specifically to health professionals giving contraceptive advice to a young person (YP) and allow advice and treatment without parental consent (see Table 11.1).

Treatment relating to sexual health can be undertaken without the knowledge or consent of an adult with parental responsibility, although their involvement should be encouraged. Children and young people have the same rights to confidentiality as other patients and this should be broken only if there are concerns that they or someone else is being harmed, or at risk of being harmed.

Table 11.1 Fraser Guidelines (YP = Young Person)

Fraser Guidelines
The YP understands the professional's advice.
The YP cannot be persuaded to inform their parents, with or without involving a doctor's help.
The YP is likely to begin or continue having sexual intercourse with or without contraceptive treatment.
Unless the YP receives contraceptive treatment, their physical or mental health, or both, are likely to suffer.
The YP's best interests require them to receive contraceptive advice or treatment with or without parental consent.

Any interaction with an adolescent patient is an opportunity to assess their risk for pregnancy. To encourage honest disclosure of sexual activity, it is essential that the adolescent is given an opportunity to see the clinician alone, without a parent or carer present. In the context of a psychosocial assessment, determine pregnancy risk and ascertain if any steps are being taken to avoid pregnancy. Assess satisfaction with their current method of contraception, if relevant, and any barriers they are experiencing to method use. The adolescent should be encouraged to choose an effective method of pregnancy and sexually transmitted infection risk reduction and empower them to follow through on their method of choice [36].

The methods of contraception suitable for adolescents are identical to those for adult women. Careful consideration should, however, be taken before use of Depot Medroxyprogesterone Acetate (DMPA) in adolescents, particularly in young women below the age of 18 years who may not have attained their peak bone mass, due to the risk of reduction of BMD with DMPA [37].

Sexual Abuse

Child sexual abuse is defined by the WHO as

> the involvement of a child in sexual activity that he or she does not fully comprehend, is unable to give informed consent to, or for which the child is not developmentally prepared and cannot give consent, or that violates the laws or social taboos of society. Child sexual abuse is evidenced by this activity between a child and an adult or another child who by age or development is in a relationship of responsibility, trust or power, the activity being intended to gratify or satisfy the needs of the other person [38].

Measurement of sexual abuse relies on retrospective self-report studies of episodes that are recalled years later by adolescents or adults. Between 5% and 10% of girls are exposed to penetrative sexual abuse during childhood, although figures that include any form of sexual abuse are much higher.

Assessment of children when there are concerns about sexual abuse requires particular expertise and is usually done in specialist centres – SARCs in the United Kingdom, child advocacy centres in the United States and child houses in Europe. It is important to note that as many as 96% of children assessed for suspected sexual abuse will have normal genital and anal examinations. A forensic interview by a trained professional, ideally a forensically trained child psychologist, must be relied on to document suspicion of abuse.

Avoidance of re-traumatization is a key principle when assessing children after suspected sexual abuse.

Many sexually abused children are also maltreated in other ways – physical and emotional abuse and/or neglect – and it is difficult to separate out the short- and long-term consequences specific to sexual abuse. Maltreatment in childhood has adverse outcomes in relation to education, mental health, physical health and violence or criminal behaviour with a substantial burden on the abused individual and on society. [39].

Transition and the Transfer to Adult Care

Transfer is the organizational shift from children's to adult healthcare and occurs for those initially seen in paediatrics. Transition is the purposeful, planned process that addresses the medical, psychosocial, educational and vocational needs of young people, as they grow up learning to live with their long-term health condition [40]. As well as those moving from child to adult services, children and young people with childhood-onset gynaecological conditions who have always received care from an adult clinician can also expect to receive 'transitional healthcare' that promotes their biopsychosocial development.

Table 11.2 Key recommendations of good practice for transition and transfer

Transition and Transfer	A care plan identifying the impact of health issues on their goals and setting out the support they require to meet these goals, from age 14
	Transition checklists can be a helpful way for identifying the young person's healthcare goals
	Routine copying of clinic letters to the young person, to help engage them in the planning process
	Involving the GP/primary care physician in planning
	Identify a coordinator within the current healthcare team in liaison with the family, to oversee the transfer of a YP with complex health needs who might be moving to multiple adult healthcare providers
	Agreeing a pathway between teams where a number of young people with the same or similar health needs move to adult services, with a clear demarcation of clinical accountability and service responsibilities
	YP should receive a detailed outline of the service(s) they will be transferring to prior to the move, and a multidisciplinary summary of the patient history should be completed and appropriately disseminated
	A clear administrative process to ensure successful transfer of patient information and to see that the YP receives their first appointment in the adult service in a timely manner

Research examines transition in health conditions such as diabetes [6] and rheumatology [41]. There are very few studies in gynaecology but the issues mirror those from other areas. For example, a review of existing studies of young people with Turner syndrome found that loss to follow-up in young adulthood was a significant issue [42]. Findings from existing research highlight the importance of attending to the impact of health upon developmental goals and needs rather than the specifics of each diagnosis, so the recommendations apply equally to this field. Recent national UK guidance is also timely and relevant [43] (Table 11.2).

As already stated, because of the current lack of focus on young people within most health professional training programmes, all clinicians working with young people will likely require further training. Mandatory safeguarding training and a working knowledge of legislation around privacy, young people's rights and confidentiality are key. The National Child and Maternal Health Intelligence Network (Public Health England) provides a useful overview of adolescent health and health transfer resources, including multidisciplinary and international online training programmes [44].

Conclusion

Gynaecological conditions in childhood and adolescence have the potential to impact upon physical well-being, social functioning, the achievement of developmental milestones such as achieving independence and developing and maintaining friendships and intimate relationships. These issues then impact upon emotional well-being and coping, and a significant issue for young people is feeling 'different' when comparing themselves to their well peers. This can impact upon a young person's developing sense of self and their esteem [45,46].

The available studies of psychological factors in adult gynaecology suggest that emotional and social issues can worsen functional impairment associated with gynaecological conditions [47]. Studies of the impacts upon children and young people with gynaecological issues is lacking and more needs to be examined about the specific treatment modalities that could be useful.

In terms of future practice, it is suggested that an integrated, multidisciplinary team approach should be fostered [47,48]. The team should include doctors, specialist nurses, a psychologist and access to other therapists, such as physiotherapists, and inclusive multidisciplinary clinics and case meetings, where psychosocial impacts are openly considered as part of management planning, are key. Direct therapeutic work could be provided by a psychologist working as part of the multidisciplinary team, and liaison and consultation with other services, such as education and voluntary agencies, could be useful, to build holistic networks of support around the family. As well as good medical and surgical practice, other key issues for the multidisciplinary team include:

- Clear information and education, as appropriate to stage of development and intellectual understanding, with frequent opportunities to revisit their understanding and health education requirements.

- Monitoring adjustment to diagnosis and coping with assessment and treatment procedures.
- Expecting anxiety to be an issue and being open to asking questions, acknowledging their concerns and offering additional discussion and support when needed.
- Considering emotional and social functioning, including impact upon self-identity and self-esteem, intimate relationships and sexual functioning.
- Asking about parental adjustment and family functioning and the need for support.
- Offering holistic pain management approaches.

Given the division of healthcare into child and adult provision, all healthcare staff working with children and young people are likely to require additional further training, to equip them with the knowledge and skills as outlined in this chapter.

Key Points

- Conditions presenting in paediatric and adolescent gynaecology (PAG) can be subdivided into general PAG, disorders of puberty and adolescence and developmental abnormalities.
- Key communication skills enable dialectical, rather than didactic, discussion with children and young people presenting in gynaecology. The child or young person has to remain central to the consultation.
- Lichen sclerosus lesions may mimic the findings of sexual abuse.
- Examination of a child when there is a disclosure or concern about sexual abuse is a specialized area and the local Sexual Assault Referral Centre or specialist service should be contacted.
- Avoidance of re-traumatization is a key principle when assessing children after suspected sexual abuse.
- Dysmenorrhoea may impact more upon physical functioning and school attendance and amenorrhoea more upon psychosocial functioning, but very little has been studied about psychosocial functioning in young people with menstrual problems and more research is needed.

- Very early puberty in girls has been associated with depressive disorders, eating disorders, advanced sexual activity and risk-taking, disruptive behaviour disorders and comorbid depression and substance disorders.
- The presenting symptom of eating disorders may be menstrual irregularity and therefore may present to the gynaecologist.
- Any interaction with an adolescent patient is an opportunity to assess their risk for pregnancy. To encourage honest disclosure of sexual activity, it is essential that the adolescent is given an opportunity to see the clinician alone, without a parent or carer present.
- Adolescents with premature ovarian failure and their parents may experience a sense of helplessness, anger, sadness and guilt which may also give rise to a negative impact on body image and perception of femininity. Evaluation by a psychologist is important to evaluate levels of depression, anxiety and coping mechanisms.
- Children and young people have the same rights to confidentiality as other patients, and this should be broken only if there are concerns that they or someone else is being harmed, or at risk of being harmed.
- Fraser Guidelines give invaluable advice for contraceptive provision in younger girls.

References

1. Department of Health, London. You're welcome: Quality criteria for young people friendly health services. www.gov.uk/government/publications/quality-criteria-for-young-people-friendly-health-services. Accessed 22 March 2017.
2. Westwood K, Irani S. What's coming through the front door? Paediatric and adolescent gynaecology in the emergency department. *Emergency Medicine Journal.* 2014; **31**(9):790.
3. Roisman G, Masten AS, Coatsworth JD, Tellegen A. Salient and emerging developmental tasks in the transition to adulthood. *Child Development.* 2004;**75**(1):123–133.
4. Colver A, Longwell S. New understanding of adolescent brain development: Relevance to transitional healthcare for young people with long term conditions. *Arch Dis Child.* 2013 November;**98**(11):902–907.
5. Lockwood G, Cooklin A, Ramsden S. Communicating a diagnosis. In Balen AH, Creighton SM, Davies

MC, MacDougall J, Stanhope R, eds. *Paediatric and Adolescent Gynaecology*. Cambridge: Cambridge University Press.2004; 193–204.

6. Dovey-Pearce G, Hurrell R, May C, Walker C, Doherty Y. Young adults' suggestions for providing developmentally-appropriate diabetes services: A qualitative study. *Health Soc Care Community* 2005 Sep;13(5):409–19.

7. Genital Examinations in Girls and Young Women: A Clinical Practice Guideline Royal Australasian College of Physicians, August 2009.

8. Garden AS, Vulvovaginitis and other common childhood gynaecological conditions *Arch Dis Child Educ Pract Ed* 2011;96:73–78.

9. Maronn ML, Esterly, NB. Constipation as a feature of anogenital lichen sclerosus in children. *Pediatrics*. 2005 Feb;115(2):e230–2.

10. Merritt DF. Genital trauma in the pediatric and adolescent female. *Obstet Gynecol Clin North Am*. 2009;36:85–98.

11. Fuqua JS. Treatment and outcomes of precocious puberty: An update. *J Clin Endocrinol Metab*. 2013;98:2198–2207.

12. Johansson T, Ritzén E. Very long-term follow-up of girls with early and late menarche, abnormalities in puberty: Scientific and clinical advances. *Endocr Dev. Basel, Karger*. 2005;8:126–136.

13. Peacock A, Alvi NS, Mushtaq T. Period problems: Disorders of menstruation in adolescents. *Arch Dis Child*. 2012;97:554–560.

14. Deligeoroglou E, Tsimaris P. Menstrual disturbances in puberty. *Best Prac Res Clin Obstet Gynaecol*. 2010;24:157–171.

15. Nur Azurah AG, Sanci L, Moore E, Grover S. The quality of life of adolescents with menstrual problems. *J Pediatr Adolesc Gynecol*. 2013; 26:102–108.

16. Knox B, Nur Azurah AG, Grover S. Quality of life and menstruation in adolescents. *Curr Opin Obstet Gynecol*. 2015;27:309–314.

17. Quint EH. Menstrual and reproductive issues in adolescents with physical and developmental disabilities. *Obstet Gynecol*. 2014;124:367–375.

18. Kirkham YA, Allen L, Kives S, et al. Trends in menstrual concerns and suppression in adolescents with developmental disabilities. *J Adolesc Health*. 2013;53:407–412.

19. Albanese A, Hopper NW. Suppression of menstruation in adolescents with severe learning disabilities. *Arch Dis Child*. 2007;92:629–632.

20. Ruuska J, Kaltiala-Heino R, Koivisto A, Rantanen P. Puberty, sexual development and eating disorders in adolescent outpatients. *Eur Child Adolesc Psychiatry* 2005 Aug;14(5):276–81.

21. Hindler CG, Crisp AH, McGuigan S, Joughin N. Anorexia nervosa: Change over time in age of onset, presentation and duration of illness. *Psychological medicine*. 1994;24:719–729.

22. Graber JA. Pubertal timing and the development of psychopathology in adolescence and beyond. *Hormones and Behavior*. 2013;64:262–269.

23. Golden NH. Eating disorders in adolescence: what is the role of hormone replacement therapy? *Curr Opin Obstet Gynecol*. 19(5):434–439.

24. Javed A, Tebben PJ, Fischer PR, Lteif AN. Female Athletic Triad and Its Components: Toward Improved Screening and Management. *Mayo Clin Proc*. 2013;88:996–1009.

25. Carlberg KA, Buckman MT, Peake GT, Riedesel ML. A survey of menstrual function in athletes. *Eur J Appl Physiol*. 1983;51:211–222.

26. Otis CL, Drinkwater B, Johnson M, Loucks A, Wilmore J. American college of sports medicine position stand: The female athletic triad. *Med Sci Sports Exerc*. 2007;39:1867–1882.

27. Fenichel RM, Warren MD. Anorexia, bulimia, and the athletic triad: Evaluation and management. *Current Osteoporosis Reports*. 2007;5:160–164.

28. Golden NH, Jacobson MS, Schebendach J, et al. Resumption of menses in anorexia nervosa. *Arch Pediatr Adolesc Med*. 1997;151:16–21.

29. Nattiv A, Loucks AB, Manore MM, et al. American college of sports medicine position stand: The female athlete triad. *Med Sci Sports Excer*. 2007;39:1867–1882.

30. Holick MF, Binkley NC, Bischoff-Ferrari HA, et al. Endocrine society: Evaluation, treatment and prevention of vitamin D deficiency: An endocrine society clinical practice guideline. *J Clin Endocrinol Metab*. 2011;96:1911–1930.

31. Nelson LM. Primary ovarian insufficiency. *N Engl J Med*. 2009;360:606–614.

32. Kalantaridou SN, Nelson LM. Premature ovarian failure is not premature menopause. *Ann N Y Acad Sci*. 2000;900:393–402.

33. Ott MA, Sucato GS. Committee on adolescence. *Contraception for adolescents. Pediatrics*. 2014;134 (4):1257–1281.

34. WHO statement on Sexual health in Young People. www.who.int/topics/sexual_health/en/. Accessed 22 March 2017.

35. www.legislation.gov.uk/ukpga/192003/42/contents.

36. Hartman LB, Monasterio MN, Hwang LY. Adolescent contraception: Review and guidance for pediatric clinicians. *Curr Probl Pediatr Adolesc Health Care.* 2012;**42**:221–263.

37. Straw F, Porter C. Sexual health and contraception. *Arch Dis Child Pract Ed.* 2012;**97**:177–184.

38. Guidelines for medico-legal care for victims of sexual violence, Chapter 7, Child Sexual Abuse, WHO, 2003 www.who.int/violence_injury_prevention/resources/publications/en/guidelines_chap7.pdf. Accessed 22 March 2017.

39. Gilbert R, Wisdom CS, Browne K et al. Burden and consequences of child maltreatment in high-income countries. *Lancet.* 2009;**37**:68–81.

40. Dovey-Pearce G, Christie D. Transition in diabetes: Young people move on – we should too. *Paediatrics and Child Health.* 2013;**23**:174–179.

41. McDonagh JE, Southwood TR, Shaw KL. The impact of a coordinated transitional care programme on adolescents with juvenile idiopathic arthritis. *Rheumatology.* 2007;**46**:161–168.

42. Davies MC. Lost in transition: The needs of adolescents with Turner syndrome. *BJOG.* 2010;**117**:134–136.

43. Transition from children's to adults' services for young people using health or social care services NICE guideline. Published: 24 February 2016. www.nice.org.uk/guidance/ng43. Accessed 22 March 2017.

44. Child and Maternal Health (CHIMAT) Intelligence Network: Knowledge hub – transitions to adulthood www.chimat.org.uk/transitions. Accessed 22 March 2017.

45. Charmaz, K. The self as habit: The reconstruction of self in chronic illness. *Occupational Therapy Journal of Research.* 2002;**22**(Suppl.):31s–41s.

46. Dovey-Pearce G, Doherty Y, May C. The influence of diabetes upon adolescent and young adult development: A qualitative study. *British Journal of Health Psychology.* 2007;**12**:75–91.

47. Bryant C, Kleinstauber M, Judd F. Aspects of mental health care in the gynaecological setting. Womens Health (Lond). 2014;**10**(3):237–254.

48. Creighton SM, Wood D. Complex gynaecological and urological problems in adolescents: Challenges and transition. *Postgraduate Medical Journal.* 2013;**89**:34–38.

Biopsychosocial Factors in Premenstrual Syndrome

Deepthi Lavu, Suman Kadian and P. M. Shaughn O'Brien

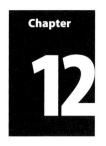

Premenstrual syndrome (PMS) is a psychological and somatic disorder which affects millions of women and their families by having a major impact on their social, occupational, academic and psychological lives [1]. Forty percent of women experience symptoms of PMS and 5%–8% suffer from severe PMS [2]. In order to differentiate physiological premenstrual symptoms from PMS, the symptoms must cause significant impairment to the individual during the luteal phase of the menstrual cycle [3]. These disorders which last from menarche to menopause did not have a clear consensus of definitive diagnostic criteria between authoritative bodies until the recent publication of the International Society for Premenstrual Disorders (ISPMD) classification. This classification now enables provision of accurate diagnosis and effective management of these disorders alongside allowing accurate epidemiological data collection [4]. The aetiology of premenstrual disorders is unknown but the symptoms are clearly related to ovulation as premenstrual disorders are not experienced before menarche, during pregnancy or post menopause. Ovarian steroids, oestrogen and progesterone, and dysfunction of neurotransmitters serotonin and gamma aminobutyric acid (GABA) are implicated in the causality of the symptoms [5]. There also appears to be a genetic link for PMS risk [6]. Licenced treatments for this condition are usually ineffective, although good effect has been achieved by the use of unlicensed approaches [7, 8, 9].

Types of Symptoms

PMS is marked by a variety of emotional, physical and behavioural symptoms, with more than 200 reported symptoms. Some of the characteristic symptoms are as follows:

Physical Symptoms

Joint pain, muscle pain, back pain
Breast tenderness or pain
Abdominal swelling or bloating
Headaches
Skin disorders
Weight gain
Swelling of extremities (hands or feet, or both)

Psychological and Behavioural Symptoms

Changes in appetite or specific food cravings
Lethargy and fatigue
Mood swings (feeling suddenly sad or crying, increased sensitivity to rejection)
Irritability
Anger
Sleep disturbances
Restlessness
Poor concentration
Social withdrawal
Not in control
Lack of interest in usual activities
Loneliness
Anxiety
Depression
Confusion
Tension
Hopelessness
Suicidal thoughts or attempts

The symptoms may be predominantly physical, predominantly psychological or both. Women with a severe form of PMS, previously known as late luteal phase dysphoric disorder, will also fulfil American Psychiatric Association's (APA) psychiatric diagnostic criteria for premenstrual dysphoric disorder (PMDD) mentioned in the Diagnostic and Statistical Manual of Mental Disorders (DSM-5) [10, 11, 12]. Severely affected women who do not fit the criteria are not eligible for treatment or reimbursement in the United States [13]. The Royal College of Obstetricians and Gynaecologists (RCOG) has relatively strict criteria but WHO in ICD-10 and the American Congress of Obstetricians and Gynaecologists (ACOG) have more liberal criteria for the diagnosis of PMS [5, 14].

Comorbidity with Other Psychiatric Conditions

Mood and anxiety disorders are prevalent in women and peak during the reproductive years [15]. Hence there is a high likelihood of comorbidity because of the frequency of mood and anxiety disorders. There is a high rate of major depressive disorder (MDD) in women and this increases the likelihood that women with MDD will have premenstrual disorders. High rates of comorbidity between premenstrual disorders and MDD have been documented by a number of groups [16]. The relationship between bipolar disorder and premenstrual disorders is not clear. Women with premenstrual disorders were found to have three to four times higher rates of obsessive compulsive disorder compared to community women [16]. Over a quarter of women with premenstrual disorders reported panic disorder and generalized anxiety disorder. There may be worsening of schizophrenia in the premenstrual period and isolated psychotic symptoms have been reported in rare instances [16].

Measurement of Symptoms

The method of retrospective diagnosis, with which most women present, was found to be unreliable when compared to a prospective symptom assessment in a large study [17]. There is no objective criterion for diagnosis of PMS and as recommended by the RCOG guidelines, the diagnosis is based on women prospectively recording their symptoms in a symptom diary over two menstrual cycles [5]. The RCOG recommends the use of the daily record of severity of problems (DRSP) tool for recording symptoms. Although the DRSP is easy to use and consistently provides a reliable and reproducible record of symptoms, this method delays diagnosis and the charts' completion and their analysis is laborious [13, 18]. An easy-to-use, commercially available diagnostic mobile phone app, PreMentricS, is now available and is currently being validated. Screening using patient history and questionnaires such as the premenstrual symptom screening tool (PSST) avoid unnecessary data collection from women in whom the diagnosis is unlikely [13, 19]. Treatment should be started only after

completion of symptom diaries for two cycles as the treatment can affect the pattern of symptoms making the charts inconclusive and diagnosis unreliable. GnRH analogues, as an un-validated diagnostic test, may be used if the completed symptom diary is inconclusive.

Diagnosis and Classification of Premenstrual Disorders

Premenstrual disorders (PMDs) were classified into Core PMD and Variant PMD by the ISPMD classification [4] (see Figure 12.1).

Core Premenstrual Disorder

Core premenstrual disorder is diagnosed based on criteria defined by the ISPMD [4]. Core PMD is precipitated by ovulation and women should have spontaneous ovulatory menstrual cycles, although ovulation does not have to be confirmed. Any number of symptoms can be present and although typical symptoms exist, the symptoms and the number are not defined. The timing of the symptoms is the key characteristic. Symptoms recur in the luteal phase and disappear by the end of menstruation, although persistence of symptoms during menstruation does not preclude the diagnosis. A clear symptom-free week should occur between menstruation and ovulation. Symptoms must be prospectively rated for two cycles and if there is any discrepancy between the two cycles then a third cycle should be rated [20]. Symptoms are not an exacerbation of an underlying psychological or physical disorder and must cause substantial impairment. The severity or impact of symptoms must (a) affect normal daily functioning (b) interfere with work, school performance or interpersonal relationships or (c) cause significant distress [4].

Variant Premenstrual Disorder

Variants of the core premenstrual disorder which do not meet the core premenstrual disorder criteria and have more complex features include the following [4]:

Premenstrual Exacerbation of an Underlying Psychological, Somatic or Medical Condition [21]

Such as depression, diabetes, migraines, epilepsy and asthma. Symptoms relevant to these conditions are

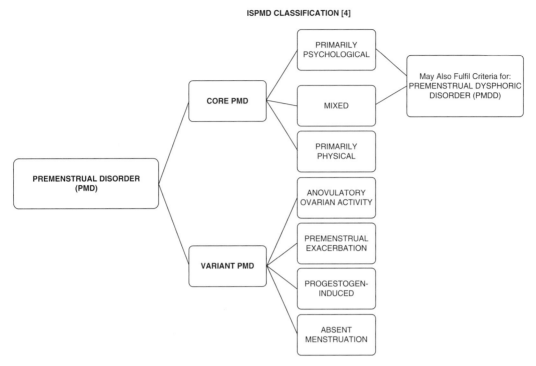

Figure 12.1

experienced throughout the menstrual cycle with exacerbation of the symptoms in the luteal phase of the cycle followed by a reduction of symptoms following menstruation.

Premenstrual Symptoms in the Absence of Menstruation

Seen in women after hysterectomy with ovarian conservation, endometrial ablation or with a levonorgestrel intrauterine system.

Progestogen-Induced Premenstrual Syndrome

Occurs during exogenous progestogen administration (cyclical hormone replacement therapy [HRT], hormonal contraception). Exogenous progesterone reintroduces symptoms in women who are sensitive to progesterone.

Non-Ovulatory Premenstrual Disorders

Symptoms are thought to be caused by unspecified non-ovulatory ovarian activity. Follicular activity of the ovary is thought to be the cause of the symptoms and is poorly understood due to lack of evidence.

Management of Premenstrual Disorders

While it seems obvious that PMD is related to ovulation, the presentation and severity of symptoms in individual women are varied and hence the management needs to be tailored to each individual. For the management plan to be successful it is crucial to ensure that the diagnosis and classification are correct. This would need a proper history of the symptoms, their duration and severity along with any treatments that may have been tried in the past along with their outcomes. The patient's lifestyle and wishes would also have a bearing on any treatment offered. Pregnancy and contraceptive needs should be considered as well. Given the impact of premenstrual disorders on a patient's psychological well-being, it is extremely important that they are involved in the decision making regarding the treatment. This not only enhances their understanding of the situation but also ensures greater compliance with the treatment. For women suffering from long-term severe symptoms an ideal set-up should include a multidisciplinary team which includes their general

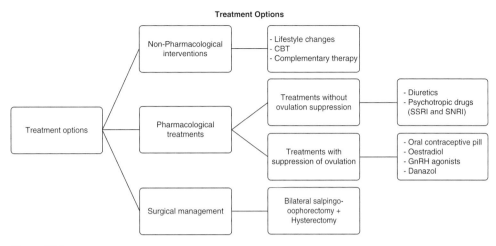

Treatment Options

Figure 12.2

practitioner, gynaecologist, psychiatrist or psychological counsellor, but this is not always possible particularly in the National Health Service.

The treatment options are broadly divided into non-surgical and surgical methods. Figure 12.2 summarizes the treatment options.

Non-Surgical Treatment

Lifestyle Changes and Education about PMD

Changes to one's lifestyle and education regarding PMD may not necessarily resolve the symptoms but often help the patient develop a better understanding of their symptoms. Regular exercise would improve general health, while knowledge of relaxation techniques may help the patient cope with the symptoms of stress better [13]. Stress reduction, improved self-care along with dietary changes and regular exercise are the first-line approach to management of premenstrual disorders and are usually recommended by the general practitioners before referral to the gynaecologists [5]. There are limitations to any science backing up these recommendations.

Complementary Therapy

Though the evidence to support the success of complementary therapy is not very robust, it is felt that a holistic approach towards treatment with the inclusion of some complementary and alternative therapies may yield good results for many women [22].

This is of particular importance to women in whom other forms of treatment like hormonal therapy or surgery may be undesirable or contraindicated.

Women should be informed of the possible treatment options after appraisal of the available evidence. Agnus castus has been used for quite a while and appears to have good-quality evidence to support its use [5]. Patients should be warned not to simultaneously take selective serotonin reuptake inhibitors (SSRIs) when using it. Other options include vitamin D or calcium supplementation [23]. Reflexology and acupuncture have also shown promise in some trials [24, 25]. Magnesium oxide, ginkgo biloba, pollen extract and isoflavones have also been explored for the management of premenstrual disorders but with limited scientific support [5].

Cognitive Behavioural Therapy

Cognitive behavioural therapy (CBT) when used by itself or in conjunction with fluoxetine has been shown to be quite effective especially in women with severe symptoms [26]. The study by Hunter et al. proposes a minimum of ten sessions and fluoxetine may be added if required. Delivery of this treatment would require expertise of a clinical psychologist. Women treated by CBT may avoid medication completely, thereby avoiding the adverse effects associated with them.

Non-Hormonal Treatment

Non-hormonal treatment includes diuretics, psychotropic drugs and anxiolytics. While there are several psychotropic and anxiolytic drugs in use, the only diuretic which has shown benefit is spironolactone. The commonly used SSRIs are fluoxetine, paroxetine, citalopram and sertraline. Venlafaxine, a serotonin and norepinephrine reuptake inhibitor (SNRI), is very effective, and the anxiolytics in use are alprazolam and buspirone [13].

SSRIs and SNRIs lead to a significant improvement in psychological symptoms and are used in lower starting doses compared to when used for depressive illnesses. These medications can be used either continuously or intermittently in the luteal phase of the cycle. The reported adverse effects of SSRIs are much less common with the lower doses and can be further reduced with intermittent use [27]. Using them this way does not appear to diminish their effectiveness in any way.

While the psychotropic drugs do not interact with oral contraceptives, they should be stopped if a pregnancy is being planned as there is some evidence to suggest that they may cause congenital cardiac septal defects [28]. Though the overall risk of congenital anomalies is extremely low, it is recommended that they be stopped pre-conceptually or if the pregnancy is unexpected, they be stopped after the first missed period.

Hormone Therapy

Suppression of ovulation by using hormones is an often-used effective form of treatment for management of PMD. Whilst GnRH agonists and danazol are also used, the mainstay of hormonal treatment has been oestrogen (combined oral contraceptive pill and non-contraceptive oestradiol).

Combined Oral Contraceptive Pills

Combined oral contraceptive pills (COCPs) have been used effectively to treat premenstrual disorders for a long time. However, some types of progestogen used in the COCPs, especially the older COCP agents, can reintroduce symptoms of premenstrual disorder in many women. The most commonly used progestogens are norethisterone, medroxyprogesterone acetate and levonorgestrel. There is evidence to suggest that the use of oral progestogens can often bring back the symptoms [8]. This limitation has been overcome to an extent with the newer preparations of COCP in which ethinylestradiol has been combined with spironolactone-derived drospirenone which is an anti-androgenic progestogen and anti-mineralocorticoid.

A recent Cochrane review showed ethinylestradiol to be effective when combined with drospirenone in resolving the symptoms of severe premenstrual disorders and is licensed in the United States for PMDD in women requiring oral contraception [29].

Combined contraceptive pills can be used in two regimens [30]. One regimen proposes using the combination for 24 days followed by 4 days of placebo. The dose of ethinylestradiol in this regimen is 20 mcg. A higher-dose regimen involves a 30-mcg ethinylestradiol and is taken in standard form with 21 days of medication followed by 7 days of placebo. The dose of drospirenone stays the same at 3 mg. The usage may be limited by adverse effects such as nausea, breast pain and breakthrough bleeding (more common with lower-dose oestrogen preparations as noted in the Cochrane review) [29]. There are data to suggest that using COCP continuously instead of cyclically brings more symptom relief in premenstrual disorders [31].

Oestradiol

Oestradiol is a very effective treatment, and women who have had hysterectomy can use it alone in the form of transdermal subcutaneous patches, implants or gel. Women who have their uterus in situ will require endometrial protection, by using progestogen, if oestrogen is being administered. The levonorgestrel intrauterine system (LNG-IUS) provides this protection without inducing (usually) progestogen-related return of premenstrual symptoms, which are likely if oral agents are used. Vaginal progesterone preparations which avoid hepatic first pass metabolism could also be better tolerated. Women should be advised that they may experience PMS type of symptoms initially when they have the LNG-IUS due to low-dose systemic absorption of progestogen [5]. Women who are extremely sensitive to progesterone may continue to experience symptoms even later due to the low doses of progestogen released by LNG-IUS. In these women natural or micronized progesterone may be tried as these may be better at avoiding progestogen-induced symptoms of premenstrual disorder [32].

The RCOG recommends that 'when treating women with percutaneous estradiol, a cyclical 12 day course of an oral progestogen or long-term progestogen with the levonorgestrel intrauterine system should be used for the prevention of endometrial hyperplasia'. Further it recommends that the LNG–IUS should be used as first line to minimise side effects. It has the additional benefit of providing contraception for women who require it. Six monthly scans to assess endometrial thickness would be advisable for women taking very low doses of oral progestogens. [5]

GnRH Agonists

GnRH analogues are highly effective in resolving symptoms of premenstrual disorders. They suppress production of ovarian steroids and bring significant relief. Their use, however, is restricted to women with severe symptoms. Long-term use (over six months) should be supplemented with – add-back HRT, as GnRH agonists work by inducing a 'medical menopause' and women may be at risk of osteoporosis in addition to suffering from menopausal symptoms like hot flushes, night sweats, nausea, mood swings, etc. which can be very disturbing. Tibolone is the most common agent used for 'add-back' HRT [33].

Danazol

Danazol is another effective treatment for PMS. Its use is restricted by its adverse effect profile caused by its irreversible androgenic properties. These include signs of virilisation like growth of excess facial and body hair, masculine voice, acne, etc. Additional contraception is advised as danazol has adverse effects on the fetus. In low-dose luteal phase administration it is effective for relief from mastalgia but has no effect on other PMS symptoms [34].

Surgery

Surgical removal of the uterus and ovaries is a reasonable option in women with severe premenstrual symptoms, where medical suppression of ovulation has brought relief in symptoms and they wish to avoid taking long-term medication especially in the form of GnRH analogues. It is the last resort in cases where medication has failed, but more acceptable where other gynaecological indications for surgery exist. A trial of GnRH is advisable if planning on surgery [13]. Surgery is not without risks and women need to be counselled regarding the surgical risks and the problems associated with induction of early menopause by this method. The latter is of major concern as women less than 50 years of age will need long-term HRT to counter the problems caused by early loss of ovarian hormones. Most women who have reached this stage of treatment will be women who are sensitive to progestogens and hysterectomy should always be considered as progestogens would otherwise be needed to counter the effects of unopposed oestrogens on the

endometrium when administering HRT, and this in turn could lead to return of symptoms [35]. Women should be made aware of possibility of loss of libido following oophorectomy. Testosterone supplements can be used to treat this problem; however, some women may not tolerate the androgenic side effects that may develop with long-term use [36].

Conclusion

Premenstrual disorders can cause substantial impairment of the lives of women and their families by causing significant social, psychological and professional disruption. The wide variety of symptoms and their varied severity cause a challenge in correct diagnosis and effective management. As the aetiology is not well defined the treatment of the condition is complex. A multidisciplinary team approach is ideal in the management of these cases. A combination of lifestyle changes alongside medical management may be effective in most cases, with surgical methods being reserved for severe premenstrual disorders. Whilst advances in electronic symptom scoring and diagnosis are being made, further research into validation of electronic diagnosis and the aetiology of premenstrual disorders is required for effective diagnosis and management of this complex condition.

Key Points

- Premenstrual syndrome is marked by a variety of emotional, physical and behavioural symptoms, with more than 200 reported symptoms.
- The International Society for Premenstrual Disorders (ISPMD) classification broadly divided the disorders into core premenstrual disorder and variant premenstrual disorders based on prospective symptom charting by women.
- The aetiology of premenstrual disorders is unknown but the symptoms are clearly related to ovulation.
- The diagnosis is based on women prospectively recording their symptoms in a symptom diary over two menstrual cycles. This could be done by means of the daily record of severity of problems (DRSP) tool or a commercially available diagnostic mobile phone app, PreMentricS.

- There is a high likelihood of comorbidity with other psychiatric conditions.
- As the presentation and severity of symptoms in individual women are varied, the management needs to be tailored to each individual. A multidisciplinary team approach is ideal.
- The treatment options are broadly divided into non-surgical (e.g. hormones, GnRH analogue, complementary therapy, cognitive behavioural therapy) and surgical (hysterectomy + bilateral oophorectomy) methods.
- A combination of lifestyle changes alongside medical management may be effective in most cases, with surgical methods being reserved for severe premenstrual disorders.

References

1. Halbreich U, Borenstein J, Pearlstein T, Kahn LS. The prevalence, impairment, impact, and burden of premenstrual dysphoric disorder (PMS/PMDD). *Psychoneuroendocrinology* 2003; **28**: 1–23.

2. Pearlstein T. Prevalence, impact, on morbidity and burden of disease. In: O'Brien PMS, Rapkin A, Schmidt P (eds.) *The Premenstrual Syndromes: PMS and PMDD*. London: Informa Healthcare. 2007; 37–47.

3. Magos AL, Studd JWW. The premenstrual syndrome. In: Studd J (ed.) *Progress in Obstetrics and Gynaecology*, Volume **4**. London: Churchill Livingstone. 1984; 334–50.

4. O'Brien PM, Bäckström T, Brown C, Dennerstein L, Endicott J, Epperson CN, et al. Towards a consensus on diagnostic criteria, measurement and trial design of the premenstrual disorders: The ISPMD Montreal consensus. *Archives of Women's Mental Health* 2011; **14** (1): 13–21.

5. Royal College of Obstetricians and Gynaecologists. *Premenstrual Syndrome. Management. Green-top guideline 48*. 2nd ed. RCOG Press, 2016. www.rcog.org .uk/globalassets/documents/guidelines/gt48manage mentpremensturalsyndrome.pdf. (Accessed 23 March 2017).

6. Gianetto-Berruti A, Feyles V. Premenstrual syndrome. *Minerva Ginecologica* 2002; **54**(2): 85–95.

7. O'Brien S, Ismail K. History of the premenstrual disorders. In: O'Brien PM, Rapkin AJ, Schmidt PJ (eds.). *The Premenstrual Syndromes: PMS and PMDD*. London: Informa Healthcare. 2007.

8. Wyatt K, Dimmock P, Jones P, Obhrai M, O'Brien S. Efficacy of progesterone and progestogens in management of premenstrual syndrome: Systematic review. *BMJ* 2001; **323**: 776.

9. Ford O, Lethaby A, Roberts H, Mol BW. Progesterone for premenstrual syndrome. *Cochrane Database Syst Rev* 2009; **2**: CD003415.

10. Premenstrual dysphoric disorder. In: *Diagnostic and Statistical Manual of Mental Disorders*. 4th ed. Washington, DC: American Psychiatric Press, 2000: 771–74.

11. American Psychiatric Association. *Diagnostic and Statistical Manual of Mental Disorders*. 3rd ed. Washington, DC: 1987.

12. American Psychiatric Association. *Diagnostic and Statistical Manual of Mental Disorders, DSM-5*. 5th ed. Arlington, VA: American Psychiatric Association Publishing: 2013.

13. O'Brien S, Rapkin A, Dennerstein L, Nevatte T. Diagnosis and management of premenstrual syndrome. *BMJ* 2011; **342**: d2994.

14. ACOG practice bulletin: Premenstrual syndrome. *Int J Gynecol Obstet* 2001; **73**: 183–91.

15. Kessler R. Epidemiology of women and depression. *J Affect Disord* 2003; **74**(1): 5–13.

16. Yonkers KA, McCunn KL. Comorbidity of premenstrual syndrome and premenstrual dysphoric disorder with other psychiatric conditions. In: O'Brien PM, Rapkin AJ, Schmidt PJ (eds.) *The Premenstrual Syndromes: PMS and PMDD*. London: Informa Healthcare. 2007.

17. Rapkin AJ, Chang LC, Reading AE. Comparison of retrospective and prospective assessment of premenstrual symptoms. *Psychol Rep* 1988; **62**: 55–60.

18. Endicott J, Nee J, Harrison W. Daily record of severity of problems (DRSP): Reliability and validity. *Archives of women's mental health* 2006; **9**: 41–49.

19. Steiner M, Macdougall M, Brown E. The premenstrual symptoms screening tool (PSST) for clinicians. *Archives of women's mental health* 2003; **6**: 203–9.

20. Nevatte T, O'Brien PMS, Bäckström T, et al. ISPMD consensus on the management of premenstrual disorders. *Archives of women's mental health* 2013; **16** (4): 279–91.

21. Case AM, Reid RL. Effects of the menstrual cycle on medical disorders. *Arch Intern Med* 1998; **158**: 1405–12.

22. Girman A, Lee R, Kligler B. An integrative medicine approach to premenstrual syndrome. *Am J Obstet Gynecol* 2003; **188**(5 suppl): S56–65.

23. Thys-Jacobs S, Starkey P, Bernstein D, Tian J. Calcium carbonate and the premenstrual syndrome: Effects on premenstrual and menstrual symptoms. *Am J Obstet Gynecol* 1998; **179**(2): 444–52.

24. Oleson T, Flocco W. Randomised controlled study of premenstrual symptoms treated with ear; hand and foot reflexology. *Obstet Gynecol* 1993; **82**: 906–11.

25. Sun Y, Guo S. Comparison of therapeutic effects of acupuncture and medicine on premenstrual syndrome. *Chinese Acupunct Moxib* 2004; **24**(1): 29–30.

26. Hunter MS, Ussher JM, Browne SJ, Cariss M, Jelley R, Katz M. A randomized comparison of psychological (cognitive behaviour therapy), medical (fluoxetine) and combined treatment for women with premenstrual dysphoric disorder. *J Psychosom Obstet Gynecol* 2002; **23**: 193–99.

27. Eriksson E, Ekman A, Sinclair S, Sörvik K, Ysander C, Mattson UB, Nissbrandt H. Escitalopram administered in the luteal phase exerts a marked and dose-dependent effect in premenstrual dysphoric disorder. *J Clin Psychopharmacol* 2008 April; **28**(2): 195–202.

28. Pedersen LH, Henriksen TB, Vestergaard M, Olsen J, Bech BH. Selective serotonin reuptake inhibitors in pregnancy and congenital malformations: Population based cohort study. *BMJ* 2009; **339**: b3569.

29. Lopez LM, Kaptein AA, Helmerhorst FM. Oral contraceptives containing drospirenone for premenstrual syndrome. *Cochrane Database of Systematic Reviews* 2012; **2**: CD006586.

30. Pearlstein TB, Bachmann GA, Zacur HA, Yonkers KA. Treatment of premenstrual dysphoric disorder with a new drospirenone-containing oral contraceptive formulation. *Contraception* 2005; **72**: 414–21.

31. Coffee AL, Kuehl TJ, Willis S, Sulak PJ. Oral contraceptives and premenstrual symptoms: Comparison of a 21/7 and extended regimen. *Am J Obstet Gynecol* 2006; **195**: 1311–19.

32. Panay N, Studd JWW. Progestogen intolerance and compliance with hormone replacement therapy in menopausal women. *Hum Reprod Update* 1997; **3**: 159–71.

33. Wyatt KM, Dimmock PW, Ismail KM, O'Brien PMS. The effectiveness of GnRHa with and without 'add-back' therapy in treating premenstrual syndrome: A meta-analysis. *Br J Obstet Gynaecol* 2004; **111**: 585–93.

34. O'Brien PM, Abukhalil IE. Randomized controlled trial of the management of premenstrual syndrome and premenstrual mastalgia using luteal phase-only danazol. *Am J Obstet Gynecol* 1999 January; **180**: 18–23.

35. Cronje WH, Vashisht A, Studd JW. Hysterectomy and bilateral oophorectomy for severe premenstrual syndrome. *Hum Reprod* 2005; **19**: 2125–5.

36. Nappi RE, Wawra K, Schmitt S. Hypoactive sexual desire disorder in postmenopausal women. *Gynecol Endocrinol* 2006; **22**: 318–23.

Chapter 13

Biopsychosocial Factors in Abnormal Uterine Bleeding

Tereza Indrielle-Kelly, Zeiad El Gizawy and P. M. Shaughn O'Brien

Introduction

Abnormal uterine bleeding (see Table 13.1) is defined as any variation in frequency or regularity of menstruation, duration or amount of blood flow [1]. There has been a trend to abandon traditional Greek and Latin terms such as 'menorrhagia' or more technical terminology such as 'dysfunctional uterine bleeding'. The psychosocial research literature still reflects this old classification; hence, for the purpose of this chapter; both new and older terminology will be used. Biopsychosocial research is mostly targeted at the two main menstrual disorders – menorrhagia (heavy menstrual bleeding) and dysmenorrhoea (painful periods).

Menstrual cycle is closely related to various body functions and mechanisms. It is known that malnutrition and obesity can cause disruption to the regularity and length of the cycle. Similar effect can be also seen in women working shifts who tend to report more often irregular periods and prolonged cycle [2]. Some menstrual disorders, mainly the length of the cycle, can be therefore regarded as physiological reaction to other conditions.

Table 13.1 Abnormal uterine bleeding. FIGO 2011

Abnormal uterine bleeding		
Onset	Acute	Episode of bleeding that requires immediate intervention to prevent further blood loss
	Chronic	Abnormal bleeding present for the majority of the last six months
Frequency	Infrequent (old term: *oligomenorrhoea*)	1–2 episodes of bleeding in 90 days
	Frequent (old term: *polymenorrhoea*)	>4 episodes of bleeding in 90 days
Regularity	Irregular	Bleeding-free interval between menses >20 days
	Absent (old: *amenorrhoea*)	No bleeding in 90 day period
Amount of blood flow	Heavy menstrual bleeding (HMB) (old: *menorrhagia*)	Excessive bleeding that interferes with quality of life (NICE)
	Heavy prolonged menstrual bleeding (HPMB)	Excessive menstrual bleeding that interferes with quality of life lasting > 8 days
	Light menstrual bleeding	
Duration of bleeding	Prolonged	Menstrual bleeding > 8 days
	Shortened	Menstrual bleeding no more than 2 days
Irregular non-menstrual bleeding	Intermenstrual	Episode of bleeding occurring between otherwise fairly normal menstrual periods
	Postcoital	Bleeding after intercourse
	Acyclic	Bleeding with no pattern, completely erratic
	Pre-/postmenstrual bleeding or spotting	Light bleeding 1 day or more before or after a recognized menstrual period

Menstrual disorders have always been a major component of referrals from the community. In 1982 gynaecologists in England and Wales performed 44,400 hysterectomies for heavy menstrual bleeding [3]. Nowadays approximately 8,000 women undergo hysterectomy and the majority of them for reasons other than heavy bleeding. This change is due to new conservative treatments that have become available, mainly levonorgestrel – releasing intrauterine device Mirena (used in Europe since 1991, approved by the United States Food and Drug Administration [FDA] in 2000).

Assessment of symptoms has also changed. While in the 1980s it was still recommended to assess blood loss objectively, nowadays the approach is more holistic and looks at the impact the menstrual bleeding has on the quality of life. According to Matteson and Clark (2010) women are not concerned about the amount of bleeding as such but about the inconvenience of menstruation, odour and social embarrassment, mostly related to staining their clothes in public. Women with abnormal uterine bleeding direct their daily activities based on their periods, for example avoiding activities where they cannot get to the bathroom promptly [4].

In the psychosocial literature menstruation was studied as a physiological phenomenon possibly influenced by personality or coping with life events. Sigmund Freud based his theories on male psyche and existence of a penis. Women were therefore regarded as sexually passive and their problems were interpreted through male psychology. Menstrual problems such as dysmenorrhoea were regarded by a young Freud as a possible result of masturbation and together with his friend, surgeon Fliess, suggested treatment through specific types of nasal surgery, as it was believed that the nose was closely connected to the uterus and vagina as it may swell or bleed during menstruation [5].

As psychoanalysis developed and became influenced by female psychologists and feminists, menstruation was no longer regarded as impure or a 'waste of potential pregnancy'. The approach to sexuality and masturbatory practice, however, continued to be of interest throughout the twentieth century (mainly as a secondary focus). It was mostly shown that women with menstrual symptomatology show a more negative attitude towards masturbation and sexual practices in general [6].

At the more scientific level doctors were searching for a link between psyche and body. It was known from times of war that stress can interfere with periods and cause amenorrhoea (war amenorrhoea). Initially the causality was attributed to malnutrition; however, the fact that even female medical staff in hospitals at that time became mostly amenorrhoeic refuted this theory.

Psychological stress was also identified as a possible cause of other menstrual disorders. 'Endocrine balance may become psychically disturbed and thus provide a vicious circle of causation for menorrhagia' [7]. This was the basis for the concept of psychogenic menorrhagia, which appears in the literature from 1930 to the 1960s, which assumed that stress and psychogenic factors increase menstrual bleeding.

Research in the second half of the twentieth century adopted more scientific approaches. Because it was still recommended in the 1980s that bleeding should be assessed objectively, many complaints were regarded as un-evidenced and 'other' reasons for complaints of menstrual problems were sought. Some authors classified menorrhagia as a psychosomatic disorder and researchers were calling for further psychological assessment as many women underwent hysterectomy with objectively normal bleeding. This was generally due to a lack of understanding of the mechanisms involved in menstrual bleeding.

Greenberg (1983) expanded on that and suggested three factors that may contribute to the generation of the complaint of menorrhagia: (1) a generally low threshold to complain due to the patient's emotional state, (2) adopting a 'sick role' as a way to express personal or emotional difficulties, and (3) general vulnerability due to a neurotic personality trait [8]. His colleagues criticized his study in that it does not leave any space for true medical causes and focusses only on psychological reasons for such a complaint.

In the twenty-first century only premenstrual syndrome is appreciated as a full biopsychosocial condition, which is also reflected in some of its treatment (SSRIs). Although there is evidence of psychosocial factors in other menstrual disorders, it is not considered robust enough to provide a platform for change of the current management.

Menorrhagia/Heavy Menstrual Bleeding

Heavy menstrual bleeding (HMB) is excessive menstrual bleeding over several consecutive cycles that interferes with the woman's physical, emotional,

Table 13.2 FIGO classification of structural and non-structural causes of abnormal uterine bleeding (2011)

Abnormal uterine bleeding (HMB and intermenstrual bleeding)	
Structural (PALM)	Non-Structural (COEIN)
P – Polyp	C – Coagulopathy
A – Adenomyosis	O – Ovulatory dysfunction
L – Leiomyoma (fibroid)	E – Endometrial
M – Malignancy and hyperplasia	I – Iatrogenic
	N – Not yet classified

social and material quality of life [9]. The old-fashioned measurement of total blood loss > 80 ml was shown to be inaccurate and clinically irrelevant (NICE), although generally women's perception of menstrual bleeding is consistent with objective measurements of blood loss [10]. The gold standard for measuring menstrual blood loss used to be alkaline haematin test, which is not suitable for routine assessment. The trend was to develop simple low-cost self-assessment tools, which could be widely used, such as pictorial charts. Objective measurement might still have place in menorrhagia management as some patients choose expectant management when their objective blood loss is shown to be within normal range [11]. Also quantification is necessary in clinical trials of treatment.

HMB affects 3% of premenopausal women, with even higher prevalence in the perimenopausal women (40–51 years) [12]. About 30% of women will experience HMB at some point in their life [9].

According to the FIGO classification (2011) (see Table 13.2) the causes of HMB can be divided into two groups – structural (PALM) and non-structural (COEIN) [1].

The treatment reflects the underlying pathology after appropriate investigations. However, if the history is not suggestive of malignancy or structural abnormality the initial treatment can be commenced 'blindly' without gynaecological investigation [9].

In the last ten years the first-line treatment has been medical. Mirena coil (levonorgestrel-releasing intrauterine system) was proved to be the most effective, reaching up to 100% decrease in monthly blood loss; it is considered in the NICE guideline to be the first-line option.

GnRH analogues are of almost equal efficacy to Mirena providing up to 95% decrease in blood loss but with a higher rate of side effects, hence are considered in treatment of fibroids, short-term preoperatively or long term when other treatment options are contraindicated. The second line of treatment after Mirena is tranexamic acid in combination with non-steroidal anti-inflammatory drugs (NSAIDs) or hormonal treatment with combined oral contraceptive. Progestogen at higher doses in oral tablets or as an implant is the third most effective medical treatment [9].

The number of hysterectomy procedures has significantly decreased since the introduction of Mirena coil in the management of menstrual disorders. Despite various lawsuits, mostly in the United States, describing the coil as a potentially dangerous device, its use has spread quickly and many women have benefitted from having virtually no periods after the initial six months. The oral selective progesterone receptor modulator, ulipristal acetate, is an effective treatment for abnormal uterine bleeding caused by fibroids.

Second-line treatment is minimally invasive surgery, including hysteroscopic resection of fibroid or polyp, endometrial ablation, uterine fibroid embolization or laparoscopic myomectomy. There are several innovative approaches that are currently under trial, such as laparoscopic or Doppler-guided transvaginal uterine artery occlusion or radiofrequency ablation of fibroids.

Third-line treatment is a hysterectomy, which can be performed laparoscopically, vaginally (with or without laparoscopic assistance) or abdominally.

Several studies addressed psychosocial factors related to the choice of treatment. Women from a poorer educational background who have severe symptoms or menstruation-related pain are likely to prefer surgical treatment. Even among women who are initially treated with a Mirena IUS, 42% of them will opt for hysterectomy during five-year follow-up [13]. Elovainio et al. (2007) found that women who were still mildly depressed after six months of treatment with Mirena were more likely to opt for hysterectomy. Depressive symptoms at the beginning of treatment were not related to increased risk of dropout. This was explained in previous research, where it was found that the depression improves significantly after the treatment of the menstrual disorder [14].

Overall we can say that pre-treatment depressive symptoms are likely to result from menstrual disorders and in turn tend to resolve with improvement of the menstrual disorder. Ongoing depressive symptoms or new onset of depression after successful treatment of menstrual disorders is more suggestive of a general mood disorder, and this tends to affect the woman's compliance and choices. It is generally considered that absorption of the levonorgestrel can result in transient or long-term mood change.

The relationship between depression and menstrual problems has been extensively studied. Strine et al. (2005) examined 11,648 American women and reported a higher incidence of anxiety, depression, insomnia and pain in women with menstrual problems. It seems that their periods also affect their self-esteem as they reported more often feeling worthless and hopeless and, possibly as a result, they showed a higher tendency to engage in smoking, excessive eating or heavy drinking [15]. This supports the assumption that gynaecological morbidity can lead to psychological disturbances. Bromberger et al. (2013) suggested opposite causality. A small number of studies had previously suggested that depression may precede the onset of menstrual problems, taking into account stress-related hypothalamic–pituitary–adrenal axis dysfunction. Bromberger therefore examined history of major depression as a predictive factor for menstrual disorders in a cohort of perimenopausal women. Past history of major depression was related to heavy bleeding symptoms independent of other risk factors, such as fibroids. They quoted other studies which confirmed that women with psychiatric disorders are twice more likely to report menstrual problems [16]. It is well known that depression is a risk factor for diabetes or cardiovascular disease, and it seems that there might be a similar connection with menstrual disorders as well.

Dysmenorrhoea/Painful Periods

Introduction

Dysmenorrhoea is pain associated with menstruation. The word derives from Greek and translates as difficult monthly flow. It is the most common gynaecological symptom with a prevalence of 45–95%, which is more pronounced in adolescents than older women. Debilitating menstrual pain, which significantly impairs daily activities, has been reported in 7–15% of women [17]. The pain typically starts a few hours

before menstrual bleeding, peaks with the highest blood flow and settles within a few days as the menses progress [18].

The pathophysiology of menstrual pain was unknown for a long time, so the initial classification reflected symptomatology rather than causality. Dalton (1969) described dysmenorrhoea as spasmodic and congestive [19]. Spasmodic typically affected women of a young age, on the first day of their period, possibly accompanied by nausea, vomiting and weakness. There are some similarities with features of primary dysmenorrhoea. Congestive dysmenorrhoea could occur anytime and was characterized by pain starting prior to the menses with physiological effects of progesterone – bloating, constipation and breast tenderness. The line between 'normal' premenstrual syndrome and congestive dysmenorrhoea was not clear.

Nowadays the classification reflects possible causes. Primary dysmenorrhoea typically starts with the onset of regular, ovulatory periods in early teenage years in the absence of any pelvic pathology. It often improves in the third decade or after childbirth. It is related to ovulatory cycles and is probably associated with prostaglandin production.

Secondary dysmenorrhoea starts after a variable length of time with painless periods, usually after the age of 25 and is typically due to underlying pathology, although normal findings do not exclude secondary dysmenorrhoea. Pain may not be related exclusively to menstruation and may persist throughout the cycle with menstrual exacerbation.

There is an argument that dysmenorrhoea should be regarded as a chronic pain or repetitive acute pain and treated as such. Pain research on dysmenorrhoea is very limited. In June 2013 only 0.1% of papers focussing on pain were dedicated to menstrual pain. It was also reflected in the grants for pain research in the United States in 2013 where only eight projects from 2,938 (0.3%) involved dysmenorrhoea [20]. At a general level it was shown that chronic pain (such as fibromyalgia, irritable bowel syndrome) is associated with widespread changes in the central nervous system's physiology and anatomy. From this perspective there is an argument to regard dysmenorrhoea as a chronic pain as it is associated with the 'typical' brain changes. Research described differences in neural function, such as abnormal cerebral metabolism (using fluorodeoxyglucose positron emission tomography) and increased neural activity induced by noxious stimuli anywhere on the skin. This means that dysmenorrhoeic women will have higher sensitivity to muscle and visceral pain in the body, even outside the pelvic region, throughout their menstrual cycle. This can explain associations of dysmenorrhoea with other types of chronic pain.

Adolescents seem to be of peripheral interest to researchers despite the fact that up to 80% of young girls experience dysmenorrhoea. Menstrual disorders play a significant role in school absenteeism [21]. There is evidence that smoking increases pain in primary dysmenorrhoea as shown by research on adolescent girls. There is similar data from older cohorts, so it probably plays a role in secondary dysmenorrhoea as well. Family history of painful periods, earlier age at menarche and prolonged and heavy periods were also associated with increased risk of dysmenorrhoea.

There has been research into other factors such as education, marital status, employment or alcohol consumption but there were no definite correlations or the results were inconclusive. Physical exercise is assumed to improve blood flow, including the pelvic region, and by release of endorphins provides some endogenous analgesia. However, the evidence for this is limited.

Causes

There have been various theories of pathophysiology of dysmenorrhoea. It is likely to be multifactorial and it is expected to show inter-individual variation. The current most prominent theory attributes dysmenorrhoea to uterine contraction and vasoconstriction.

A drop in progesterone leads to disintegration of endometrial cells, which releases prostaglandins PGF2a and PGE2. Prostaglandins induce prolonged uterine contraction, which decreases blood flow and causes an ischaemic type of pain. This was supported in research where it was shown that an abnormal pattern of uterine contractions and higher levels of prostaglandins in the endometrial fluid correlate to the severity of pain during menstruation.

Complementary to this theory, researchers argued that the increased pain can be due to abnormal stimulation of pain fibres. During these ischaemic episodes the anaerobic metabolites within the tissues stimulate type C neurons, which leads to greater pain perception.

Other substances were shown to play a role in uterine stimulation and are therefore thought to be related to dysmenorrhoea. Leukotrienes increase uterine contractions and induce vasoconstriction. It is possible that they constitute an alternative pathway of pain induction as research has shown that women who fail to respond to prostaglandin inhibitors have high levels of leukotrienes and should respond to leukotriene synthesis inhibition. It was also suggested that they play a role in higher sensitivity of C neurons.

Treatment

The first option is medication, which reduces cyclooxygenase activity, thereby inhibiting prostaglandin production, such as paracetamol, aspirin and NSAIDs. The second option is inhibition of ovulation, typically by oral contraceptives. Mirena coil (LNG-IUCD) does not suppress the ovulation, but its effect on the endometrium and significant decrease of blood flow offers another therapeutic option for dysmenorrhoeic patients.

Approximately 10–20% of women with primary dysmenorrhoea do not respond or have contraindications to those treatments. There is evidence on the effectiveness of thiamine, pyridoxine, magnesium and fish oil in relieving menstrual pain, but their use might be affected by the side effects (constipation with magnesium, nausea and worsening acne with fish oil).

Surgical management in primary dysmenorrhoea is a last-resort treatment, and its effectiveness is uncertain. The first procedure is presacral neurectomy, which, according to a Cochrane review (2005), is associated with some improvement in the long term but not short term. The second procedure is laparoscopic uterosacral nerve ablation, which was not proved to make any significant difference in pain and hence is no longer used [22].

Hysterectomy is a possibility for women with refractory severe dysmenorrhoea whose reproductive plans are complete and who are fully counselled on risks of the procedure.

Secondary dysmenorrhoea is most commonly caused by endometriosis. It is not clear how the ectopic endometrial tissue increases menstrual pain, but some studies have suggested that women with endometriosis have increased levels of prostaglandins and or inflammatory substances such as cytokines. This would translate into greater pain during menstruation.

The mechanism of pain perception in endometriosis is generally poorly understood. It is evident from the research and clinical practice that the extent and location of lesions do not correspond to the magnitude of the pain. Also reappearance of the

Table 13.3 Causes/associations of secondary dysmenorrhoea

Most common	• Endometriosis
	• Chronic inflammatory disease
	• Adenomyosis
Common	• Intrauterine polyps
	• Intrauterine contraceptive devices (though progestogen-containing IUS may improve)
	• Submucous fibroids
Uncommon	• Uterine retroversion (only when fixed and associated with endometriosis)
	• Asherman syndrome
	• Ovarian cysts and tumours

pain after the treatment is not always associated with recurrence of the lesions [23].

Adenomyosis is thought to cause tonic contractions of the uterus by endometrial gland destruction within the myometrium. Dysmenorrhoea secondary to chronic pelvic inflammatory disease is probably caused by abnormal uterine contractions and scar tissue formation. Any abnormal content of the uterine cavity – intrauterine devices, submucous fibroids or polypi – can cause dysmenorrhoea by increased uterine activity in an attempt to expel these. There are other less common causes of secondary dysmenorrhoea – see Table 13.3.

The treatment options for secondary dysmenorrhoea include primarily dealing with the cause. There are, however, certain mechanisms that overlap, as many women with secondary dysmenorrhoea react well to the medical treatment targeted at reducing uterine contractions and vasoconstriction.

Psychosocial Aspects

Chronic pain syndromes have been extensively studied in psychology. The second half of the twentieth century was marked by extensive research in personality traits in the hope of finding the type of 'dysmenorrhoeic women' and including these findings in the treatment. Due to the limited medical knowledge, many gynaecological problems were thought to be fully or partially attributed to psychosomatic disorders. Wittkower and Wilson (1940) suggested that dysmenorrhoea sufferers give a history of maladjustment four times greater than women with normal periods [24]. This maladjustment might be related to the hypersensitivity established in neurological studies, which subjects them to experiencing pain more intensely than others. Dysmenorrhoea is also associated with greater somatization, i.e. complaining of symptoms with minimal or no medical cause. This type of behaviour can be attributed, according to some authors, to greater attention-seeking behaviour [25].

The personality trait traditionally associated with dysmenorrhoea is neuroticism. It is one of the Big Five personality traits used in psychology. Such individuals show a tendency to be emotionally less stable, experiencing high levels of anxiety, guilt or depressed moods. Indeed, some papers concluded that dysmenorrhoeic women are more depressed, anxious and withdrawn, but these were mostly from studies published in the 1980s with various methodological flaws. At that time it was assumed that dysmenorrhoea resulted from hormonal imbalance, and the higher score in neuroticism was therefore attributed to it. The mechanism of dysmenorrhoea is, however, no longer regarded as hormonal imbalance, so the explanation for higher neuroticism probably lies within the experience of the pain itself.

Influenced by the work of Sigmund Freud, psychologists attempted to describe a potential link between femininity and menstrual problems. The concept was mainly rejection of one's femininity leading to the psychosomatic symptom of suffering for it. This was never fully proven in the research. Woods et al. (1979) described for example congestive dysmenorrhoea patients as scoring high on masculinity [26], while Dalton (1969) described them as desiring large families and in possession of marked maternal instincts [19]. Overall it is understandable that women will have mixed feelings towards menstruation if it causes them regular distress. Holmlund (1990) reported that dysmenorrhoeic girls aged 15 showed significantly lower self-esteem than the controls. He described them as conventionally more feminine than the controls. In the ten-year follow-up the researcher looked at their initial behaviour and linked it to the school achievements. The dysmenorrhoeic cohort was more successful in regard to education performance than the participants with painless periods. This led him to a hypothesis that dysmenorrhoeic girls show initially lower self-esteem, but in time they compensate for it by bigger effort and greater school achievements [27].

Research into the relationships of dysmenorrhoeic women with their mothers found a correlation with unpleasant, humiliating or unloving relationships [28]. From the views of psychoanalysts this corresponds to adverse feelings towards the 'world of women'. This refers to the concept of parents representing the 'worlds' of opposite sexes. If the relationship with mother is troublesome the daughter does not want to associate with being a woman, i.e. being what her mother is. This controversial approach clashes with her female identity and, as menstruation is taken as a sign of being a woman, her body also develops adverse (painful) reaction to being a woman.

University female students with primary dysmenorrhoea showed higher scores on paternal dominance and maternal abuse in family relationship questionnaires [29], which is again suggestive that dysmenorrhoeic girls are more likely to be suppressed in their personal development as women.

As for relationships with males, dysmenorrhoea seems to affect women in their marital functioning. Mathur et al. (1988) found that dysmenorrhoeic women have lower coital frequency with half the frequency of orgasms than subjects with normal periods [30]. From research in chronic pain it is also evident that certain aspects of marital relationship affect chronic pain. For example marital satisfaction has been found to be related to the severity of depressive symptoms from chronic pain. Spousal solicitousness also adversely affects coping with chronic pain [31]. On the other hand negative spouse response to pain increases anxiety symptoms and low marital satisfaction increases depressive symptoms [32]. There is some evidence from randomized controlled trials that behavioural interventions like biofeedback, relaxation therapy and exercise may be effective. However, results should be interpreted with care. The studies varied between trials, which were of small trial size, poor methodological quality and most were old studies [22].

Summary

At the beginning of the twentieth century menstrual disorders were mostly regarded as psychosomatic conditions, partially or completely caused by psychological stress. With the advances in medicine and identification of pathophysiological mechanisms involved in menstruation, the current approach to abnormal uterine bleeding is purely medical.

Limited research suggests that psychosocial factors play a role in heavy bleeding and painful periods; they are, however, not regarded as relevant in the management of such conditions.

Key Points

- In the FIGO classification, causes of abnormal uterine bleeding are divided into two groups – structural (PALM) and non-structural (COEIN).
- There is a higher incidence of anxiety, depression, insomnia and pain in women with menstrual problems. On the other hand, a past history of major depression is a risk factor for menstrual problems.
- Smoking, a family history of painful periods, earlier age at menarche and prolonged and heavy periods are associated with increased risk of dysmenorrhoea.
- Research suggests that dysmenorrhoeic women have higher sensitivity to muscle and visceral pain in the body, even outside the pelvic region, throughout their menstrual cycle.
- Both prostaglandins and leukotrienes increase uterine contractions and induce vasoconstriction, and are probably involved in the pathogenesis of dysmenorrhoea – women with dysmenorrhoea who fail to respond to prostaglandin inhibitors have high levels of leukotrienes.

References

1. Fraser IS, Critchley HOD, Broder M, Munro MG. The FIGO recommendations on terminologies and definition for normal and abnormal uterine bleeding. *Seminars in Reproductive Medicine* 2011; **29**: 383–390.

2. Baker FC, Driver HS. Circadian rhythms, sleep, and the menstrual cycle. *Sleep Med* 2007; **8**: 613–622.

3. McPherson R. The response to hysterectomy: A case study. *Update* 1983; **24**: 332–334.

4. Matteson KA, Clark MA. Questioning our questions: Do frequently asked questions adequately cover the aspects of women's lives most affected by abnormal uterine bleeding? Opinions of women with abnormal uterine bleeding participating in focus group discussions. *Womens Health* 2010; **50**: 195–211. DOI: 10.1080/03630241003705037.

5. Lupton MJ. *Menstruation and psychoanalysis*. Urbana: University of Illinois Press, 1993.

6. Granleese J. Personality, sexual behaviour and menstrual symptoms: Their relevance to clinically presenting with

menorrhagia. *Personality Individual Differences* 1989; **11**: 379–390.

7. Miller GS. The primate basis of human sexual behavior. *Quarterly Review of Biology* 1931; **6**: 379–410.

8. Greenberg M. The meaning of menorrhagia: An investigation into the association between the complaint of menorrhagia and depression. *Journal of Psychosomatic Research* 1983; **27**: 209–214.

9. National Institute for Health and Care Excellence (NICE) *Heavy menstrual bleeding. NICE clinical guidelines 44*, 2007. London; NICE.

10. Lukes AS, Baker J, Eder S, Adomako TL. Daily menstrual blood loss and quality of life in women with heavy menstrual bleeding. *Women's Health* 2012; **5**: 503–511.

11. Magnay JL, Navette T, Seitz C, O'Brien PMS. A new menstrual pictogram for use with feminine products that contain superabsorbent polymers. *Fertil Steril* 2013; **100**: 1715–1721.

12. Royal College of Obstetricians and Gynaecologists. Abnormal uterine bleeding. STRATOG Core training modules. https://stratog.rcog.org.uk/tutorial/abnormal-uterine-bleeding. Accessed 22 March 2017.

13. Hurskainen R, Teperi J, Rissanen P, Aalto AM, Grenman S, Kivela A. Clinical outcomes and costs with the levonorgestrel-releasing intrauterine system or hysterectomy for treatment of menorrhagia – randomised controlled trial. 5 – year follow – up. *Journal of the American Association* 2004; **291**: 1456–1463.

14. Elovainio M, Teperi J, Aalto, AM, Grenman S, Kivela A, Kujansuu E, Vuorma S, Yliskoski M, Paavonen J, Hurskainen R. Depressive symptoms as predictors of discontinuation of treatment of menorrhagia by levonorgestrel-releasing intrauterine system. *International Journal of Behaviour Medicine* 2007; **14**: 70–75.

15. Strine TW, Chapman DP, Ahluwalia IB. Menstrual-related problems and psychological distress among women in the United States. *Women's Health* 2005; **14**: 16–23.

16. Bromberger JT, Schott LL, Matthews KA, Howard M, Kravitz DO, Randolph JF, Harlow S, Crawford S, Green R, Joffe H. Association of past and recent major depression and menstrual characteristics in midlife: Study of Women's Health Across the Nation. *Menopause* 2012; **19**: 959–966.

17. Harlow SD, Ephross SA. Epidemiology of menstruation and its relevance to women's health. *Epidemiology review* 1995; **17**: 265–286.

18. National Institute for Health and Care Excellence (NICE) Clinical Knowledge Summary Dysmenorrhea. NICE 2014. http://cks.nice.org.uk/dysmenorrhoea#!topicsummary. Accessed 22 March 2017.

19. Dalton RA. *The Menstrual Cycle*. New York: Pantheon Books, 1969.

20. Berkley KJ. Primary dysmenorrhea: An urgent mandate. *Pain: Clinical Updates* 2013; **3**: 1–8.

21. Knox B, Azurah AG, Grover SR. Quality of life and menstruation in adolescents. *Curr Opin Obstet Gynecol* 2015; **27**: 309–3014.

22. Proctor M, Murphy PA, Pattison HM, Suckling JA, Farquhar C. Behavioural interventions for dysmenorrhoea. *Cochrane Database of Systematic Reviews* 2007, Issue 3. Art. No.: CD002248. DOI: 10.1002/14651858.CD002248.pub3.

23. Stratton P, Berkley KJ. Chronic pelvic pain and endometriosis: Translational evidence of relationship and implications. *Human Reproduction Update* 2011; **17**: 327–346.

24. Wittkower E, Wilson AT. Dysmenorrhoea and sterility: Personality studies. *Br. Med. J.* 1940; **2**: 586–589.

25. Godlstein-Feber S, Granot M. The association between somatization and perceived ability: Roles in dysmenorrhea among Israeli Arab adolescents. *Psychosomatic Medicine* 2006; **68**: 136–142.

26. Woods DJ, Launius A. Type of menstrual discomfort and psychological masculinity in college women. *Psychological Reports* 1979; **44**: 257–258.

27. Holmlund U. The experience of dysmenorrhea and its relationship to personality variables. *Acta Psychiatrica Scandinavia* 1990; **82**: 182–187.

28. Shainess N. A re-evaluation of some aspects of femininity through a study of menstruation: A preliminary report. *Comprehensive Psychiatry* 1961; **2**: 20–26.

29. Xu K, Chen L, Fu L, Mao H, Liu J, Wang W. Stressful parental bonding exaggerate the functional and emotional disturbances of primary dysmenorrhea. *European Journal of Psychotraumatology* 2014; **5**: 26532 http://dx.doi.org/10.3402/ejpt.v5.26532. Accessed 22 March 2017.

30. Mathur CN, Prabha J, Lall SB. Psychometric studies on the possible relationship between sexual orgasm and primary dysmenorrhea in Indian women. *Indian Journal of Psychological Medicine* 1988; **11**: 17–20.

31. Kerns RD, Hayworthwaite J, Southwick S, Giller Jr. WL. The role of marital interaction in chronic pain and depressive severity. *Journal of Psychosomatic Research* 1990; **34**: 401–408.

32. Cano A, Gillis M, Heinz W, Geisser M, Foran H. Marital functioning, chronic pain and psychological distress. *Pain* 2004; **107**: 99–106.

109

Biopsychosocial Aspects of Infertility

Lamiya Mohiyiddeen and Christian Cerra

Introduction

This chapter will cover different aspects concerning the impact that diagnosis, investigation and treatment of infertility has on patients. It aims to explore the psychological burden of subfertility on couples, from both female and male perspectives, the latest research on stress and infertility, and the differences between medical and social infertility, as well as issues surrounding third-party reproduction and surrogacy. Finally, in order to help address these issues, the latest clinical practice guidelines on psychosocial care for fertility patients are discussed.

The Impact of Infertility and Its Treatment on Couples

Infertility is defined as 'the inability of a couple to achieve conception or to bring a pregnancy to term after a year or more of regular, unprotected intercourse' (WHO-ICMART glossary). It affects up to 10–15% of couples of reproductive age worldwide, or 48.5 million women worldwide. The cause may be attributed to male factor, female factor or both. For a significant proportion the cause will be unexplained.

Social factors such as delayed childbearing age in women and lifestyle factors (smoking, obesity) coupled with an increased awareness of treatments available have resulted in an unprecedented demand for fertility services [1]. Only recently have such services started to explore the psychosocial aspects of infertility: its mental health burden on patients, their psychological needs and effective psychotherapeutic interventions.

A distinction is made between 'medical' and 'social' infertility. Medical infertility results from a known or unknown disease, whereas social infertility may be age-related infertility, single women or same-sex couples aspiring to parenthood.

Social infertility more than medical infertility has the added concerns about donors, the wish for phenotypic similarities with recipient parents, as well as concerns over family and friends' perception and disclosure or non-disclosure to them. However, socially infertile individuals, especially single mothers accessing assisted reproductive techniques (ART), appear to also have better coping strategies and self-esteem to deal with the added stresses [2]. The genetic link with the child appears more important for heterosexual couples compared to those affected by social infertility [2].

For those with unsuccessful treatment, the realization that their life goal of parenthood can no longer be fulfilled may lead to anger, anxiety and depression, marital problems, a sense of inadequacy, sexual dysfunction, social pressure and isolation, and low self-esteem [1].

Infertility treatments are characterized by cycles of hope and disappointment, posing very significant stress and emotional burden on the general psychological well-being of the individuals involved, both female and male [3, 4].

Infertility treatment is a significant source of stress and emotional distress, with higher reported rates of depression after each ART cycle failure [5, 6].

Psychological stress and depression are highly prevalent among women with recurrent pregnancy loss [7].

Although infertile women have been found to have slightly raised anxiety traits compared to fertile controls [8, 9], couples seeking treatment are on the whole psychologically well-adjusted [9–11]. This may be simply a reflection of a self-selection bias in which well-adjusted couples would be more likely to seek fertility treatment which is in itself a problem-solving strategy. Such strategies may work in controllable situations; however, over time couples will realise they have little control over the outcome of fertility treatment. The series of interventions such as frequent scans and other investigations, sample provision, and daily hormonal injections may cause anxiety, especially during particular steps of the process, such as waiting for news on treatment outcomes at different stages of the process (awaiting news on successful implantation being a critical and particularly stressful step for couples).

Decision making is also stressful at every stage. For example in choosing between conventional in vitro fertilization (IVF) and natural cycle IVF, different elements need to be taken into account, i.e. invasiveness, cost, side effects, pregnancy rate and time to pregnancy. Whilst the last two factors would favour conventional IVF, lower-risk natural cycle IVF confers advantages on all the other aspects, with reduced psychological stress, as well as being ethically suitable for those with concerns regarding embryo selection and storage.

Unsuccessful outcomes trigger reactions of sadness and anger and often lead to lasting clinical depression, in 66% of females and 40% of the men followed up for 18 months after treatment [12].

After a failed IVF cycle, women experience an increase in depressive symptoms and lower levels of self-esteem than they did prior to the treatment cycle. A problem-solving coping strategy was associated with better psychological adjustment, while the use of avoidance coping and social isolation had the opposite effect; hence, behavioural strategies may help these patients deal with their loss of control [13].

Another stressful aspect associated with the IVF treatment process is the side effects and risks involved, such as ovarian hyperstimulation syndrome (OHSS). Side effects from ovulation induction with clomiphene include hot flushes, nausea, weight gain, OHSS, anxiety and depression. Hormonal treatments can generally affect emotional stability.

Although couples that are unsuccessful following treatment are more likely to be emotionally distressed and have difficult marital adjustments [14], couples that are successful may also be affected – they have higher rates of psychological problems and mental stress during pregnancy than couples who conceived naturally [15], and have higher levels of reported anxiety about losing the pregnancy, about fetal wellbeing (see Chapter 28 for the effect on the maternal-fetal relationship) and traumatic childbirth. However, male partners may perceive the pregnancy as more special than fathers of naturally conceived babies, and similarly mothers see the delivery as an exceptional event.

Parents of IVF-conceived children have been reported to have closer emotional attachment and better parent–child relationship as well as marital relationships compared to normally fertile parents; however, this may be the result of bias to positive self-reporting [16].

Does Stress Cause Infertility or Does Infertility Cause Stress?

The psychology of infertility emerged from what Berg and Wilson [17] later named the psychogenic model of infertility, which proposed psychopathology as an aetiological factor in infertility. This psychogenic model was introduced in the 1930s to account for infertility that had no identifiable biomedical cause [18].

We have thankfully now moved on from a psychogenic model, due to better diagnosis and decreased proportion of unexplained infertility, and it is generally agreed that long-standing infertility is unlikely to be caused solely by psychological problems. However, some old-fashioned attitudes remain, leading to a treatment process and research focus which revolves still mostly around women alone as the cause of infertility, and to unhelpful advice to 'relax and wait', which further delays couples seeking treatment in a situation that is already age- and time-critical.

Studies have been carried out to investigate the effect of psychosocial factors on fertility and on fertility treatment outcomes. A 'hostile' mood state and higher trait anxiety were associated with a lower cumulative pregnancy rate in a study by Sanders et al. 1999. In a study of 330 women by Thiering et al. depressed women exhibited a lower pregnancy rate for the first treatment cycles than non-depressed women [19]. A history of depressive symptoms has been associated with a doubled risk of developing infertility in another study [20]; however, lifestyle factors such as smoking, body mass index [BMI] and alcohol use were not taken into account.

Although higher levels of anxiety and stress have been associated with a lower chance of conception, it is unclear whether they are the causal factor or a consequence [21]. Any speculative statements on causality between the two would need to take into account factors which may be spuriously correlated, for example general health affecting both mood and fertility. A subsequent study by the same group failed to find an association between prolactin levels (considered a surrogate for stress) and outcome of IVF.

The impact of psychological and psychosocial interventions on fertility treatment outcome is still hotly debated with some investigators proposing an effect and others not [22–24].

Studies have shown a possible association between stress reduction exercises and the probability of conception [25]. More prospectively designed studies investigating whether psychological factors can predict fertility and fertility treatment outcomes are required.

Whilst financial considerations or clinical reasons are often the reason for dropping out of fertility treatment among private care service users, psychological factors have also been implicated [26]. A lack of psychological support and patient-centred care is often a common reason for discontinuing ART treatments and low levels of patient satisfaction [22].

Results from a recent couple-based prospective cohort study showed that pre-conception stress increases the risk of infertility [27]. After adjustment for confounders, women with high levels of salivary alpha-amylase (associated with adrenergic activity/stress response) had a 29% decreased odds of pregnancy compared to women with low levels (greater than twofold increased risk of infertility in that group). However, no association was seen when using salivary cortisol levels as biomarker of stress. Possible mechanisms have been postulated to explain this association: stress causing decreased libido/intercourse frequency, delay or inhibition of the LH surge in ovulation, hyposecretion of corticotropin-releasing hormone, resulting in changes in the uterine autoimmune environment.

Similarly, a study by Pal et al. found that chronic lifetime psychosocial stressors (such as a personal history of abuse, or personal or family history of recreational drug use) were associated with diminished ovarian reserve when serum FSH levels are used as a marker [28]. Current stresses in terms of mood scores and serum cortisol levels did not correlate to ovarian reserve markers. Hypothalamic-adreno–cortical axis over-activation may be a possible mechanism affecting ovarian function. However, the study sample was small and other confounding lifestyle, environmental and biological factors (only family history of early menopause, BMI, age and ethnicity were taken into account), which may coincide with those chronic stressors, may be implicated in the results.

It is more likely that stress effects do not affect reproductive physiology or hormones directly, but are mediated by patient behaviour, for example lifestyle factors mentioned previously which could affect fertility [29].

Male Aspects of Infertility

Among couples undergoing IVF treatment, females experienced higher levels of anxiety states and anxiety traits as well as depression compared to male partners [10]. This observed gender difference may be due to the women's greater physical involvement in the IVF process, as well as possible hormonal effects on the CNS of the treatment itself. Levels of anxiety and depression only start to rise considerably compared to normative data once repeated IVF procedures are unsuccessful, probably as a result of an initial optimistic view and unrealistic high expectation on the chances of success from IVF treatment [30, 31].

Although levels of clinical depression in the male fertility patient population are no different from the general population, unsuccessful treatment can lead to poorer long-term mental health in this population compared to males who manage to become fathers, highlighting an obvious grieving process of lost parenthood [32].

Interestingly, Hjelmstedt et al. found that, as a result of worrying for their partners, for many men unsuccessful treatment may even lead to enhanced personal maturity and closer marital relationship. Indeed, a large proportion of men (47.3%) have been found to be confiding only in their spouse for support, making them less likely to discuss infertility and its treatment with others [33].

This may be due to perceived vulnerability to being subject of humiliation from other males questioning masculinity and conflating infertility with impotence.

Men prefer to receive information and emotional support from the infertility clinician rather than from friends or mental health professionals and support groups. Hence infertility clinicians should in the first instance explore themselves any psychological and emotional needs of male patients as part of their fertility treatment, rather than delegate this to other colleagues. The only exception seems to be the need for more structured support as well as more informal sharing of experiences within support groups for those men who require donor sperm, to address issues such as anonymity [34].

Gender roles appear to influence the way in which women with endometriosis and their partners adjust to living with endometriosis. The role of men as partners of women with endometriosis (a known cause of subfertility, pelvic pain and dyspareunia) has been studied. In line with dominant masculine norms, men tend to take control not only when they provide support to women from a treatment process point of view (attending clinic, helping with decisions, care after surgery) but also practically, by managing everyday tasks at home, and contributing financially if partners need to take time off work. Finally they provide emotional support for those women with endometriosis who, drawing on conventional feminine norms, feel anxious or guilty about their fertility, or the lack of sexual intimacy or their inability to perform household tasks [35].

Taking these roles may reinforce traditional masculine identities, with possible strains on their relationship, as they may also feel frustrated, isolated and helpless. Consultations should be inclusive of the impact of endometriosis on quality of life on women, as well as on their partners and their relationship. Referral should be considered to specialist services (pain clinics, psychosexual counselling) with clear signposting of women and couples to appropriate support services and organizations [36].

Psychosocial Care for Fertility Patients in Practice

Fertility clinics should address the psychosocial and emotional needs of their patients as well as their medical needs.

Specifically, from staff, patients appear to value sensitive interactions, tailored psychological support, involvement of both partners in the treatment process and decision making.

Clinic characteristics valued by patients include the opportunity to share experiences with others through access to support groups, as well as personalized care and continuity of care.

Patients value written, preparatory customized information about treatment and significance of results.

In terms of patient-specific needs, these can be subdivided into cognitive (imparting knowledge and addressing concerns), behavioural (lifestyle and behaviour change advice, exercise and nutrition compliance advice), relational and social (support in the relationship with partner, family and social network) and emotional (coping with anxiety and/or depression) [37].

These domains can be addressed before, during and after treatment (whether this is successful or not). Online assessment tools and information leaflets exploring and addressing these needs are useful before starting treatment.

During treatment, support and advice with regard to issues such as non-compliance, low social support and absence from work are required. Couples also need psychological support to deal with anticipatory anxiety as well as distress after failure. Whilst stress from repeated attempts and unsuccessful treatment leads to increased rates of depression, couples should also be aware of the self-reported experiences of increased relationship quality following treatment failure.

Couples may need access to a variety of psychosocial services to help them cope with the challenge of an infertility diagnosis, such as couples counselling, a peer education mentor system to share experiences and coping strategies, and easy to understand leaflets with information about the physical and emotional demands of infertility treatment. A brief questionnaire to assess patients' mental health state and support needs may help identify which local support services they need to be referred to.

Unfortunately, only 10–34% of patients seek counselling services, with the uptake rate among men being especially poor [38–40].

Further research focussing on routine patient-centred psychosocial care is required, although by definition tailored individualized care will place more constraints on collecting eligible data for comparison.

The European Society for Human Reproduction and Embryology (ESHRE) has produced guidelines offering best practice advice on how to incorporate psychosocial care in infertility care and medically assisted reproduction (ESHRE Psychology and Counselling Guideline Development Group, March 2015). As described in the work by Boivin et al., this aim can be achieved by ensuring that psychosocial care is delivered on three complementary levels of psychosocial care: routine psychosocial care (e.g. provision of information, self-help, support interventions), infertility counselling (e.g. crisis intervention, grieving support, implications counselling) and psychotherapy (e.g. support for patients with diagnosed mental health disorders) [41].

Routine psychosocial care should be provided by all fertility staff in contact with infertile patients (doctors, nurses, counsellors, social workers, psychologists, embryologists and administrative staff).

The guidelines highlight that whilst patient consultations in other areas of obstetrics and gynaecology traditionally focus on a specific symptom or disease, infertility consultations differ in several ways [42]:

(1) The focus is on an unfulfilled wish or goal in life, the severity of which can be very subjective.

(2) The wished child cannot be included in the decision-making process or the treatment. This situation poses ethical dilemmas in terms of what constitutes best interest of the child, and in terms of the type of family into which the child conceived by the use of assisted reproduction will be born, and potential discrepancies between the choices of the parents and the presumed interests of the child.

(3) The investigation and treatment of infertility can be very invasive physically and emotionally for a couple and affect its dynamics and sexuality; hence, these effects and the couple's ability to cope with them must be taken into account in the treatment decisions.

(4) The processes involved with fertility investigation and treatment can impact on relationship intimacy and sexuality, and a couple's resilience to withstand these stressors must be taken into account.

The infertility treatment journey is a stepwise process beginning with the initiation of the therapeutic relationship and terminating with the outcome of the treatment received. The guidelines state how each step in the cycle will have a *purpose* and a set of *objectives* and each step will present *typical issues* and will require specific *communication skills*. Doctors can provide their medical perspective through a patient-centred approach. Furthermore, specific psychosocial needs can be better addressed by providing tailored counselling. The clinician will provide patient-centred care by building a relationship (e.g. by remembering their names, professions and previous interactions in clinic) and by giving a helpful and competent impression when explaining treatment options and evaluating treatment outcomes (e.g. a failed treatment cycle), exploring patients' ideas, concerns and expectations and making patients feel understood, respected and reassured.

'Patient-centred care' is defined by the guidelines as 'the psychosocial care provided as part of routine services at the clinic'. This is provided and expected by all members of the medical team. 'Counselling', on the other hand, 'involves the use of psychological interventions based on specific theoretical frameworks', usually delivered by a mental health professional with relevant training in psychology, social work or counselling. Patients should receive patient-centred care as well as be able to access counselling services [42].

Patient-centred care can be enhanced through adjunct psychosocial services. Table 14.1 presents some of the objectives and typical issues that might arise from using these additional psychosocial services.

Counselling, on the other hand, focusses on meeting patients' needs outside the routine care/treatment process. 'Counselling might include individual and couple therapy and/or professionally facilitated support groups. The content of counselling may differ depending on the patient and the treatment choice but will usually involve at least some form of information and implication counselling, and support or therapeutic counselling. Information and implication counselling might focus on ensuring that individuals understand the different psychosocial issues involved in their treatment choice, whereas therapeutic counselling might involve an understanding of the emotional consequences of childlessness' [42].

Three different groups of patients may benefit from counselling. The first group comprises the majority of patients seen by the counsellor – patients who experience very high levels of distress they can no longer cope with. Although these patients form a significant proportion of those seen by counsellors, they make up only ~20% of all infertility patients. Some personal characteristics (such as preexisting anxiety and depression) may place patients at increased risk of extreme levels of stress, as well as specific situations, such as treatment failure. These special situations may require specific counselling to address the specific issues which arise from them (Table 14.2).

The second group of patients requiring counselling services are couples considering 'third party reproduction': i.e. recipient of donated gametes, and patients requiring surrogacy and/or adoption to achieve parenthood. The psychosocial issues affecting these patients are summarized by the guideline in Table 14.3, and are further discussed in the next section of

Table 14.1 Objectives when using adjunct (additional) psychosocial services

Adjunct services	Objectives
Written (or video) information, telephone counselling *(Boivin, Section 6.1)*	• Supplement existing psychosocial care and counselling • Provide information on common emotional/psychological reaction to infertility and information about coping with this condition • Normalize patients' experiences with services such as telephone counselling providing information and emotional support • Provide psychosocial information in a format that is cost-effective and widely accessible • Information must be provided in such a way that patients do not feel excluded if their own experiences differ from the experiences described
Self-help groups *(Thorn, Section 6.2)*	• Empower patients and increase patients' autonomy through the proactive nature of the self-help group structure where each member contributes to the success of the group • Provide medical information and normalize the experiences of the patient • Provide emotional support and coping information
Professionally facilitated group work *(Thorn, Section, 6.3)*	• Inform and educate patients about infertility and the psychosocial and legal aspects of family building using different medical and non-medical options • Explore underlying intra- and interpersonal issues surrounding reactions to infertility • Help couples resolve and come to terms with the failure of treatment and the prospect of a life without children

Note: Boivin J, Appleton TC, Baetens P, et al. European Society of Human Reproduction and Embryology. Guidelines for counselling in infertility: Outline version. Hum Reprod. 2001;16(6):1301–4.

this chapter. A newly contentious issue is the debate on provision of donor information to gamete recipients, in particular how much information couples want/should receive about gamete donors.

An interesting finding is that some of the gamete recipients in the study by Rubin et al. 2015 report that having too much information about possible oocyte donors can actually make their decision more difficult than with only limited details about the donor provided [43]. Less information may leave more space to the imagination for the gamete-receiving couple but it also means less access to information for the child who may want to find out about their donor once grown up. Such dilemmas reinforce the importance of appropriate counselling for gamete recipient couples before the decision to use gamete donation, and the need for counselling to continue once couples go through the donor selection process (Table 14.3).

Lastly, the third group of patients who may need non-routine psychological counselling are patients who require assisted reproductive techniques as a result of social circumstances. There are additional issues surrounding 'social infertility', which affects single women and lesbian couples who require sperm donation, and gay men who build their family through surrogacy. The individuals included in this category will also be affected by the issues described in Table 14.3. Same-sex couples may, for example, seek counselling surrounding the setting of family structure and parental responsibilities, and the assignment of parental roles, the legal status of the child and nonbiological mother/father, or addressing the absence of a mother or father figure in the child's development. This issue may also affect single mothers choosing to start their parenting experience at an older age in most cases. These women may also be interested in discussing social and economic implications of single parenting in later life [42].

Psychosocial Aspects of Surrogacy

The Human Fertilisation and Embryology Authority code of conduct for clinics in the United Kingdom states that surrogacy should be considered only when it is 'physically impossible or highly undesirable for medical reasons for the commissioning mother to carry the child'.

Table 14.2 Counselling objectives in special situations

Special situations	Counselling objectives
Patients experiencing high distress (Boivin, Section 2.3)	• Enable the expression of emotions • Identify the cause(s) of distress • Provide intervention(s) to minimize distress and help patients better manage distress • Discuss high-risk personal, situational, social and treatment-linked factors which may predispose or trigger high distress • Help the individual cope with [repeated] treatment failure
Pregnancy after infertility (Baetens, Section 4.1)	• Facilitate transition from infertile patient to pregnant patient • Normalize feelings of disbelief and ambivalence about the pregnancy, the child and future ability to parent
Multiple pregnancy (McWhinnie, Section 4.2)	• Provide a realistic picture of what it would be like to parent two or three children of identical age • Prepare patients for the emotional consequences of using fetal reduction
Facing the end of medical treatment (Wischmann, Section, 4.3)	• Help couples end treatment despite availability of medical treatments • Discuss the personal meaning of the loss of an important life goal • Address differences between spouses in readiness to end treatment
Sexuality (Darwish, Section 4.4)	• Systematically open up discussion of sexual issues • Evaluate the significance and severity of any sexual problems for the couple and identify factors which may contribute to the problem (e.g. depression, side effects of medication). • Address relationship issues which may arise from discussion of sexual issues • Help patients rebuild their sexuality as a source of pleasure
Patients in migration (Kentenich, Section 4.5)	• Make diagnosis and therapy accessible by ensuring medical practice is respectful of patients' sociocultural background • Facilitate communication between patients and the medical team by exploring and understanding the meaning of infertility from the perspective of the couple's culture • Discuss how continued childlessness affects the way the couple, especially the woman, are perceived in their community • Discuss cultural pressure to perceive infertility as a woman's problem

Note: Boivin J, Appleton TC, Baetens P, et al. European Society of Human Reproduction and Embryology. Guidelines for counselling in infertility: Outline version. Hum Reprod. 2001;16(6):1301–4.

The clinical use of surrogacy obviously involves ethical and moral dilemmas and psychosocial implications. Although the use of surrogacy in some cases may be more acceptable by society, for example if a woman requires it following a hysterectomy due to malignancy, commercial surrogacy (which is illegal in the United Kingdom) may not receive the same acceptance at a societal level. In commercial surrogacy a commissioning couple/intending parents require a woman to initiate the pregnancy, and carry the pregnancy until delivery in return for a financial compensation. Non-commercial gestational surrogacy, on the other hand, receives less criticism compared with genetic surrogacy [44, 45].

Surrogate and intended mothers appear to reconcile their unconventional choice through a process of cognitive restructuring, whereby an initial discrepancy between their beliefs and actions is rebalanced from a cognitive dissonance to one of cognitive consonance [46], and the result of this cognitive appraisal will influence disclosure of their choice to others. Surveys of the general population, on the contrary, show less acceptance for third-party reproduction, as there is no personal need to reconsider their beliefs and therefore remain in their normative cognitively consonant state [44].

The expecting parents as well as the surrogate mother who is to conceive purposefully with the intention to relinquish the baby after delivery require

Table 14.3 Counselling objectives in third-party reproduction

Third-party reproduction (gamete and embryo donation, surrogacy) *(Daniels, Section 5.1; Baetens, Section 5.2; Appleton, Sections 5.3 and 5.4; Baron, Section 5.5)*	• Help couples acknowledge and come to terms with the implications of using third-party reproduction as an alternative to family creation. • Address the gender difference in willingness to use third-party reproduction • Assess the suitability of recipient couples, donors and/or surrogates for treatment (e.g. mental health screening, drug addiction) • Ensure the well-being of the parent who will not be genetically related to the child • Counsel on secrecy/openness towards the future child and social network about the use of third-party reproduction. • Address lack of support some individuals may encounter about being part of third-party reproduction arrangements • Discuss the legal issues, medical risks and religious and cultural considerations of using third-party reproduction. • Ensure the decision to donate or become a surrogate was free from coercion (familial, financial)
Oocyte donation *(Baetens, Section 5.2)*	• In egg-share programmes donors need to be prepared for possibility that the recipient will become pregnant with their oocytes but the donor will not. • Recipients need to be prepared for the long waiting list in egg-share programmes, the high risk of drop-out by voluntary donors and the possibility that scarcity of donors means donors can only be matched on ethnicity.
Embryo donation *(Appleton, Section 5.3)*	• Couples donating embryos must resolve their feelings about the embryos and be certain they would not want to use them in future. • Help couples come to terms with the possibility that other children born from their gametes may exist in their community.
Surrogacy *(Appleton, Section 5.4)*	• Evaluate reasons for needing surrogacy (i.e. absence of uterus vs. busy lifestyle) and motives for becoming a surrogate (altruistic vs. financial) • Discuss legal issues concerning the nature of the contract between surrogate and commissioning couple and the legal status of any future child • Address difficulty in defining parenthood in surrogacy especially if social parents are not genetically related to the child.
Adoption *(Baron, Section 5.5)*	• To make an informed decision on whether or not to pursue adoption and the implications of being a parent for an adopted child • Help couples make the transition from using medical treatment to achieve parenthood to choosing adoption • Inform couples of state/country practice and the effect of the limited number of children available for adoption on time to adopt • Discuss issues involved in integrating adopted child into families where other children already exist

[42].

extensive counselling, as all individuals involved, including the offspring, will need to be prepared psychologically to face the potential long-term psychosocial consequences.

It is likely that infertile couples who choose to opt for surrogacy will have put a lot of thinking into what kind of family they would raise, again going through a cognitive appraisal from cognitive dissonance to cognitive consonance [44].

Recipient parents may have concerns over accusations of financial exploitation; medicalisation; fear of non-relinquishment by the surrogate mother; legal, emotional and social stigma; genetic links and baby worries. Despite these concerns, studies have shown that the psychological well-being of the parents was good [47, 48].

Baslington in 1996 interviewed 19 surrogate mothers and found them to be assertive and not medically or otherwise controlled. In the latter study, genetic surrogates in particular felt in control.

Few women choose to become surrogates for financial motivation, and the majority said they do it for altruistic reasons. Most surrogates enjoyed pregnancy and childbirth, and reported increased self-esteem, and the wish to develop meaningful relationships in their life with the commissioning parents. Relinquishment of the baby was a happy event for most surrogates, although some said they felt relief at the end of the gestation [44].

Maternal attachment to their baby is supposed to start prenatally and continue after birth. However, a number of factors affect attachment, such as maternal age and attitude towards the pregnancy. These factors may help explain how surrogates are able to relinquish the baby to the recipient parents following delivery; surrogate mothers tend to be old enough for them to believe they have completed their family [49].

A study based in the United Kingdom following up the relationship between children born through surrogacy and their recipient parents found overall good family functioning and child development compared to conventional families [48].

These parents will obviously benefit from counselling to help them decide how and when to disclose the surrogacy to their children [50]. Parents will have to cope with the uncertainty of future arrangements as in the United Kingdom and many other countries there cannot be any legally binding contracts about future arrangements for the child, as the surrogate is legally the mother of the child, even if the child is the genetic child of the commissioning couple.

Conclusion

Infertility care, perhaps more than any other area of obstetrics and gynaecology, involves psychosocial implications which require appropriate support to reduce patient distress and help them come to terms with their situations and make important life decisions. Training aimed at recognising and managing these biopsychosocial aspects of infertility and assisted reproduction should be part of training requirements for generalists and subspecialists. This should include psychosexual counselling, the role of cognitive

behavioural therapy and issues relating to same-sex partnerships, single parenthood, gender identity, gamete preservation and surrogate motherhood.

Clinicians should be prepared to confront and address these issues not only by using a patient-centred holistic approach in all interactions and at each step of the investigation and treatment process but also through referral to tailored counselling services in specific situations which require a trained mental health professional.

Key Points

- Emotions and psychological problems associated with infertility include hope, disappointment, anger, anxiety, depression, sense of inadequacy, sexual dysfunction, social pressure and isolation, low self-esteem and marital discord.
- Anxiety levels and stress have been linked to a lower chance of conception, but it is unclear whether they are the causal factor or a consequence of subfertility.
- Chronic lifetime psychosocial stressors (such as a personal history of abuse, or personal or family history of recreational drug use) have been shown to be associated with diminished ovarian reserve.
- Generally, men prefer to receive information and emotional support from the infertility clinician rather than from friends or mental health professionals and support groups.
- Couples undergoing fertility treatment value sensitive interactions, tailored psychological support, continuity of care and involvement of both partners in the treatment process and in decision making. Their needs can be subdivided into cognitive, behavioural, emotional and relational/social domains.
- The initial assessment of infertility patients should include assessment of their mental health state and support needs. A brief questionnaire may be helpful in determining what referrals to local services may be necessary.
- Guidelines published by the European Society for Human Reproduction and Embryology (ESHRE) describe three complementary levels of psychosocial care: routine psychosocial care, infertility counselling and psychotherapy.

- Health professionals providing care to infertility patients should develop skills for 'patient-centred care'. Those involved in surrogacy arrangements should be familiar with the pertinent psychosocial issues.

References

1. Deka P, Sarma S. Psychological aspects of infertility. *BJMP.* 2010;**3**(3):a336.

2. Diaz DG. Psychosocial differences between medical and social infertility. Presented at European Society of Human Reproduction annual meeting, Lisbon 2015.

3. Cousineau TM, Domar AD. Psychological impact of infertility. *Best Pract Res Clin Obstet Gynaecol.* 2007;**21**(2):293–308.

4. Dhillon R, Cumming CE, Cumming DC. Psychological well-being and coping patterns in infertile men. *Fertility and Sterility.* 2000;**74**(4):702–6.

5. Donarelli Z, Lo Coco G, Gullo S, Marino A, Volpes A, Allegra A. Are attachment dimensions associated with infertility-related stress in couples undergoing their first IVF treatment? A study on the individual and cross-partner effect. *Hum Reprod.* 2012;**27**(11):3215–25.

6. Holter H, Anderheim L, Bergh C, et al. First IVF treatment–short-term impact on psychological well-being and the marital relationship. *Hum Reprod.* 2006;**21**(12):3295–302.

7. AM Kolte, EM Mikkelsen, LK Egestad, et al. Psychological stress and moderate/severe depression are highly prevalent among women with recurrent pregnancy loss. Presented at European Society of Human Reproduction annual meeting, 2014. www.eshre.eu/Education/epresentations/ESHRE-2014-Webcasts/Webcast-Monday.aspx. (Accessed 22 March 2017.)

8. Eugster A, Vingerhoets AJ. Psychological aspects of in vitro fertilization: A review. *Soc Sci Med.* 1999;**48**(5):575–89.

9. Hearn MT, Yuzpe AA, Brown SE, et al. Psychological characteristics of in vitro fertilization participants. *American Journal of Obstetrics and Gynecology.* 1987;**156**:269–274.

10. Shaw P, Johnston M, Shaw R. Counselling needs, emotional and relationship problems in couples awaiting IVF. *Journal of Psychosomatic Obstetrics and Gynecology.* 1988;**9**:171–80.

11. Newton CR, Hearn MT, Yuzpe AA. Psychological assessment and follow-up after in vitro fertilization: Assessing the impact of failure. *Fertility and Sterility.* 1990;**54**:879–86.

12. Baram D, Tourtelot E, Muechler E, et al. Psychosocial adjustment following unsuccessful in vitro fertilization. *Journal of Psychosomatic Obstetrics and Gynecology.* 1988;**9**:18–90.

13. Hynes GJ, Callan VJ, Terry DJ, et al. The psychological well-being of infertile women after a failed IVF attempt: The effects of coping. *British Journal of Medical Psychology.* 1992;**65**:269–78.

14. Slade P, Emery J, Lieberman BA. A prospective, longitudinal study of emotions and relationships in in vitro fertilization treatment. *Human Reproduction.* 1997;**12**:183–90.

15. van Balen F, Naaktgeboren N, Trimbos-Kemper TC. In-vitro fertilization: The experience of treatment, pregnancy and delivery. *Hum Reprod.* 1996;**11**(1):95–8.

16. van Balen F, Trimbos-Kemper TC. Involuntarily childless couples: Their desire to have children and their motives. *J Psychosom Obstet Gynecol.* 1995;**16**(3):137–44.

17. Berg BJ, Wilson JF. Psychological functioning across stages of treatment for infertility. *J Behav Med.* 1991;**14**:11–26.

18. Boivin J, Gameiro S. Evolution of psychology and counseling in infertility. *Fertil Steril.* 2015;**104**(2):251–59.

19. Thiering P, Beaurepaire J, Jones M, et al. Mood state as a predictor of treatment outcome after in vitro fertilization/embryo transfer technology (IVF/ET). *Journal of Psychosomatic Research.* 1993;**37**:481–91.

20. Lapane KL, Zierler S, Lasater TM, et al. Is a history of depressive symptoms associated with an increased risk of infertility in women? *Psychosom Med.* 1995;**57**(6):509–13.

21. Demyttenaere K, Nijs P, Koninckx PR, et al. Anxiety and conception rates in donor insemination couples. *Journal of Psychosomatic Obstetrics and Gynecology.* 1988;**8**:175–81.

22. Boivin J. A review of psychosocial interventions in infertility. *Soc Sci Med.* 2003;**57**:2325.

23. Frederiksen Y, Farver-Vestergaard I, Skovgård NG, et al. Efficacy of psychosocial interventions for psychological and pregnancy outcomes in infertile women and men: A systematic review and meta-analysis. *BMJ Open.* 2015;**5**:e006592.

24. Haemmerli K, Znoj H, Barth J. The efficacy of psychological interventions for infertile patients: A meta-analysis examining mental health and pregnancy rate. *Hum Reprod Update.* 2009;**15**:279–95.

25. Domar AD, Seibel MM, Benson H. The Mind/Body program for infertility: A new behavioral treatment approach for women with infertility. *Fertility and Sterility.* 1990;**53**:246–49.

26. Olivius C, Fridén B, Borg G, Bergh C. Why do couples discontinue in vitro fertilization treatment? A cohort study. *Fertility and Sterility.* 2004;**81**:258–61.

27. Lynch CD, Sundaram R, Maisog MJ, et al. Preconception stress increases the risk of infertility: Results from a couple-based prospective cohort study, the LIFE study. *Hum Reprod.* 2014 May;**29**(5):1067–75. Presented at European Society of Human Reproduction annual meeting, Lisbon 2015. www.eshre.eu/en/Education/epresentations/ESHRE-2015-Webcasts.aspx. (Accessed 12 April 2017.)

28. Pal L, Bevilacqua K, Santoro NF. Chronic psychosocial stressors are detrimental to ovarian reserve: A study of infertile women. *J Psychosom Obstet Gynecol.* 2010;**31**(3):130–9.

29. Boivin J, Griffiths E, Venetis CA. Emotional distress in infertile women and failure of assisted reproductive technologies: Meta-analysis of prospective psychosocial studies. *BMJ.* 2011;**342**:d223.

30. Beaurepaire J, Jones M, Thiering P, et al. Psychosocial adjustment to infertility and its treatment: Male and female responses at different stages of IVF/ET treatment. *Journal of Psychosomatic Research.* 1994;**38**:229–40.

31. Collins A, Freeman EW, Boxer AS, Tureck R. Perceptions of infertility and treatment stress in females as compared with males entering in vitro fertilization treatment. *Fertility and Sterility.* 1992;**57**, 350–56.

32. Ware JE, Kosinski M, Keller SD. A 12-item short-form health survey: Construction of scales and preliminary results of reliability and validity. *Med Care.* 1996;**34**:220–33.

33. Hjelmstedt A, Andersson L, Skoog-Svanberg A, Bergh T, Boivin J et al. Gender differences in psychological reactions to infertility among couples seeking IVF- and ICSI-treatment. *Acta Obstet Gynecol Scand.* 1999;**78**:42–8.

34. Eisenberg ML, Smith JF, Millstein SG, Walsh TJ, Breyer BN et al. Perceived negative consequences of donor gametes from male and female members of infertile couples. *Fertility and Sterility.* 2010;**94**:921–6.

35. Hudson N, Culley L, Mitchell H, Law C, Denny E, Raine-Fenning N. Men living with endometriosis: Perceptions and experiences of male partners of women with the condition. European Society of Human Reproduction annual meeting, 2015. www.eshre.eu/en/Education/epresentations/ESHRE-2015-Webcasts.aspx. (Accessed 12 April 2017.)

36. Fisher JR, Hammarberg K. Psychological and social aspects of infertility in men: An overview of the evidence and implications for psychologically informed clinical care and future research. *Asian J Androl.* 2012;**14**(1):121–9.

37. Gameiro S, J Boivin, E Dancet, et al. ESHRE guideline: Psychosocial care in infertility and medically assisted reproduction. Presented at European Society of Human Reproduction annual meeting, 2014. www.eshre.eu/en/Education/epresentations/ESHRE-2014-Webcasts.aspx. (Accessed 12 April 2017.)

38. Read SC, Carrier ME, Boucher ME, et al. Psychosocial services for couples in infertility treatment: What do couples really want? *Patient Educ Couns.* 2014;**94**(3):390–5.

39. Wischmann T, Scherg H, Strowitzki T, Verres R. Psychosocial characteristics of women and men attending infertility counselling. *Hum Reprod.* 2009;**24**:378–85.

40. Boivin J, Scanlan LC, Walker SM. Why are infertile patients not using psychosocial counselling?. *Hum Reprod.* 1999;**14**:1384–91.

41. ESHRE Psychology and Counselling Guideline Development Group. Routine psychosocial care in infertility and medically assisted reproduction – A guide for fertility staff, ESHRE March 2015.

42. Boivin J, Appleton TC, Baetens P, et al. European Society of Human Reproduction and Embryology. Guidelines for counselling in infertility: Outline version. *Hum Reprod.* 2001;**16**(6):1301–4.

43. Rubin LR, Melo-Martin I, Rosenwaks Z, et al. Once you're choosing, nobody's perfect: is more information necessarily better in oocyte donor selection? *Reprod. Biomed. Online* 2015;**30**(3):311–18.

44. van den Akker OB. Psychosocial aspects of surrogate motherhood. *Hum Reprod Update.* 2007;**13**(1):53–62.

45. BMA. Changing Conceptions of Motherhood. *The Practice of Surrogacy in Britain.* British Medical Association: London, UK, 1996.

46. Festinger L. *A Theory of Cognitive Dissonance.* Stanford University Press: Stanford, USA, 1957.

47. van den Akker OBA. Coping, Quality of Life and psychiatric morbidity in 3 groups of sub-fertile women: Does process or outcome affect psychological functioning? *Patient Educ Couns.* 2005;**57**:183–89.

48. Golombok S, Murray C. Families created through surrogacy: Parent-child relationships in the first year of life. *Fertility and Sterility.* 2004;**80**:133.

49. Siddiqui A, Hagglof B, Eisemann M. An exploration of prenatal attachment in Swedish expectant women. *J Reprod Infant Psychol.* 1999;**17**:369–80.

50. Edelmann R. Surrogacy: The psychological issues. *J Reprod Infant Psychol.* 2004;**22**(2):123–36.

Chapter 15

Psychological and Social Aspects of Reproductive Life Events among Men

Jane R. W. Fisher and Karin Hammarberg

Investigations of the psychological and social aspects of reproductive life events and reproductive health have focussed predominantly on women, but in the most recent decade there has been an increased focus on the needs and experiences of men. This body of evidence has been derived from secondary analyses of national data, quantitative self-report surveys and qualitative investigations based on interviews and group discussions. Some research has been designed specifically to investigate men, and some has investigated men as members of couples or as fathers. The research evidence has been generated predominantly in high-income countries; there is less evidence about these experiences among men living in resource-constrained low- and lower-middle income nations.

Unintended Pregnancy

Decisions to have intercourse, use or not use contraception, or whether or not to continue a pregnancy are generally not made by women alone, but much less is known about men's, than women's, contraceptive behaviours and experiences of unintended (mistimed or unwanted) pregnancies. Kågesten et al. undertook secondary analyses of data from the population-based FECOND survey in France that used random digit dialling to recruit 8,675 people (3,373 men) aged 15–49 years [1]. Questions about pregnancy intention (whether or not it was wanted, and timing) were asked of participants who reported a pregnancy in the prior five years. Overall 5% of the heterosexually active participants reported an unintended pregnancy in the ascertainment period. Risks were higher among those who were younger, whose financial circumstances were insecure and whose relationships were fragile or ending. Although 72% of men in this circumstance reported that they (or their sexual partner) had been using contraception, more than half (58%) considered that their use of contraceptives had been inconsistent

(had not used a condom all the time) or that it had failed (oral contraceptive pills had been missed or condoms had slipped or broken). More than half believed that their partner had been using contraception and they had not themselves taken contraceptive steps.

Questions about pregnancies and pregnancy prevention were also asked in the Understanding Fertility Management in Contemporary Australia national survey that was completed anonymously by 2,234 people (691 men) aged 18–50 selected randomly from the electoral roll [2]. Detailed follow-up questioning was not possible, but 23% of the men indicated a lifetime experience of at least one 'acci-accidental pregnancy'. Only 17.6% of male respondents were aware of the fertile period of the menstrual cycle, and about 10% were using withdrawal to avoid pregnancy. Although most felt comfortable talking to a sexual partner about contraception (90.6%) and believed that contraception should be a shared responsibility (92.7%), less than a third (29.3%) recalled being taught about pregnancy prevention in school sex education. The unintended pregnancy was attributed to contraceptive failure by 15.3%, forgetting to use contraception by 21.6% and withdrawing too late by 10.8% of men.

Fatherhood: Attitudes, Intentions and Aspirations

The desire to have a child is multifactorially determined, including by age, marital status, parity, gender, culture, religious beliefs and the degree of reproductive autonomy and access to contraception in a particular setting [3]. In most high-income countries there has been a rapid increase in the average ages at which men father children, and at which women first give birth; there is also a decrease in the total fertility rate and average family size.

Fatherhood Aspirations among Men Who Are Presumed to Be Fertile

There are relatively few population-based investigations of the aspirations, expectations and desires to have children among men. Thompson and Lee surveyed 382 childless single men who were taking a first-year psychology subject at an Australian university and had self-identified as wanting to have a child at some point in the future [4]. Most wanted to father a child by their late twenties or early thirties, and the circumstances in which they wished this to occur was within a stable and loving partnership, when qualifications were completed, and when personal maturity had been achieved. Preferences were expressed for fatherhood to occur within a married, rather than a non-married but stable relationship and when a permanent job and dependable income had been secured. The preferences were explored in further semi-structured interviews about general life aspirations, including fatherhood by the age of 40 years, with 16 of these men aged between 18 and 22 years [5]. Marriage and having children (in general two or three) were widely described as fundamental to lifetime contentment and fulfilment. A tension was identified between the traditional view that men should be the main financial providers for their families and the contemporary ideal that fathers need to be competent and available caregivers who share household work with their partners. Few contemplated part-time employment in order to share the care of dependent children, and it was concluded that few had role models to follow in which income-generating and unpaid care-giving work had been shared equitably between partners who were parents. Some acknowledged that realizing the circumstances essential to being able to contemplate parenthood might narrow the life window in which this goal was possible.

Using random-digit dialling, Roberts et al. recruited 495 biologically childless men aged 20–45 years living in Calgary, Canada, who completed a structured interview about their plans for parenthood and factors associated with the decision to have a child [6]. A third were partnered and almost all (86%) wanted to have a child; 6.3% were trying actively to conceive. Like the younger Australian men in Thompson et al.'s studies, this Canadian group as a whole identified financial security as an important precondition, but also the partner's desire for children and her 'suitability' as a potential co-parent. They also found, however, that men who were in the older age group (35–45 years) were significantly less likely than younger men (20–24 years) to regard financial security as a precondition for fatherhood, and more likely to acknowledge that they were experiencing a 'biological clock', suggesting that there is more adaptation to the reality that there are rarely perfect circumstances in which to have a child, as they aged. Kessler et al. (2013) analysed the data from the 6,168 childless men aged 15–44 years collected in the US 2006–2010 National Survey of Family Growth among a representative sample of more than 22,000 American people. Most (88%) wanted to have a child in the future, with proportions expressing this wish declining with age.

Attitudes and motives influencing the desire to have or not to have children were examined in community-based surveys in Germany [7] and England [8]. Overall, desire for children among childless women and men aged at least 30 years was equal and linked to wishes to create new life, form a household and experience love, and was lowered by financial concerns.

Fatherhood Aspirations among Men Who Are Gay

There is a small literature describing aspirations for fatherhood and intentions to become a parent among gay men. In Italy, where people in same-sex relationships only recently acquired rights to form civil partnerships, but only in rare circumstances to adopt children, a small proportion (10%) of gay men have children, most born in prior heterosexual relationships. Baiocco and Laghi compared the parenting intentions and aspirations among 930 childless heterosexual and homosexual people, including 199 gay men [9]. Fewer gay (51.8%) than heterosexual men (81.0%) wanted to have children, and even fewer (30.2%), compared to 73.1% described an intention to become a parent. In the United States, Riskind and Patterson analysed data from the 2002 National Survey of Family Growth of 12,571 people (103 gay men), to investigate the same questions [10]. Findings were very similar to the Italian study, including that desires and intentions to become a parent were lower among homosexual than heterosexual men and lesbian women. In both studies, however, a substantial proportion did want to become parents, and Riskind and Patterson noted that valuing of parenthood was the same among heterosexual and homosexual participants [10]. Baiocco and Laghi interpreted their findings as reflecting the contextual barriers of lack of access to surrogacy or adoption for men in same-sex partnerships [9].

Fatherhood Aspirations among Men Who Are Experiencing Fertility Difficulties

Stereotypically, women are presumed to desire children and therefore to experience grief when the life goal of motherhood is unrealized, but men, having more diverse life opportunities, have been described as being 'disappointed but not devastated' by being unable to have a child [11]. Desire for fatherhood has also been investigated among men diagnosed as infertile or whose partners are infertile or who have unexplained infertility as a couple. Edelmann et al. conducted a postal survey of emotional distress among 205 couples belonging to the National Association for the Childless in the United Kingdom in which the male partner was infertile [12]. Levels of distress were higher than in the general community and similar among men and women, suggesting that men do not experience infertility as merely 'disappointing'. Dyer et al. found among 50 couples attending public infertility treatment clinics in South Africa that men and women desired children with similar intensity [13].

Longer-term attitudes towards parenthood were surveyed among 112 Australian men who had been diagnosed as infertile five years earlier [14]. Of these participants 84% reported that they desired parenthood as much as their partner did; fewer than half agreed that it would be more disappointing for a woman than a man not to have a child. In the Netherlands 108 infertile couples who had not become parents, on average 8.6 years after treatment initiation, completed self-report questionnaires. Men were less likely than women to 'think often' about having children, but they were equally likely (86%) still to want a child and to identify happiness as the main motive to seek parenthood [15].

Age, Health and Fertility among Men

Age

The consequences of chronological age for female fertility, including increased time to pregnancy and higher rates of chromosomal abnormalities that are associated with reduced conception and increased spontaneous abortion, from the mid-thirties are well established [16]. Fertility among men also declines with age, with increasing proportions of morphologically abnormal sperm and higher mutation rates in genetic material carried within the sperm of older compared to younger men. While conceptions can occur between a man in his fifties and a younger woman, in general infertility rates increase among men from the late thirties [17]. In a recent review of the evidence about the impact of paternal age on the health and development of offspring, Lawson and Fletcher found that when maternal age is controlled, rates of stillbirth are higher when the father is aged over 40 years and increase further when he is over 50 years [18]. While overall rates are low, they also found that there are increased risks of autism spectrum disorders, bipolar affective disorders and schizophrenia among the offspring of older, than younger, fathers.

Mental Health

There have been substantial investigations in recent decades into whether semen quality at a population level is changing in response to factors other than chronological age. Psychological stress, long thought to be a factor contributing to unexplained infertility among women, has been investigated in relation to men but, most commonly using semen samples from men in couples seeking fertility treatments and thus not representative of men in the general population. Gollenberg et al. assessed experiences of major adverse life events in the prior three months (the period of spermatogenesis) and standard parameters of semen quality among 744 fertile men who, with their pregnant partners, were participants in the Study for Future Families, conducted in five US major cities [19]. They found that those reporting two or more recent challenging events were twice as likely to have sperm classified as below-normal standard international criteria for concentration, motility and morphology than those who reported fewer than two such events, including when alcohol, tobacco and illegal substance abuse was controlled for in analyses. These authors propose an endocrine pathway with increased stress hormones leading to reduction in essential precursors for sperm production. Li et al. undertook a review of 57 cross-sectional studies with a total participant pool of almost 30,000 men from 26 nations, which had investigated associations between psychological, social or behavioural factors and semen parameters [20]. Meta-analyses of the impact of age, body mass index, smoking, alcohol and coffee consumption and self-reported psychological stress were conducted. They concluded that although there might be interactions among them, higher age, smoking, alcohol consumption and psychological stress were all risk factors for poorer semen quality and therefore for male fertility.

Cancer and Cancer Therapies

One of the most clearly established risks to fertility is cancers, some of which have a direct impact on reproductive organs, and the cytotoxic chemotherapies or radiotherapy required for cancer treatment [21]. There have been quite extensive investigations of the psychological and social consequences of fertility difficulties related to cancer experienced during childhood or reproductive life, synthesized in recent systematic and narrative reviews [22, 23].

People in this circumstance experience the complex psychological demands of adjustment to a potentially life-limiting condition, which might require treatments with the potential side effect of loss of fertility, including removal of malignant tissues, and adjuvant treatments to prevent recurrence. Tschudin and Bitzer reviewed 24 studies, which had used interviews or surveys to assess the psychological aspects of fertility preservation among men and women in the context of cancer [23]. They identified the contrasting psychological processes of fear, loss and despondency that might accompany cancer, and of joy and optimism that are associated with fertility, and suggested that fertility preservation could be experienced as providing hope in an otherwise bleak situation. However, they also found that while clinicians were in general in favour of sperm banking for all men experiencing cancer, some oncology specialists lacked personal knowledge of the techniques, relationships with clinicians specialized in fertility preservation, or access to services, to offer it and were hesitant to raise the topic in consultations. In general patient perspectives were that they wanted to preserve future fertility but did not want it to involve delays in initiating cancer treatment.

Goossens et al. reviewed 27 papers reporting investigations of fertility-related information needs and preferences, and experiences of clinical consultations from the perspectives of people who had experienced cancer, and healthcare providers [24]. People

with cancer, in particular those who are young, do not yet have children, or who have plans for further children want fertility-related information, but there is great variation in the proportion (0–85%) who receive it. Younger patients were more likely than those who were older, to report unmet information needs. Barriers to the provision of such information identified by healthcare providers included prioritization of survival over other concerns, and self-appraised lack of knowledge and skills about fertility preservation. Similar conclusions had been reached by Quinn et al. in their review of 29 papers about fertility decision-making in the context of paediatric cancers [25]. They found consistent evidence that adolescents experiencing cancer want to participate in fertility decision-making and do not want decisions made in their interests by either treating clinicians or their parents.

Crawshaw elaborated these findings in a narrative review of the fertility preservation needs of adolescents and young adults experiencing cancer [26]. She concluded that 'professional gate-keeping' related to inadequate knowledge or perceptions that patients are too young, or too sick, or have too limited a prognosis, or that risk of damage to fertility is low, or unease in discussing sexual or reproductive matters can lead clinicians not to provide information or invite discussion with young people in this predicament or their families. Fertility preservation was more likely to be discussed with people who were childless, graduates, Caucasian and heterosexual than others. Parents too can feel awkward about discussing fertility preservation with young men, in particular as collection of semen requires masturbation.

As survival rates following testicular cancer are generally high and life expectancy is not necessarily reduced, Carpentier and Fortenberry argued there are needs to consider long-term as well as the immediate and medium-term impacts of survivorship among adolescents and young men [22]. In their review of 37 studies they found that the mental health, including self-esteem, of men who were in committed romantic relationships at point of diagnosis was protected. However, men who were single were especially vulnerable to subsequent lasting anxiety about sexual functioning and fear that disclosure of having experienced cancer would limit future intimate partnerships. Although some studies reported that there was little evidence that sexual interest, functioning and pleasure changed after treatment for testicular cancer, others reported that anxiety about sexual performance began during treatment and was enduring.

Overall, conclusions were that providing clinical care in this situation is especially difficult because it involves not only the transfer of information about cancer and cancer treatments but also about future fertility, each with ethical complexities [23]. It requires sustained emotional support and consideration of existential meanings all bound by the time constraints of commencement of oncology treatment. Crawshaw highlights the importance of taking a life course approach, which incorporates awareness that from the point of cancer diagnosis onwards, future hopes, aspirations and expectations both in the immediate and longer term are altered [26]. She concludes that consideration of fertility, including fertility preservation, is intrinsic to comprehensive cancer care and should be included routinely as a best practice.

Fertility-Related Knowledge, Attitudes and Behaviours

In addition to social and economic circumstances, the achievement of desired goals of family formation requires knowledge of fertility, fertility management and both contraception- and fertility-promoting behaviours that can reflect personal values and attitudes.

Knowledge of Factors That Influence Fertility

Knowledge of the associations among aging, health-related behaviours and fertility was assessed in a population-based telephone interview survey initiated by the Fertility Coalition, a consortium of agencies in Australia [27]. Participants were English-speaking adults aged 18–45 years who wished to have a child in the future. While the recruitment fraction was quite low (18% of eligible respondents), 462 people (45% men) provided complete data. Among male participants, 35% believed that male fertility begins to decline at the age of 50 years and 23% that it is unaffected by age. They were significantly more likely than female participants to state either that they did not know at what age fertility begins to decline, or that age does not affect fertility. Among men who had not completed secondary schooling 19% believed that female fertility is unaffected by age, compared to only 2% of those with post-secondary education.

Fewer respondents believed that male obesity (30%) or smoking (36%) influences men's fertility compared with the equivalent beliefs about the adverse impact of female obesity or smoking (both 59%) on fertility. Higher proportions of men than women believed that obesity and smoking have no influence at all on male fertility. Only a third were accurately informed about the time during a woman's menstrual cycle when conception is most likely to occur.

In order to assess knowledge about fertility among younger people who had received sexual and reproductive health education at school, Ekelin et al. surveyed 274 18- to 20-year-olds (146 young men) in two Swedish schools [28]. Most wanted to have children in the future. The males believed that female fertility begins to decline markedly at the age of 47.5 years (significantly older estimated age than among female respondents), and fewer of them were aware that conception is most likely to occur mid-menstrual cycle, and that age or high or low body mass index influences fertility, than women.

Understanding and knowledge of fertility treatment using assisted reproductive technologies (ART) was assessed among 599 childless Canadian men aged 20–50 years who were presumed to be fertile, using a male adaptation of the Fertility Awareness Survey and compared to equivalent data from women by Daniluk and Koert [29]. Overall 53% were assessed as having some knowledge and 13% as being fairly knowledgeable about ART. However, answers to the 20 information-based questions suggested major knowledge gaps, and 81% believed that general health and physical fitness are better indicators of fertility than age among women older than 30 years. Their overall knowledge levels were significantly worse among men than the comparison population of childless women.

Bunting et al. investigated related questions among 10,045 people (1,690 men) aged 18–50 years from 79 countries who had been trying actively to conceive for at least six months [30]. Their International Fertility Decision Making Study used an online survey to investigate aspects of decisions to have a child and what to do if attempts to conceive spontaneously were unsuccessful. Men, in particular those without post-secondary education, who were not employed or lived in a rural area had lower knowledge than women on fertility knowledge questions which included awareness of indicators for reduced fertility and misconceptions about fertility.

Experiences of Pregnancy and Early Adjustment to Parenthood

Psychological aspects of pregnancy, childbirth and the early postpartum period have been investigated extensively among women, in particular in high-income countries. Condon et al. completed one of the first prospective cohort investigations of psychological symptoms, sexual satisfaction and alcohol use among 312 men without children, but who were partners in a pregnancy. Repeat assessments were undertaken from about 23 weeks' gestation until the end of the first postpartum year [31]. They found that the highest level of symptoms of depression and anxiety was in mid-pregnancy, and that these diminished and thereafter remained stable from advanced pregnancy. In mid-pregnancy, 5.2% of men scored in the clinical range (> 12) on the Edinburgh Postnatal Depression Scale (EPDS), but at all subsequent assessments about 1% scored at this level. Of greatest concern was that at all assessment points about one in four men reported using alcohol (Alcohol Use Disorders Identification Test score > 7) at harmful levels. Proportions of men reporting low sexual satisfaction increased from 27% in mid-pregnancy to 37% a year postpartum, and for up to half of them frequency of intercourse was lower than had been anticipated at each assessment point. The authors concluded that contrary to their expectations, pregnancy was more stressful for men making the transition from being childless to becoming a parent than the postpartum year but that overall, men appeared to be underprepared for the impact of parenthood on their lives.

Wynter et al. assessed the period prevalence of common mental disorders in a community cohort of 172 couples in the six months after the birth of a first child [32]. They found that no men met diagnostic criteria for major or minor depression, but that experiences of anxiety were more common. In total 13% experienced an adjustment disorder with anxiety and 4% an anxiety disorder. They found in further analyses that higher levels of depressive symptoms (EPDS scores) were reported by both men and women who experienced their intimate partners as critical and controlling [33]. Symptoms worsened if the baby was unsettled with unsoothable crying or difficulties settling to sleep or if they had coincidental adverse life events.

Fisher et al. completed a cross-sectional survey of a randomly selected sample of 231 men whose wives were >28 weeks' pregnant or mothers of 4- to 6-week-old babies in rural and urban communes in northern Vietnam [34]. As has been found among women, prevalence of common mental disorders was much higher in this lower-middle-income nation than that found in high-income countries. Overall, 17.7% were diagnosed with a depressive or anxiety disorder and 33.8% with harmful alcohol use. Perinatal common mental disorders among men were associated with experiencing coincidental life adversity (most commonly poverty and food insecurity), intimate partner violence, an unwelcome pregnancy and primiparity. Alcohol misuse was more common among men with low education, living in the poorest households and in unskilled work.

Humberd et al. used in-depth interviews to investigate how 36 American men established their identities as fathers in the context of changes in social expectations of the roles and responsibilities of parents and traditional workplaces [35]. They concluded that a strong and widely held cultural belief prevailed that there would be little change in any aspect of a man's employed role or income-generating activities once he became a father. They also concluded that there was little appreciation within organizations, or among colleagues, that fathers of young children needed flexibility in order to fulfil care-giving obligations and that this constitutes a significant structural barrier to more equitable gender roles and division of labour.

Experiences of Infertility and Infertility Treatment

In high-income countries about 15% of heterosexual couples experience difficulties conceiving when pregnancy is desired and in up to half of these couples infertility is attributable to male factors [36]. In low-income settings prevalence is thought to be higher in particular where undetected and untreated reproductive tract infections are common [37]. Men are affected by infertility either through being diagnosed as infertile themselves, being the partner of a woman who is infertile, or by being a member of a couple with unexplained infertility. Fisher and Hammarberg reviewed 73 papers which reported data about the psychological and social aspects of diagnosis, ART treatment and unsuccessful treatment among men with fertility difficulties [38]. Although the research is diverse in theoretical conceptualizations, research designs, study settings, inclusion criteria for participants and data sources, there is general consistency of findings. These indicate that diagnosis and initiation of treatment are associated with elevated infertility-specific anxiety and that unsuccessful treatment can lead to a state of lasting sadness, but rates of clinically significant mental health problems are no higher among them than among men in the general population. Infertile men who are socially isolated, have an avoidant style and appraise stressful events as overwhelming are vulnerable to more severe anxiety. Men prefer oral to written treatment information and to receive emotional support from infertility clinicians rather than from mental health professionals, self-help support groups or friends.

Summary and Implications for Policy and Practice

Overall therefore the evidence indicates that most young and older men with and without fertility difficulties express a desire to have children. It is possible that there is some idealization of the potential to achieve the circumstances in which they want to do this, including establishment of an occupational identity, security of employment and income, and finding a partner with desired qualities to be a co-parent to their child. Despite these aspirations, unintended and unwelcome pregnancies occur related to inconsistent or incorrect use of contraception, use of less effective methods like withdrawal and inaccurate presumptions that contraception is a woman's responsibility. Using likelihood estimations, Kessler et al. ascertained the chance that men childless at a specific age would actually achieve fatherhood [17]. They concluded that by the age of 45 more than one in seven would remain childless and that 'Miscalculation in the postponement of fatherhood is one of the most likely causes of involuntary childlessness among men'. In the context of cancer the available evidence is that semen quality is broadly similar among males with and without malignancies, but deteriorates rapidly after a single cycle of cytotoxic treatment [39]. Sperm can be stored and pregnancies occur using frozen sperm, but decisions first to store and then to use sperm for conception in this context remain complex for men who are affected, their families and treating clinicians [21]. Together

these have major implications for policies and clinical practices about reproductive events and reproductive health among men.

Policy

Policies to promote reproductive autonomy and the realization of reproductive aspirations have to include strategies both to reduce unintended and unwanted pregnancies and to preserve and promote fertility. Each requires approaches that address the information needs of boys and men as well as girls and women and the interpersonal skills to negotiate fertility decision-making. Kågesten et al. argue that 'male-oriented strategies are needed to help men take control over their reproductive goals' [1]. These include school-based and public education programs about contraceptive behaviours and skills to negotiate use of contraception, including to avoid presumptions that it is a female responsibility. Hammarberg et al. concluded that a high proportion of men and women of reproductive age in Australia lack knowledge about the potentially modifiable factors that affect fertility [27]. They advocate a 'broad-based approach' to improve knowledge, which should be integrated into school-based sexual and reproductive health curricula and public health education, in particular using online resources and social media (e.g. yourfertility.org.au).

Clinical Practice

Each clinical encounter is an opportunity to assess knowledge, address information gaps, assist behaviour change and model interpersonal skills. Kågesten et al. advocate that all family planning should be 'gender-inclusive' and engage men and women as individuals with reproductive rights, aspirations and health needs in which each should participate actively [1].

Ginsberg et al. and Crawshaw conclude that storage of sperm should be offered to all boys and men who experience cancers while of reproductive age [39, 40]. The discussion should be initiated by the oncology clinicians and is assisted by the availability of clear pathways to fertility preservation services. Among adolescents and young men, this discussion has to include their parents (on whom most adolescents rely for assistance with interpretation of information) who are usually more conscious of the impact of potentially compromised fertility than the young people themselves. They also found that the order of presenting information was crucial: people hearing the risks before the benefits are more likely to accept fertility preservation than when it is presented in the reverse order, in particular if their parents have a good understanding of the process and the potential outcomes.

Fisher and Hammarberg conclude that comprehensive clinical care within infertility services is of particular importance to the protection of emotional well-being among men affected by infertility [38]. As men appear to be more likely to confide in and want information and emotional support from infertility clinicians, than from friends or mental health professionals, explicit assessment of the emotional well-being of men at initial assessment and during treatment might be beneficial.

Key Points

- Stereotypically, women are presumed to desire children and therefore to experience grief when the life goal of motherhood is unrealized, while men in the same position have been described as being 'disappointed but not devastated', Studies have shown, however, that men do not experience infertility as merely 'disappointing', and that men and women desire children with similar intensity.
- A substantial proportion of homosexual men want to become parents and valuing of parenthood has been found to be the same among heterosexual and homosexual persons. Although desires and intentions to become a parent are lower among homosexual than heterosexual men and lesbian women, this probably reflects the contextual barriers of lack of access to surrogacy or adoption for men in same-sex partnerships.
- When maternal age is controlled, rates of stillbirth are higher when the father is aged over 40 years and increase further when he is aged over 50 years. While overall rates are low, there are increased risks of autism spectrum disorders, bipolar affective disorders and schizophrenia among the offspring of older, than younger, fathers.
- Although there might be interactions among them, higher age, smoking, alcohol consumption and psychological stress are all risk factors for poorer semen quality and therefore for male fertility.

- Adolescents experiencing cancer want to participate in fertility decision-making and do not want decisions made on their behalf by either treating clinicians or their parents.
- The achievement of desired goals of family formation requires knowledge of fertility, contraception- and fertility-promoting behaviours that can reflect personal values and attitudes. Men are less informed about these aspects of their reproductive lives and health than women are. A higher proportion of men than women believe that obesity and smoking have no influence at all on male fertility, and only a third of men are accurately informed about the time during a woman's menstrual cycle when conception is most likely to occur.

References

1. Kågesten A, Bajos N, Bohet A, Moreau C. Male experiences of unintended pregnancy: Characteristics and prevalence. *Human Reproduction* 2015;**30**:186–96.

2. Rowe H, Holton S, Kirkman M, Bayly C, LJordan L, McNamee K, *et al.* Prevalence and distribution of unintended pregnancy: The Understanding Fertility Management in Australia National Survey. *Australian and New Zealand Journal of Public Health* 2016;**40**:104–109.

3. Hadley R, Hanley T. Involuntarily childless men and the desire for fatherhood. *Journal of Reproductive and Infant Psychology* 2011;**29**:56–68.

4. Thompson R, Lee C. Sooner or later? Young Australian men's perspectives on timing of parenthood. *Journal of Health Psychology* 2011;**16**:807–18.

5. Thompson R, Lee C, Adams J. Imagining fatherhood: Young Australian men's perspectives on fathering. *International Journal of Men's Health* 2013;**12**:150–65.

6. Roberts E, Metcalfe A, Jack M, Tough SC. Factors that influence the childbearing intentions of Canadian men. *Human Reproduction* 2011;**25**:1202–8.

7. Stöbel-Richter Y, Beutel ME, Finck C, Bräler E. The 'wish to have a child', childlessness and infertility in Germany. *Human Reproduction* 2005;**20**:2850–7.

8. Langdridge D, Sheeran P, Connolly K. Understanding the reasons for parenthood. *Journal of Reproductive and Infant Psychology* 2005;**23**:121–33.

9. Baiocco R, Laghi F. Sexual orientation and the desires and intentions to become parents. *Journal of Family Studies* 2013;**19**:90–8.

10. Riskind RG, Patterson CJ. Parenting intentions and desires among childless lesbian, gay, and heterosexual individuals. *J Fam Psychol* 2010;**24**:78–81.

11. Greil A, Slauson-Blevins K, McQuillan J. The experience of infertility: A review of recent literature. *Sociology of Health & Illness* 2010;**32**:140–62.

12. Edelmann RJ, Humphry M, Owens DJ. The meaning of parenthood and couples' reactions to male infertility. *British Journal of Medical Psychology* 1994;**67**:291–9.

13. Dyer S, Mokoena N, Maritz J, van der Spuy Z. Motives for parenthood among couples attending a level 3 infertility clinic in the public health sector in South Africa. *Human Reproduction* 2008;**23**:353–7.

14. Fisher J, Baker H, Hammarberg K. Long-term health, well-being, life satisfaction, and attitudes towards parenthood in men diagnosed as infertile: Challenges to gender stereotypes and implications for practice. *Fertility and Sterility* 2010;**94**:574–80.

15. van Balen F, Trimbos-Kemper TCM. Involuntary childless couples: Their desire to have children and their motives. *Journal of Psychosomatic Obstetrics and Gynecology* 1995;**16**:137–44.

16. Sauer MV. Reproduction at an advanced maternal age and maternal health. *Fertility and Sterility* 2015;**103**: 1136–43.

17. Kessler LM, Craig BM, Saigal C, Quinn GP. Starting a family: Characteristics associated with men's reproductive preferences. *American Journal of Men's Health* 2013;**7**:198–205.

18. Lawson G, Fletcher R. Delayed fatherhood. *Journal of Family Planning and Reproductive Health Care* 2014;**40**:283–8.

19. Gollenberg AL, Liu F, Brazil C, Drobnis E, Gizick D, Overstreet JW et al. Semen quality in fertile men in relation to psychosocial stress. *Fertility and Sterility* 2010;**93**:1104–11.

20. Li Y, Lin H, Li Y, Cao J. Association between socio-psycho-behavioral factors and male semen quality: A systematic review and meta-analyses. *Fertility and Sterility* 2011;**95**:116–23.

21. Pacey AA. Fertility issues in survivors from adolescent cancers. *Cancer Treatment Reviews* 2007;**33**:646–55.

22. Carpenter MY, Fortenberry JD. Romantic and sexual relationships, body image, and fertility in adolescent and young adult testicular cancer survivors: A review of the literature. *Journal of Adolescent Health* 2010;**47**: 115–25.

23. Tschudin S, Bitzer J. Psychological aspects of fertility preservation in men and women affected by cancer and other life-threatening diseases. *Human Reproduction Update* 2009;**15**:587–97.

24. Goossens J, Delbaere I, Van Lancker Al, Beeckman D, Verhaeghe S, Van Hecke A. Cancer patients' and professional caregivers' needs, preferences and factors associated with receiving and providing fertility-related information: A mixed-methods systematic review. *International Journal of Nursing Studies* 2014;**51**:300–19.

25. Quinn GP, Murphy D, Knapp C, Stearsman DK, Bradley-Klug KL, Sawczyn K et al. Who decides? Decision making and fertility preservation in teens with cancer: A review of the literature. *Journal of Adolescent Health* 2011;**49**:337–46.

26. Crawshaw M. Psychosocial oncofertility issues faced by adolescents and young adults over their lifetime: A review of the research. *Human Fertility* 2012;**16**:59–63.

27. Hammarberg K, Setter T, Norman R, Holden C, Michelmore J, Johnson L. Knowledge about factors that influence fertility among Australians of reproductive age: A population-based survey. *Fertility and Sterility* 2013;**99**:502–7.

28. Ekelin M, Akesson C, Angerud M, Kvist L. Swedish high school students' knowledge and attitudes regarding fertility and family building. *Reproductive Health* 2012; **9**:6, DOI: 10.1186/1742-4755-9-6

29. Daniluk JC, Koert E. The other side of the fertility coin: A comparison of childless men's and women's knowledge of fertility and assisted reproductive technology. *Fertility and Sterility* 2013;**99**:839–46.

30. Bunting L, Tsibulsky I, Boivin J. Fertility knowledge and beliefs about fertility treatment: Findings from the International Fertility Decision-making Study. *Human Reproduction* 2013;**28**:385–97.

31. Condon JT, Boyce P, Corkindale CJ. The first-time fathers study: A prospective study of the mental health and wellbeing of men during the transition to parenthood. *Aust N Z J Psychiatry* 2004;**38**:56–64.

32. Wynter K, Rowe H, Fisher J. Common mental disorders in women and men in the first six months after the birth of their first infant: A community study in Victoria, Australia. *Journal of affective disorders* 2013;**151**:980–5.

33. Wynter K, Rowe H, Fisher J. Interactions between perceptions of relationship quality and postnatal depressive symptoms in Australian, primiparous women and their partners. *Australian Journal of Primary Health* 2014;**20**:174–81.

34. Fisher J, Tran T, Nguyen T, Tran T. Common perinatal mental disorders and alcohol dependence in men in northern Viet Nam. *Journal of affective disorders* 2012;**140**:97–101.

35. Humberd B, Ladge J, Harrington B. The 'New' dad: Navigating fathering identity within organizational contexts. *J Bus Psychol* 2015;**30**:249–66.

36. Skakkebaek N, Giwercman A, de Kretser D. Pathogenesis and management of male infertility. *The Lancet* 1994;**343**:1473–9.

37. Inhorn MC. Right to assisted reproductive technology: Overcoming infertility in low-resource countries. *International Journal of Gynecology&Obstetrics* 2009;**106**:172–4.

38. Fisher J, Hammarberg K. Psychological and social aspects of infertility in men: An overview of the evidence and implications for psychologically informed clinical care and future research. *Asian Journal of Andrology* 2012;**14**:121–9.

39. Ginsberg JP, Ogle SK, Tuchman LK, Carlson CA, Reilly MM, Hobbie WL *et al.* Sperm banking for adolescent and young adult cancer patients: Sperm quality, patient, and parent perspectives. *Pediatric Blood & Cancer* 2008;**50**:594–8.

40. Crawshaw M. Male coping with cancer-fertility issues: Putting the 'social' into biopsychosocial approaches. *Reproductive Biomedicine Online* 2013;**27**:261–70.

Chapter 16

Biopsychosocial Factors in Chronic Pelvic Pain

Linda McGowan

Introduction

The aim of this chapter is to provide an overview of chronic pelvic pain utilizing a biopsychosocial framework. A broad perspective is provided to support the rationale for using this framework in both clinical and research settings. Emphasis is placed on research which informs the biopsychosocial approach, and treatments/interventions which are underpinned by this model.

Background

Chronic pelvic pain (CPP) is a surprisingly common condition that is challenging for both women and their health professionals. CPP is a worldwide phenomenon affecting all ethnic groups and countries [1]. Community surveys conducted in the United Kingdom and the United States report between 15 and 24% of women aged 18–50 report experiencing CPP within the last three months [2, 3]. In the United Kingdom, CPP accounts for approximately 38 per 1,000 visits to primary care services; a rate similar to that of asthma and chronic back pain [4]. In addition, CPP is the reported reason for 20–40% of all gynaecology outpatient appointments in the United Kingdom (RCOG, Green Top Guidelines) [5].

The aetiology of persistent pelvic pain is complex and poorly understood; common diagnoses include endometriosis, infection, adhesions and irritable bowel syndrome (IBS); the aetiology may be related to musculoskeletal and neurological conditions. [6] The most frequently reported comorbid conditions include dysmenorrhoea, dyspareunia and IBS [7]. Early work suggested that pelvic vein incompetence may be an important cause of CPP [8]; it has been suggested that this could be missed at diagnostic laparoscopy, as patients are tilted head down which causes the dilated veins to empty (McCollum – personal communication). Given the complexity of CPP it is not surprising that standardized guidance for clinicians is more helpful in cases where there is a definitive diagnosis or a more complete workup of presenting symptoms (Royal College of Obstetricians and Gynaecologists [RCOG]; European Association of Urology; American College of Obstetricians and Gynecologists [ACOG]) [5, 9, 10].

The majority of women who suffer CPP are in their reproductive years. Living with persistent lower abdominal pain has an adverse effect on women's quality of life, including coping with pain, psychological distress and difficulties with personal relationships and sexual functioning. [11, 12] There is limited research into the effect CPP has on personal relationships [13], although one study has noted the impact of endometriosis for women in heterosexual relationships had significant implications for the male partner and for the couple's relationship. This was not just confined to sex and intimacy but also affected areas such as communication, negotiating healthcare and support and planning for and having children.

The true economic cost of CPP is hard to quantify due to the lack of current data. Annual direct treatment costs in the United Kingdom have been estimated at £158 million, with indirect costs of £24 million [14]. The economic burden was higher in women who undergo multiple evaluations. In the United States reported costs of managing CPP were estimated at $100 billion/year in 1998.

Facilitating a Diagnosis

Laparoscopy is the most common surgical technique used by gynaecologists to facilitate making the diagnosis, and as a means of excluding more serious underlying pathology. When identifiable pathology is found at laparoscopy (e.g. endometriosis, adhesions, pelvic congestion syndrome), then guidance for clinical management is available (RCOG; ACOG) [5, 10]. However, laparoscopy fails to identify underlying pathology in up to 35% (range 3–92%) of women

[15]. This means that many women do not receive a medical explanation to account for their pain. Subsequently, many women enter a cycle of re-investigation and re-referral in a search for an explanation for their pain [12, 16]. Some even undergo hysterectomy which often fails to relieve their symptoms [17].

Ghaly and Chien [18] aptly referred to CPP as the 'clinician's dilemma or clinician's nightmare' as women who present with this problem pose a major challenge to a range of health professionals and services. Both gynaecologists and GPs have described women with CPP as 'heartsink' patients as they were considered to be difficult to manage and treat, and referral options were limited [19, 20]. This was most evident in cases without a medical explanation, where management was varied and idiosyncratic [21]. Interviews with women, 18 months post negative laparoscopy, indicate that they remained anxious and were dissatisfied with their care; some women disengage from healthcare despite remaining symptomatic [22].

Current Approaches to Treatment and Intervention

Two recent systematic reviews have comprehensively assessed current evidence on treatment and interventions for CPP. Andrews et al. [7] addressed the comparative effectiveness of therapies for noncyclical pelvic pain. They included a total of 36 studies which used a range of designs (18 RCTs; 3 cohort; 15 cross-sectional) to address a series of research questions. These covered both surgical and non-surgical interventions and the prevalence of comorbidities.

The most common non-surgical treatment to date has been hormonal therapy, usually for the management of endometriosis. Comparisons of various agents were of similar effectiveness. However, an RCT of raloxifene (selective oestrogen receptor modulator) versus placebo noted that pain returned earlier in the raloxifene group. The lack of studies of hormonal therapy on women with CPP without endometriosis makes it difficult to assess whether this would be an option for this subgroup. Surgical approaches included laparoscopic uterosacral nerve ablation which was no more effective than simple diagnostic laparoscopy. In addition, studies found no evidence of treatment benefit of lysis for adhesions for pain

reduction or improved quality of life. There was insufficient evidence to support hysterectomy as an ultimate option for women with intractable pain.

Various studies have reported significant clinical improvement in the majority of women undergoing embolization for pelvic venous incompetence [23].

Given the lack of good evidence for both surgical and medical treatments, it is surprising that only a limited number of studies (n=4) were included in the review which evaluated other approaches. One study which used a musculoskeletal approach compared distension of the pelvic floor muscles and joint between the coccyx and the rectum; this was compared with counselling. The 'distension' group reported reduced pain. A further two studies utilized common diagnostic techniques – ultrasound and laparoscopy. Ghaly [24] combined ultrasound and counselling with expectant management and reported reduced pain scores in the ultrasound group. In an attempt to share the visualization of results with women, Onwude et al. (2004) [25] showed women photographs taken at laparoscopy. The aim was to reinforce the clinical messages from the investigation. Unfortunately, no differences were found between women who received photographic evidence and those who did not. Peters et al. [26] used a more integrative approach which draws on the biopsychosocial approaches used in pain management programmes. Consultations gave equal focus to potential explanations for the pain including biological, psychological, posture and lifestyle with laparoscopy included if indicated versus usual clinical workup with laparoscopy. The intervention group reported a significant improvement in pain and reduction of associated symptoms, and less interruption of daily activities.

The interventions outlined previously describe some interesting yet diverse approaches which provide promising lines of enquiry. However, it should be noted that these are single studies that require further replication.

The quality of included studies was variable. The authors note that only a few intervention studies obtained a quality rating of good or fair, and many of the comparison studies did not include a placebo. Therefore, treatment effects are likely to be inflated. In addition, there was a paucity of reporting of harms data.

The lack of effective surgical interventions for CPP has led to a resurgence of interest in developing appropriate non-surgical and psychosocial interventions (sometimes in combination). Cheung et al. [27] conducted a systematic review to assess the effectiveness and safety of non-surgical interventions. The authors included randomized controlled trials which addressed a range of non-surgical interventions including medical, physical, lifestyle and psychological approaches. Thirteen RCTs were identified for inclusion in the review.

The main findings were similar to the Andrews et al. [7] review in that hormonal treatment (high-dose progesterone) had the greatest impact on pain reduction at baseline and up to nine months. Side effects include bloating and weight gain; however, these appeared to be tolerated by some women. Head-to-head comparison showed that women taking goserelin (GnRH analogue) had greater improvement in pelvic pain score at one year than those taking progestogen – but this evidence was from a single study, and the study did not report on adverse effects [27].

Interventions which included a psychological component showed some promising effects on pain scores. For example, as already noted, when ultrasound scan was combined with counselling this has benefits over a 'wait and see' policy.

One interesting study identified by Cheung et al. [27] involved the use of writing therapy [28]. This study was based on the premise that written disclosure about emotional problems and concerns may be a useful approach to stress management. This research is based on the seminal work of Pennebaker and Beall [29], who demonstrated a link between writing about traumatic or stressful events and physical health. The aim of the study [27] was to identify potential moderators of the effects of disclosure since previous work has shown that some participants gain more benefit than others when using this approach. Forty-eight women with CPP were included in a prospective RCT; those in the disclosure group were asked to write about stressful consequences of their pain, whilst the comparison group were asked to record positive events over a three-day period. Health status was measured at baseline and two months after the writing exercise. Whilst the results did not show a range of significant differences (women in the disclosure group reported less pain intensity but no differences on sensory or affective pain, disability or mood), they did identify a group of women who appeared to benefit the most. Rather counterintuitively this group of women were those who were most ambivalent about emotional disclosure at baseline. Whilst this study clearly needs replication, it does suggest the need to be cognizant of the various subgroups within CPP which researchers and clinicians should take into account when designing interventions and treatments.

Again, the authors note that the quality of included studies is an issue. The randomization process was often not fully described, and participants were not always adequately blinded. Attrition rates across studies were high. Taken together these reviews confirm the paucity of research relating to non-surgical interventions for CPP. In both reviews the authors caution about the quality of the research to date; it is not robust with issues relating to limited power, inadequate comparators and flawed designs.

Both reviews note other potential barriers to developing tailored and effective treatments for women with CPP. Within the existent literature CPP as a condition is ill-defined and there is a lack of clear diagnostic and treatment pathways. Andrews et al. [7] state that better characterization of CPP would inform the development of effective and acceptable interventions. Related to this is the need for better outcome measures particularly relating to quality-of-life outcomes to assess the impact of interventions on women's lives. In order to capture the biopsychosocial aspects of CPP, Cheung et al. [26] note the need for future research studies to incorporate a combination of both objective and patient-related outcome measures [30, 31].

Emergence of a Biopsychosocial Approach

Lack of effective treatments and the increasing acknowledgement of women's dissatisfaction with their care have prompted both clinicians and researchers to acknowledge that a biopsychosocial approach to management is needed.

The reliance on laparoscopy, as both a clinical and research tool, to assign women with CPP into known pathology versus unknown pathology categories has led to the emergence of an oversimplified, dualistic model of these complex pain phenomena. A study which analysed the stories and trajectories of women with CPP noted that this dualistic approach can lead women to continue the search for a diagnosis, and they view the laparoscope as an 'all seeing camera' that will provide them with a definitive answer [12]. When the laparoscopy is negative and no diagnosis is made, women often feel disbelieved by their doctors. Gaining a diagnosis is seen as validation for their pain and symptoms; if investigations are negative, this can have a lasting impact on how women make sense of their condition. This difference in world views is illuminated by the following quote, where, for one woman, her distress at being informed that her laparoscopy is 'negative' appears to be compounded by the 'delight' of her gynaecologist:

> Gynaecologist No. 2 booked me for a scan and a laparoscopy, he was delighted to inform me that there was nothing of any relevance inside. How could I be in so much pain with nothing causing it? I was devastated. [12, p 269]

This suggests that the way negative laparoscopy results are communicated can impact on the way women perceive their pain. This in turn can give women a sense that their accounts are not believed. In an attempt to draw on people's own views, rather than questionnaires, a recent study looked at the effects of being disbelieved when you have a chronic pain condition (the study included accounts from women with chronic pelvic pain). This suggests that a sense of being disbelieved, or that your condition is not a valid one, can affect personal relationships and leave people feeling stigmatized, isolated and distressed [32]. The juxtaposition of these opposing world views can lead to difficult and unsatisfactory consultations and misunderstandings by both women and their doctors [19, 20, 21].

According to Grace [33] the dominance of the medical paradigm has promoted the 'failure to develop understandings of the subjective aspects of pain, the tendency to reduce causal processes to mechanisms, and the tendency to consider the psychosocial as purely reactive to the biological' (p. 525). Indeed, Souza et al. [16] argue for more qualitative research to be conducted to provide the basis for a biopsychosocial approach to women who present with CPP. They contend that in order to understand the complexity of conditions like CPP researchers and clinicians need to understand how women construct their pain, and that this is achieved only by considering the meanings, attitudes, aspirations, beliefs and values. The authors note that the majority of research in this area has focussed on the 'biological' with limited emphasis on the 'psychological' and the 'social' from the women's own unique perspectives. This has led to a dominance of quantitative methods. The inclusion of women's voices, captured by

qualitative inquiry, will strengthen the design of future interventions and improve services and facilities where women access treatment and care. The authors conclude their paper with a call for more psychological approaches for CPP, including cognitive behavioural therapy.

Some researchers have brought attention to the gendered nature of pelvic pain [34]. The majority of research has focussed on women, with CPP in men being acknowledged only recently (usually as a result of chronic prostatitis). This has meant that CPP has been considered to be a condition suffered exclusively by women. It has been argued that pelvic pain in women can be normalized if it is associated with hormonal disturbances, menstruation or the menopause [16]. Thus, CPP can be downgraded as a pain condition and viewed as a problem commonly associated with being female.

More recent qualitative research has shed further light on the lived experience of women who suffer with CPP. Toye et al. [35] used a meta-ethnographic approach to synthesize qualitative research on the views and understandings that women who suffer with CPP may hold. This overview revealed that the ongoing search for an answer for their pain leaves many women struggling to construct their pain experience as 'real'. The sense of not being believed was apparent across studies, and this was compounded by lack of awareness of the condition by both health professionals and family and friends. The authors describe a 'culture of secrecy' in reference to the fact that 'women's problems' remain hidden. This has an isolating effect on women and can affect how, when and to whom they disclose their experience of living with 'relentless and overwhelming pain'. In their synthesis Toye et al. [35] propose a conceptual model which represents women's struggle to construct their CPP as 'real'. This analysis of qualitative research to date reinforces that the labelling of pain of 'real' versus 'not real' only goes to perpetuate the legitimacy of women's symptoms, and this has an adverse effect on women's quality of life as a whole.

Toward Supportive Self-Management

Although multidisciplinary approaches to CPP, and other similar conditions, are to be recommended, the cost (or lack of cost effectiveness data) and the availability of few published studies on effectiveness mean that these services are not widely available in healthcare systems. This has led to a focus on the role of self-management and self-care in people with long-term conditions. In the United Kingdom the NHS Plan [36] promotes a model of care for patients with long-term conditions whereby patients are encouraged to self-manage their conditions, alongside medical management and support. Evidence suggests that self-management of conditions plays an essential part in minimizing patients' symptoms. For example, it is asserted that supported self-help in patients with IBS reduced the number of primary care consultations and the perceived severity of symptoms [37]. The evidence-based self-help package consisted of advice on lifestyle, diet and pharmacological and alternative therapies and was informed by patients' own experiences. It is therefore plausible that women with CPP, a condition with a similar profile to IBS, might benefit from such an approach.

However, self-management should not become self-burden. Seear [38] notes that women with endometriosis who become experts of their own condition see this as being a 'third shift'. That is a form of work which adds to women's roles of both paid and unpaid workers. Self-management support needs to be designed based on current evidence and in the context of the healthcare systems in which it will be situated. It is feasible that such self-management packages would require a facilitator to support women with the process. In the United Kingdom, interviews with GPs and practice nurses concluded that GPs would be best placed to facilitate self-management, since practice nurses reported feeling uncomfortable with those women who did not have a definitive diagnosis [21]. Women with PPS often become engaged in a process of re-investigation and referral during the trajectory of their condition. Supported self-management earlier in the process of care has the potential to prevent women disengaging from care and also to feel comfortable to manage their symptoms earlier in the time course of their illness.

Who facilitates self-management, as in those with long-term conditions, has been much debated and lack of facilitation can be perceived as a barrier to self-care [39]; hence, adequate training and support of this group of peers is essential. Evaluations of peer support models are most prevalent in mental health, where there is some evidence of benefit; however, more quality randomized trials are needed [40]. There is the possibility to harness peer support from other women who have had direct experience of CPP. Women may also use other information sources such as the Internet and patient representative organizations as a resource and gain support from other women who have direct experience of CPP. These organizations are of particular importance in less well-understood conditions such as CPP as they provide information which takes the women's perspectives into account. In addition, they help to reassure women that there are other women who are suffering with CPP which has the potential to reduce feelings of isolation. Examples in the United Kingdom are Pelvic Pain Support Network UK (PPSN UK) (www.pelvicpain.org.uk/) and in the United States the International Pelvic Pain Society (IPPS) (http://pelvicpain.org/home.aspx) [41, 42]. Both organizations contribute and support research in pelvic pain, and the IPPS also has information for clinicians and healthcare providers.

Summary

Chronic pelvic pain is a multifaceted condition that is often difficult to treat and manage. As argued by Edozien [43] there is a need to adopt a biopsychosocial approach to gynaecology service provision, which includes conditions such as CPP. As this chapter has shown, the separating of the biological from the psychosocial has led to inadequate treatments for women with CPP and has held back more innovative approaches. Treating the pain alone is often inadequate, and a more multidisciplinary approach is required [44]. Findings from interventions which have used a multidisciplinary model show promise and some benefits [26]. Whilst a multidisciplinary approach to the treatment and care of women with CPP would seem most appropriate, the lack of evidence on effective treatment approaches and associated cost effectiveness of data acts as a barrier to the commissioning of services.

Research to date has been of varying quality, and there is an urgent need for more randomized and controlled trials of treatments which include medical, lifestyle and psychological. It is also important that those approaches which have shown some benefits are replicated to assess the strength of the evidence. In parallel, robust and in-depth qualitative research should continue to illuminate the views, beliefs and experiences of women who live with CPP, and address the acceptability of new ways of treating and managing this condition.

CPP is a prevalent condition which adversely affects the quality of the lives of women across several domains. Given that research has shown that only 20% of women respond to treatment over a three-year period [45], it is important that both clinicians and researchers work together to identify and develop new interventions that incorporate a biopsychosocial approach to improve the lived experience of women who suffer with CPP.

Key Points

- Living with persistent lower abdominal pain has an adverse effect on women's quality of life, including coping with pain, psychological distress and difficulties with personal relationships and sexual functioning.
- Laparoscopy fails to identify underlying pathology in about 35% of women with chronic pelvic pain (CPP). This means that many women do not receive a medical explanation to account for their pain and they remain anxious and dissatisfied with their care.
- The way that negative laparoscopy results are communicated can impact on how women perceive their pain.
- There is a lack of good evidence for both surgical and medical treatments (such as laparoscopic uterosacral nerve ablation, adhesiolysis and raloxifene). The lack of effective surgical interventions for CPP has led to a resurgence of interest in developing appropriate non-surgical and psychosocial interventions, but there remains a paucity of robust research data pertaining to non-surgical interventions for CPP.
- The reliance on laparoscopy to assign women with CPP into known versus unknown pathology categories has led to the emergence of an oversimplified, dualistic model of these complex pain phenomena which often leaves women anxious as they continue to search for a diagnosis.
- In order to understand the complexity of conditions like CPP researchers and clinicians need to understand how women construct their pain, and that this is achieved only by considering the meanings, attitudes, aspirations, beliefs and values.

References

1. Latthe P, Latthe M, Say L, Gulmezoglu M, Khan KS. WHO systematic review of prevalence of chronic pelvic pain: A neglected reproductive health morbidity. *BMC Public Health* 2006; **6**: doi: 10.1186/1471-2458-6-177.
2. Mathias S, Kuppermann M, Liberman R, Lipschutz R, Steege J. Chronic pelvic pain: Prevalence, health-related quality of life, and economic correlates. *Obstetrics & Gynecology* 1996; **87**(3): 321–7.
3. Zondervan KT, Yudkin PL, Vessey MP, Jenkinson CP, Dawes MG, Barlow, DH, et al. The community prevalence of chronic pelvic pain in women and associated illness behaviour. *British Journal of General Practice* 2001; **51**: 541–47.
4. Zondervan KT, Yudkin PL, Vessey MP, Dawes MG, Barlow DH, Kennedy SH. Prevalence and incidence of chronic pelvic pain in primary care: Evidence from a national general practice database. *British Journal of Obstetrics and Gynaecology* 1999; **106**: 1149–55.
5. Royal College of Obstetricians and Gynaecologists. Chronic Pelvic Pain, Initial Management (Green-top Guideline No. 41). Updated December 2014. www.rcog.org.uk/en/guidelines-research-services/guidelines/gtg41/. Accessed 22 March 2017.
6. Bruckenthal, P. Chronic pelvic pain: Approaches to diagnosis and treatment. *Pain Management Nursing* 2011; **12**(1): S4–10.
7. Andrews J, Yunker A, Reynolds WS, Likis FE, Sathe NA, Jerome RN. Noncyclic Chronic Pelvic Pain Therapies for Women: Comparative Effectiveness. Comparative Effectiveness Review No. 41. (Prepared by the Vanderbilt Evidence-Based Practice Center under Contract No. 290-2007-10065-I.) AHRQ Publication No. 11(12)-EHC088-EF. Rockville, MD: Agency for Healthcare Research and Quality. January 2012. http://effectivehealthcare.ahrq.gov/index.cfm/search-for-guides-reviews-and-reports/?productid=931&pageaction=displayproduct.
8. Beard RW, Highman JH, Pearce S, Reginald PW. Diagnosis of pelvic varicosities in women with chronic pelvic pain. *Lancet* 1984; **2**(8409): 946–9.
9. European Association of Urology. Guidelines on Chronic Pelvic Pain. 2012. www.pelvicpain.org.uk/uploads/EAU-%20CPP%20guideline%202012.pdf. Accessed 22 March 2017.
10. American College of Obstetricians and Gynecologists (ACOG). Chronic pelvic pain. FAQ099. August 2011. Available at www.acog.org/Patients/FAQs/Chronic-Pelvic-Pain. Accessed 22 March 2017.
11. Souza PP, Romao APMS, Nakano AMS, Rosa-e-Silva JC, Candido-dos-Reis, Nogueira AA, Poli-Neto OB. Biomedical perspectives about women with

chronic pelvic pain: A qualitative analysis. *International Journal of Clinical Medicine* 2012; **3**: 411–18.

12. McGowan L, Luker K, Creed F, Chew-Graham C. 'How do you explain a pain that can't be seen?' The narratives of women with chronic pelvic pain and their disengagement with the diagnostic cycle. *British Journal of Health Psychology* 2007; **12**(2): 261–74.

13. Culley L, Hudson N, Mitchell, H, Law C, Denny E, Raine-Fenning N. Endometriosis: improving the wellbeing of couples. Summary report and recommendations. October 2013. www.dmu.ac.uk/do cuments/research-documents/health-and-life-sciences /reproduction-research/endopart/endopart-study-summary-report-and-recommendations.pdf. Accessed 22 March 2017.

14. Stones RW, Selfe SA, Fransman S, Horn SA. Psychosocial and economic impact of chronic pelvic pain. *Baillieres Clinical Obstetrics and Gynaecology* 2000; **14**(3): 415–31.

15. Howard FM. The role of laparoscopy in chronic pelvic pain: Promise and pitfalls. *Obstetrical & Gynecological Survey* 1993; **48**: 357–87.

16. Souza PP, Romao APMS, Nakano AMS, Rosa-e-Silva JC, Candido-dos-Reis, Nogueira AA, Poli-Neto OB. Qualitative research as the basis for a biopsychosocial approach to women with chronic pelvic pain. *Journal of Psychosomatic Obstetrics and Gynecology* 2011; **32**(4): 165–72.

17. Lamvu G. Role of hysterectomy in the treatment of chronic pelvic pain. *Obstetrics and Gynecology* 2011; **117**(5): 1175–8.

18. Ghaly AFF, Chien PFW. Chronic pelvic pain: Clinical dilemma or clinician's nightmare. *Sex Transm Inf* 2000; **76**: 419–25.

19. Selfe SA, Van Vugt M, Stones RW. Chronic gynaecological pain: An exploration of medical attitudes. *Pain* 1998; **77**(2): 215–25.

20. McGowan L, Pitts MK, Clark-Carter D. Chronic pelvic pain: The general practitioners' perspective. *Psychology, Health & Medicine* 1999; **4**(3): 303–17.

21. McGowan L, Escott D, Luker K, Creed F, Chew-Graham C. Is chronic pelvic pain a comfortable diagnosis for primary care practitioners: A qualitative study. *BMC Family Practice* 2010: **11**(7): doi: 10.1186/ 1471-2296-11-7.

22. Savidge CJ, Slade P, Stewart P, Li TC. Women's perspectives on their experiences of chronic pelvic pain and medical care. *J Health Psychol* 1998; **42**: 103–16.

23. Venbrux AC, Sharma GK, Jackson ET, Harper AP, and Hover L. In Ignacio EA and Venbrux AC (eds.), *Women's Health in Interventional Radiology*, doi:

10.1007/978–1-4419-5876-1_2, New York: Springer, 2012.

24. Ghaly AFF. The psychological and physical benefits of pelvic ultrasonography in patients with chronic pelvic pain and negative laparoscopy. A random allocation trial. *Journal of Obstetrics and Gynaecology* 1994; **14**: 269–71.

25. Onwude JL, Thornton JG, Morley S, et al. A randomised trial of photographic reinforcement during postoperative counselling after diagnostic laparoscopy for pelvic pain. *Eur J Obstet Gynecol Reprod Biol*. 2004 January 15; **112**(1): 89–94.

26. Peters AAW, van Dorst E, Jellis B, van Zuuren E, Hermans J, Trimbos JB. A randomized clinical trial to compare two different approaches in women with chronic pelvic pain. *Obstetrics and Gynecology* 1991; **77** (5): 740–4.

27. Cheung YC, Smotra G, de C Williams A. Non-surgical interventions for the management of chronic pelvic pain. Cochrane Review. Updated February 2014. doi: 10.1002/14651858.CD008797.pub2.

28. Norman SA, Lumley MA, Dooley JA, Diamond MP. For whom does it work? Moderators of the effects of written emotional disclosure in a randomised trial among women with chronic pelvic pain. *Psychosomatic Medicine* 2004; **66**: 174–83.

29. Pennebaker JW, Beall SK. Confronting a traumatic event. Toward an understanding of inhibition and disease. *Journal of Abnormal Psychology* 1986; **95**: 274–81.

30. Dworkin RH, Turk DC, Farrar JT, Haythornthwaite JA, Jensen MP, Katz NP, et al. Core outcome measures for chronic pain clinical trials: IMMPACT guidelines. *Pain* 2005; **113**: 9–19.

31. Dworkin RH, Turk DC, Peirce-Sandner S, Baron R, Bellamy N, Burke LB, et al. Research design considerations for confirmatory chronic pain clinical trials: IMMPACT recommendations. *Pain* 2010; **149**: 177–93.

32. Newton BJ, Southall JL, Raphael JH, Asford RL, LeMarchand K. Narrative review of the impact of disbelief in chronic pain. *Pain Management Nursing* 2013; **14**(3): 161–71.

33. Grace VM. Pitfalls of the medical paradigm in chronic pelvic. *Baillière's Clinical Obstetrics and Gynaecology* 2000; **14**(3): 525–39.

34. Grace VM, MacBride-Stewart S. Women get this: Gendered meanings of chronic pelvic pain. *Health* 2007; **11**(1): 47–67.

35. Toye F, Seers K, Barker K. A meta-ethnography of patients' experiences of chronic pelvic pain: Struggling to construct chronic pelvic pain as 'rea'. *Journal of Advanced Nursing* 2012; **70**(12): 2713–27.

36. NHS England. Everyone counts: Planning for patients for 2014/15 to 2018/19. www.england.nhs.uk/wp-content/uploads/2013/12/5yr-strat-plann-guid-wa.pdf. Accessed 22 March 2017.

37. Robinson A, Lee V, Kennedy A, Middleton L, Rogers A, Thompson DG, Reeves D. A randomised controlled trial of self-help interventions in patients with a primary care diagnosis of irritable bowel syndrome. *Gut* 2006; **55**: 643–48.

38. Seear K. The third shift: Health, work and expertise among women with endometriosis. *Health Psychology Review* 2009b; **2**: 194–206.

39. Nagelkerk J, Reick K, Meengs L. Perceived barriers and effective strategies to diabetes self-management. *Journal of Advanced Nursing* 2006; **54**(2): 151–58.

40. Pitt V, Lowe D, Hill S, Prictor M, Hetrick SE, Ryan R, Berends L. Involving adults who use mental health services as providers of mental health services to others. 28 March 2013. Cochrane Review. http://onlinelibrary.wiley.com/doi/10.1002/14651858.CD004807 .pub2/abstract;jsessionid=032E702FC10D4F808F4B2 F300F085939.f03t03. Accessed 22 March 2017

41. Pelvic Pain Support Network UK. www.pelvicpain.org .uk/. Accessed 22 March 2017.

42. International Pelvic Pain Society. http://pelvicpain.org /home.aspx. Accessed 22 March 2017.

43. Edozien LC. Beyond biology: The biopsychosocial model and its application in obstetrics and gynaecology. *BJOG An International Journal of Obstetrics & Gynaecology* 2015; **122**(7): 900–3.

44. Miller-Matero LR, Saulino C, Clark S, Bugenski M, Eshelman A, Eisenstein, D. When treating the pain is not enough: A multidisciplinary approach for chronic pelvic pain. *Archives of Women's Mental Health* epub ahead of print 5 May 2015.

45. Weijenborg PT, Greeven A, Dekker FW, Peters AAW, ter Kuile MM. Clinical course of chronic pelvic pain in women. *Pain* 2007; **132**(1): S117–23.

Biopsychosocial Factors in Emergency Gynaecology

Olanike Bika

Introduction

Psychosocial, psychological, sociocultural, ethical and other aspects of social functioning and behaviour have a significant impact on the perception, presentation and management of gynaecological emergencies. The association and health outcomes may not be a direct causal relationship but may reflect the confounding effects that the physical, social and psychological environment can have on objective measures of physical health [1].

The coping mechanisms and mental resilience to physical disease vary greatly from person to person. Women with mental health disorders often present with physical symptomatology because the latter carries fewer stigmas. Another reason for psychosomatic presentations is those women tend to find it easier to describe physical, rather than psychological, symptoms to their health professionals. Health professionals find it easier to treat physical symptoms, so women who present with physical symptoms that have strong psychosocial undercurrents often receive incomplete or inappropriate treatment.

Patients with depressive disorder are more likely to have somatic complaints, including chronic pain resulting in more frequent visits to the emergency unit, and prognosis tends to worsen in women with gynaecological problems who also have an untreated depressive disorder.

This chapter discusses the psychological and psychosocial domains of common diagnoses encountered in the emergency gynaecology unit and emphasizes the importance of a holistic approach to diagnosis and treatment.

Common Gynaecology Emergencies

Gynaecological emergencies (see Table 7.1) are disease conditions of the female reproductive system that can threaten the quality of life of the woman, her existence, her sexual function and her fertility. Gynaecological

Table 17.1 Gynaecology emergencies

Examples of common Gynaecology emergencies
Acute on chronic pelvic pain
Acute pelvic inflammatory disease (PID)
Complications arising from ovarian cysts
Complications arising from tumours
Complications following artificial reproductive techniques
Complications of early pregnancy (miscarriage, ectopic)
Menstrual problems
Post-surgical complications

emergencies, including life-threatening ones, require not only appropriate and rapid clinical decision-making but also an understanding of the emotional implications for the patient, family and staff.

Complications of Early Pregnancy

Miscarriage

Problems encountered from complications arising in early pregnancy can have significant psychosocialproblems on women, and this needs to be sensitively-handled. About a quarter of pregnancies end in miscarriage with a psychological aftermath which may last for a number of months. Miscarriage can mean different things to different women, but it is usually a personal and emotional experience. While some women will adjust without distress, others will experience it as the loss of a baby with all of the sadness and grief that this entails. Many women who suffer a miscarriage will feel not just the loss of the pregnancy but also a loss of self-confidence, hopes and dreams. The psychological aftermath includes avoidance, grief, guilt, anger, anxiety and depression. About 15% of women experience clinical depression and or anxiety for up to three years after a miscarriage. The range and severity of the symptoms may vary; some women may continue to mourn their lost baby even after the subsequent birth of a healthy child [2]. Because of the suddenness and urgency associated with miscarriage there is often little time to prepare for the loss and its impact. Many women report a sense of chaos – on one hand everything happens so quickly and yet, at the same time, the world stands still for them. There is often inadequate time to assimilate events and adjust on a psychological and emotional level. However, the majority of studies show that levels of anxiety and depression reported were generally within a range considered normal, indicating most women do not experience significant anxiety and depression following miscarriage. There is no confirmation of an association between the gestation age at miscarriage and intensity of grief, anxiety or depression. The underlying psychosocial risk factors predisposing a miscarrying woman to psychological morbidity include a history of psychiatric illness, infertility, childlessness, conception by assisted reproduction, lack of social support or poor marital adjustment, prior pregnancy loss and abortion and poor coping mechanism [3]. Simple and effective screening measures of psychological morbidity in the context of miscarriage have not been well established, although some studies have highlighted that psychological follow-up was highly desired by miscarrying women, and that psychological intervention was potentially beneficial [4].

Women do not experience miscarriage as a routine complication; medicalisation is both resisted and desired and, for some women, more support and information are needed to assist their search for meaning [5]. Attributing pregnancy loss to medical causes may be associated with lower levels of anxiety and identifying the cause of fetal loss may reduce the feelings of self-blame. Whether a woman declines or engages in therapy, a key component of all communications to couples who miscarry is that they are not alone [6]. Psychological debriefing processes may have a positive influence on emotional adaptation. A study looking at women debriefed and assessed at one week and four weeks after miscarriage showed a positive influence on emotional adaption when the Hospital Anxiety and Depression Scale and Impact of Events Scale were used. Half of the women who also received psychological debriefing at two weeks showed the following: Intrusion and avoidance scores were initially high but had significantly decreased by four months. Depression was not detected at any time point, but anxiety was significantly higher than community sample estimates at one week and four months. Psychological debriefing was perceived to be helpful but did not influence emotional adaptation [7].

Holistic management following a miscarriage should address women's different needs, such as understanding the reasons for the loss of their pregnancy as well as the emotional side. Miscarriage should be conceptualized not as a trigger to psychological morbidity but as a process involving the stages of turmoil, adjustment and resolution [8]. Miscarriage has been considered as a pivotal point in the lives of some women resulting in the reassessment of both their past and future experiences.

Holistic management also engages the partner as a major source of support.

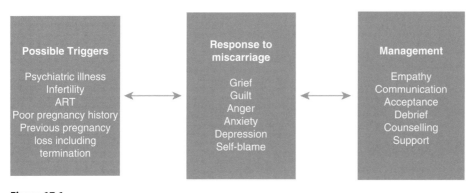

Figure 17.1

Table 17.2 Complications of ART

Complications of ART Joanne McManus, 2003 [9]
Miscarriage
Ectopic pregnancy
Ovarian hyperstimulation syndrome
Thromboembolism
Bleeding
Bowel injury
Infection
Adnexal torsion
Anaesthetic complications

Complications Following Assisted Reproductive Technologies (ART)

Fertility treatment is stressful because of the emotional roller coaster of expectations, disappointment and the marked hormonal changes that occur during the cycle of treatment (see also Chapter 14. The most dreaded misfortunes (see Table 17.2) for couples who want children following successful ART are miscarriage (29%) and ectopic pregnancy (2–11%, including heterotopic, interstitial and cervical ectopic pregnancies). Four deaths were directly attributed to ART in the 2009–2012 UK Confidential Enquiry into Maternal Deaths. The higher miscarriage rate following ART is attributed to characteristics of the population concerned. Notably, the older women are at increased risk of having an early miscarriage due to chromosomal abnormalities.

Ovarian hyperstimulation syndrome (OHSS) can be mild/moderate or severe with incidences of 3–6% and 0.3–0.5% respectively and manifests with bilateral ovarian enlargement by multiple cysts, third-spacing of fluids and clinical findings ranging from gastrointestinal discomfort to life-threatening renal failure and coagulopathy. Enlarged, hyperstimulated ovaries are at risk of torsion. Clinical symptoms are often nonspecific, and ovarian torsion should be excluded in any female patient undergoing infertility treatment who presents with significant abdominal pain [10]. Managing the clinical aspects all of these complications should go hand in hand with managing the pertinent psychosocial issues. Steps for re-engaging in life, clarifying one's values, modifying unhelpful thinking, communicating effectively, solving problems and

achieving acceptance are useful. Women and their partners would have been fully counselled prior to commencing fertility treatment, but this is not a substitute for managing the aftermath of failed pregnancy.

Ectopic Pregnancy

Ectopic pregnancy accounts for 1–2% of all pregnancies and is potentially life-threatening and should be managed promptly [11]. This event also represents the loss of a pregnancy and may additionally have longer-term consequences for fertility. Fear and panic are therefore understandable emotional responses from women in these circumstances [12]. Hospital staff coping with the clinical demands of a gynaecological emergency such as an ectopic pregnancy may feel that, particularly with a very acute situation, there is little time to offer these women the psychological support they need – empathy, explanation, time and support. In another study, the calculated rates of attempted suicide and mortality due to suicide in these patients were 3.75% and 0.625% respectively. The combination of failure of pregnancy, trauma of surgery and threat to future reproduction can lead to a breaking point and an insult to self-image [13]. The psychosocial aspect should be recognized as part of clinical management of any early pregnancy loss, regardless of how this loss has occurred. Health professionals can play a critically important role in helping families begin the long and difficult journey to recovery and, where necessary, referral for professional psychological intervention should be offered. The importance of good communication and an understanding of patients' responses and reactions to events cannot be overemphasized. All women should be treated with dignity and respect, and all women should be given information and support in a sensitive manner, taking into account their individual circumstances and emotional response. Caring attitudes convey professionals' understanding that surgical intervention in miscarriage and ectopic pregnancy is more than just a procedure.

Hyperemesis Gravidarum

The assumption is frequently made that women with severe nausea and vomiting during pregnancy are manifesting psychological distress as physical symptoms, but there is little evidence for this hypothesis (see Chapter 21). The exact pathophysiological mechanism is unknown. There is some evidence that sociocultural factors are largely responsible for symptoms and resulting complications. There are suggestions that psychological responses to pregnancy may become entrenched, or conditioned [14] [15].

Hyperemesis gravidarum has been shown to be associated with stress, anxiety and depression. In some cases the physical and psychological burden has resulted in elective termination of the pregnancy. Prompt recognition and treatment (pharmacological and non-pharmacological) of hyperemesis gravidarum are essential to minimize associated maternal and fetal morbidity. Care of a woman with hyperemesis gravidarum requires compassion and acknowledgement of individual needs and responses to interventions. Communication, support, the importance of validating their condition and the perception that the severity of their condition is believed by health professionals may contribute positively to the management of these women [16].

Pelvic Pain Unrelated to Pregnancy

Pelvic pain is the most common reason for urgent laparoscopic examination in the United Kingdom and elsewhere. Pelvic pain may be accompanied by other symptoms such as abnormal vaginal bleeding, lower back pain and vaginal discharge; these are important clues in identifying the possible aetiology. All of these symptoms can be alarming to women. Sometimes pain as a presenting symptom can uncover deeper psychological issues. Often the fear of surgery, the apparent loss of control or the state of being in hospital induces the patient to reflect on personal issues that were not previously addressed.

Diagnosing the underlying cause of pelvic pain can be challenging because the presenting symptoms and signs are often non-specific and non-diagnostic. It has been argued that psychological and social factors may contribute to 'unexplained' pain. Several gynaecological, gastroenterological, surgical and psychosocial factors are strongly associated with pelvic pain, and more randomized controlled trials of interventions targeting these potentially modifiable factors are needed to assess their clinical relevance [17]. In one study the diagnosis of the cause of nonspecific abdominopelvic pain was established in only 45% of women compared with 79% of women randomized to the laparoscopy arm for definitive diagnosis, exemplifying the diagnostic challenge of acute pelvic pain in

women [18]. To some women, the inability to establish a diagnosis may heighten psychosocial issues.

Chronic Pelvic Pain

There is a strong and consistent association between chronic pelvic pain and the presence of pelvic pathology, history of abuse and coexistent psychological morbidity (see Chapter 16). These key gynaecological and psychosocial factors may provide potential targets for new therapeutic strategies for treating women with this disabling condition, for which current treatment options provide little relief. Child sex exploitation and abuse may initiate a cascade of events or reactions which makes an individual more vulnerable to the development of chronic pelvic pain as an adult. Women who continue to be abused were particularly at risk. An integrated approach to management in this group of women includes paying attention to psychological factors in the presence of a negative diagnostic laparoscopy [19].

Endometriosis

Endometriosis is a chronic condition affecting between 2% and 17% of women of reproductive age. There is considerable negative impact of this condition on women's quality of life, especially in the domains of pain and psychosocial functioning. Women with endometriosis can have debilitating pelvic pain and present with acute pelvic pain and have somewhat more severe pain and greater social dysfunction than those with unexplained pain [20]. Their symptoms can be difficult to control despite endocrine treatment, surgery and pain management. Mood disorder and social dysfunction appear to be at least as important in patients with proven endometriosis as in those with unexplained pain. The disruption in their quality of life, social functioning and mental health can be significant, hence the importance of a holistic approach to addressing the psychosocial impact of pelvic pain and management of these women.

Women are often aware of these psychosocial and psychological influences on pelvic pain and may choose not to discuss them, fearing that their pain will be dismissed as psychological or that non-gynaecological symptoms will be considered irrelevant. We should offer women an integrated approach to clinical and possible psychosocial issues.

Menstrual Problems

Menorrhagia can present as an emergency and require resuscitation, reduction of blood loss and correction of anaemia. Massive vaginal bleeding can be frightening and overwhelming to the affected woman. Psychosocial factors can have an influence on the perception of heavy periods and may disrupt a woman's life in major ways [21]. The psychosocial impact of heavy and/or painful periods should be taken into account and managed sensitively alongside the clinical presentation. Better understanding of factors which can explain why women with normal periods complain of menorrhagia could improve both medical and psychosocial outcomes (see also Chapter 13).

Dysmnenorrhoea affects up to 80% of reproductive age women and in many cases causes sufficient pain to dramatically affect social and occupational roles. The prevalence varies across ethnic groups, which in part may reflect varying cultural attitudes towards women and menstruation. Risk factors for dysmenorrhea include age of menarche, body mass, dietary habits, associated uterine bleeding disorders, comorbid pelvic pathology and psychosocial problems. Mood changes are related to menorrhagia, dysmenorrhea and abnormal menstrual cycles. Adolescent girls with dysmenorrhea have an increased risk of depression and anxiety [22]. It is important to emphasize the significance of a multidisciplinary approach to primary dysmenorrhea, follow-up and treatment.

Pelvic Inflammatory Disease

Pelvic inflammatory disease (PID) is a condition that affects mostly young sexually active, reproductive-age women. Most cases are considered to be the sequelae of the sexually transmitted pathogens. Classic PID presents as abdominal pain, fever, vaginal discharge and abnormal vaginal bleeding. The intensity and character of the pain varies greatly and tends to be bilateral. These symptoms are not altogether specific to PID, and the initial diagnosis may be subjective. Women are treated for presumed acute PID at presentation because of the long-term tubal complications associated with untreated PID. Nearly all women experience some sort of distress when they receive the diagnosis and empirical treatment for PID. At the time of diagnosis most women have little or no knowledge of the condition. It can generate emotions such as anger, shock and sadness, and can have an impact on sexual behaviour and intimacy [23]. Tubo-ovarian abscess is a significant acute complication of PID. It is estimated to occur in up to one-third of women hospitalized with acute PID, and it is characterized by an inflammatory mass that involves the fallopian tube, ovary and often adjacent structures (e.g. bowel and pelvic peritoneum). Tubal factor infertility, ectopic pregnancy and chronic pelvic pain constitute the large portion of the sequelae of PID. The possible psychosocial implication of PID and its sequelae should also be addressed sensitively with the woman by offering appropriate lines of communication, explanation of PID and follow-up by the genitourinary medical team who are appropriately trained to support and manage these women.

Female Genital Tract Tumours

Tumours of the female genital tract may cause significant acute pain or bleeding. They may undergo torsion or rupture and present in the gynaecology emergency setting. The common cases presenting as emergencies are ovarian cysts which are a particular source of worry for patients because of the perceived link to cancer. Women with ovarian cysts may present with pelvic pain, bloating, back pain and nausea or vomiting. Many women believe ovarian cysts will grow into ovarian cancer and adding to this anxiety may be the need for emergency surgery when they present with acute symptoms. A laparoscopy is required to excise cysts and prevent severe vascular compromise, peritonitis or tissue necrosis. Laparoscopy may need to be upgraded to a laparotomy when malignancies are suspected or if complications occur.

Nothing prepares one for the diagnosis of cancer, and ovarian malignancy is one of the deadliest of all gynaecology cancers, greatly impacting the psychosocial health of survivors. An increase in awareness of psychosocial health among survivors themselves, their social support system and their healthcare providers is necessary to adequately address their unique needs [24]. Psychosocial factors have previously been linked with clinical outcomes in a variety of cancer populations recognizing the protective role of social support in mortality outcomes. Many cancers are treatable when diagnosed and treated early; however, it may be difficult to distinguish between cancerous and noncancerous tumours at presentation. Women experience mild to moderate symptoms of depression and anxiety, as well as impairment of vocational, domestic and sexual functioning when diagnosed with cancer. The psychological and psychosocial impact of such a diagnosis cannot be overemphasized, hence the multidisciplinary management for women with gynaecological cancer (see also Chapter 20).

Summary

Psychosocial interventions have so far shown little effect on objective physical health outcomes; however, there is also no evidence to suggest otherwise. A more critical and evidence-based approach is needed.

Psychosocial explanations of health are viewed as different processes that cannot be fully captured by a single measure because of differences in perceptions and psychological processes. On the other hand, a pill or surgical operation cannot solve every ailment and there is growing evidence that a healthy mind is just as important for the prevention and management of diseases. Therefore, the concept of psychosocial health, a state of mental, emotional, social and spiritual well-being, deserves a better look and should be part and parcel of clinical management.

Understanding the interplay between body, mind and the environment plays an important part in the provision of holistic management. It is important to look at the whole person, including their physical, nutritional, environmental, emotional, social, spiritual and lifestyle values. The biopsychosocial approach encompasses all stated modalities of diagnosis and treatment including drugs and surgery as well as lifestyle and social support interventions.

To most lay people and many health professionals, psychosomatic per se means malingering or 'all in the mind'. Telling patients that they have a psychosomatic disorder is usually the first step towards a deteriorating doctor–patient relationship [25]. Doctors and nurses working in emergency gynaecology should explore and manage the psychosocial issues associated with their patients' clinical presentation without dismissing symptoms as 'all in the mind'.

A small proportion of women seen in the emergency gynaecology unit will need formal psychological counselling. For the vast majority of women what is needed is empathy, tailored information giving and other emotional support, all of which can be provided by any healthcare professional attuned to the biopsychosocial approach.

Key Points

- Women with mental health disorders may present to the emergency gynaecology unit with physical symptoms. On the other hand, women with primary physical disorders may have secondary psychological sequelae.
- Many women who suffer a miscarriage or an ectopic pregnancy will feel not just the loss of the pregnancy but also a loss of self-confidence, hopes and dreams. The psychological aftermath includes avoidance, grief, guilt, anger, anxiety and depression.
- The grief reaction after early pregnancy loss is similar to that which occurs after loss of a child.
- Pelvic pain may be an expression of deeper psychological or psychosocial issues.
- Women presenting with gynaecological emergencies need urgent clinical care, but they also need empathy, tailored information giving and other emotional support, all of which can be provided by any healthcare professional attuned to the biopsychosocial approach.

References

1. Macleod J, Smith GD. Psychosocial factors and public health: A suitable case for treatment? *J Epidemiol Community Health*. 2003; **57**: 565–70.

2. Blackmore ER, Côté-Arsenault D, Tang W, et al. Previous prenatal loss as a predictor of perinatal depression and anxiety. *The British Journal of Psychiatry*. 2011; **198**(5): 373–8. DOI: 10.1192/bjp. bp.110.083105.

3. Brier N. Understanding and managing the emotional reactions to a miscarriage. *Obstet Gynecol*. 1999; **93**(1): 151–5.

4. Lok IH, Neugebauer R. Psychological morbidity following miscarriage. *Best Pract Res Clin Obstet Gynaecol*. 2007; **21**(2): 229–47.

5. Simmons RK, Singh G et al. Experience of miscarriage in the UK: Qualitative findings from the National Women's Health Study. *Social Science & Medicine*. 2006; **63**: 1934–46.

6. Nikcevic AV, Tinkel SA, Kuczmierczyk AR, Nicolaides KH: Investigation of the cause of miscarriage and its influence on women's psychological distress BJOG. *An International Journal of Obstetrics & Gynaecology*. 1999; **106**(8): 808–13. DOI: 10.1111/j. 1471-0528.1999.tb08402.x.

7. Lee C, Slade P, Lygo V. The influence of psychological debriefing on emotional adaptation in women following early miscarriage: A preliminary study. *British Journal of Medical Psychology.* 1996; **69**(1): 47–58.

8. Maker C, Ogden J. The miscarriage experience: More than just a trigger to psychological morbidity? *Psychology & Health.* 2003; **18**(3): 403–15.

9. McManus J, Neil McClure N. Complications of assisted reproduction. *The Obstetrician & Gynaecologist.* 2002; **4**(3): 124–9.

10. Baron KT, Babagbemi KT, Arleo EK, et al. Emergent complications of assisted reproduction: Expecting the unexpected. *Radiographics.* 2013; **33**(1): 229–44.

11. National Collaborating Centre for Women's and Children's Health (UK). Ectopic Pregnancy and Miscarriage: Diagnosis and Initial Management in Early Pregnancy of Ectopic Pregnancy and Miscarriage. NICE Clinical Guidelines, No. 154. London: RCOG; December 2012.

12. Lasker JN, Toedter LJ. The impact of ectopic pregnancy: A 16 year psychosocial follow-up study. *Health Care Women Int.* 2003; **24**(3): 209–20.

13. Farhi J. Suicide after Ectopic Pregnancy. *N Engl J Med.* 1994; 330: 714.

14. Munch S. Chicken or the egg? The biological-psychological controversy surrounding hyperemesis gravidarum. *Soc Sci Med.* 2002; **55**(7): 1267–78.

15. Buckwalter JG, Simpson SW. Factors in the aetiology and treatment of severe nausea and vomiting in pregnancy. *AJOG.* 2002; **186**(5), Supplement 2, Pages S210–14.

16. Castillo MJ, Phillippi JC. Hyperemesis gravidarum: A holistic overview and approach to clinical assessment and management. *J Print Neonatal Nurs.* 2015; **29**(1): 12–22.

17. Latthe P, Gray R, Hills R, et al. Factors predisposing women to chronic pelvic pain: Systematic review. *BMJ.* 2006; **332**(7544): 749–55.

18. Morino M, Pellegrino L, Castagna E, et al. Acute nonspecific abdominal pain: A randomised, controlled trial comparing early laparoscopy versus clinical observation. *Ann Surg.* 2006; **244**(6): 881–8.

19. Peters AA, Van Dorst E, Jellis B, et al. A randomised clinical trial to compare two different approaches in women with chronic pelvic pain. *Obstet Gynecol.* 1991; 77: 740–4.

20. Peveler R, Edwards J, Daddow J, et al. Psychosocial factors and chronic pelvic pain: A comparison of women with endometriosis and with unexplained pain. *J. Psychosom Res.* 1996; **40**(3): 305–15.

21. Hurskainen R, Aalto AM, Teperi J, et al. Psychosocial and other characteristics of women complaining of menorrhagia, with and without actual increased menstrual blood loss. *BJOG.* 2001; **108**(3): 281–5.

22. Balık G, Ustüner I. Is there a relationship between mood disorders and dysmenorrhea? *Pediatr Adolesc Gynecol.* 2014; **27**(6): 371–4.

23. Hocking J, Newton D, Bayly C, et al. The impact of pelvic inflammatory disease on sexual, reproductive and psychological health. *Sex Transm Infect* 2011; **87**: A318. DOI: 10.1136/sextrans – 2011 – 050108. 533.

24. Roland KB, Rodriguez JL, Patterson JR, et al. A literature review of the social and psychological needs of ovarian cancer survivors. *Psychooncology.* 2013; **22**(11): 2408–18.

25. Simon W, Peter D. White. There is only one functional somatic syndrome. *The British Journal of Psychiatry,* 2004; **185**(2): 95–6. DOI: 10.1192/bjp.185.2.95.

Biopsychosocial Factors in Urinary Incontinence

Caroline E. North and Jason Cooper

Introduction

The definition of 'urinary incontinence' has varied over time. The currently accepted definition, used by the International Continence Society, is the complaint of involuntary loss of urine [1]. This definition embraces the concept that such urinary loss is without or against conscious will or control. Urinary incontinence is rarely the result of life-threatening pathology. However, it is a common symptom in women and can cause considerable embarrassment as well as having a negative impact on their physical, psychological and social well-being.

The severity and nature of such impact is highly individual and will be affected by a woman's pre-existing state of physical and mental health as well as her social relationships, employment, independence, personal beliefs and relationship to her environment. This complex concept is often termed 'quality of life'. The World Health Organization defines this as 'an individual's perception of their position in life in the context of the culture and value systems in which they live and in relation to their goals, expectations, standards and concerns' [2]. The assessment of quality of life and its improvement is, therefore, the primary aim of healthcare professionals who care for women with urinary incontinence. This is exemplified by the International Continence Society which describes its very purpose as striving 'to improve the quality of life' for people affected by pelvic floor disorders, including urinary incontinence.

There is, therefore, a degree of understanding that urinary incontinence can have psychological and social affects as well as the biological, and that this interaction is complex, with psychological and social factors also affecting urinary incontinence. This complex interaction influences the presentation of urinary incontinence in women, its impact upon them and how interventions to improve urinary incontinence are best delivered.

Urinary Continence

Having control of our bladder, and bowels (being continent), is fundamental to our culture. Society expects individuals to gain this control and empty their bladder and bowels at a socially acceptable time and place. The bladder is an unusual viscus in that it is dependent upon the central nervous system and is voluntarily controlled. This is a learned behaviour, developed by 'toilet training' in early childhood which overcomes the filling and emptying of babies' bladders which occur independently of cortical control. Failure of such bladder control in older children and adults is taboo. It is a source of censure, ridicule and, even, illegality. For those affected, it is a source of considerable distress and impaired quality of life.

Neural control of normal bladder function is complex and involves a sophisticated interaction between the peripheral nervous system, central nervous system (CNS), bladder and urethral sphincter mechanism. Autonomic (sympathetic and parasympathetic) and somatic neurones are involved. Sympathetic efferent neurones exit the thoracolumbar outflow of the cord, whereas parasympathetic efferents exit from the sacral cord. Somatic fibres arise in the S2–S4 motor neurones of Onuf's nucleus and travel in the pudendal nerve. Afferent fibres also travel in these nerves. Sympathetic neurones synapse with β-adrenergic inhibitory receptors in the detrusor muscle (preventing contraction) and with α-adrenergic excitatory receptors in the urethra and bladder neck (keeping it closed). Uninhibited parasympathetic stimulation leads to detrusor contraction which is mediated mainly by M3 muscarinic cholinergic receptors.

Most of the time, the bladder is filling. It is highly compliant, such that during this period there is little change in intra-vesical pressure. In order for continence to be maintained, there must be no detrusor contraction and the sphincter mechanism must remain closed. As the bladder fills, sensory stimulation is received and transmitted to the spinal cord via the pelvic and hypogastric nerves. These synapse both with interneurons, involved in spinal reflexes, and spinal tract neurones projecting to the higher centres of the CNS. The detection of filling and sensory mechanism within the bladder is not well understood. Some detection of filling is provided by stretching of the compliant bladder wall. However, the urothelium is not a simple lining. In the sub-urothelial layer there is a dense nexus of sensory nerves, most prominent at the bladder neck [3, 4]. Non-neuronal cells also have a role in providing sensory information about the condition of the bladder, and multiple complex chemical interactions have been described [5].

Afferent information ascends in the dorsal column and the spinothalamic tract. The afferent activity occurring during filling leads to inhibition of the parasympathetic innervation to the detrusor muscle and activation of the striated parts of the urethral sphincter. This gradual recruitment of muscle increases sphincter resistance and is known as the guarding reflex. The efferent pathway is inactive [6].

At some point the bladder will reach 'capacity' and a desire to void will be experienced. Normal, functional capacity (experienced normally, outwith urodynamic testing) varies but is usually between 300 and 400 ml [7]. In continent, healthy women voiding is under voluntary control and no void occurs without cortical 'permission'. Despite the close proximity of the afferent and efferent neurones in the cord, coordination occurs in the pontine tegmentum and caudal brainstem [8]. The higher centres of the brain have overall control over voiding and allow continence to be maintained.

The periaqueductal grey (PAG) receives ascending afferent signals and passes this into the higher cortex, primarily prefrontal cortex [9], where conscious awareness of a full bladder is interpreted. The PAG then receives input from the higher cortex and controls the input to the area of the pontine tegmentum responsible for control of voiding, known as the pontine micturition centre (PMC) [6]. The cerebral cortex can suppress excitatory signals to the PMC until voiding is desired. Activation of the PAG during bladder filling can be seen on functional magnetic resonance imaging [10].

Normal female voiding is not well understood. However, when voiding is desired, descending pathways are activated, causing inhibition of sympathetic excitation of the sphincter mechanism. A reduction in urethral pressure is the first sign of normal voiding

[11], but it is unclear whether this is a passive or active process. Active relaxation of smooth muscle in the proximal urethra may be mediated by nitric oxide [12]. Activation of sacral parasympathetic neurones is then responsible for sustained detrusor contraction. However, some women may void by gravity alone once the sphincter is relaxed, with no identifiable detrusor contraction [11].

Following the void, there is a switch back to sympathetic mediated inhibition of detrusor contraction and excitation of the sphincter mechanism, restoring continence and allowing bladder filling once again. In addition to the PMC, a pontine storage centre, located more ventrally and laterally in the pontine tegmentum, has been described, which is responsible for this part of the bladder cycle [8]. Despite its close proximity to the PMC, the two may not be interconnected.

Incontinence

We have mentioned that urinary incontinence is the complaint of involuntary loss or urine. In women there are two main types of incontinence: stress urinary incontinence (SUI) and urgency urinary incontinence (UUI). Urinary symptoms, including these, have been defined by the International Urogynecological Association/International Continence Society joint statement on the terminology for female pelvic floor dysfunction [1]. Stress urinary incontinence is defined as the involuntary loss of urine on effort or physical exertion, for example with exercise or coughing. It is commonly related to pelvic floor injury such as that resulting from childbirth. Urgency urinary incontinence is defined as the complaint of involuntary loss of urine associated with urgency to void. It is most commonly idiopathic.

A combination of both SUI and UUI is called mixed urinary incontinence (MUI). Other types of incontinence defined include postural urinary incontinence (involuntary loss of urine associated with a change in position, e.g. rising from a lying or sitting position); nocturnal enuresis (involuntary urinary leakage which occurs whilst asleep); continuous urinary incontinence (continuous involuntary loss of urine); insensible urinary incontinence (when the woman is unaware of how it occurred) and coital urinary incontinence (involuntary loss of urine with coitus) [1].

Urinary incontinence is very common in women; however, accurate epidemiological data with regard to the prevalence of incontinence is unavailable. There is considerable variation in the reported rates which depend on the population studied (particularly their age), the definitions of incontinence applied and how the population were surveyed. A prevalence of approximately 35% has been suggested for urinary incontinence in women; however, this will depend on age with the prevalence increasing with advancing age [13]. Prevalence also varies depending on the type of urinary incontinence, with a prevalence of 40–50% for SUI, 10–20% for UUI and 20–40% for MUI [14]. However, this may include a proportion of women with mild symptoms, who are not bothered by them and will never seek medical help. When bother and severity are taken into account, the prevalence of bothersome urinary incontinence is estimated to be between 3 and 17% [5].

Biopsychosocial Impact of Incontinence

Although there is some understanding that urinary incontinence can have negative psychological and social effects, there is a paucity of research evidence with regard to the exact nature of this relationship. There has been development and utilization of condition-specific tools to measure quality of life and well-being which, for example, include the impact of incontinence on daily activities. Condition-specific questionnaires to investigate the impact on sexual function are also now widely available. The emotional impact of urinary incontinence and its impact on how women feel about themselves are less well studied.

Qualitative studies often do not differentiate between SUI, UUI and MUI. Conditions which may not include leakage, such as 'urethral syndrome', may be included. Some studies describe a population with 'pelvic floor dysfunction' and include a mixed group of women with symptoms of incontinence, prolapse or both.

However, the current data suggests an impact of incontinence on psychological/social well-being and an association with poor psychological health, including depression and anxiety. What is not clear is whether incontinence causes psychosocial ill-health or whether psychosocial ill-health may cause or exacerbate incontinence symptoms. Such associations are likely to be complex; for example, some conditions are known to be associated with lack of psychosocial well-being and incontinence, such as fibromyalgia.

General Quality of Life

Urinary incontinence, although a benign condition in the vast majority of women, has a negative effect on well-being. Women report that urinary incontinence interferes with their daily life [15] and, in a survey of over 9,000 European women, over 60% were moderately or extremely bothered by their incontinence symptoms [16].

Several condition-specific questionnaires have been developed to measure the impact of urinary incontinence on well-being, and to demonstrate change over time such as following treatment. These include the incontinence impact questionnaire (IIQ) [17], the King's Health Questionnaire (KHQ) [18], the Incontinence Quality of Life instrument (I-QOL) [19] and the electronic Personal Assessment Questionnaire – Pelvic Floor (ePAQ-PF) [20]. Such condition-specific tools demonstrate that both stress and urge incontinence impair quality of life and that quality of life can be improved by treating these conditions [21].

Treatment-Seeking Behaviour

There is a large hidden need for incontinence treatment. Despite its prevalence and impact on quality of life, women with urinary incontinence may not seek treatment for their incontinence or may delay seeking advice for many years [22, 23]. Women who avoid seeking treatment for their incontinence do more readily seek help with other medical conditions [24] and, therefore, it does not reflect a habitual pattern of reluctance to seek treatment. Instead, the reasons for delay or avoidance in seeking assistance for urinary incontinence are varied, and the woman's personality has an impact [25].

Some women perceive urinary incontinence as a normal part of aging and a normal consequence of childbirth [23–31]. Urinary incontinence may be considered as inevitable [24] and the perception of normality is reinforced by women's awareness of how common such symptoms are among their peers [28]. Providing information in pregnancy about urinary incontinence encourages women to seek help postnatally if they develop symptoms [32] and may help to alter this ingrained perception that women who have babies should expect to develop urinary incontinence as part of the package.

Women may not believe incontinence is actually a medical problem [25] for which consultation with a healthcare professional would be appropriate or they may prioritize other medical problems [33]. Feelings of shame [24, 34], humiliation [30] or embarrassment [24–26, 28, 31] about their incontinence are identified by women as a barrier to seeking treatment. Beliefs that incontinence cannot be effectively treated [25–27] also prevent women from seeking help from a healthcare professional, rather than trying to cope alone. Women report feeling shy [29] and therefore avoid raising the issue with a healthcare professional. They may have a preferred healthcare professional with whom they wish to discuss their incontinence. For example, they may not seek advice if it means seeing a male healthcare provider [31] and preferred providers with whom they had already established a relationship [28]. Not being able to consult with their preferred provider or difficulty scheduling an appointment acted as a barrier to seeking treatment [28, 30]. Preferred providers were reported to often be busy with less availability for women to disclose their incontinence symptoms [2, 28]. An open environment and a willingness of the healthcare provider to listen to women's symptoms and concerns increased treatment-seeking behaviour [30].

Generational [24, 31] and cultural [31] differences are reported to affect treatment-seeking behaviour for incontinence and may lead to reluctance in disclosing health problems perceived to be 'personal matters'. This needs to be considered when providing services, including the provision of patient information. Culturally sensitive information should be available and differing formats may be preferred [31].

Women may not know who to approach for help with urinary incontinence [35]. Initial attempts to voice concerns about continence and seek help may be made towards professionals outside a traditional model of healthcare, such as social workers [36]. Women with urinary incontinence report wishing that their healthcare professional had asked them directly whether they had symptoms rather than having to raise it themselves [30] and, therefore, an approach of actively screening women for urinary symptoms has been proposed with the aim of increasing those accessing treatment [27].

Women may seek help for their incontinence in subtle ways. Even casual references to incontinence or jokes about it may indicate that incontinence is affecting their psychological health and should prompt further enquiry [37].

The severity of the incontinence [38–41] and the greater the bother it causes women [42] are, unsurprisingly, the greatest predictors of treatment-seeking behaviour. Women who perceive their incontinence as mild or not bothersome do not seek treatment. However, many women reporting the most severe incontinence still do not seek treatment [39, 40]. Most studies do not differentiate between types of incontinence, although those suffering with UUI may be more likely to seek treatment than those women with other forms of incontinence [40, 41]. When women do choose to seek help with regard to their urinary incontinence, it is important that their symptoms are investigated and managed appropriately and empathetically. Unfortunately, not all women are satisfied with the outcome of their consultation [41], and this may depend upon the patient's prior expectations of treatment [44].

Coping Strategies

Coping strategies for urinary incontinence are practical approaches taken by women to attenuate the impact of their leakage. They include reducing fluid intake, staying close to a toilet, prioritizing finding the location of toilets when out of the house (toilet mapping) and the use of containment products such as pads. Coping strategies are common [27, 33, 41, 42] and usually tried before seeking help from a healthcare professional [46]. The use of these strategies is more common in women than in men with urinary incontinence [42]. It is motivated by a desire to maintain a normal lifestyle [47].

Despite this, the use of coping strategies may be unhelpful in treating the incontinence and may actually worsen the condition. Where pads are used they may be unsuitable for the intended purpose [46]. Frequent voiding may exacerbate symptoms of overactive bladder and UUI by encouraging a small capacity [33, 43]. Women may also need to manage their urinary incontinence by trying to exercise the pelvic floor [33, 43, 45]. Although pelvic floor muscle training is an effective treatment for urinary incontinence, unsupervised exercises are less effective and can even be harmful with up to one-third of women generating a Valsalva manoeuvre rather than contracting their pelvic floor [48, 49].

Although coping strategies are frequently employed prior to seeking help from a healthcare professional, it is unclear whether their use encourages or prevents women from eventually seeking assistance [24, 25]. Some women report feeling expected to cope without 'resorting' to medical professionals and that seeking help was 'giving in' to their incontinence [28].

Self/Body Image

Urinary incontinence affects how women feel about themselves as people as well as their previously held beliefs about their body. Feeling that they are less attractive or unattractive as a result of their leakage is common; reported in up to two-thirds of women [50–52]. Concerns about unpleasant odour as a result of incontinence are common. The authors' experience is certainly that many women in clinic express horror at the thought of becoming a 'smelly old lady'. Worries or concerns about unpleasant odour are reported in up to two-thirds of women [50], with many reporting this to be their major concern about their incontinence [53].

Sometimes the change in feelings about self are less defined and are described as feeling 'odd' or 'different' [52] or as a loss of control [51]. Urinary incontinence is associated with a reduction in both self-confidence [54] and self-esteem [55, 56]. Women may even report that urinary incontinence has caused them to feel a reduced purpose in life and a loss or impairment of their personal growth [56].

Relationships

Urinary incontinence also affects women's ability to emotionally connect with others. Positive relationships with other people may be impaired [56], or they may feel other people avoid them [52]. Women may also avoid others because of their incontinence [52]. Women with urinary incontinence report that it has an adverse impact on making new friends and their family life [57]. Single women report their leakage has a negative effect on finding a partner [5, 51].

Urinary incontinence commonly has a negative impact on established relationships for women with a husband or partner [58, 59]. A reduction in intimacy between partners is reported [58, 60] as well as impairment to the usual levels of affection and warmth between the couple [58]. Partners of women with urinary incontinence may develop emotions such as embarrassment, anxiety, anger, worry, frustration and sympathy [61] which are likely to affect their interactions with their partner.

Exercise and Obesity

Women with incontinence spend fewer hours walking and more hours watching television compared to continent women [62]. Incontinence is reported as a moderate or substantial barrier to taking exercise, with less exercise taken as the severity of the leakage increases [63, 64]. Urinary incontinence and pelvic organ prolapse commonly coexist and, for these women, there appears to be a greater interference with exercise or recreation [65].

Obese women are significantly more likely to have urinary incontinence and symptoms worsen with increasing episodes of incontinence as weight increases [66, 67]. In contrast, weight loss can improve symptoms [68]. Reduced activity levels in women with incontinence may lead to further weight gain, therefore worsening symptoms.

Employment and Finances

Urinary incontinence is common in women working outside the home [69]. Incontinence has a detrimental impact on women's employment [34, 52, 57, 69]. Women with urinary incontinence spend fewer hours in employment per week compared with their continent colleagues [62]. Those with more severe symptoms reported a greater impact on work activities, such as concentration, the ability to perform physical tasks and their ability to complete tasks at work without interruption [70]. Although incontinence has been shown to increase work disability, it does not appear to increase exit from employment [71]. Interestingly, urinary incontinence may affect work outside the home less than household work [65].

Incontinence is significantly associated with financial problems [72], although the reasons for this are unclear.

Travel and Social Activities

Urinary incontinence has a negative effect on women's ability to participate in their usual social activities outside the home [16, 45, 51, 73]. This is not limited to those women with more severe symptoms as the degree of incontinence may not relate to the degree of social disability [73]. The degree to which women feel socially isolated is independent of any depressive feelings which may be associated with their incontinence [74].

Incontinence in women is associated with a reduction in travel [45, 61, 75] which is most marked in older women (aged over 65 years) compared to younger women [75]. The reasons for this are complex and are likely to be influenced by the impact of incontinence on self-image and relationships with others, as described previously. Women also report wanting to remain close to home [76] which may be the ready access to toilet and washing facilities, containment products and a change of clothing. Women also report avoiding public transport [52]. The impact on travel affects not just women with incontinence but also their families with their partners reporting that it also limits their travel plans [61].

Sleep

Incontinence is significantly associated with fatigue and sleeping disorders [51, 57, 72]. Although SUI has demonstrated an association with sleep disturbance [77], women are more likely to report disturbed sleep with UUI [78]. Nocturia (being woken from sleep with the desire to pass urine) disturbs sleep, and this has an impact on daytime quality of life for both the affected woman [79] and her partner [61]. Both duration and quality of sleep may be improved by treating nocturia [80].

Ageing and Care in Later Life

Age is a risk factor for urinary incontinence, with the prevalence increasing with increasing age. Urinary incontinence has an anthropological significance as it is perceived as an inevitable and irreversible part of ageing and a sign of incompetence. Incontinence has, thus, become a cultural symbol of old age [81]. Women may be concerned about the meaning of incontinence for their overall and future health, and this is an important reason for seeking treatment for their symptoms [82].

Older women (aged 65–84 years) with incontinence are more socially isolated than younger women [78]. Older women who describe themselves as being in poor health are more likely to have urinary incontinence [83]. The impact of incontinence is greater in those older adults who have other health problems. It is proposed that this results from there being a 'functional threshold' after which the additional distress of incontinence is severe [84]. For older women, urinary incontinence is associated with an increase in their informal care needs and additional care costs [85]. As a result, urinary incontinence leads to an early decision to institutionalize elderly relatives as their relatives have difficulty coping [86]. Urinary incontinence is a significant independent indicator of institutionalism [87] and increases the risk of both hospitalization and admission to a nursing home. This effect is independent of age and the presence of other disease conditions [88]. The prevalence of urinary incontinence is, therefore, much higher in nursing home residents than would be expected in the general population of the same age [89].

Overactive bladder and UUI are associated with a greater risk of falls and fractures in older women [90]. They are also associated with an increased risk of urinary tract and skin infection [90, 91]. However, despite the increase in risk of other negative health outcomes urinary incontinence has little overall effect on mortality [88].

Sexual Function

Urinary incontinence has a negative impact on sexual function. Although sexual dysfunction is common in women, it is more common in those with urinary incontinence [92]. Women with incontinence report avoiding intercourse [52, 93]. Of those women who continue to be sexually active, up to half report urinary incontinence has a negative impact on their sexual function [50]. It is unclear whether sexual dysfunction is more likely depending on the type of urinary incontinence, with studies reporting very different results.

Coital incontinence is common, affecting up to two-thirds of women with urinary incontinence [50, 94]. Those women who don't experience coital incontinence may still worry about potential leakage during sexual activity [50]. Although sexual dysfunction is more common in women with incontinence compared to age-matched controls, age may be a bigger predictor of sexual activity [93].

Validated questionnaires are available to measure the impact of urinary incontinence on sexual function. Generic sexual function questionnaires, such as the Female Sexual Function Index (FSFI), demonstrate significantly poorer outcomes in women with urinary incontinence [95]. Condition-specific tools have also been developed, with sexual function included in some quality-of-life questionnaires, such as ePAQ-PF. The Pelvic Organ Prolapse/Incontinence Sexual Questionnaire (PISQ) is a condition-specific tool used to measure the impact of prolapse and/or incontinence on sexual function [96].

Both generic and condition-specific questionnaires have demonstrated improvement in sexual function following treatment of UUI with antimuscarinic medication [97, 98]. Urinary incontinence occurring at orgasm, which is particularly associated with UUI [94], responds less well [99]. Generic and condition-specific questionnaires have also been utilized to measure change in sexual function following treatment for SUI. Studies employing PISQ have given variable results [100–102].

Psychological Morbidity

The impact of urinary incontinence on psychological health and the impact of psychological health on continence are not well studied. In clinical practice, psychosocial factors may be overlooked or missed [103, 104]. Women with urinary incontinence appear to have abnormal psychological test results reflecting moodiness, feelings of helplessness and sadness, pessimism and general hypochondriasis/somatization compared to women without incontinence. These abnormalities appear to be specifically associated with urinary incontinence rather than with other diseases of the urinary tract [92]. It is unclear whether this association is causal or a result of living with incontinence as this interrelationship is complex and highly individual [105].

Effect of Incontinence on Mental Health

Urinary incontinence has a negative effect on mental health with almost half of women screening positive for psychiatric morbidity [106]. Urinary incontinence is associated with negative feelings such as shame [34], humiliation [72], embarrassment [73], lack of satisfaction with life [107] and worry [108]. Women with urinary incontinence also report feeling lonely or sad [109]. It is associated with an increased risk of depression [16, 56, 57, 62, 71, 107, 110], although the criteria by which authors determine the presence of 'depression' vary. Where women have other medical conditions which affect their mental health, additional problems with incontinence may add further psychological morbidity [111, 112].

Increased risk of anxiety is also reported with urinary incontinence [16, 113] with leakage that leads to a change in day-to-day activities or routines being more likely to be associated with an anxiety disorder [114]. It is unclear whether such relationships are causal; however, it is reported that the onset of anxiety disorder is predicted by incontinence associated with functional loss [115]. Anxiety, urge incontinence and frequency may interact and exacerbate each other [116]. In women for whom incontinence causes loss of normal functioning, psychological distress is greater, even in the absence of an anxiety disorder [117, 118]. This effect may be seen particularly in younger women for whom incontinence causes impaired sexual function [34]. One study found that women who felt their incontinence made their life intolerable were as anxious, depressed and phobic as a group of psychiatric inpatients [119]. However, psychological distress may not be proportionate to objective severity of leakage [17].

Data vary as to whether one form of urinary incontinence has a greater effect on psychiatric morbidity than others. Some report UUI worse than SUI in terms of emotional disturbance [78, 110], whereas other studies demonstrate no difference between types of urinary incontinence [92, 120]. Women with SUI or MUI have reported an increased conviction of illness during personality assessment [121]. Women with urinary incontinence can be stigmatized by their condition and even those who are not experience a detrimental effect on their self-esteem [122]. Personality also has an effect on psychosocial response to urinary incontinence. Personality testing in women with urinary incontinence has demonstrated an association with anger [121], neuroticism [123], hypochondriasis [92, 121] and hysteria [92, 113, 119].

Women's mental health is influenced by not only having to live with incontinence but also the treatment (or lack of treatment) they are offered. Fear and concerns about possible incontinence treatments [23, 30, 34, 52] contribute to delays in seeking help. The attitude of others, including health professionals, towards incontinence also affects women's feelings about their continence [124]. Women themselves may then behave in ways that make their fears come true [122]. For example, 'my incontinence will never get any better, so there's no point seeing anyone about it' then means it never gets better because no help is sought.

Effect of Mental Ill-Health on Continence

Not only can incontinence have an adverse impact on mental health, coexisting mental ill-health may have a negative impact on incontinence and its treatment. Qualitative studies have added to the understanding of the relationship between incontinence and psychological/psychiatric ill-health; however, they have included a variety of conditions causing lower urinary tract symptoms, which may not include incontinence such as 'urethral syndrome'. In a thematic analysis of 15 studies, none had the investigation of living with incontinence as a primary outcome [124]. However, incontinence appears to be associated with a number of psychological issues and those women with UUI are more likely to have underlying mental illness [125].

Women with depression are more socially isolated, less likely to use health services and less likely to seek help for their incontinence than those who enjoy good mental health. Despite this, women with depression report poorer quality of life and an increased perception of the severity of their incontinence [124]. Their lack of treatment-seeking behaviour, therefore, does not appear to be a result of perceiving a lack of bother from their incontinence.

Major depressive and panic disorders are highly prevalent in women with urinary incontinence. Major depressive illness impacts on symptom reporting, condition-specific quality-of-life scores and functional status [125]. Major depressive illness predicts the onset of urinary incontinence, whereas incontinence does not predict the onset of major depressive illness [126], suggesting that this does not represent the impact of incontinence on mood. Schizophrenia is also associated with urinary incontinence, particularly UUI and detrusor overactivity on cystometry investigations. It has been suggested that this may be an integral part of the disease process [127].

Mind-Body Therapies

Emotional states, behavioural disposition and psychological stresses have the ability to influence health and, therefore, it may be possible to improve some ill-health by utilizing the link between body and mind. Mind-body therapies encompass a group of interventions that are employed to facilitate conscious influence over the body and, therefore, manage symptoms (see Chapter 7). Sometimes termed 'psychosocial-mind-body interventions', they include techniques such as cognitive behavioural therapies, biofeedback, imagery and relaxation. There is evidence that such mind-body therapies are effective adjuncts in the management of other medical conditions such as headache, insomnia and low back pain. They

have also been used to improve outcomes following surgery [128].

In urogynaecology, mind-body therapy interventions have been employed for symptomatic pelvic floor dysfunction, including urinary incontinence, mild uterovaginal prolapse and obstructive defecation. Pelvic floor muscle training and 'bladder retraining' are effective and are recommended in the management of urinary incontinence.

Pelvic floor muscle training as a treatment for SUI was popularized by Kegel [129]. To be most effective, this should be supervised by a trained healthcare professional such as a physiotherapist. Bladder retraining is a form of biofeedback to improve UUI, MUI and overactive bladder without incontinence. Initially described as an inpatient treatment over seven to ten days, bladder retraining is now performed as an outpatient. It utilizes imagery, relaxation techniques, voluntary pelvic floor contraction and distraction to reduce bladder urgency and allow the bladder to fill, increasing bladder capacity. This improves symptoms of urgency, frequency and nocturia and reduces UUI. Such techniques were initially described as 'bladder drill'. At the time, it was suggested that the success of bladder drill resulted from the psychosomatic origin of overactive bladder/urinary urgency [130]. That these symptoms originate in the mind remains, almost 40 years later, a current hypothesis [131], although the mind is more likely to have a role in the exacerbation or prolongation of symptoms rather than being the initial cause.

Conclusion

Urinary incontinence in women is a common symptom that, although seldom associated with life-threatening pathology, does cause psychosocial harm. It impairs women's quality of life and mental health, affecting all aspects of their life, including their personal and sexual relationships. In addition, urinary incontinence also has a negative effect on those closest to them: their partners, family and carers. The economic and social impact of incontinence has wider implications for society, especially as the population ages.

Women may avoid seeking help for their incontinence for many years, despite the availability of effective treatment. Doctors may not feel comfortable enquiring about incontinence and may feel they don't know what to do should patients disclose they are suffering with urinary incontinence [132]. However, it is important that such symptoms are identified to minimize the biopsychosocial harm caused by the condition. Doctors and other healthcare professionals play an important role in education and encouraging disclosure of incontinence, and must be mindful that women's feelings of shame or fear about their symptoms can be improved or worsened by the attitude of their healthcare professional [30].

Key Points

- Urinary incontinence negatively affects women's self-confidence, body image, relationships, sleep patterns, employment, social life, travel activities and sexual function.
- Women with urinary incontinence report wishing that their healthcare professional had asked them directly whether they had symptoms rather than having to raise it themselves and, therefore, an approach of actively screening women for urinary symptoms may facilitate access to treatment.
- Women with urinary incontinence appear to have abnormal psychological test results reflecting moodiness, feelings of helplessness and sadness, pessimism and general hypochondriasis/somatization compared to women without incontinence. It is unclear whether this association is causal or a result of living with incontinence as this relationship is complex and highly individual.
- Psychological distress may not be proportionate to objective severity of leakage.
- Validated questionnaires are available to measure the impact of urinary incontinence on sexual function. These include generic sexual function questionnaires, such as the Female Sexual Function Index (FSFI), and condition-specific tools such as the Pelvic Organ Prolapse/Incontinence Sexual Questionnaire (PISQ).
- Women with urinary incontinence adopt coping strategies – such as reducing fluid intake, toilet mapping and use of containment products – to attenuate the impact of their leakage, but some strategies may be unhelpful in treating the incontinence and may actually worsen the condition.

- Women may also need to manage their urinary incontinence by trying to exercise the pelvic floor. Pelvic floor muscle training is an effective treatment for urinary incontinence, but unsupervised exercises are less effective and can even be harmful.
- Mind-body therapy interventions have been employed for symptomatic pelvic floor dysfunction, including urinary incontinence. 'Bladder retraining' is effective. These interventions may be combined with specific drug treatment.

References

1. Haylen BT et al. An International Urogynecological Association (IUGA)/International Continence Society (ICS) joint report on the terminology for female pelvic floor dysfunction. *Neurourol Urodyn.* 2010;**29**(1):4–20.

2. World Health Organisation. Constitution of the World Health Organization, 1946 www.who.int/en/.

3. Wiseman OJ, et al. The ultrastructure of bladder lamina propria nerves in healthy subjects and patients with detrusor hyperreflexia. *J Urol.* 2002;**168**:2040–45.

4. Gabella G, Davis C. Distribution of afferent axons in the bladders of rats. *J Neurocytol.* 1998;**27**:141–55.

5. Apodaca G. The uroepithelium: Not just a passive barrier. *Traffic.* 2004;**5**:117–28.

6. Fowler CJ, Griffiths D, de Groat WC. The neural control of micturition. *Nat Rev Neurosci.* 2008;**9**(6):453–66.

7. Fitzgerald MP, Stablein U, Brubaker L. Urinary habits among asymptomatic women. *Am J Obstet Gynecol.* 2002 **187**;(5):1384–88.

8. Blok BFM, Holstege G. Two pontine micturition centers in the cat are not interconnected directly: Implications for the central organization of micturition. *J Comp Neurol.* 1999;**403**(2):209–18.

9. Holstege G. Micturition and the soul. *J Comp Neurol.* 2005;**493**(1):15–20.

10. DasGupta R, Kavia RB, Fowler CJ. Cerebral mechanisms and voiding function. *BJU International.* 2007;**99**:731–34.

11. Hinman F Jr, Miller GM, Nickel E. Normal micturition – certain details as shown by serial cystograms. *Calif Med.* 1955;**82**:6–7.

12. Bennet BC, Vizzard MA, Booth AM. Role of nitric oxide in reflex urethral sphincter relaxation during micturition. *Soc Neurosci Abstr.* 1993;**19**:511.

13. Luber KM. The definition, prevalence and risk factors for stress urinary incontinence. *Rev Urol.* 2004;**6**(Suppl 3):S3–S9.

14. Nitti VW. The prevalence of urinary incontinence. *Rev Urol.* 2001;**3**(Suppl 1):S2–S6.

15. Ouslander JG, Zarit SH, Orr NK, Muira SA. Incontinence among elderly community-dwelling dementia patients. *J Am Geriatr Soc.* 1990;**38**:440–45.

16. Monz B, et al. Patient-reported impact of urinary incontinence – results from treatment seeking women in 14 European countries. *Maturitas.* 2005;**30**(52 Suppl 2):S24–34.

17. Wyman JF, Harkins SW, Choi SC, Taylor JR, Fantl JA. Psychosocial impact of urinary incontinence in women. *Obstet Gynecol.* 1987;**70**(3 Pt 1):378–81.

18. Kelleher CJ, Cardozo LD, Khullar V, Salvatore S. A new questionnaire to assess the quality of life of urinary incontinent women. *Br J Obstet Gynaecol.* 1997;**104**(12):1374–79.

19. Wagner TH, Patrick DL, Bavendam TG, Martin ML, Buesching DP. Quality of life of persons with urinary incontinence: Development of a new measure. *Urology.* 1996;**47**(1):67–71.

20. Radley SC, Jones GL, Tanguy EA, Stevens VG, Nelson C, Mathers NJ. Computer interviewing in urogynaecology: Concept, development and psychometric testing of an electronic pelvic floor assessment questionnaire in primary and secondary care. *BJOG.* 2006;**113**(2):231–38.

21. Khullar V, Chapple C, Gabriel Z, Dooley JA. The effects of antimuscarinics on health-related quality=of life in overactive bladder: A systematic review and meta-analysis. *Urology.* 2006;**68** (2 Suppl):38–48.

22. Shaw C, et al. The extent and severity of urinary incontinence amongst women in UK GP waiting rooms. *Fam Pract.* 2006;**23**(5):497–506.

23. Cooper J, Annappa M, Quigley A, Dracocardos D, Bondili A, Mallen C. Prevalence of female urinary incontinence and its impact on quality of life in a cluster population in the United Kingdom (UK): A community survey. *Prim Health Care Res Dev.* 2015;**16**(4):377–82.

24. Horrocks S, Somerset M, Stoddart H, Peters TJ. What prevents older people from seeking help for urinary incontinence? A qualitative exploration of barriers to the use of community continence services. *Fam Pract.* 2004;**21**(6):689–96.

25. Shaw C. A review of the psychosocial predictors of help-seeking behaviour and impact on quality of life in people with urinary incontinence. *J Clin Nurs.* 2001;**10**(1):15–24.

26. Perera J, Kirthinanda DS, Wijeratne S, Wickramarachchi TK. Descriptive cross sectional study on prevalence, perceptions, predisposing factors and health seeking behaviour of women with stress urinary incontinence. *BMC Women's Health.* 2014;**14**:78.

27. Visser E, de Bock GH, Kollen BJ, Meijerink M, Berger MY, Dekker JH. Systematic screening for urinary incontinence in older women: Who could benefit from it? *Scand J Prim Health.* 2012;**30**(1):21–8.

28. Hale S, Grogan S, Willott S. 'Getting on with it': Women's experience of coping with urinary tract problems. *Qual Res Psych.* 2009;**6**(3):203–18.

29. Kumari S, Singh AJ, Jain V. Treatment seeking behavior for urinary incontinence among north Indian women. *Indian J Med Sci.* 2008;**62**(9):352–56.

30. Hägglund D, Wadenstein B. Fear of humiliation inhibits women's care-seeking behaviour for long-term urinary incontinence. *Scand J Caring Sci.* 2007;**21**(3): 305–12.

31. Doshani A, Pitchforth E, Mayne CJ, Tincello DG. Culturally sensitive continence care: A qualitative study among South Asian Indian women in Leicester. *Fam Pract.* 2007;**24**(6):585–93.

32. Ruiz de Viñaspre Hernández R, Tomás Aznar C, Rubio Aranda E. Factors associated with treatment-seeking behavior for postpartum urinary incontinence. *J Nurs Scholarsh.* 2014;**46**(6):391–97.

33. Andersson G, Johansson JE, Nilsson K, Sahlberg-Blom E. Accepting and adjusting: Older women's experiences of living with urinary incontinence. *Urol Nurs.* 2008;**28**(2):115–21.

34. Margalith I, Gillon G, Gordon D. Urinary incontinence in women under 65: Quality of life, stress related to incontinence and patterns of seeking health care. *Qual Life Res.* 2004;**13**(8):1381–90.

35. Buckley BS, Lapitan MC. Prevalence of urinary and faecal incontinence and nocturnal enuresis and attitudes to treatment and help-seeking amongst a community-based representative sample of adults in the United Kingdom. *Int J Clin Pract.* 2009;**63**(4):568–73.

36. Sanders S, Bern-Klug M, Specht J, Mobily PR, Bossen A. Expanding the role of long-term care social workers: Assessment and intervention related to urinary incontinence. *J Gerontol Soc Work.* 2012;**55**(3): 262–81.

37. Saiki LS, Cloyes KG. Blog text about female incontinence: Presentation of self, disclosure and social risk assessment. *Nurs Res.* 2014;**63**(2):137–42.

38. Jimenez-Cidre M, Costa P, Ng-Mak D, Sahai A, Degboe A, Smith CP, Tsai K, Herschorn S. Assessment of treatment-seeking behavior and healthcare utilization in an international cohort of subjects with overactive bladder. *Curr Med Res Opin.* 2014;**30**(8): 1557–64.

39. Hannestad YS, Rortveit G, Hunskaar S. Help-seeking and associated factors in female urinary incontinence.

The Norwegian EPICONT study. Epidemiology of incontinence in the county of Nord-Trøndelag. *Scand J Prim Health Care*. 2002;**20**(2):102–7.

40. Seim A, Sandvik H, Hermstad R, Hunskaar S. Female urinary incontinence – consultation behaviour and patient experiences; an epidemiological survey in a Norwegian community. *Fam Pract*. 1995;**12**(1):18–21.

41. Sandvik H, Kveine E, Hunskaar S. Female urinary incontinence. *Scand J Car Sci*. 1993;**7**:53–56.

42. Irwin DE, Milsom I, Kopp Z, Abrams P; EPIC Study Group. Symptom bother and health care-seeking behavior among individuals with overactive bladder. *Eur Urol*. 2008;**53**(5):1029–37.

43. Hägglund D, Walker-Engstrom ML, Larsson G, Leppert J. Reasons why women with long-term urinary incontinence do not seek professional help: A cross-sectional population-based cohort study. *Int Urogynecol J Pelvic Floor Dysfunct*. 2003;**14**(5):296–304.

44. Marschall-Kehrel D, Roberts RG, Brubaker L. Patient-reported outcomes in overactive bladder: The influence of perception of condition and expectations for treatment benefit. *Urol*. 2006;**68**(2):29–37.

45. Johnson TM, Kincade JE, Bernard SL, Busby-Whitehead J, DeFriese GH. Self-care practices used by older men and women to manage urinary incontinence: Research from the national follow-up survey on self-care and ageing. *J Am Ger Soc*. 2000;**48**(8):894–902.

46. Anders K. Coping strategies for women with urinary incontinence. *Best Prac Res Clin Obstet Gynaecol*. 2000;**14**(2):355–61.

47. Milne JL, Moore KN. Factors impacting self-care for urinary incontinence. *Urol Nurs*. 2006;**26**(1):41–51.

48. Bump RC, Hurt WG, Fantl JA, Wyman JA. Assessment of Kegel pelvic muscle exercise performance after brief verbal instructions. *Am J Obstet Gynecol*. 1991;**165**(2):322–29.

49. Bø K, et al. Knowledge about and ability to correct pelvic floor exercises in women with stress urinary incontinence. *Neurourol Urodyn*. 1988;**69**:261–62.

50. Nilsson M, Lalos O, Lindkvist H, Lalos A. How do urinary incontinence and urgency affect women's sexual life? *Acta Obstet Gynecol Scand*. 2011;**90**:621–28.

51. Brown JS, Subak LL, Gras J, Brown BA, Kuppermann M, Posner SF. Urge incontinence: The patient's perspective. *J Women's Health*. 1998;**7**(10):1263–69.

52. Norton PA, MacDonald LD, Sedgwick PM, Stanton SL. Distress and delay associated with urinary incontinence, frequency and urgency in women. *BMJ*. 1988;**297**(6657):1187–89.

53. Lagro-Janssen T, Smits A, VanWeel C. Urinary incontinence in women and the effects on their lives. *Scand J Prim Health Care*. 1992;**10**(3):211–16.

54. Fultz NH, Burgio K, Diokno AC, Kinchen KS, Obenchain R, Bump RC. Burden of stress urinary incontinence for community-dwelling women. *Am J Obstet Gynecol*. 2003;**189**(5):1275–82.

55. Woods NF, Mitchell ES. Consequences of incontinence for women during the menopausal transition and early postmenopause: Observations from the Seattle midlife women's health study. *Menopause*. 2013;**20**(9):915–21.

56. Heidrich SM, Wells TJ. Effects of urinary incontinence: Psychological well-being and distress in older community-dwelling women. *J Gerontol Nurs*. 2004;**30**(5):47–54.

57. Yeung CK, Sihoe JD, Sit FK, Bower W, Sreedhar B, Lau J. Characteristics of primary nocturnal enuresis in adults: An epidemiological study. *BJU Int*. 2004;**93**(3):341–45.

58. Nilsson M, Lalos A, Lalos O. The impact of female urinary incontinence and urgency on quality of life and partner relationship. *Neurourol Urodyn*. 2009;**28**(8):976–81.

59. Yip SK, Chan A, Pang S, Leung P, Tang C, Shek D, Chung T. The impact of urodynamic stress incontinence and detrusor overactivity on marital relationship and sexual function. *Am J Obstet Gynecol*. 2003;**188**(5):1244–48.

60. Cassells C, Watt E. The impact of incontinence on older spousal caregivers. *J Advan Nurs*. 2003;**42**:607–16.

61. Coyne KS, Matza LS, Brewster-Jordan J. 'We have to stop again?!': The impact of overactive bladder on family members. *Neurourol Urodyn*. 2009;**28**(8):969–75.

62. Fultz NH, Fisher GG, Jenkins KR. Does urinary incontinence affect middle-aged and older women's time use and activity patterns? *Obstet Gynecol*. 2004;**104**(6):1327–34.

63. Nygaard I, Girts T, Fultz NH, Kinchen K, Pohl G, Sternfeld B. Is urinary incontinence a barrier to exercise in women? *Obstet Gynecol*. 2005;**106**(2):307–14.

64. Brown WJ, Miller YD. Too wet to exercise? Leaking urine as a barrier to physical activity in women. *J Sci Med Sport*. 2001;**4**(4):373–78.

65. Nygaard I, et al. Physical activity in women planning sacrocolpopexy. *Int Urogynecol J Pelvic Floor Dysfunct*. 2007;**18**(1):33–37.

66. Subak LL, Richter HE, Hunskaar S. Obesity and urinary incontinence: Epidemiology and clinical research update. *J Urol.* 2009;**182**(6 Suppl):S2–S7.

67. Dwyer PL, Lee ETC, Hay DM. Obesity and urinary incontinence in women. *BJOG.* 1988;**95**:91–96.

68. Wing RR, et al. Effect of weight loss on urinary incontinence in overweight and obese women: Results at 12 and 18 months. *J Urol.* 2010;**184**(3): 1005–10.

69. Fitzgerald ST, Palmer MH, Kirkland VL, Robinson L. The impact of urinary incontinence in working women: A study in a production facility. *Women Health.* 2002;**35**(1):1–16.

70. Fultz N, Girts T, Kinchen K, Nygaard I, Pohl G, Sternfeld B. Prevalence, management and impact of urinary incontinence in the workplace. *Occup Med (London).* 2005;**55**(7):552–57.

71. Hung KJ, Awtrey CS, Tsai AC. Urinary incontinence, depression, and economic outcomes in a cohort of women between the ages of 54 and 65. *Obstet Gynecol.* 2014;**123**(4):822–27.

72. Franzén K, Johansson JE, Andersson G, Pettersson N, Nilsson K. Urinary incontinence in women is not exclusively a medical problem: A population-based study on urinary incontinence and general living conditions. *Scand J Urol Nephrol.* 2009;**43**(3):226–32.

73. Norton C. The effects of urinary incontinence in women. *Int Rehab Med.* 1982;**4**(1):9–14.

74. Yip SO, Dick MA, McPencow AM, Martin DK, Ciarleglio MM, Erekson EA. The association between urinary and fecal incontinence and social isolation in older women. *Am J Obstet Gynecol.* 2013;**208**(2):146. e1–7.

75. St John W, Griffiths S, Wallis M, McKenzie S. Women's management of urinary incontinence in daily living. *J Wound Ostomy Cont.* 2013;**40**(5):524–32.

76. Engberg SJ, McDowell BJ, Burgio KL, Watson JE, Belle S. Self-care behaviors of older women with urinary incontinence. *J Geront Nurs.* 1995;**21**(8):7–14.

77. Ornat L, Martínez-Dearth R, Chedraui P, Pérez-López FR. Assessment of subjective sleep disturbance and related factors during female mid-life with the Jenkins sleep scale. *Maturitas.* 2014;**77**(4):344–50.

78. Grimby A, Milsom I, Molander U, Wiklund I, Ekelund P. The influence of urinary incontinence on the quality of life of elderly women. *Age Ageing.* 1993;**22**(2):82–89.

79. Bliwise DL, Rosen RC, Baum N. Impact of nocturia on sleep and quality of life: A brief, selected review for the International Consultation on Incontinence Research Society (ICI-RS) nocturia think tank. *Neurourol Urodyn.* 2014;**33**:S15–18.

80. Takao T, et al. Solifenacin may improve sleep quality in patients with overactive bladder and sleep disturbance. *Urology.* 2011;**78**(3):648–52.

81. Mitteness LS, Barker JC. Stigmatizing a 'normal' condition: Urinary incontinence in late life. *Med Anthropol Quar.* 1995;**9**(2):188–210.

82. Kinchen KS, Burgio K, Diokno AC, Fultz NH, Bump R, Obenchain R. Factors associated with women's decisions to seek treatment for urinary incontinence. *J Women's Health (Larchmt).* 2003;**12**(7):687–98.

83. Park J, Hong GR, Yang W. Factors associated with self-reported and medically diagnosed urinary incontinence among community-dwelling older women in Korea. *Int Neurourol J.* 2015;**19**(2):99–106.

84. Dugan E, et al. The quality of life of older adults with urinary incontinence: Determining generic and condition-specific predictors. *Qual Life Res.* 1998;**7**(4): 337–44.

85. Langa KM, Fultz NH, Saint S, Kabeto MU, Herzog AR. Informal caregiving time and costs for urinary incontinence in older individuals in the United States. *J Am Geriatr Soc.* 2002;**50**(4):733–37.

86. Miner PB Jr. Economic and personal impact of fecal and urinary incontinence. *Gastroenterology.* 2004;**126** (1 Suppl):S8–13.

87. Nuotio M, Tammela TL, Luukkaala T, Jylhä M. Predictors of institutionalization in an older population during a 13-year period: The effect of urge incontinence. *J Gerontol A Biol Sci Med Sci.* 2003;**58**(8): 756–62.

88. Thom DH, Haan MN, Van Den Eeden SK. Medically recognized urinary incontinence and risks of hospitalization, nursing home admission and mortality. *Age Ageing.* 1997;**26**(5):367–74.

89. Offermans MP, Du Moulin MF, Hamers JP, Dassen T, Halfens RJ. Prevalence of urinary incontinence and associated risk factors in nursing home residents: A systematic review. *Neurourol Urodyn.* 2009;**28**(4): 288–94.

90. Brown JS, McGhan WF, Chokroverty S. Comorbidities associated with overactive bladder. *Am J Manag Care.* 2000;**6**(11 Suppl):S574–79.

91. Ouslander JG, Kane RL, Abrass IB. Urinary incontinence in elderly nursing home patients. *JAMA.* 1982;**248**(10):1194–98.

92. Walters MD, Taylor S, Schoenfeld LS. Psychosexual study of women with detrusor instability. *Obstet Gynecol.* 1990;**75**(1):22–26.

93. Barber MD, et al. Sexual function in women with urinary incontinence and pelvic organ prolapse. *Obstet Gynecol.* 2002;**99**(2):281–89.

94. Hilton P. Urinary incontinence during sexual intercourse: A common, but rarely volunteered, symptom. *Br J Obstet Gynaecol.* 1988;**95**(4):377–81.

95. Sen I, et al. The impact of urinary incontinence on female sexual function. *Adv Ther.* 2006;**23**(6):999–1008.

96. Rogers RG, Kammerer-Doak D, Villarreal A, Coates KW, Qualls C. A new instrument to measure sexual function in women with urinary incontinence or pelvic organ prolapse. *Am J Obstet Gynecol.* 2001;**184**(4):552–58.

97. Rogers RG, Bachmann G, Jumadilova Z, Sun F, Morrow JD, Guan Z, Bavendam T. Efficacy of tolterodine on overactive bladder symptoms and sexual and emotional quality of life in sexually active women. *Int Urogynaecol J Pelvic Floor Dysfunct.* 2008;**19**(11):1551–57.

98. Hajebrahimi S, Azaripour A, Sadeghi-Bazargani H. Tolterodine immediate release improves sexual function in women with overactive bladder. *J Sex Med.* 2008;**5**(12):2880–85.

99. Serati M, et al. Urinary incontinence at orgasm: Relation to detrusor overactivity and treatment efficacy. *Euro Urol.* 2008;**54**(4):911–17.

100. Rogers RG, Kammerer-Doak D, Darrow A, Murray K, Olsen A, Barber M, Qualls C. Sexual function after surgery for stress urinary incontinence and/or pelvic organ prolapse: A multicenter prospective study. *Am J Obstet Gynecol.* 2004;**191**(1):206–10.

101. Brubaker L, et al. The impact of stress incontinence surgery on female sexual function. *Am J Obstet Gynecol.* 2009;**200**(5):562.e1–7.

102. Jha S, Moran P, Greenham H, Ford C. Sexual function following surgery for urodynamic stress incontinence. *Int Urogynaecol J Pelvic Floor Dysfunct.* 2007;**18**(8):845–50.

103. Levinson W, Gorawara-Bhat R, Lamb J. A study of patient clues and physician responses in primary care and surgical settings. *JAMA.* 2000;**284**(8):1021–27.

104. Hall JA, Andrzejewski SA, Yopchick JE. Psychosocial correlates of interpersonal sensitivity: A meta-analysis. *J Nonverb Behav.* 1999;**33**(3):149–80.

105. Wyman JF. The psychiatric and emotional impact of female pelvic floor dysfunction. *Curr Opin Obstet Gynecol.* 1994;**6**(4):336–39.

106. Morrison LM, Morrison M, Small DR, Glen ES. Psychiatric aspects of female incontinence. *Int Urogynecol J.* 1991:**2**(2):69–72.

107. Herzog AR, Fultz NH, Brock BM, Brown MB, Diokno AC. Urinary incontinence and psychological distress among older adults. *Psych Ageing.* 1988;**3**(2):115–21.

108. Brocklehurst JC. Urinary incontinence in the community: Analysis of a MORI poll. *BMJ.* 1993;**306**:832.

109. Fultz NH, Herzog AR. Self-reported social and emotional impact of urinary incontinence. *J Am Geriat Soc.* 2001;**49**(7):892–99.

110. Zorn BH, Montgomery H, Pieper K, Gray M, Steers WD. Urinary incontinence and depression. *J Urol.* 1999;**162**(1):82–84.

111. Sung V, et al. Association between urinary incontinence and depressive symptoms in overweight and obese women. *Am J Obstet Gynecol.* 2009;**200**(5):557.e1–557.e5.

112. Merell J, Brethauer S, Windover A, Ashton K, Heinberg L. Psychosocial correlates of pelvic floor disorders in women seeking bariatric surgery. *Surg Obesity Rel Dis.* 2012;**8**(6):792–96.

113. Macaulay AJ, Stern RS, Stanton SL. Psychological aspects of 211 female patients attending a urodynamic unit. *J Psychosom Res.* 1991;**35**:1–10.

114. Bogner HR, et al. Urinary incontinence and psychological distress in community-dwelling older adults. *J Am Geriat Soc.* 2002;**50**(3):489–95.

115. Bogner HR, O'Donnell AJ, de Vries HF, Northington GM, Joo JH. The temporal relationship between anxiety disorders and urinary incontinence among community-dwelling adults. *J Anxiety Dis.* 2011;**25**(2):203–8.

116. Perry S, McGrother CW, Turner K and the Leicestershire MRC Incontinence Study Group. An investigation of the relationship between anxiety and depression and urge incontinence in women: Development of a psychological model. *Br J Health Psych.* 2006;**11**(3):463–82.

117. de Vries HF, Northington GM, Bogner HR. Urinary incontinence (UI) and new psychological distress among community dwelling older adults. *Arch Gerontol Geriat.* 2012;**55**(1):49–54.

118. Bogner HR, Gallo JJ. Anxiety disorders and disability secondary to urinary incontinence among adults over age 50. *Int J Psychiatry Med.* 2002;**32**(2):141–54.

119. Macaulay AJ, Stern RS, Holmes DM, Stanton SL. Micturition and the mind: Psychological factors in the aetiology and treatment of urinary symptoms in women. *BMJ.* 1987;**294**:540.

120. Norton KR, Bhat AV, Stanton SL. Psychiatric aspects of urinary incontinence in women attending an outpatient urodynamic clinic. *BMJ.* 1990;**301**(6746):271–72.

121. Chiara G, Piccioni V, Perino M, Ohlmeier U, Fassino S, Leombruni P. Psychological investigation in female patients suffering from urinary incontinence. *Int Urogynecol J.* 1998;**9**(2):73–77.

122. Garcia JA, Crocker J, Wyman JF. Breaking the cycle of stigmatization: Managing the stigma of incontinence in social interactions. *J Wound Ostomy Cont Nurs.* 2005;**32**:38–52.

123. Morrison LM, Eadie AS, McAllister A, Glen ES, Taylor J, Rowan D. Personality testing in 226 patients with urinary incontinence. *BJU Int.* 1986;**58**:387–89.

124. Avery JC, et al. Identifying the quality of life effects of urinary incontinence with depression in an Australian population. *BMC Urol.* 2013;**13**:11.

125. Melville JL, Walker E, Katon W, Lentz G, Miller J, Fenner D. Prevalence of comorbid psychiatric illness and its impact on symptom perception, quality of life and functional status on women with urinary incontinence. *Am J Obstet Gynecol.* 2002;**187**(1):80–87.

126. Melville JL, Fan MY, Rau H, Nygaard IE, Katon WJ. Major depression and urinary incontinence in women: Temporal associations in an epidemiologic sample. *Am J Obstet Gynecol.* 2009;**201**(5):490.

127. Bonney WW, Gupta S, Hunter DR, Arndt S. Bladder dysfunction in schizophrenia. *Schizophrenia Research.* 1997;**25**(3):243–49.

128. Austin JA, Shapiro SL, Eisenberg DM, Forys KL. Mind-body medicine: State of the science, implications for practice. *J Am Board Fam Pract.* 2003;**16**(2):131–47.

129. Kegel AH. Stress incontinence of urine in women; physiologic treatment. *J Int Coll Surg.* 1956;**25**(4 part 1):487–99.

130. Frewen WK. An objective assessment of the unstable bladder of psychosomatic origin. *B J Urology.* 1978;**50** (4):249–49.

131. Debus G, Kästner R. Psychosomatic aspects of urinary incontinence in women. *Geburtshilfe Frauenheilkunde.* 2015;**75**(2):165–69.

132. Jirschele K, Ross R, Goldberg R, Botros S. Physician attitudes toward urinary incontinence identification. *Female Pelvic Med Reconstr Surg.* 2015;**21**(5):273–76.

Chapter 19

Biopsychosocial Perspectives on the Menopause

Myra S. Hunter and Melanie Smith

Menopause: A Biopsychosocial Transition

Menopause occurs on average between the ages of 50 and 51, for women living in western countries, and literally refers to a woman's last menstrual period. The menopause is a fairly universal experience for women if they live long enough; for some the process of menopause is influenced by surgery or disease, for example oophorectomy or breast cancer treatment. However, the last menstrual period takes place within a gradual process of physiological change, occurring concurrently with age and developmental changes, and within varied psychosocial and cultural contexts [1].

Definitions

Menopause literally is typically defined on the basis of menstrual changes and is said to have occurred when there has been one year without a menstrual period, although endocrine changes occur over a number of years. The definition of the menopause, which has been widely used, is based on that of the World Health Organization [2], which refers to the menopause as the 'permanent cessation of menstruation resulting from loss of ovarian follicular activity'. The following stages of the menopause transition and postmenopause are based on menstrual patterns:

Premenopause is defined by regular menstruation. *Perimenopause* includes the phase immediately prior to the menopause and the first year after menopause and is defined by changes in the regularity of menstruation during the previous 12 months. Women who have not menstruated during the past 12 months are defined as *postmenopausal*. Some women who have undergone hysterectomy or those who are taking hormone therapy may be difficult to classify within these definitions and are typically classified separately. Moreover, the classification of postmenopause can only be made retrospectively, since it is impossible to know which menstruation will be the last.

More recently, the Stages of Reproductive Ageing Workshop (STRAW) created a staged model to reflect parallel changes in menstruation and hormonal changes across women's lifespan [3]. Using the final menstrual period as an anchor (0), STRAW proposed five main stages preceding this point and two following. Stages –5 to –3 encompass the reproductive phases (menarche and regular menstruation), -2 early menopause transition (regular menstruation but change in cycle length), -1 late menopause transition (two or more missed menstrual periods and at least one intermenstrual interval of 60 days or more), +1a and +1b (early postmenopause) refers to the two years following the last menstrual period, +1c refers to 3–6 years following the last menstrual period and +2 (late postmenopause) the subsequent years. The stages of early and late menopause transition and the first year after the last menstrual period (−2 to +1a) correspond to the 'perimenopause'.

Related broader terms, such as 'climacteric syndrome' and 'menopause syndrome', have been used to refer to a wide variety of physical and emotional experiences that may or may not be related to hormone or menstrual changes, including hot flushes, vaginal dryness, loss of libido, depression, anxiety, irritability, poor memory, loss of concentration, mood swings, insomnia, tiredness, aching limbs, loss of energy and dry skin. 'The change' or 'change of life' is a commonly used colloquial term in western cultures that reflects the view that the menopause often occurs in parallel with other psychological and social adaptations during midlife. For example, there may be coincidental changes in personal and social roles and relationships, such as dealing with illness, caring for parents, dealing with adolescent children or children leaving home, as well as perceived personal and social consequences of reaching the age of 50. The impact of these changes and the extent to which they are attributed to the menopause will vary with the social and cultural context.

Cross-cultural studies have challenged the concept of the menopause as a universal phenomenon since there are wide variations in the reports of symptoms in women of different ethnic origins living in different countries [4]. Cultural explanations of these differences need to include lifestyle (diet, exercise, social factors, as well as reproductive patterns), which can affect biological processes, population differences in biology, as well as beliefs and attitudes to the menopause and the social status of mid-aged and older women – hence the need for a biopsychosocial understanding of the menopause.

Biological Influences

Physiological Changes

The function of the ovaries and hormone secretion is regulated by the hypothalamo-pituitary-ovarian axis. The primary factor influencing the transition from regular menstruation to the perimenopause appears to be the number of ovarian follicles. While at birth there are approximately 700,000 follicles in a woman's ovaries, the numbers reduce markedly in the decade before the menopause and, at the time of the last menstrual period, few follicles remain. Follicle-stimulating hormone (FSH) concentrations gradually increase and serum inhibin concentrations reduce in the years leading up to the perimenopause. These are now regarded as useful indices of the number and/or quality of follicles remaining in the ovary [5, 6]. During the reproductive years oestradiol is the main type of oestrogen produced but after the menopause oestrogen production does not cease because another oestrogen, oestrone, is produced. This arises from three main sources: the adrenal cortex, indirectly from the body's fat cells which convert androstenedione to oestrone, and from the ovaries which continue to produce small quantities of androgens which are converted to oestrogens. Testosterone levels stay at approximately the same level after the menopause, being produced by the adrenal glands and by conversion of other hormones.

The average age of menopause is estimated to be 50–51 years in most western countries but tends to be earlier in some developing countries and is associated with poverty and nutrition. Current smokers experience their last menstruation on average two years earlier than non-smokers and women who have a hysterectomy tend to have an earlier menopause even when their ovaries are conserved. In the US Study of Women's Health Across the Nation (SWAN), ethnic differences in hormone levels were found. Some of this was explained by smoking and body mass index (BMI), but differences in FSH (highest in Hispanic and African American and lowest in Japanese women) and testosterone (highest in Hispanic and African American and lowest in Japanese women) were evident when confounding factors were controlled [7]. The Melbourne Women's Midlife Health Project [8] similarly documented the biological and subjective changes experienced by women during the menopause transition. The main hormone changes were increases in FSH and decreases in oestradiol occurring during the menopause transition and early postmenopause, with maximum change two years before the last menstrual period. Oestradiol reached a stable lower level (below 20 pmol/l) between two and five years after the last menstrual period. Nevertheless, defining stages of menopause in clinical settings generally relies on age and menstrual criteria rather than measuring hormone levels [9].

Vasomotor Symptoms

Hot flushes and night sweats or vasomotor symptoms (VMS) are the most characteristic symptom of the menopause. Women living in North America and Europe tend to report more VMS than those living in China, Japan and the Indian subcontinent. They are reported by 60–80% of menopausal women in western cultures and are problematic for approximately 20–25% [10], having a negative impact on quality of life, largely due to discomfort, social embarrassment and disrupted sleep [11]. Recent studies suggest that the duration of VMS is longer (lasting up to ten years for some) than previously believed [12, 13].

Hot flushes are commonly described as sensations of heat in the face, neck and chest, frequently accompanied by perspiration and/or shivering, and often accompanied by increases in skin conductance and finger temperature as well as peripheral blood flow and heart rate. The exact aetiology is unknown, but they appear to be associated with the rate of change of plasma oestrogen, which influences the thermoregulatory system via the hypothalamus [6, 14]. Hot flushes are also more prevalent following rapid withdrawal of oestrogen, for example following surgical menopause or adjuvant chemotherapy for breast cancer. Alterations in oestrogen levels (but not absolute oestrogen levels) and neurotransmitters, such as

161

norepinephrine and serotonin, and their subsequent impact on thermoregulatory homeostasis, have been widely implicated in the pathogenesis of vasomotor symptoms [6]. Freedman [14] proposes that there is a narrowed thermoneutral zone in women who have hot flushes, such that hot flushes are triggered by small elevations in core body temperature, caused by changes in ambient temperature or other environmental triggers, including stress.

In general, it is how problematic or bothersome VMS are that is associated with quality of life and help seeking, rather than frequency of VMS [11, 15, 16]. Problematic or bothersome VMS are more likely to be associated with surgical menopause (bilateral oophorectomy or hysterectomy), higher BMI and chronicity of VMS [6, 16]. Breast cancer patients also have more severe and chronic VMS because of the acute loss of ovarian function associated with cancer therapies [17].

Psychosocial Perspectives

Attitudes and Beliefs

Psychological perspectives on menopause include the meanings and definitions of menopause, appraisals and attributions of symptoms to menopause, as well as cognitive, affective and behavioural reactions to the menopause. Social factors include socioeconomic and demographic variables, lifestyle and work settings, as well as roles and stressful life events.

The meaning of menopause and attitudes towards treatment are influenced by religion, ethnicity and personal values [18]. In western societies menopause tends to be associated with emotional and physical symptoms, ageing and uncertainty, while in many developing countries menopause is not regarded as a medical condition and thus may be better accepted as a natural part of life, with less focus on 'symptoms'. There are also cultural differences in women's attributions of different types of symptoms to the menopause, which in turn could result in some women not seeking or receiving appropriate advice and healthcare [19]. Negative beliefs and attitudes, and expectations held before the menopause predict symptom experience during the menopause [20]; it is therefore important not to generalize from those women who seek help with problematic symptoms to the majority for whom menopause is more manageable. In general, women tend to be pleased not to have menstrual period or

the need for contraception but are troubled if VMS are severe and also by negative attitudes and social images of mid-aged and older women which can affect self-esteem [21, 22]. Negative beliefs and cognitive appraisals (perceptions and interpretations) of VMS (social embarrassment, feeling out of control and frustration) and behavioural reactions (avoiding social situations) are in turn associated with more problematic VMS [16, 23].

Menopause and Mood

The menopause transition is not necessarily associated with psychological symptoms in healthy women. Therefore, depressed mood should not be attributed automatically to the menopause. Past depression is the main predictor of depressive symptoms during the menopause and psychosocial factors are also highly relevant. Age is another strong predictor in that low mood is more prevalent during midage; in general psychological distress tends to rise during adulthood to middle age before declining and levelling off in old age and, after the age of 55, women generally report improvements in mood [24]. Interestingly in this study of over 90,000 women in England, the midlife increase in distress (for both men and women) applied only to the lower-income groups (bottom 20% of the income groups) [24]. These findings are consistent with other data showing that financial and social pressures may lead to increased stress in other areas of life.

In a more detailed study of specific changes that occur for women across the menopause transition (The Medical Research Council National Survey of Health and Development, known as the 1946 British birth cohort study) [25], for most women, overall, psychological symptoms (depression and anxiety) generally tended to stay the same, with some increases and decreases, across the menopause transition. However, there was a proportion of women, estimated to be about 10%, who tend to be at a higher risk of psychological symptoms, including depressed mood, during the menopause transition. Factors found to be associated with psychological symptoms and depressed mood include past history of depression and psychological problems, social factors (educational and occupational status), poor health, surgical menopause, stressful life events, cigarette smoking, attitudes to menopause and ageing and early life circumstances and experiences [25, 26]. Overall, the experience of psychosocial factors has been found to have a much stronger association with psychological symptoms than the stage of menopause.

Mood and Vasomotor Symptoms

There are complex and bidirectional relationships between hot flushes and mood [27]. For example, anxiety reported before the menopause is a predictor of VMS during the menopause [28], and concurrent depressed mood and anxiety are associated with more problematic VMS [16, 23]. In turn, having troublesome VMS can lead to low mood and psychological symptoms if they affect sleep and interfere with quality of life [29].

It is important to consider the psychosocial context and interactions between specific psychosocial factors and menopause-specific changes. For example, mid-aged women report more work-related stress than mid-aged men or women of other age groups [30]; studies suggest that there are complex relationships between reports of work-related stress and menopausal symptoms; again there are likely to be two-way interactions [31].

A Biopsychosocial Approach

This approach takes into account the impact of hormone changes, a woman's beliefs and attitudes, mood, social context and past experiences, as well as her preferences. The attribution of symptoms to menopause is important since, apart from VMS, other 'menopausal symptoms' may well have other causes or are likely to interact with other factors. For example, memory and concentration are influenced by stress and ageing, and sleep can be disrupted by night sweats, as well as stress and unhelpful sleep habits. Similarly, sexual functioning is very much a biopsychosocial issue. Sexual interest (libido) in general tends to reduce with age and across the stages of the menopause, but is highly variable between women and is associated with ageing, stress, relationship issues, negative beliefs about ageing and sexuality, partners' sexual functioning, poor body image and certain medications that can contribute to a reduction in libido. However, vaginal dryness is associated with lower levels of oestrogen and is reported more commonly by postmenopausal women. This can have a significant impact in increasing the likelihood of intercourse being painful which in turn can reduce enjoyment and desire for sex (see NICE 2015 [9]). But there is wide variation between women; some even

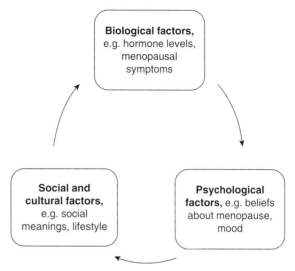

Figure 19.1 A biopsychosocial model of factors influencing experience of the menopause

report an increase in libido and enjoyment as they no longer have to worry about contraception.

A collaborative approach, discussing the relevant factors relating to menopause for an individual using the biopsychosocial model (Figure 19.1), can be helpful and can avoid mind–body dualism, which can be a barrier to doctor–patient relationships. Similarly, most parameters of the menopause transition vary considerably between women, so it is difficult to generalize, for example in relation to how long it might last, and attitude to sexual relationships.

A cognitive behavioural model of VMS has been proposed to understand the possible role of psychosocial factors in the experience of hot flushes [16] (Figure 19.2). Biological factors are included, such as the impact of reduced oestrogen levels on the thermoneutral zone, which in turn interacts with concurrent stress, mood, and negative beliefs and behaviours leading to problematic hot flushes. Environmental factors such as rushing, spicy food and alcohol might trigger hot flushes and cognitive reactions, can exacerbate distress. Negative thoughts and beliefs about VMS (relating to social embarrassment, disgust, feeling out of control and worry about sleep) and certain behavioural reactions, such as avoiding social situations, are associated with problematic VMS. On the other hand, calm thoughts and behaviours, such as using calm breathing, accepting the symptoms and not reacting with frustration or anxiety, are associated with less problematic VMS [32, 33].

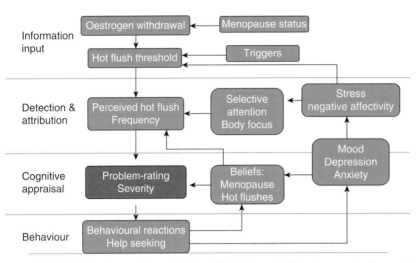

Figure 19.2 A cognitive behavioural model of hot flushes and night sweats

Hunter & Mann (2010) Journal of Psychosomatic Research

If women think that they are 'unattractive', 'not needed' or 'unsuccessful' during flushes – thoughts, which are associated with negative stereotypes about menopause in general – they are more likely to feel distressed [34]. Low mood and low self-esteem increase symptom perception, and the extent to which the symptoms are perceived as a problem is less associated with VMS frequency or duration but more with cognitions (perceptions of ability to control and cope), mood (depressed mood, anxiety) [23, 35]. Consequently assessing VMS using daily dairies and rating scales can provide information about both frequency and severity or problem-ratings; for example, the Hot Flush Rating Scale (HFRS) is a short scale which measures hot flush and night sweat frequency and 'problem-rating' (3 items including distress, extent to which a problem and interference with daily routine) [36].

A Biopsychosocial Approach to Treatment

Lifestyle Advice

There is some evidence that women who participate in psychoeducational and health promotion programmes have more accurate knowledge, more positive attitudes regarding menopause, less discomfort associated with changes at these stages and more frequent engagement in healthy habit levels than women who do not participate in these programmes [37]. Menopause may offer an important opportunity for healthcare professionals to encourage positive health-related behaviours (smoking cessation, physical activity and stress reduction), as women frequently seek information and advice at this stage. Physically active women tend to report higher quality of life and fewer VMS compared to inactive women. However, a recent Cochrane review found inadequate evidence to support exercise alone as an effective intervention for problematic hot flushes [38]. Weight tends to increase with age and, while there tends to be a redistribution of fat during the menopause to the abdomen, weight gain is not a necessary consequence of menopause. However, weight loss (using a healthy diet and exercise) can lead to improvements in quality of life and also improvements in VMS [39]. Such changes might benefit women during menopause transition but also offer prevention of longer-term health problems.

Treatment Approaches for VMS

It has been estimated that approximately 75% of women seek information and advice about menopause, usually through their general practitioner, in the United Kingdom. There are several categories of treatment options for VMS which can be discussed taking account of the women's values, situation and preferences: hormone therapies, non-hormonal pharmacological treatments, complementary therapies and non-hormonal therapies. Current guidance is available [9, 40] and a 'Practitioner's Toolkit for Managing the Menopause' [41] offers algorithms for treatment decision-making, hormonal and non-hormonal treatment options, symptom management and patient review.

Hormonal Therapies

Hormone therapy (HT) is a highly effective treatment for menopausal VMS and is available in different regimes [9, 40] (for full detail, see NICE, 2015). The publication of prospective data from the Women's Health Initiative and the Million Women Study cast doubt on the long-term safety of HT, and led to a decline in its use. Women who stop taking HT often experience a return of menopause symptoms [42]. Women who have an early menopause are encouraged to have HT until the age of natural menopause [9]. HT is generally contraindicated for women who have a history of breast cancer, patients, for whom safe and effective options are more limited.

Non-Hormonal Pharmacological Treatments

There is a growing evidence base for the efficacy of selective serotonin reuptake inhibitors and serotonin–norepinephrine reuptake inhibitors (SSRIs and SNRIs) for the reduction of VMS, such as citalopram and venlafaxine, although the long-term efficacy of these interventions has been questioned and side effects are reported. Paroxetine is not recommended for breast cancer patients due to its interactions with tamoxifen. A Cochrane review of non-hormonal medications identified that certain SSRIs/SNRIs (e.g. Venlafaxine), antihypertensives (e.g. clonidine) and anticonvulsants (e.g. gabapentin) demonstrated a modest reduction in symptoms but that side effects can limit use [43].

Complementary Therapies and Non-Hormonal Therapies

Complementary or alternative therapies are popular, for example vitamin E, oil of evening primrose, black cohosh, soy foods and red clover. However, several reviews conclude that there is little consistent benefit for botanical or dietary supplements and that further well-controlled studies of complementary therapies and herbal remedies are needed [9, 44]. There is rather more evidence that 'mind–body' and psychosocial interventions, such as relaxation, hypnosis, mindfulness and cognitive behavioural therapy, have beneficial effects on menopausal symptoms and quality of life [37, 45].

Cognitive Behavioural Approaches

Cognitive behavioural therapy (CBT) has been developed specifically for the treatment of VMS based on the CBT model [16] and can be delivered, with positive outcomes, in a self-help format and in groups over four or six weeks [46, 47]. The CBT interventions significantly reduced the impact (problem-rating) of VMS in three randomized controlled trials, including well women and breast cancer patients, with improvements being maintained at a six-month follow-up [48–50]. Interestingly the self-help format (book and CD) was as effective in reducing VMS as the group intervention. The CBT targets beliefs and behaviours and provides strategies to deal with stress, hot flushes, night sweats and sleep. Women reported feeling more in control of their VMS, and there were additional benefits to quality of life, i.e. social and physical functioning.

Conclusions

Women's experiences of the menopause are highly varied. They are influenced by biological (hormone changes, VMS, general health) and psychosocial factors (culture, early life adversity and concurrent life stress, past anxiety and depression, current mood, beliefs and expectations and socioeconomic factors). Consequently, a biopsychosocial approach is needed to understand the range of influences on a woman's presenting problems and to engage in a collaborative discussion of these. Women tend to seek help during the menopause when having difficulty in coping with problematic VMS, together with the menopause and life stresses. There is a range of evidence-based options available to meet women's varied needs during the menopause, depending on their personal preferences, medical history and possible contraindications. Menopause also offers an important opportunity for healthcare professionals to encourage positive health-related behaviours (smoking cessation, physical activity and stress reduction), as women frequently seek information and advice at this life stage.

Key Points

- The menopause often occurs in parallel with psychological and social adaptations during midlife. The impact of these changes and the extent to which they are attributed to the menopause will vary with the social and cultural context.
- In general, it is how problematic or bothersome vasomotor symptoms (VMS) are that is associated with quality of life and help seeking, rather than frequency of VMS. Problematic or bothersome VMS are associated with surgical menopause (bilateral oophorectomy or hysterectomy), higher body mass index, mood, beliefs and chronicity of VMS.
- Psychological perspectives on menopause include the meanings and definitions of menopause, appraisals and attributions of symptoms to menopause, as well as cognitive, affective and behavioural reactions to the menopause. Social factors include socioeconomic and demographic variables, lifestyle and work settings, as well as roles and stressful life events.
- The biopsychosocial approach takes into account the impact of hormone changes, a woman's beliefs and attitudes, mood, social context and past experiences, as well as her preferences.
- The attribution of symptoms to menopause should be carefully considered since, apart from vasomotor symptoms, 'menopausal symptoms' may well have other causes or are likely to interact with other factors.
- Assessing VMS using daily dairies and rating scales (such as the Hot Flush Rating Scale) can provide information about both frequency and severity or problem-ratings.
- Women who participate in psychoeducational and health promotion programmes have more accurate knowledge of the menopausal transition, more positive attitudes, less discomfort and more frequent engagement in healthy habits levels than women who do not participate in these programmes.
- A cognitive behavioural model of VMS has been proposed to understand the possible role of psychosocial factors in the experience of hot flushes

- There is evidence that 'mind–body' and psychosocial interventions, such as hypnosis, mindfulness and cognitive behavioural therapy, have beneficial effects on menopausal symptoms and quality of life.

References

1. Hunter MS, Rendall M. Bio-psycho-socio-cultural perspectives on menopause. *Best Practice & Research Clin Obstet & Gynaecol* 2007; 21(2): 261–274.

2. World Health Organisation. Research on Menopause. Report of a WHO Scientific group. WHO technical report N670. WHO, Geneva, 1981.

3. Harlow SD, Gass M, Hall JE, Lobo R, Maki P, Rebar RW, et al. Executive summary of the Stages of Reproductive Aging Workshop+ 10: Addressing the unfinished agenda of staging reproductive aging. *Climacteric* 2012; 15: 105–114.

4. Freeman EW, Sherif K. Prevalence of hot flushes and night sweats around the world: A systematic review. *Climacteric* 2007; 10(3): 197–214.

5. Richardson S. The biological basis of the menopause. In: Burger HG, ed. *The Menopause: Clinical Endocrinology and Metabolism*. London, Bailliere Tindall. 1993; 1–16.

6. Archer DF, Sturdee DW, Baber R, De Villiers TJ, Pines A, Freedman RR, et al. Menopausal hot flushes and night sweats: Where are we now? *Climacteric* 2011; 14(5): 515–528.

7. Sowers MF, Crawford SL, Sternfeld B, Morgenstein D, Gold EB, Greendale GA, et al. SWAN: A multi-center, multi-ethnic, community-based cohort study of women and the menopause transition. In: Lobo RA, Kelsey J & Marcus R, eds. *Menopause: Biology and Pathobiology*. San Diego, Academic Press. 2000; 175–188.

8. Guthrie JR, Dennerstein L, Taffe JR, Lehert P, et al. The menopause transition: A 9 year prospective population-based study. The Melbourne Women's Midlife Health Project. *Climacteric* 2004; 7: 375–389.

9. National Institute for Health and Care Excellence (NICE) *Diagnosis and management of menopause guideline*. October 2015.

10. Porter M, Penney GC, Russell D, Russell E, Templeton A. A population based survey of women's experience of the menopause. *Brit J Obstet Gynaecol* 1996; 103: 1025–1028.

11. Ayers B, Hunter MS. Health-related quality of life of women with menopausal hot flushes and night sweats. *Climacteric* 2013; 16: 235–239.

12. Hunter MS, Gentry-Maharaj A, Ryan A, Burnell M, Lanceley A, Fraser L, et al. Prevalence, frequency and problem rating of hot flushes persist in older postmenopausal women: Impact of age, BMI, hysterectomy, lifestyle and mood in a cross sectional cohort study of 10,418 British women aged 54–65. *Brit J Obstet & Gynaecol* 2012; 119: 40–50.

13. Avis NE, Crawford SL, Greendale G, Bromberger JT, Everson-Rose SA, Gold EB, et al. Duration of menopausal vasomotor symptoms over the menopause transition. *JAMA Int Med* 2015; 175(4): 531–539.

14. Freedman RR, Krell, W. (1999). Reduced thermoregulatory null zone in postmenopausal women with hot flashes. *Am J Obstet Gynecol* 1999; 181(1): 66–70.

15. Rand KL, Otte JL, Flockhart D, et al. Modeling hot flushes and quality of life in breast cancer survivors. *Climacteric* 2011; 13: 171–180.

16. Hunter MS, Mann E. A cognitive model of menopausal hot flushes and night sweats. *J Psychosom Research* 2010; 69(5): 491–501.

17. Mom CH, Buijs C, Willemse PHB, Mourits MJE, et al. Hot flushes in breast cancer patients. *Crit Rev Oncol/Haem* 2006; 57: 63–77.

18. Sievert LL. Menopause across cultures: Clinical considerations. *Menopause* 2014; 21(40): 421–423.

19. Hunter MS, Gupta P, Papitsch-Clarke A, Sturdee D. Mid-aged Health in Women from the Indian Subcontinent (MAHWIS): A quantitative and qualitative study of experience of menopause in UK Asian women, compared to UK Caucasian and women living in Delhi. *Climacteric* 2009; 12(1): 26–37.

20. Ayers B, Fisher M, Hunter MS. A systematic review of the role of attitudes to the menopause upon experience of menopause. *Maturitas* 2010; 65: 28–36.

21. Hunter MS, O'Dea I. Menopause: Bodily changes and multiple meanings. In: Ussher JM, ed. *Body Talk: The Material and Discursive regulation of Sexuality, Madness and reproduction.* UK and New York, Routledge. 1997; 199–222.

22. Hvas L. Menopausal women's positive experience of growing older. *Maturitas* 2006; 54: 245–251.

23. Hunter MS, Chilcot J. Testing a cognitive model of menopausal hot flushes and night sweats. *J Psychosom Res* 2013; 74(4): 307–312.

24. Lang IA, Llewellyn DJ, Hubbard RE, et al. Income and midlife peak in common mental disorder prevalence. *Psychol Med* 2011; 41: 1365–1372.

25. Mishra GD, Kuh D. Health symptoms during midlife in relation to menopausal transition: British prospective cohort study. *Brit Med J* 2012; 344: e402.

26. Vivian-Taylor J, Hickey M. Menopause and depression: Is there a link? *Maturitas* 2014; 79: 142–146.

27. Thurston RC, Bromberger JT, Joffe H, Avis NE, Hess R, Crandall CJ, et al. Beyond frequency: Who is most bothered by vasomotor symptoms? *Menopause* 2008; 15(5): 841.

28. Freeman EW, Sammel MD, Lin H, Gracia CR, Kapoor S, Ferdousi T. The role of anxiety and hormonal changes in menopausal hot flashes. *Menopause* 2005; 12(3): 258–266.

29. Worsley R, Bell R, Kulkarni J, Davis SR. The association between vasomotor symptoms and depression during perimenopause: A systematic review. *Maturitas* 2014; 77(2): 111–117.

30. Griffiths A, Knight A, Mahudin D. *Ageing, Work-related Stress & Health.* Age Concern & TAEN (Age UK), 2009. www.taen.org.uk/uploads/resources/24455_TAEN_Work_Related_Stress_32pg1.pdf Accessed 23 March 2017.

31. Matsuzaki K, Uemura H, Yasui T. Associations of menopausal symptoms with job-related stress factors in nurses in Japan. *Maturitas* 2014; 79: 77–85.

32. Rendall MJ, Simonds LM, Hunter MS. The Hot Flush Beliefs Scale: A tool for assessing thoughts and beliefs associated with the experience of menopausal hot flushes and night sweats. *Maturitas* 2008; 60(2): 158–169.

33. Hunter MS, Ayers B, Smith M. The Hot Flush Behaviour Scale: A measure of behavioural reactions to menopausal hot flushes and night sweats. *Menopause* 2011; 18(11): 1178–1183.

34. Reynolds F. Exploring self-image during hot flushes using a semantic differential scale: Associations between poor self-image, depression, flush frequency and flush distress. *Maturitas* 2002; 42: 201–207.

35. Norton S, Chilcot J, Hunter MS. Cognitive behaviour therapy for menopausal symptoms (hot flushes and night sweats): Moderators and mediators of treatment effects. *Menopause* 2014; 21 (6): 574–578.

36. Hunter MS, Liao KLM. A psychological analysis of menopausal hot flushes. *Br J Clin Psychol* 1995; 34: 589–599.

37. Toral MV, Godoy-Izquierdo D, García AP, Moreno RL, Ladrón de Guevara NM, Ballesteros AS, et al. Psychosocial interventions in perimenopausal and postmenopausal women: A systematic review of randomised and non-randomised trials and non-controlled studies. *Maturitas* 2014; 77: 93–110.

38. Daley A, Stokes-Lampard H, Thomas A, MacArthur C. Exercise for vasomotor menopausal symptoms. *Cochrane Database of Systematic Reviews*, 2014; 11. Art. No.: CD006108.

39. Davis SR, Castelo-Branco C, Chedrui P, Lumsden MA, Nappi RE, Shah D, et al. Understanding weight gain at menopause, *Climacteric* 2012; 15(5): 419–429.

40. Shifren JL, Gass ML. NAMS Recommendations for Clinical Care of Midlife Women Working Group. The North American Menopause Society recommendations for clinical care of midlife women. *Menopause*, 2014; 21(10): 1038–1062.

41. Jane FM, Davis SR. A practitioner's toolkit for managing the menopause. *Climacteric* 2014; 17: 564–579.

42. Gentry-Maharaj A, Karpinskyj C, Glazer C, Burnell M, Ryan A, Fraser L, et al. Use and perceived efficacy of complementary and alternative medicines after discontinuation of hormone therapy: A nested United Kingdom Collaborative Trial of Ovarian Cancer Screening cohort study. *Menopause*, 2015; 22(4): 384–390.

43. Rada G, Capurro D, Pantoja T, et al. Non-hormonal interventions for hot flushes in women with a history of breast cancer. *The Cochrane Library*, 2010; (9).

44. Drewe J, Bucher KA, Zahner C. A systematic review of non-hormonal treatments of vasomotor symptoms in climacteric and cancer patients. *SpringerPlus*, 2015; 4 (1): 65.

45. Tremblay A, Sheeran L, Aranda SK. Psychoeducational interventions to alleviate hot flashes: A systematic review. *Menopause* 2008; 15(1): 193–202.

46. Hunter MS, Smith M. *Managing Hot Flushes and Night Sweats: A Cognitive Behavioural Self-Help Guide to the Menopause.* UK and New York: Routledge, 2014.

47. Hunter MS, Smith M. *Managing Hot Flushes with Group Cognitive Behaviour Therapy: An Evidence Based Treat Manual for Health Professionals.* UK and New York, NY: Routledge, 2014.

48. Ayers B, Smith M, Hellier J, Mann E, Hunter MS. Effectiveness of group and self-help cognitive behavior therapy in reducing problematic menopausal hot flushes and night sweats (MENOS 2): A randomized controlled trial. *Menopause* 2012; 19 (7): 749–759.

49. Mann E, Smith MJ, Hellier J, Balabanovic JA, Hamed H, Grunfeld EA, et al. Cognitive behavioural treatment for women who have menopausal symptoms after breast cancer treatment (MENOS 1): A randomised controlled trial. *The Lancet Oncol* 2012; 13(3): 309–318.

50. Duijts SF, van Beurden M, Oldenburg HS, Hunter MS, Kieffer JM, Stuiver MM, et al. Efficacy of cognitive behavioral therapy and physical exercise in alleviating treatment-induced menopausal symptoms in patients with breast cancer: Results of a randomized, controlled, multicenter trial. *J Clin Oncol* 2012; 30(33): 4124–4133.

Chapter 20

Biopsychosocial Factors in Gynaecological Cancer

Laura E. Simonelli and Amy K. Otto

Gynaecological Cancer Statistics

Global statistics on the prevalence of gynaecological cancers as a group are limited. In the United States, gynaecological cancers – which include cancers of the cervix, ovary, uterus, vagina and vulva – account for 11% of all cancers diagnosed in women, affecting approximately 90,000 women each year [1]. Cervical cancer is the most common type of gynaecological cancer worldwide and is the fourth most common cancer in women, affecting over half a million women each year [2]. Cervical cancer alone represents approximately 7.9% of all cancers in women [2]. Endometrial cancer and ovarian cancer are the next most common types of gynaecological cancer, accounting for 4.8% and 3.6% of all cancers in women, respectively [2].

Survival rates for gynaecological cancer vary greatly by country, as well as site and stage of cancer. About 7.5% of female cancer deaths worldwide are due to cervical cancer, with the vast majority of cervical cancer cases and deaths occurring in less-developed countries [2]. The five-year survival rate for cervical cancer is around 60–70% worldwide, but ranges from as low as 46% in India to as high as 77% in South Korea [2,3]. Globally, the five-year survival rates for endometrial and ovarian cancer are approximately 69% and 30–50%, respectively [2]. Worldwide survival rates for less-common gynaecological cancers are limited, but in the United States the five-year relative survival rate is about 50% for vaginal cancers and 16–86% for vulvar cancers, although these figures depend largely on cancer stage [3].

Treatments for Gynaecological Cancer

Treatment for gynaecological cancers will vary depending on the site and stage of the disease, but most commonly involve surgery, chemotherapy and radiation therapy. Surgery often includes total abdominal hysterectomy (including removal of the uterus and cervix), bilateral salpingo-oophorectomy (removal of both ovaries and fallopian tubes) and potentially resection of additional organs and lymph nodes [4]. Chemotherapies including platinum drugs (e.g. cisplatin) and taxanes (e.g. paclitaxel) are often used in the treatment of gynaecological cancers [5]. Finally, radiation therapy is used in the treatment of approximately 40% of gynaecological cancers as an adjunct to surgery [5].

Quality of Life

The gynaecological cancer patient's physical and emotional symptom burden negatively impacts health-related and overall quality of life [4,6]. Quality of life concerns in gynaecological cancer vary by disease site and can include issues related to physical functioning (e.g. urinary and faecal incontinence, sexual dysfunction, lymphoedema) and psychosocial functioning (e.g. body image concerns, role changes, anxiety, depression, sexual dysfunction), which are reviewed in greater detail subsequently in this chapter. Among women treated with radiation therapy for gynaecological cancers, nearly all report some negative change in quality of life, specifically physical, sexual and/or social functioning [7]. Within this population, pain, dyspareunia and decreased interest in sex specifically have been associated with decreased quality of life in physical, psychological or social domains [8]. Among gynaecological cancer patients treated with chemotherapy, nausea and vomiting have been negatively associated with quality of life [9]. More broadly, urinary incontinence [10] and sexual morbidity [4,11] in particular have been found to predict poorer short-term and long-term quality of life and are associated with anxiety and depression.

Biological Factors

Physical Sequelae

The physical sequelae of gynaecological cancers include both acute side effects (e.g. fatigue, gastrointestinal problems, alopecia) and long-term/late effects of disease and treatment. Late effects of treatment can appear months to years after cancer treatment completion. Common, late effects of gynaecologic cancer include cognitive changes, sexual side effects, changes in bowel patterns, peripheral neuropathy and skin changes [12].

Neurological Effects

Neurological and central nervous system effects may include pain, neuropathy, cognitive changes, fatigue and sleep disturbance. Both acute and chronic pain are common in cancer patients. Gynaecological cancer pain may include both neuropathic pain, as discussed next, and nociceptive pain, which results from tissue damage and is described as sharp, aching or throbbing [6]. Unfortunately, there are no evidence-based guidelines for treating pain in gynaecological cancer specifically, and pain is often inadequately managed. Treatment for pain related to gynaecological cancer typically follows guidelines established for cancer pain or general pain management; analgesics are traditionally used, ranging from non-opioid analgesics (e.g. nonsteroidal anti-inflammatory drugs [NSAIDs]) for milder pain to full opioid agonists (e.g. fentanyl) for more severe pain [6].

Peripheral neuropathy occurs in 5–38% of patients treated with chemotherapy, and the co-administration of platinum and taxane chemotherapies increases the likelihood of neurotoxic sequelae sevenfold [5]. Some patients will experience a reduction in neuropathy post treatment, while others will deal with it as a long-term effect. Pharmacotherapy including NSAIDs, tricyclic antidepressants and GABA agonists such as pregabalin and gabapentin may be used to target neuropathy, though with varying success and undesirable secondary side effects [5]. Physical therapy including gait training and lower body strengthening to improve balance [13] and alternative therapies including acupuncture may also offer some relief [5].

Cognitive changes such as memory loss, short-term memory impairment and difficulty concentrating or learning new skills are common following treatment for gynaecological cancers [12]. Though there is limited research on the occurrence of 'chemo-brain' specifically within a gynaecological cancer population, there is evidence to support changes in brain function following chemotherapy in other cancers [14,15]. There is evidence that cognitive skills

such as attention, processing speed and reaction time decline during the course of chemotherapy for ovarian cancer [16]. There is also evidence that other factors such as fatigue, sleep disturbance, anxiety and depression may also contribute to cognitive changes, as some cognitive changes have been noted before the initiation of chemotherapy treatment [17]. Treatments may target the multifactorial nature of cognitive changes after cancer through use of cognitive behavioural therapy, exercise, brain-training and pharmacological interventions including antidepressants or central nervous system stimulants (e.g. Provigil, Ritalin).

Fatigue is almost ubiquitous among cancer patients, with prevalence rates of up to 96% [6]. Fatigue often persists and is a top survivorship concern with up to 30% of survivors reporting fatigue one year post treatment [6]. An interplay of multiple factors including cancer disease and treatment directly, nutrition, anaemia, anxiety, depression and sleep disturbance exacerbate this common concern. Multidisciplinary approaches to managing fatigue include pharmacotherapy, nutrition, treating sleep disturbance and psychological comorbidities, and exercise, though optimal type, timing and intensity of the latter have not been determined [6]. One small study investigated the use of a psychostimulant (methylphenidate) twice per day in women treated for recurrent gynaecological cancer and found significant improvement in fatigue, mood and quality of life [18].

Most of the research on sleep disturbance in gynaecological cancer has been conducted in women with ovarian cancer. Sleep disturbance or poor sleep quality was endorsed by almost 70% of patients with ovarian cancer both during and after treatment, and almost half used sleep medication during the month prior to responding [19]. Additionally, poor sleep quality is associated with reduction in all quality-of-life domains and increased depression [19]. Sleep disturbance also appears to persist at least a year after treatment, and factors such as depression, use of pain medication and premenopausal status may contribute to this [20]. Cognitive behavioural therapy, including sleep hygiene, stimulus control, cognitive restructuring and relaxation training, is effective in treating sleep disturbance [11]. Pharmacological agents (e.g. benzodiazepines, antidepressants, hypnotic medications or melatonin), though often prescribed, do not appear to adequately help with this issue [20].

Lymphatic System Effects

Lymphoedema – a condition where fluid is blocked from properly draining in the lymphatic system and builds up in body tissue – is caused by surgery, radiation or metastases in women with gynaecological cancer. It is most common in vulvar cancer patients (35–47%), followed by cervical cancer (12–17%), uterine (8–17%) and ovarian cancer (4–7%) [6]. Lymphoedema can result in considerable fluid accumulation and impacts on patients' appearance, body image and mobility. Lymphoedema is a chronic condition requiring lifelong, consistent management. Treatment for lymphoedema includes use of compression garments, lymphatic drainage massage and physical therapy [6].

Gastrointestinal and Genitourinary Effects

Acute effects of radiation therapy may include damage to intestinal mucosa resulting in diarrhoea, nausea, and stomach cramps, while long-term and late effects may include enteritis, bowel obstruction or fistula formation, often leading to the need for additional surgeries and related comorbidities [5]. Faecal incontinence is also a significant concern for survivors of gynaecologic cancer [21]. Additionally, there is a high prevalence of intestinal obstruction symptoms near the end of life [6].

Pelvic floor dysfunction includes bladder storage and voiding problems, urinary and faecal incontinence and sexual dysfunction. Survivors of gynaecologic cancer are significantly more likely than non-cancer controls to have urinary storage issues, including nocturia, urinary urgency, urinary leakage and bladder pain [22]. They are also significantly more likely than controls to have urinary incontinence issues, including urge, stress, mixed and nocturnal enuresis [22]. Approximately two out of three women with gynaecologic cancer will suffer from pre-existing urinary incontinence, pelvic organ prolapse or both before cancer treatment, though it may be possible to surgically address these concerns in the course of cancer treatment [23]. Physical therapy in the form of pelvic floor training may benefit gynaecologic cancer survivors with pelvic floor dysfunction by strengthening the pelvic floor muscles and in turn reducing incontinence and improving sexual functioning [24]. The combination of pelvic floor therapy and behavioural therapy including urinary incontinence management advice (e.g. avoiding bladder irritants, optimal balance of fluid intake) may also hold

promise as demonstrated in gynaecologic cancer survivors [25].

Endocrine and Sexual Functioning Effects

Surgery, chemotherapy and radiation therapy contribute to sexual morbidity. Surgery for vaginal, vulvar and cervical cancers may alter anatomy, including loss of clitoral tissue. Surgery and radiation therapy also contribute to vaginal stenosis and related dryness, loss of elasticity and resilience, and scar tissue [26]. Chemotherapy can contribute to menopause and the resulting loss of oestrogen leading to vaginal atrophy, dryness and dyspareunia [26]. Additionally, cytotoxic effects of chemotherapy, including fatigue, nausea, pain, and early menopause, may affect a woman's libido [26]. Abbott-Anderson and Kwekkeboom [27] categorized quality-of-life concerns related to sexual function into three main dimensions: physical (including dyspareunia, changes in the vagina, and decreased sexual activity), psychological (including 'decreased libido, alterations in body image, anxiety related to sexual performance') and social ('difficulty maintaining previous sexual roles, emotional distancing from partners, perceived change in partner's level of sexual interest') [p. 477].

In order to help address sexual dysfunction among cancer survivors, an open dialogue between patients and their providers is helpful. Providers can assess sexual health history and include sexual health in routine review of systems [26]. Assessment measures are also available; the Female Sexual Functioning Index demonstrates sound psychometric properties for measuring sexual functioning in cancer survivors [28]. Once concerns are identified, multidisciplinary treatment approaches including medical, physical therapy and psychological management may help with sexual functioning changes. For example, non-hormonal lubricating agents such as Replens can relieve vaginal dryness and reduce pain during sexual activity, and vaginal dilators may help with stenosis [26]. While using hormones to address sexual concerns among gynaecological cancer survivors is still of some debate, vaginal oestrogen may be an option for some women to relieve dryness and thinning of the vaginal area. There is also some evidence that hormone replacement therapy to treat menopausal symptoms does not increase risk of recurrence for women with endometrial, epithelial ovarian, cervical, vaginal and vulvar cancers [29]. Physical therapy including pelvic floor therapy can address sexual dysfunction related to weak pelvic floor muscles [24]. Psychotherapy can target body image concerns, communication, arousal problems and depression and anxiety symptoms leading to sexual dysfunction by using education and cognitive behavioural interventions [30].

Treatment for gynaecologic cancers can impact fertility in women of childbearing age. Surgical resection of cancer or disease staging typically involves the removal of organs necessary for reproduction, including the uterus, ovaries, fallopian tubes and cervix. Fertility-sparing procedures, though not always possible, may include trachelectomy for early-stage cervical cancer, and uterine and contralateral ovarian preservation for good-prognosis ovarian tumours and the latter early-stage uterine and cervical cancers [31]. Progestational agents might also be used for treatment of early-stage uterine cancer, though more research is needed. If ovarian- or cervical-sparing treatments are not an option, oocyte or embryo cryopreservation may still allow for future childbearing if the uterus is maintained [32]. Chemotherapy can contribute to infertility via damage to oocytes; this impact is variable depending on the chemotherapeutic agent and dosage, patient age and ovarian functioning. Similarly, radiation therapy may damage oocytes, in addition to the effects in the uterus and hypothalamic-pituitary axis. Ovarian transposition is one option for protecting the ovaries from radiation in treating cervical, vaginal and uterine cancers [32]. Nonetheless, fertility-sparing options are not always possible, and the resulting psychosocial impact can be enormous.

Psychological Factors

The physical sequelae of gynaecological cancer often contribute to symptoms of depression and anxiety [33,34]. Interestingly, women who receive more extensive treatments consistently report higher distressed mood and anxiety and lower quality of life but do not report higher levels of depression overall when compared to women who received less extensive treatment [35]. Among survivors who have undergone more extensive treatment, those who use more avoidant coping strategies (e.g. denial) tend to report higher levels of depression and distressed mood and lower quality of life than those who use more engagement-based coping strategies like positive reframing [35]; this relationship was not found, though, among women who received shorter, less extensive treatments.

Depression

Although about a quarter of all cancer patients experience depression, few are offered treatment for their depressive symptoms [6]. A limited amount of research has specifically examined depression among gynaecological cancer patients. In a sample of low-income, ethnic-minority women in the United States who were being treated for gynaecological or breast cancer, approximately 17% reported at least moderate levels of depressive symptoms, yet only a minority received treatment for their depression in the form of antidepressant medication (12%) or counselling/support groups (5%) [36]. Among these women, those who reported greater economic stress experienced even greater rates of depression and poorer quality of life [37]. The substantial number of untreated depression cases among gynaecological cancer patients is thought to be due to the underestimation of depressive symptoms on the part of providers [36] as well as the expectation among both patients and providers that depression is a normal part of the cancer experience [6]. Unmet survivorship needs (e.g. need for help reducing overall stress in life) among gynaecological cancer survivors have been associated with increased symptoms of depression [38].

Increased physical sequelae of treatment, especially menopausal symptoms and sexual dysfunction, have also been linked to increased depressive symptoms [39]. Side effects of treatment like fatigue may inhibit participation in usual activities and mirror somatic symptoms of depression, which may also make the identification of depression in cancer patients more challenging [6]. However, the relationship between physical sequelae of treatment and distress has been found to be moderated by social support such that patients with greater support experience fewer depressive symptoms and traumatic stress [40].

Anxiety

Anxiety is another common issue among cancer patients, with approximately one-fifth of all cancer patients reporting significant anxiety symptoms [6] and up to about 60% wanting help with management [41]. As with depression, little research has focussed on anxiety among gynaecologic cancer patients and survivors specifically. One study found that nearly one-third of survivors endorse clinically significant levels of anxiety, and these survivors are three times more likely to report anxiety symptoms than the general population [38]. Some side effects of treatment like lymphoedema have also been suggested to trigger increased anxiety, as some patients wrongly attribute these symptoms to disease recurrence or progression [4]. As with depression, anxiety often goes undiagnosed and untreated among cancer patients due to incorrect beliefs that anxiety is normal in the context of cancer, or that anxiety symptoms stem directly from the cancer or its treatment [6].

For many cancer patients, anxiety is often focussed around fear of cancer recurrence; in fact, it is often comorbid with anxiety disorders like generalized anxiety disorder, although it is a distinct construct from generalized anxiety [42]. Fear of cancer recurrence has been found to be the most common need for supportive care among women with gynaecological cancers, endorsed by about one-quarter of survivors [38]; however, comparatively little work has examined this construct among survivors. More advanced disease, as may be the case among many ovarian cancer survivors, is associated with greater and more persistent levels of fear of cancer recurrence over time [43]. Unfortunately, this is a realistic fear for many survivors, as many gynaecological cancers, particularly ovarian cancer, have very high recurrence rates (70–90% over five years) [44]. Psychosocial factors, such as exaggerated perception of disease severity, are also strong predictors of fear of cancer recurrence [43]. Recently, an increasing amount of research has investigated potential interventions specifically for fear of cancer recurrence such as cognitive-existential group therapy, which has shown promising results in breast and ovarian cancer survivors [45].

Aside from fear of cancer recurrence, the presence of other unmet survivorship needs has been significantly correlated with anxiety, depression and post-traumatic stress symptoms, and those with advanced disease reported more unmet needs [38,46].

Concerns about Death/Dying

Many gynaecologic cancer patients experience worry and concerns related to death and dying at diagnosis and throughout treatment [47], although some research has suggested that death anxiety may decrease with time following diagnosis [48]. Many women respond to worries about death with avoidance strategies like distraction; others take a more task-oriented approach, making lists and getting legal documentation in order, or an emotion-oriented approach, using positive self-talk and relying on 'inner psychological strength' to cope [47].

Along with worry about death itself, another common fear among gynaecological and other cancer survivors is becoming physically/mentally incapacitated and dependent on others towards the end of life [47]. Utilization of palliative and hospice care earlier in the illness trajectory has been encouraged, which can improve symptom management and patient and family satisfaction [49], as the value that patients place on survival is generally tempered by the desire for good quality of life [50].

General Loss and Grief

Infertility is often an unfortunate outcome associated with treatment of cancer among women of reproductive age. It is often associated with increased feelings of grief and sadness, and decreased quality of life, even beyond a year after completing treatment [31]. In some women, the loss of childbearing ability compounds the stress of the cancer diagnosis and effectively creates a 'double trauma', which can lead to poorer long-term outcomes such as prolonged grief and poor coping strategies [31]. However, research has suggested that receipt of support and information about reproductive issues may help reduce levels of anxiety and emotional distress among cancer survivors [31].

For women dealing with the many and varied physical problems of gynaecologic cancer and resulting physical or functional losses (e.g. disability, infertility, loss of energy, loss of role functioning), one's sense of meaning or purpose in life may change [51]. Survivors may have difficulty making sense of their cancer experience, and this loss of meaning can exacerbate depressive symptoms in survivorship [51].

Body Image Issues

Appearance and functional changes are common among gynaecological cancer survivors. Body image concerns including hair loss, weight change, loss of female organs, changes to vaginal and vulvar areas, functional urinary and bowel changes, and ostomies may also contribute to changes in a woman's sexual self-schema and libido [52], especially among younger patients [53]. Swelling caused by lymphoedema may also contribute to changes in body image and often necessitates changes to the patient's usual clothing choices [4].

Social Factors

Role Changes and Social Isolation

Impaired social functioning is associated with increased distress and decreased quality of life. Survivors with more social contacts and social support have been found to be less negatively affected by their cancer, reporting fewer symptoms of anxiety and depression, better role functioning, more energy and better health than those who are more socially isolated [40].

Patients often experience significant interference to their social activities and family life. Many of the physical sequelae of treatment can impact daily activities, ability to work and body image. For example, urinary incontinence [10], lymphoedema [54] or cognitive impairment [5] can create feelings of embarrassment or decreased self-confidence and are associated with social withdrawal. Fertility issues, sexual dysfunction and menopausal symptoms stemming from cancer treatment leave some patients feeling like 'damaged goods', which may also contribute to social isolation [31]. Reducing or stopping work may result in disconnection from social contacts as well. Although cancer survivors in general are at an elevated risk of unemployment compared to healthy individuals, gynaecologic (and breast) cancer survivors are even more likely to choose to stop working or reduce their work hours than other cancer survivors [53]. Younger survivors in particular appear to report greater interference in their social and family lives; however, they report better role functioning than older survivors, as measured by limitations on work, daily activities and pursuing hobbies [53].

Changes in Sexual Relationships

Partners of women with gynaecological cancer are also affected by loss of sexuality and intimacy. Resentment, withdrawal and relationship conflict can develop due to partner's mixed responses, including worrying about the patient's health, and desiring sexual activity but feeling guilty [30]. Conversely, some research has suggested that patients' feelings of intimacy during sexual activity may actually increase following their diagnosis [28].

Health Disparities

Additional social factors such as income and racial disparities can impact cancer outcomes. As already mentioned, gynaecological cancer rates and mortality are higher in less-developed regions of the world [2]. In the United States, low-income and minority women are less likely to receive adjuvant treatment, less likely to adhere to treatment and more likely to die from gynaecologic cancers [37]. Low-income women with gynaecologic cancer report greater unmet supportive care needs related to physical/daily living and practical concerns, and African-American women report greater unmet sexuality and psychological needs compared to their Caucasian counterparts [55]. Patient navigation [37] and multidisciplinary care, including psychology, physical therapy, and social work [55], to target unmet needs may improve adherence and subsequent outcomes.

Summary

The biopsychosocial and quality-of-life impairment of gynaecological cancer is extensive, from multisystem physical sequelae, to depression and anxiety, to role and relationship changes and social isolation. As summarized, some of these issues can be addressed with multidisciplinary approaches including medical, physical therapy and psychological treatments, whilst others have fewer approaches available. Research has been less devoted to gynaecological cancers compared to other cancers affecting women, and a more concentrated effort at the many and sometimes unique issues gynaecologic cancer survivors face is warranted. Additionally, since many survivors do not have access to or awareness of the full range of resources available, research should also continue to examine health disparities and develop outreach options for underdeveloped regions and underserved populations.

Key Points

- Gynaecological cancers account for 11% of all cancers diagnosed in women.
- The gynaecological cancer patient's physical and emotional symptom burden negatively impacts health-related and overall quality of life.
- Quality-of-life concerns in gynaecological cancer vary by disease site and can include issues related to physical functioning (e.g. urinary and faecal incontinence, dyspareunia, lymphoedema) and psychosocial functioning (e.g. body image concerns, role changes, anxiety, depression, sexual dysfunction).

- Cognitive changes such as memory loss, short-term memory impairment and difficulty concentrating or learning new skills are common following treatment for gynaecological cancer.
- For many cancer patients, anxiety is often focussed around fear of cancer recurrence.
- Although about a quarter of all cancer patients experience depression, few are offered treatment for their depressive symptoms. This is thought to be due to the underestimation of depressive symptoms on the part of providers as well as the expectation among both patients and providers that depression is a normal part of the cancer experience.
- Many women respond to worries about death with avoidance strategies like distraction; others take a more task-oriented approach, making lists and getting legal documentation in order, or an emotion-oriented approach, using positive self-talk and relying on 'inner psychological strength' to cope.
- Psychosocial assessment should be part of the routine care of women with gynaecological cancer. Tools for doing this are available. Multidisciplinary approaches including medical, physical therapy and psychological treatments are associated with improved quality of life.

References

[1] Centers for Disease Control and Prevention. Inside Knowledge: Get the Facts About Gynecologic Cancer. 2015; Available at: www.cdc.gov/cancer/gynecologic/. Accessed 23 March 2017.

[2] Ferlay J, Soerjomataram I, Ervik M, Dikshit R, Eser S, Mathers C, et al. GLOBOCAN 2012 v1.1, Cancer Incidence and Mortality Worldwide: IARC CancerBase No. 11 [Internet]. Lyon, France: International Agency for Research on Cancer; 2014. Available at: http://globocan.iarc.fr. Accessed 23 March 2017.

[3] American Cancer Society. Learn About Cancer. 2015; Available at: www.cancer.org/cancer/index. Accessed 23 March 2017.

[4] Carter J, Stabile C, Gunn A, Sonoda Y. The physical consequences of gynecologic cancer surgery and their impact on sexual, emotional, and quality of life issues. J Sex Med 2013;10(S1):21–34.

[5] Andrews S, von Gruenigen VE. Management of the late effects of treatments for gynecological cancer. Curr Opin Oncol 2013 September;25(5):566–570.

[6] Casey C, Chen L, Rabow MW. Symptom management in gynecologic malignancies. Expert Rev Anticanc 2011;11(7):1079–1091.

[7] Mirabeau-Beale KL, Viswanathan AN. Quality of life (QOL) in women treated for gynecologic malignancies with radiation therapy: A literature review of patient-reported outcomes. Gynecol Oncol 2014;134(2):403–409.

[8] Vaz AF, Conde DM, Costa-Paiva L, Morais SS, Esteves SB, Pinto-Neto AM. Quality of life and adverse events after radiotherapy in gynecologic cancer survivors: A cohort study. Arch Gynecol Obstet 2011;284(6):1523–1531.

[9] Perwitasari DA, Atthobari J, Mustofa M, Dwiprahasto I, Hakimi M, Gelderblom H, et al. Impact of chemotherapy-induced nausea and vomiting on quality of life in Indonesian patients with gynecologic cancer. Int J Gynecol Cancer 2012 January;22(1):139–145.

[10] Skjeldestad FE, Rannestad T. Urinary incontinence and quality of life in long-term gynecological cancer survivors: A population-based cross-sectional study. Acta Obstet Gynecol Scand 2009;88(2):192–199.

[11] Salani R. Survivorship planning in gynecologic cancer patients. Gynecol Oncol 2013;130(2):389–397.

[12] Grover S, Hill-Kayser CE, Vachani C, Hampshire MK, DiLullo GA, Metz JM. Patient reported late effects of gynecological cancer treatment. Gynecol Oncol 2012;124(3):399–403.

[13] Stubblefield MD, Burstein HJ, Burton AW, Custodio CM, Deng GE, Ho M, et al. NCCN task force report: Management of neuropathy in cancer. Journal of the National Comprehensive Cancer Network 2009;7(Suppl 5):S1–S26.

[14] Craig CD, Monk BJ, Farley JH, Chase DM. Cognitive impairment in gynecologic cancers: A systematic review of current approaches to diagnosis and treatment. Support Care Cancer 2014;22(1):279–287.

[15] Kaiser J, Bledowski C, Dietrich J. Neural correlates of chemotherapy-related cognitive impairment. Cortex 2014;54:33–50.

[16] Hess LM, Chambers SK, Hatch K, Hallum A, Janicek MF, Buscema J, et al. Pilot study of the prospective identification of changes in cognitive function during chemotherapy treatment for advanced ovarian cancer. J Support Oncol 2010;8(6):252–258.

[17] Cimprich B, Hayes D, Askren M, Jung M, Berman M, Ossher L, et al. Neurocognitive impact in adjuvant

chemotherapy for breast cancer linked to fatigue: A prospective functional MRI study. *Cancer Res* 2012;**72**(24 Supplement):S6–3.

[18] Johnson RL, Block I, Gold MA, Markwell S, Zupancic M. Effect of methylphenidate on fatigue in women with recurrent gynecologic cancer. *Psycho-Oncol* 2010;**19**(9):955–958.

[19] Sandadi S, Frasure HE, Broderick MJ, Waggoner SE, Miller JA, von Gruenigen VE. The effect of sleep disturbance on quality of life in women with ovarian cancer. *Gynecol Oncol* 2011;**123**(2):351–355.

[20] Clevenger L, Schrepf A, DeGeest K, Bender D, Goodheart M, Ahmed A, et al. Sleep disturbance, distress, and quality of life in ovarian cancer patients during the first year after diagnosis. *Cancer* 2013;**119**(17):3234–3241.

[21] Rutledge TL, Heckman SR, Qualls C, Muller CY, Rogers RG. Pelvic floor disorders and sexual function in gynecologic cancer survivors: A cohort study. *Obstet Gynecol* 2010;**203**(5):514.e1–514.e7.

[22] Donovan KA, Boyington AR, Judson PL, Wyman JF. Bladder and bowel symptoms in cervical and endometrial cancer survivors. *Psycho-Oncol* 2014;**23**(6):672–678.

[23] Thomas SG, Sato HR, Glantz JC, Doyle PJ, Buchsbaum GM. Prevalence of symptomatic pelvic floor disorders among gynecologic oncology patients. *Obstet Gynecol* 2013 November;**122**(5):976–980.

[24] Yang EJ, Lim J, Rah UW, Kim YB. Effect of a pelvic floor muscle training program on gynecologic cancer survivors with pelvic floor dysfunction: A randomized controlled trial. *Gynecol Oncol* 2012;**125**(3):705–711.

[25] Rutledge TL, Rogers R, Lee S, Muller CY. A pilot randomized control trial to evaluate pelvic floor muscle training for urinary incontinence among gynecologic cancer survivors. *Gynecol Oncol* 2014;**132**(1):154–158.

[26] Dizon DS, Suzin D, McIlvenna S. Sexual health as a survivorship issue for female cancer survivors. *Oncologist* 2014;**19**(2):202–210. DOI: 10.1634/theoncologist.2013-0302

[27] Abbott-Anderson K, Kwekkeboom KL. A systematic review of sexual concerns reported by gynecological cancer survivors. *Gynecol Oncol* 2012;**124**(3):477–489.

[28] Baser RE, Li Y, Carter J. Psychometric validation of the Female Sexual Function Index (FSFI) in cancer survivors. *Cancer* 2012;**118**(18):4606–4618.

[29] Michaelson-Cohen R, Beller U. Managing menopausal symptoms after gynecological cancer. *Curr Opin Oncol* 2009;**21**(5):407–411.

[30] Ratner ES, Foran KA, Schwartz PE, Minkin MJ. Sexuality and intimacy after gynecological cancer. *Maturitas* 2010;**66**(1):23–26.

[31] Carter J, Lewin S, Abu-Rustum N, Sonoda Y. Reproductive issues in the gynecologic cancer patient. *Oncology* 2007;**21**(5):598–609.

[32] Noyes N, Knopman JM, Long K, Coletta JM, Abu-Rustum NR. Fertility considerations in the management of gynecologic malignancies. *Gynecol Oncol* 2011;**120**(3):326–333.

[33] Koch L, Bertram H, Eberle A, Holleczek B, Schmid-Höpfner S, Waldmann A, et al. Fear of recurrence in long-term breast cancer survivors – still an issue. Results on prevalence, determinants, and the association with quality of life and depression from the Cancer Survivorship – a multi-regional population-based study. *Psycho-Oncol* 2014;**23**(5):547–554.

[34] Suzuki N, Ninomiya M, Maruta S, Hosonuma S, Nishigaya Y, Kobayashi Y, et al. Psychological characteristics of Japanese gynecologic cancer patients after learning the diagnosis according to the hospital anxiety and depression scale. *J Obstet Gynaecol Res* 2011;**37**(7):800–808.

[35] Costanzo ES, Lutgendorf SK, Rothrock NE, Anderson B. Coping and quality of life among women extensively treated for gynecologic cancer. *Psycho-Oncol* 2006;**15**(2):132–142.

[36] Ell K, Sanchez K, Vourlekis B, Lee PJ, Dwight-Johnson M, Lagomasino I, et al. Depression, correlates of depression, and receipt of depression care among low-income women with breast or gynecologic cancer. *J Clin Oncol* 2005 May 1;**23**(13):3052–3060.

[37] Ell K, Vourlekis B, Xie B, Nedjat-Haiem FR, Lee P, Muderspach L, et al. Cancer treatment adherence among low-income women with breast or gynecologic cancer. *Cancer* 2009;**115**(19):4606–4615.

[38] Hodgkinson K, Butow P, Fuchs A, Hunt GE, Stenlake A, Hobbs KM, et al. Long-term survival from gynecologic cancer: Psychosocial outcomes, supportive care needs and positive outcomes. *Gynecol Oncol* 2007;**104**(2):381–389.

[39] Carter J, Sonoda Y, Baser RE, Raviv L, Chi DS, Barakat RR, et al. A 2-year prospective study assessing the emotional, sexual, and quality of life concerns of women undergoing radical trachelectomy versus radical hysterectomy for treatment of early-stage cervical cancer. *Gynecol Oncol* 2010;**119**(2):358–365.

[40] Carpenter KM, Fowler JM, Maxwell GL, Andersen BL. Direct and buffering effects of social support among gynecologic cancer survivors. *Ann Behav Med* 2010;**39**(1):79–90.

[41] Steele R, Fitch MI. Supportive care needs of women with gynecologic cancer. *Cancer Nurs* 2008;**31**(4):284–291.

[42] Thewes B, Bell M, Butow P, Beith J, Boyle F, Friedlander M, et al. Psychological morbidity and stress but not social factors influence level of fear of cancer recurrence in young women with early breast cancer: Results of a cross-sectional study. *Psycho-Oncol* 2013;**22**(12):2797–2806.

[43] Savard J, Ivers H. The evolution of fear of cancer recurrence during the cancer care trajectory and its relationship with cancer characteristics. *J Psychosom Res* 2013;**74**(4):354–360.

[44] Armstrong D. Treatment of Recurrent Disease Q & A. 2002; Available at: http://ovariancancer.jhmi.edu/recurrentqa.cfm. Accessed 23 March 2017.

[45] Lebel S, Maheu C, Lefebvre M, Secord S, Courbasson C, Singh M, et al. Addressing fear of cancer recurrence among women with cancer: A feasibility and preliminary outcome study. *J Cancer Surviv* 2014;**8**(3):485–496.

[46] Urbaniec OA, Collins K, Denson LA, Whitford HS. Gynecological cancer survivors: Assessment of psychological distress and unmet supportive care needs. *J Psychosoc Oncol* 2011;**29**(5):534–551.

[47] Kim H. *Understanding Death Anxiety in Women with Gynecologic Cancer.* 2009.

[48] Sigal JJ, Ouimet MC, Margolese R, Panarello L, Stibernik V, Bescec S. How patients with less-advanced and more-advanced cancer deal with three death-related fears: An exploratory study. *J Psychosoc Oncol* 2007;**26**(1):53–68.

[49] Lopez-Acevedo M, Lowery WJ, Lowery AW, Lee PS, Havrilesky LJ. Palliative and hospice care in gynecologic cancer: A review. *Gynecol Oncol* 2013;**131**(1):215–221.

[50] Havrilesky LJ. Palliative services enhance the quality and value of gynecologic cancer care. *Gynecol Oncol* 2014;**1**(132):1–2.

[51] Simonelli LE, Fowler J, Maxwell GL, Andersen BL. Physical sequelae and depressive symptoms in gynecologic cancer survivors: Meaning in life as a mediator. *Ann Behav Med* 2008;**35**(3):275–284.

[52] Andersen BL, Woods XA, Copeland LJ. Sexual self-schema and sexual morbidity among gynecologic cancer survivors. *J Consult Clin Psychol* 1997;**65**(2):221–229.

[53] Bifulco G, De Rosa N, Tornesello M, Piccoli R, Bertrando A, Lavitola G, et al. Quality of life, lifestyle behavior and employment experience: A comparison between young and midlife survivors of gynecology early stage cancers. *Gynecol Oncol* 2012;**124**(3):444–451.

[54] Carter J, Penson R, Barakat R, Wenzel L. Contemporary quality of life issues affecting gynecologic cancer survivors. *Hematol Oncol Clin North Am* 2012;**26**(1):169–194.

[55] Simonelli LE, Pasipanodya E. Health Disparities in Unmet Support Needs of Women with Gynecologic Cancer: An Exploratory Study. *J Psychosoc Oncol* 2014;**32**(6):727–734.

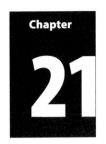

Chapter

21

Assessment and Management of Women with Nausea and Vomiting during Pregnancy
A Biopsychosocial Approach

David McCormack and Leroy C. Edozien

Introduction

Nausea and vomiting are very common symptoms experienced during pregnancy, with approximately 80% of pregnant women experiencing some vomiting and/or nausea and 52% having both nausea and vomiting [1]. A smaller number of pregnant women, approximately 0.3 to 1.5%, will experience hyperemesis gravidarum (HG), which is a severe and intractable form of nausea and vomiting during pregnancy (NVP), typically starting between the fourth and sixth weeks of gestation and resolving before the end of the 22nd week, with around 13% reporting it as lasting beyond 20 weeks' gestation [1–3]. NVP is associated with negative physical, social and psychological effects [4–6]. Severe and persistent vomiting, particularly if left untreated, can lead to maternal weight loss, dehydration and electrolyte imbalance; if electrolyte disturbance occurs, there is some evidence that this presents an elevated risk of lower birth weight and fetal anomalies [7–9].

Aetiology of Nausea and Vomiting during Pregnancy

At present the precise aetiology of NVP is unknown, and the exact relationship between mild-moderate symptoms (i.e. typical NVP) and the more uncommon severe and persistent presentation of symptoms (i.e. HG) is unclear. There have been many aetiological theories proposed including genetic, biochemical, immunological and conceptualizing it as being fetoprotective or a by-product of maternal-embryo conflict [10–12]. In addition, psychological theories have been advanced [13].

Psychological theories range from viewing NVP as a form of conversion/somatization disorder through

to seeing it as a result of behavioural conditioning. The psychological approach conceptualizing NVP as a form of conversion disorder is underpinned by the assumption that the symptoms observed are the physical manifestation of ambivalence of attitude from the mother towards her developing baby (i.e. fetus), and/or overwhelming psychical conflict or dysphoric affect [14]. Despite a number of nuanced theoretical accounts and research carried out in this area, there is little evidence to support the conversion/somatization theory [15, 16].

Another notable psychological theory, the behavioural conditioning formulation, attempts to account for persistent NVP by proposing that stimuli which would not normally trigger NVP, such as, food, places, people and normal physiologic symptoms (i.e. unconditioned stimuli), become 'conditioned stimuli' after repeated episodes of typical NVP. That is, food, places, people etc. through repeated pairings/association with NVP become by themselves capable of inducing nausea and vomiting (i.e. the unconditioned stimuli become conditioned stimuli). As a consequence, nausea and vomiting becomes more frequent and persistent [17]. The explanation as to why all women with NVP do not develop more severe and persistent symptoms rests on the assumption that some women are more susceptible to conditioning than others (e.g. individual differences in autonomic nervous system functioning, particularly having a more reactive sympathetic nervous system). There is some limited evidence to support this assumption, for example an interesting small non-prospective study found that pregnant women with HG were more hypnotizable (i.e. more prone to conditioning) than pregnant women without HG [18]. Preliminary data showing that hypnosis may be effective at reducing NVP for some women appears to lend further support to the role of conditioning; however, fully powered and methodologically rigorous research studies are needed to confirm this [19]. Overall, while the behavioural conditioning theory may help explain why some pregnant women with mild nausea and vomiting of pregnancy go on to develop more severe symptoms, it does not provide a persuasively robust aetiological account for why the symptoms occur in the first place.

The majority of the research supporting a psychogenic origin of NVP and HG suffers from methodological problems. Typically, published studies in this area seldom include control comparison groups, are not prospective, and most of the studies are cross-sectional in design. As a consequence, based on present data, the direction of effect is difficult to establish. That is, are psychological effects the cause of nausea and vomiting or the result? There is growing evidence that psychological effects are secondary to NVP and HG [20].

Currently there appears to be insufficient evidence for a psychogenic origin. However, it does appear as though NVP can negatively impact on the psychological and emotional well-being of pregnant women, and it seems theoretically plausible that psychological distress and behavioural conditioning could play a role in exacerbating symptoms for some women [21].

At present pursuing a biological line of enquiry and studying the role of hormones such as oestrogen, progesterone and particularly human chorionic gonadotropin (hCG) may prove fruitful in better understanding the aetiology of NVP and HG. While hCG seems very likely to play an important role in the aetiology of NVP and HG, there is insufficient evidence that it is causal. For example, some women who do not experience NVP have been found to have elevated levels of hCG [22]. This has led some to speculate that this may be attributable to biological activity of different isoforms of hCG in addition to individual differences among women regarding their sensitivity to emetogenic stimuli [23]. It has also been theorized that hCG may play a role in increasing the production of prostaglandin E2 and this then is a key factor in what causes NVP [24].

It seems likely that what causes and maintains NVP may turn out to be multifactorial and that there may be slightly different variables at play depending on the individual woman and her present circumstances. That is, similar to other medical conditions (e.g. chronic pelvic pain [25], see Chapter 16), psychological, environmental and social factors may unhelpfully interact with

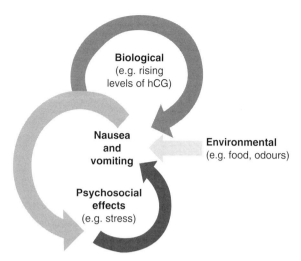

Figure 21.1 A biopsychosocial model of nausea and vomiting of pregnancy

physiological processes, which may then exacerbate symptoms and negatively affect functioning and quality of life. Taking this more complex multifactorial view of what causes and maintains NVP has led some researchers to propose that a biopsychosocial approach be adopted [26]. Informed by this approach a simple hypothetical model is presented in Figure 21.1.

Within this model the hypothesized driver for the symptoms is biological (e.g. rising levels of hCG), which increases the risk of NVP. Triggers for NVP episodes may be internal (e.g. physiological) or external (e.g. environmental – such as food odours) and/or a complex interplay of both internal and external factors. Within this model resultant NVP then effectively becomes a psychological and social stressor, contributing to psychological distress and negative social effects. The negative social effects may include challenges in performing occupational duties, and placing a strain on relationships leading to insufficient social support being available [6]. It seems plausible that social effects and psychological distress could then negatively interact with one another (e.g. strained relationships may increase anxiety and in turn anxiety contributes to making relationships with others more strained), and these psychosocial effects, particularly stress and anxiety, may then further increase the risk of nausea and vomiting and/or exacerbate symptoms [27].

Taking a biopsychosocial approach may prove a useful paradigm to use both in the search for what causes and maintains NVP and as a framework for its assessment and management.

Assessment

In line with the biopsychosocial approach we will firstly outline how to carry out a biopsychosocial assessment of NVP and HG. We will start out with the medical assessment before moving on to look at how to assess the psychological and social aspects.

Medical

The first step is to take a careful history which includes assessing the onset of symptoms, the typical duration and severity of nausea and vomiting, and asking the patient about any associated symptoms (e.g. weight loss, abdominal pain) and/or other conditions that they may have (e.g. diabetes). Examination and investigation should then be guided by history and include taking the patient's temperature, pulse, blood pressure and testing the urine for ketones, and looking for signs of dehydration.

It is crucial before diagnosing NVP that other causes for the symptoms are excluded; this is particularly relevant when symptoms commence after week ten of gestation and when attendant symptoms other than fatigue are present [23]. Making a diagnosis of NVP involves a process of exclusion. As NVP might not be directly related to the pregnancy itself, it is routine practice to exclude other causes, including gastroenteritis, metabolic disorders, thyroid and other endocrine conditions, appendicitis, nephrolithiasis etc. [28–32].

Once NVP is confirmed it is important to then establish if the symptoms suggest typical NVP (i.e. mild-moderate symptoms) or HG (i.e. severe and persistent symptoms) with or without metabolic imbalance. The use of a standardized measure is recommended; for instance, the Pregnancy-Unique Quantification of Emesis (PUQE) is a brief validated measure which enables symptoms to be classed as mild, moderate or severe [33]. ICD-10 defines HG as severe and persistent NVP starting before the end of the 22nd week of gestation [3] (ICD-10, code 021.1). It is associated with dehydration, ketonuria and weight loss [32].

Psychological

There is evidence that NVP / HG negatively impact on functioning and is associated with psychological and emotional difficulties [5,20]. As a result one should sensitively enquire as to how the patient is coping, how they feel generally and when they experience symptoms, if their daily activities are affected by their symptoms and/or how they are feeling emotionally. This should help gain some understanding of their social functioning and emotional well-being.

The Whooley questions, while primarily intended to screen for depression, can be helpful to facilitate discussion of emotional issues generally [34]. They consist of the following:

(1) During the past month have you been bothered by feeling down, depressed or hopeless?

(2) During the past month, have you been bothered by having little interest or pleasure in doing things?

As the Whooley questions do not assess other common psychological and emotional difficulties associated with NVP and HG (e.g. anxiety problems), it is important to enquire about such symptoms.

National Institute for Health and Care Excellence (NICE) guidance for antenatal and postnatal mental health recommends when assessing depression and anxiety to also consider using the 2-item Generalized Anxiety Disorder scale (GAD-2) [35]:

(1) Over the last two weeks, how often have you been bothered by feeling nervous, anxious or on edge?

Not at all (score = 0) Several days (score = 1) More than half the days (score = 2) Nearly every day (score = 3)

(2) Over the last two weeks, how often have you been bothered by not being able to stop or control worrying.

Not at all (score = 0) Several days (score = 1) More than half the days (score = 2) Nearly every day (score = 3)

If the patient answers yes to either of the Whooley questions and/or scores 3 or more on the 2-item anxiety scale (GAD-2) [36], it would likely be helpful to assess her past and current mental health in more detail. Administering standardized measures, such as the EPDS [37] or PHQ-9 [38] to screen for depression and/or GAD-7 [39] to further screen for anxiety, may also prove useful.

If psychological and emotional difficulties are identified, it is worth asking the patient, 'is this something you feel you need help with?' (the 'Arrol' question). After discussing this with the patient you may consider that a referral to a clinical psychologist or psychiatrist is warranted.

It is very important when working with a patient with NVP, and particularly when discussing issues around mental health, that it is done sensitively, and that one makes an active attempt to carefully listen and empathize with the patient. If a patient is treated unsympathetically it risks worsening her psychological and emotional well-being [40]. If she is found to be experiencing mental health difficulties, where possible try to help normalize what she is experiencing and reassure her (e.g. let her know that such problems are common) and try to instil hope that something can be done to help ameliorate and manage her difficulties.

Social

Assessing whether the patient has adequate social support and is aware of sources of help is an important part of the assessment process. Women with NVP and HG, just like everyone, are members of dynamic social systems (e.g. families, workplaces, medical teams) and are influenced by these cognitively, emotionally and behaviourally – that is, the individuals affect the systems they are in and these systems affect the individuals. The impact on the individual can be positive (e.g. she feels supported) or negative (e.g. the person experiences low mood because of how she is treated by others). One needs to be mindful when working with a patient with NVP/HG to consider her social context, the systems she inhabits. NVP and particularly HG can negatively impact on the woman's well-being, functioning and her social support system [26]. How well a woman is supported may in turn affect her general well-being, how well she copes and manages with nausea and vomiting and adapts to pregnancy [27].

A number of questionnaires have been developed to assess social functioning and/or the social support needs of pregnant women; for example, the Social Functioning Questionnaire [41] assesses social functioning in a number of situations (e.g. functioning at work and home, financially and in relationships). The Short Form Social Support Questionnaire assesses perceived social support [42], and a brief Maternity Social Support Scale has also been developed [43]. These measures have their advantages; for example, they can give a quick snapshot of social functioning and/or social support needs, and they are often quicker to administer and score than conducting a verbal assessment.

However, there are a number of shortcomings; for instance, they lack specificity and may miss out on details that can emerge during a conversation between the doctor and patient – with these details, tailored follow-up questions can then be asked to highlight specific unmet needs which can be addressed.

Asking patients questions about their social support and functioning should help gain an insight into their present circumstances and enable an assessment of whether they require input regarding this (e.g. having additional social support put in place). Aspects of social support and functioning that may be helpful to ask about include (1) do they feel that they are getting the support that they need from others (e.g. partner/family); (2) is there anyone in particular that they can rely on when they need practical help; (3) is there anyone who provides them with emotional support; (4) are they having any difficulties at home (e.g. with partner, children, finances); (5) if they are working, are they having any problems at work and do they feel well supported by colleagues and/or management; and (6) how satisfied are they with the support that they are receiving from others. It is important to be mindful that some women might find talking about such issues to be irrelevant to their symptoms and/or distressing to talk about. Providing the woman with a brief rationale as to why you are asking such questions, being warm and empathic, and tailoring the questions to make them relevant to her situation may diffuse such problems and lead to a meaningful and useful conversation.

Formulation of the Assessment

After carrying out a biopsychosocial assessment the doctor should be in a position to formulate what the main difficulties are and to have ascertained what is likely contributing to the nausea and vomiting and/or making it particularly challenging to cope with (e.g. if secondary psychological distress is present and/or there is insufficient social support). Sharing this formulation with patients increases the likelihood that they will feel heard and understood and it also provides an opportunity to see what their views are. Any differences of opinion can then be discussed and ideally, a shared understanding of what has caused and is maintaining/contributing to the symptoms can be reached. This is an important step before moving on to agreeing to a management

---

BOX 21.1 Regime of Antiemetic Therapies Recommended by the Royal College of Obstetricians and Gynaecologists [48]

First Line
Cyclizine 50 mg PO, IM or IV 8 hourly
Prochlorperazine 5–10 mg 6–8 hourly PO; 12.5 mg 8 hourly IM/IV; 25 mg PR daily
Promethazine 12.5–25 mg 4–8 hourly PO, IM, IV or PR
Chlorpromazine 10–25 mg 4–6 hourly PO, IV or IM; or 50–100 mg 6–8 hourly PR

Second Line
Metoclopramide 5–10 mg 8 hourly PO, IV or IM (maximum 5 days' duration)
Domperidone 10 mg 8 hourly PO; 30–60 mg 8 hourly PR
Ondansetron 4–8 mg 6–8 hourly PO; 8 mg over 15 minutes 12 hourly IV

Third Line
Corticosteroids: hydrocortisone 100 mg twice daily IV and once clinical improvement occurs, convert to prednisolone 40–50 mg daily PO, with the dose gradually tapered until the lowest maintenance dose that controls the symptoms is reached.
   IM intramuscular; IV intravenous; PO by mouth; PR by rectum.

---

plan because if the woman and her doctor have a shared understanding of the illness it should hopefully improve her satisfaction with the care provided [44]. This then will facilitate development of a comprehensive mutually-agreed management plan that should address the woman's symptoms and any secondary difficulties.

Management

The management of NVP and HG should be guided and informed by the assessment. In line with the biopsychosocial approach we will describe both the medical treatment of NVP/HG, and how to manage psychosocial aspects.

Medical Management

NVP – Mild to Moderate Symptoms

Most women with mild to moderate NVP should be able to be cared for in the community by primary care teams. Pharmacological treatments include antiemetics, such as promethazine or cyclizine, as there is some evidence that these are both safe and effective [45–47]. Cyclizine is both an anticholinergic drug and an antihistamine (H1 receptor blocker). The phenothiazines (promethazine, prochlorperazine) are dopamine receptor antagonists. Promethazine is also an antihistamine. Metoclopramide is a dopamine receptor antagonist but also has a direct action on the gastrointestinal tract. Drug-induced extrapyramidal symptoms and oculogyric crises can occur with the use of phenothiazines and metoclopramide. If this occurs, there should be prompt cessation of the medications. To minimize this risk, high-dose treatment should be avoided. Metoclopramide should not be prescribed for more than five days. Combinations of different drugs should be used in women who do not respond to a single antiemetic. A recommended regime of antiemetic therapy is reproduced in Box 21.1.

Regarding non-pharmacological treatments, there is also some equivocal evidence that ginger and acupuncture/acupressure may be beneficial [45]. Some women may also find that dietary and lifestyle modifications and avoidance of triggers may help (see Box 21.2). Some general advice in this regard may include that the woman tries eating bland food little and often until she can tolerate a normal well-balanced diet, that she remembers to stay hydrated, take rest when it is necessary, and if required temporarily avoid triggers, such as foods and odours.

For women with persistent or severe HG who are unable to tolerate oral medication, the parenteral or rectal route may be necessary. Inpatient care should be considered when primary/outpatient care has failed, when symptoms are severe and persistent and/or ketonuria and weight loss greater than 5% of body weight occurs and/or when severe abdominal pain is present.

BOX 21.2 Triggers of NVP/HG

Environmental

Stuffy room; humidity

Perfume, food, smoke and other odours

Noise and other abrasive auditory stimuli

Flickering lights and similar visual challenges

Excessively stressful situations

Mealtime Habits and Diet

Spicy, high-fat and acidic foods

Lying down soon after eating and lying on the left side (both of which delay gastric emptying)

Foods with a strong odour

HG – Severe and Persistent Symptoms

Those with severe and persistent symptoms will require more care and monitoring. Nonetheless where possible even a woman with HG should be provided with care in the community particularly when suitable outpatient services are available, as this will avoid the inconvenience of hospital admission. Treatment should include vitamin supplements (thiamine, folic acid) and antiemetics as well as careful assessment and close monitoring. When dehydration, significant weight loss or electrolyte imbalance is detected, hospital admission is required.

If inpatient care is required treatment should commence by promptly addressing any signs of dehydration and electrolyte imbalance. Treatment should start with intravenous fluid (normal saline or Hartmann's solution) and electrolyte replacement [49] and include first-line antiemetics and ondansetron (a serotonin antagonist). The overall risk of birth defects associated with ondansetron exposure appears to be low, but there may be a small increase in the incidence of cardiac abnormalities, so ondansetron should be used as a second-line treatment [50]. Corticosteroids should be considered only if symptoms do not respond to standard treatment, and should be avoided in the first trimester [51].

Some women with HG will develop a transient hyperthyroidism, due to the thyroid-stimulating activity of hCG. This is a self-limiting condition, and treatment should not be offered unless there is other evidence (goitre or thyroid autoantibodies) of thyroid disease.

The patient should be carefully monitored and, when suitable for discharge, they should be provided with symptom management advice (e.g. continue with medications and basic advice regarding diet and lifestyle modifications). Before the woman is discharged if any additional specialist support is required she should be appropriately referred/signposted to services (e.g. if a social work or a clinical psychology/psychiatry referral is required).

Psychosocial Management

Whether NVP symptoms are mild to moderate or severe and persistent, as in the case with HG, one should be mindful of the impact that symptoms can have on a woman's well-being and quality of life. After carrying out the psychosocial assessment and sharing a formulation of the assessment (*see the assessment section earlier in this chapter*), it should be clear to what extent nausea and vomiting are impacting on psychological and social functioning and the role that these may be playing in contributing to symptoms.

If the patient is found to have any psychological and emotional difficulties and/or insufficient social support (e.g. the relationship with her partner is strained as a result of the symptoms), then this should guide where psychosocial interventions are targeted. For example, if anxiety problems seem to be contributing to the symptoms or making them more challenging to manage and cope with, then these should be addressed by providing evidence-based interventions, such as, cognitive behavioural therapy for anxiety secondary to medical problems [52]. If insufficient social support and/or relationship difficulties are present, some counselling could be provided to both the woman and her partner and/or additional social supports identified. It may prove useful to consult with one of the hospital clinical psychologists or social workers when psychosocial problems are present.

Regarding psychological treatments to treat NVP and HG symptoms directly, a number of approaches have been developed, including behavioural therapy and hypnosis [13, 19, 26]. However, these treatments have not yet been subjected to sufficient rigorous scientific study (e.g. randomized control trials). Given this lack of data it is not possible to recommend any specific psychosocial treatment that directly treats the symptoms of NVP and HG. The use of psychological therapy for directly treating nausea and vomiting of pregnancy should be regarded as being an experimental treatment until well-conducted studies (e.g. randomized control trials) find support for the efficacy of such therapies. While there is insufficient evidence for the routine use of psychological interventions at present to directly treat NVP or HG, there are scenarios where psychological therapy may be indicated, for example to treat secondary anxiety and depression. Effective evidence-based interventions to treat these difficulties should be used (e.g. interpersonal therapy, cognitive behavioural therapy). As there is evidence that negative psychosocial effects may continue even after symptoms have resolved and into the postnatal period, close monitoring is advised, as is ensuring an adequate psychological and social support plan is in place.

Summary

Nausea and vomiting are common symptoms experienced during pregnancy with approximately 52% having both nausea and vomiting [1]. A smaller number of pregnant women, approximately 0.3 to 1.5%, will experience hyperemesis gravidarum, which is a severe and persistent form of NVP [1, 2]. NVP is associated with negative physical, social and psychological effects [5,6,20]. It seems likely that what causes and maintains the symptoms is multifactorial and taking a biopsychosocial approach is recommended [22, 26]. Within the hypothetical model presented in this chapter the main aetiological factor is assumed to be biological (e.g. rising levels of hCG), and psychological and social effects are seen as secondary to the nausea and vomiting. These negative psychosocial effects may potentially play a role in maintaining and exacerbating nausea and vomiting for some women. The biopsychosocial approach is a useful framework to apply in both the assessment and management of NVP. After carrying out a biopsychosocial assessment it is recommended that a formulation of the assessment (i.e. a synthesis of the

information gathered during the assessment) is shared with the woman. Management should be guided and informed by assessment and adhere to clinical guidelines [22, 45, 48]. Interventions should be matched to the severity of symptoms. When possible care should be provided at a primary care or outpatient level, with hospital admission reserved for severe cases. A parsimonious approach to psychosocial input should be applied; interventions should be evidence-based and targeted to address specific problems. As negative effects may continue even after symptoms have resolved, it is recommended that an adequate psychosocial care plan should be in place for the postnatal period.

Key Points

- The aetiology of nausea and vomiting during pregnancy (NVP) is uncertain. The majority of the research supporting a psychogenic origin of NVP suffers from methodological problems.
- The cause of NVP is probably multifactorial, and there may be slightly different variables at play depending on the individual woman and her biological, psychological and social circumstances.
- NVP can negatively impact on the psychological and emotional well-being of pregnant women, and it seems theoretically plausible that psychological distress and behavioural conditioning could play a role in exacerbating symptoms for some women.
- Making a diagnosis of NVP involves a process of exclusion.
- The Pregnancy-Unique Quantification of Emesis (PUQE) is a brief validated measure which enables symptoms to be classed as mild, moderate or severe.
- The Social Functioning Questionnaire can be used to assess functioning at work and home, financially and in relationships. The Short Form Social Support Questionnaire and the Maternity Social Support Scale assess perceived social support. These measures have their advantages but they lack specificity and may miss out on details that can emerge during a conversation between the doctor and patient.
- If the woman and her doctor have a shared understanding of the illness, it should hopefully improve her satisfaction with the care provided.

- Where possible women with NVP/HG should be provided with care in the community or managed as outpatients.
- Medical treatment comprises antiemetic drugs, acid-reducing drugs, rehydration and electrolyte replacement. Antiemetic drugs include antihistamines (cyclizine), dopamine antagonists (e.g. prochlorperazine, metoclopramide) and serotonin antagonist (ondansetron).
- Psychotherapy, behavioural therapy and hypnosis could be beneficial, but these treatments have not yet been subjected to sufficient rigorous scientific study.
- While there is insufficient evidence for the routine use of psychological interventions at present to directly treat NVP or HG, there are scenarios where psychological therapy may be indicated, for example to treat secondary anxiety and depression.

References

1. Gadsby R, Barnie-Adshead AM, Jagger C. A prospective study of nausea and vomiting during pregnancy. *Br J Gen Pract. Royal College of General Practitioners*; 1993;**43**(371):245–8.

2. Verberg MFG, Gillott DJ, Al-Fardan N, Grudzinskas JG. Hyperemesis gravidarum, a literature review. *Hum Reprod Update*. 2005;**11**(5):527–39.

3. World Health Organization (WHO). *International Statistical Classification of Diseases and Related Health Problems*, ICD-10 XV;021. Geneva: WHO 2016.

4. O'Brien B, Naber S. Nausea and Vomiting During Pregnancy: Effects on the Quality of Women's Lives. *Birth* 1992;**19**(3):138–43.

5. McCormack D, Scott-Heyes G, McCusker CG. The impact of hyperemesis gravidarum on maternal mental health and maternal-fetal attachment. *J Psychosom Obstet Gynecol*. 2011;**32**(2):79–87.

6. Swallow BL, Lindow SW, Masson EA, Hay DM. Psychological health in early pregnancy: Relationship with nausea and vomiting. *J Obstet Gynaecol*. 2004;**24**(1):28–32.

7. Dodds L, Fell DB, Joseph KS, Allen VM, Butler B. Outcomes of pregnancies complicated by hyperemesis gravidarum. *Obstet Gynecol*. 2006; **107** (2 Pt 1): 285–92.

8. Gross S, Librach C, Cecutti A. Maternal weight loss associated with hyperemesis gravidarum: A predictor of fetal outcome. *Am J Obstet Gynecol*. 1989;**160**(4):906–9.

9. Chin RK, Lao TT. Low birth weight and hyperemesis gravidarum. *Eur J Obstet Gynecol Reprod Biol*. 1988;**28**(3):179–83.

10. Forbes S. Pregnancy sickness and parent-offspring conflict over thyroid function. *J Theor Biol*. 2014;**355**: 61–7. doi: 10.1016/j.jtbi.2014.03.041.

11. Weigel MM, Reyes M, Caiza ME, Tello N, Castro NP, Cespedes S, et al. Is the nausea and vomiting of early pregnancy really feto-protective? *J Perinat Med*. 2006;**34**(2):115–22.

12. Lee NM, Saha S. Nausea and vomiting of pregnancy. *Gastroenterol Clin North Am*. 2011;**40**(2):309–34–vii.

13. Buckwalter JG, Simpson SW. Psychological factors in the etiology and treatment of severe nausea and vomiting in pregnancy. *Am J Obstet Gynecol*. 2002;**186**(5 Suppl Understanding):S210–4.

14. Chertok L, Mondzain ML, Bonnaud M. Vomiting and the wish to have a child. *Psychosom Med*. 1963;**25**:13–8.

15. Simpson SW, Goodwin TM, Robins SB, Rizzo AA, Howes RA, Buckwalter DK, et al. Psychological factors and hyperemesis gravidarum. *J Women's Health Gend Based Med*. 2001;**10**(5):471–7.

16. Munch S. Chicken or the egg? The biological-psychological controversy surrounding hyperemesis gravidarum. *Soc Sci Med*. 2002;**55**(7): 1267–78.

17. Matteson S, Roscoe J, Hickok J, Morrow GR. The role of behavioral conditioning in the development of nausea. *Am J Obstet Gynecol*. 2002;**186**(5 Suppl Understanding):S239–43.

18. Apfel RJ, Kelley SF, Frankel FH. The Role of Hypnotizability in the Pathogenesis and Treatment of Nausea and Vomiting of Pregnancy. *J Psychosom Obstet Gynaecol*. 2009;**5**(3):179–86.

19. McCormack D. Hypnosis for hyperemesis gravidarum. *J Obstet Gynaecol*. 2010;**30**(7):647–53. doi: 103109/014436152010509825.

20. McCarthy FP, Khashan AS, North RA, Moss-Morris R, Baker PN, Dekker G, et al. A Prospective Cohort Study Investigating Associations between Hyperemesis Gravidarum and Cognitive, Behavioural and Emotional Well-Being in Pregnancy. Wang H, editor. *PLOS ONE. Public Library of Science* 2011;**6**(11): e27678.

21. King TL, Murphy PA. Evidence-Based Approaches to Managing Nausea and Vomiting in Early Pregnancy. *Journal of Midwifery & Women's Health* 2009;**54**(6): 430–44.

22. McCarthy FP, Lutomski JE, Greene RA. Hyperemesis gravidarum: Current perspectives. *International Journal of Women's Health*. 2014;**6**:719–25.

23. Jueckstock JK, Kaestner R, Mylonas I. Managing hyperemesis gravidarum: A multimodal challenge. *BMC Medicine* 2010;**8**(1):46.

24. Gadsby R, Barnie-Adshead A, Grammatoppoulos D, Gadsby P. Nausea and vomiting in pregnancy: An association between symptoms and maternal prostaglandin E2. *Gynecol Obstet Invest.* 2000;**50**(3): 149–52.

25. Moore J, Kennedy S. Causes of chronic pelvic pain. *Best Practice & Research Clinical Obstetrics & Gynaecology* 2000;**14**(3):389–402.

26. Swallow BL. Nausea and vomiting in pregnancy. *The Psychologist. (Journal of the British Psychological Society)* 2010;**23**:206–209.

27. Chou FH, Avant KC, Kuo S-H, Fetzer SJ. Relationships between nausea and vomiting, perceived stress, social support, pregnancy planning, and psychosocial adaptation in a sample of mothers: A questionnaire survey. *International Journal of Nursing Studies.* 2008;**45**(8):1185–91.

28. Davis M. Nausea and Vomiting of Pregnancy: An Evidence-based Review. *The Journal of Perinatal & Neonatal Nursing.* 2004;**18**(4):312.

29. Koch KL. Gastrointestinal factors in nausea and vomiting of pregnancy. *Am J Obstet Gynecol.* 2002;**186** (5):S198–203.

30. Arsenault M-Y, Lane CA, MacKinnon CJ, Bartellas E, Cargill YM, Klein MC, et al. The management of nausea and vomiting of pregnancy. *Journal of Obstetrics and Gynecology Canada JOGC.* 2002; **24** (10):817–31–quiz832–3.

31. American College of Obstetrics and Gynecology. ACOG Practice Bulletin No. 153: Nausea and Vomiting of Pregnancy. *Obstetrics and Gynecology.* 2015;.**126**:687–8. doi: 10.1097/01. AOG.0000471177.80067.19.

32. National Collaborating Centre for Women's and Children's Health (UK). *Antenatal Care: Routine Care for the Healthy Pregnant Woman.* London: RCOG Press; 2008 Mar.

33. Koren G, Boskovic R, Hard M, Maltepe C, Navioz Y, Einarson A. Motherisk-PUQE (pregnancy-unique quantification of emesis and nausea) scoring system for nausea and vomiting of pregnancy. *Am J Obstet Gynecol.* 2002;**186**(5 Suppl Understanding): S228–31.

34. Scottish Intercollegiate Guidelines Network (SIGN). Management of perinatal mood disorders. A national clinical guideline. SIGN publication no. 127 Edinburgh (Scotland): SIGN; 2012 Mar.

35. National Collaborating Centre for Mental Health (UK). Antenatal and Postnatal Mental Health: Clinical Management and Service Guidance: Updated edition.

NICE Clinical Guidelines, No. 192. Leicester (UK): British Psychological Society; 2014 Dec.

36. Kroenke K, Spitzer RL, Williams JBW, Monahan PO, Löwe B. Anxiety disorders in primary care: Prevalence, impairment, comorbidity, and detection. *Ann Intern Med.* 2007;**146**(5):317–25.

37. Cox JL, Holden JM, Sagovsky R. Detection of postnatal depression. *Development of the 10-item Edinburgh Postnatal Depression Scale. Br J Psychiatry.* 1987;**150**: 782–6.

38. Kroenke K, Spitzer RL, Williams JB. The PHQ-9: Validity of a brief depression severity measure. *J Gen Intern Med.* 2001;**16**(9):606–13.

39. Spitzer RL, Kroenke K, Williams JBW, Löwe B. A brief measure for assessing generalized anxiety disorder: The GAD-7. *Arch Intern Med.* 2006;**166**(10):1092–7.

40. Poursharif B, Korst LM, Fejzo MS, MacGibbon KW, Romero R, Goodwin TM. The psychosocial burden of hyperemesis gravidarum. *J Perinatol.* 2008;**28**(3): 176–81.

41. Tyrer P, Nur U, Crawford M, Karlsen S, McLean C, Rao B, et al. The Social Functioning Questionnaire: A rapid and robust measure of perceived functioning. *Int J Soc Psychiatry.* 2005;**51**(3):265–75.

42. Sarason IG, Sarason BR, Shearin EN, Pierce GR. A Brief Measure of Social Support: Practical and Theoretical Implications. *Journal of Social and Personal Relationships.* 1987;**4**(4):497–510.

43. Webster J, Linnane JW, Dibley LM, Hinson JK, Starrenburg SE, Roberts JA. Measuring social support in pregnancy: Can it be simple and meaningful? *Birth.* 2000;**27**(2):97–101.

44. Munch S, Schmitz MF. Hyperemesis gravidarum and patient satisfaction: A path model of patients' perceptions of the patient-physician relationship. *J Psychosom Obstet Gynaecol.* 2006;**27**(1):49–57.

45. Matthews A, Haas DM, O'Mathúna DP. Interventions for nausea and vomiting in early pregnancy. *Database Syst Rev.* 2014.

46. Gill SK, Einarson A. The safety of drugs for the treatment of nausea and vomiting of pregnancy. *Expert Opin Drug Saf.* 2007;**6**(6):685–94.

47. Magee LA, Mazzotta P, Koren G. Evidence-based view of safety and effectiveness of pharmacologic therapy for nausea and vomiting of pregnancy (NVP). *Am J Obstet Gynecol.* 2002;**186**(5 Suppl Understanding): S256–61.

48. RCOG. 2016. The Management of Nausea and Vomiting (Green-top 69). Available at: www.rcog.org .uk/globalassets/documents/guidelines/green-top-guidelines/gtg69-hyperemesis.pdf. (Accessed 23 March 2017).

49. Jarvis S, Nelson-Piercy C. Management of nausea and vomiting in pregnancy. *BMJ*. 2011;**342**:d3606–6ss.

50. Carstairs SD. Ondansetron Use in Pregnancy and Birth Defects: A Systematic Review. *Obstetrics & Gynecology* 2016;**127**:878–83. doi: 10.1097/AOG.0000000000001388.

51. Nelson-Piercy C, Fayers P, Swiet M. Randomised, double-blind, placebo-controlled trial of corticosteroids for the treatment of hyperemesis gravidarum. *BJOG: An International Journal of Obstetrics & Gynaecology*. 2001;**108**(1):9–15.

52. Butler AC, Chapman JE, Forman EM, Beck AT. The empirical status of cognitive-behavioral therapy: A review of meta-analyses. *Clin Psychol Rev*. 2006;**26**(1):17–31.

Chapter 22

Psychosexual Disorders

Claudine Domoney and Leila Frodsham

Introduction

Psychosexual disorders demonstrate the clear link between mind and body. Somatization of distress is a common feature of sexual dysfunction in general, even if the primary cause is a physical one. Both men and women will present with sexual problems that are contextualized as a physical entity, although their psychological reaction to them may be unrecognized. The skills of psychosexual medicine seek to understand the combination of physical and psychological and therefore within the therapeutic relationship between healthcare professional (HCP) and patient, to achieve understanding of both conscious and unconscious responses. Presentation may be overt or covert. The experienced professional can reduce the exposure of the patient to unnecessary interventions and encourage more rapid resolution of symptoms. It is common that women presenting with dyspareunia or pelvic pain are subjected to a number of invasive investigations without any further understanding of their symptoms or their causes. Others with vulval pain are sent to clinics for specialist help that may not achieve a return to a normal quality of life until the impact on sexual life is acknowledged and addressed. Sexual problems presenting to the doctor, nurse, midwife or physiotherapist can be examined and treated using eyes and emotions as well as ears and hands.

Prevalence

Sexual difficulties are common in both men and women. A frequently cited paper from the United States reported a sexual dysfunction rate of 43% in women and 31% in men aged 18 to 59, yet this is frequently criticized as medicalizing normal, temporary changes in sexual function. The Diagnostic and Statistical Manual of Mental Disorders (DSM-5) [4] published in 2013 categorizes gender-specific sexual dysfunctions with a duration of at least six months with a frequency of 75–100%. This precise diagnostic definition has not been used for most prevalence studies but does aim to reduce the burden of disease that should ideally encourage greater health service engagement.

Most studies, whether in general or disease-specific populations, report high levels of sexual disorder that impact on well-being, contributing to and/or secondary to other mental health disorders. The questionnaire used in any study is crucial to addressing the appropriateness of many factors. These include recall period, validity in the study population, language used, degree of anonymity and assessment of degree of distress felt by the responder.

The National Attitudes to Sex and Lifestyle surveys of the United Kingdom, initially undertaken at decade intervals from 1990, have shown significant changes in sexual behaviours, with recent additional assessment of older age groups from 45 to 74. Expectations also alter with changing behaviours, and measurement of sexual disappointment or anxiety is an important part of managing the presentation of sexual problems. In the most recent survey published in 2013, one in six men and women reported a health condition that affected their sex life in the last year but only 24% of men had reported this to a HCP and only 18% of women [1]. With increasing age, sexual dysfunction may maintain similar prevalence rates, but this appears to be explained by the decline in activity and distress associated [2].

Key to determining the prevalence of sexual dysfunction is an estimate of distress and persistence. Female sexual dysfunction (FSD) studies reassessed using a sexual distress scale to estimate a more realistic prevalence of clinically relevant sexual difficulties indicate much lower rates of dysfunction. It is clear that asking patients about their sexual life is generally welcomed and increases the diagnostic rate [3]. The opportunity to understand the true complaint of a patient who is unable to voice their fears and anxieties can raise the same feelings in the HCP.

However, in clinical practice, treating the patient who reports distress and offering a therapeutic approach to the holistic management of problems is to be expected in twenty-first-century healthcare.

Psychogenic Aetiology of Psychosexual Disorders

Sex is a mind–body activity – a psychosomatic event. Even in the absence of a partner, disruption can have a major impact on quality of life and sense of self-worth. Perception of difficulties can restrict an individual's ability to engage in relationships, yet sometimes therapeutic interventions can be limited without a partner. Fears and problems encountered in a sexual relationship may be controlled by a defensive retreat into single status.

A normal sexual response involves evoking feelings that are usually suppressed in a vulnerable, intimate situation requiring an ability to let go and cope with loss of control. Demonstrating emotions and allowing the powerful mix of them to cause disorder of the self can be difficult for those uncomfortable with disarray or frightened or overwhelming feelings. The tolerance of these feelings may not be fully conscious. Psychological defences to protect the individual from harm are normal and can lead to sexual difficulties that then become pathological.

Emotional development may be influenced by temperament, but the natural progression of a child learning to be independent involves dealing with pain, fear, guilt, shame, anxiety and conflict. Difficulty with expressing these feelings may readily be acted out in sexual relationships and result in long-standing problems.

Presentation of Common Sexual Problems in Women

Women may present directly with specific complaints of low libido, loss of sensation or satisfaction, inability to orgasm or pain. They may test out the health professional's receptivity with a 'calling card' of another less sensitive complaint or an oblique approach to asking about a sexual problem or 'hand on the door' question (so doctor or patient can escape if the query is not received well).

Arousal and Desire Disorders

Female hypoactive desire dysfunction and female arousal disorder have been combined by DSM-5 [4]

to sexual interest/arousal disorder as they are so often coexistent. For women, desire disorders or loss of/low libido is a common endpoint of other sexual problems, as it is a defensive mechanism to prevent psychological and/or physical pain. It also is a common consequence of partner factor sexual difficulties when a woman may consciously or subconsciously protect her partner from the disappointment and distress the problem causes both of them.

> *I have found my mojo again. I lost myself for a while as sex has always been important to my husband and I. But we sprinkled some fairy dust when we started talking again.*

A perimenopausal woman coming to terms with her bodily changes but unable to discuss with her fearful husband.

> *I have blossomed again – I was a husk but now my ears of corn are plump and ripening. I am sexy again.*

A tall, pale perimenopausal woman single for years before finding both hormone replacement and a respectful partner.

Yet making assumptions about sexuality based on a medical model can disempower the woman who has her own construct of sexual identity.

> *I'm so worried about my increase in libido.*

An unusual complaint in gynaecology clinics but she was seven years post diagnosis and treatment of ovarian cancer. However, explaining her reasoning, she admitted she thought sexual feelings came from her hormones which in turn were produced from ovarian tissue – the logical conclusion for her was a recurrence of disease.

Hypoactive sexual desire disorder (HSDD) as described in DSM-IV [5] is the persistent or recurrent deficiency or absence of sexual desire or sexual fantasies or thoughts, and/or the desire for or receptivity to sexual activity which causes distress. The emphasis on causing distress and focus on sexual thoughts allows the flexibility of definition to include those who are not in a relationship or have lost their relationships secondary to HSDD. Arousal disorder was persistent or recurrent inability to attain or maintain sexual excitement causing personal distress, which may be described as subjective feelings and/or lack of physical changes. Women will complain of loss of desire or lack of sensation. Specific physical problems such as lack of lubrication are easier to treat, but often the primary physical cause may be forgotten over the passage of time. It is important to evaluate any specific somatic causes. Many drugs, including some contraceptives (particularly hormonal), antidepressants, antihypertensives, etc., may have an effect on arousal and libido. Postnatally, breastfeeding and menopause are times of hormonal fluctuation and changes in the pelvic floor that can impact on the physical elements of sexual response. Understanding the impact these conditions may have on the psychosexual functioning of an individual will inform the therapeutic pathway.

Orgasmic Disorders

This is the absence of, or persistent or recurrent difficulty in achieving, orgasm following sufficient stimulation and arousal. It may follow from both desire and arousal disorders or be truly independent. Lifelong or primary anorgasmia may be due to suppression of feelings – sexual or otherwise. The inability to 'let go' or excessive control or composure can be the focus of attention. Secondary anorgasmia occurs in response to physical (endocrine, neurological, dermatological, pharmaceutical) causes, relationship issues or other psychosexual causes. Major life events may be associated with a change in orgasmic potential – sexual abuse, sexual violence and gynaecological operations or conditions. Traditionally primary anorgasmia is considered more difficult to treat due to deep underlying psychological problems that are often difficult to elicit. The perception of orgasm as a definitive physical event can lead to unrealistic expectations in some women. What is imagined may be an altered state that is formed by imagined experiences read about or seen acted out in films rather than a physical reflex chain of reactions accompanied by excitement. How women experience orgasm is more varied and less measurable than in men.

Dyspareunia and Vaginismus

These conditions were formerly separate conditions in DSM-IV, but DSM-5 has combined them to genito-pelvic pain/penetration disorder. Dyspareunia is the medical label for pain during sex described by the patient. This can be pain felt psychologically and/or in the pelvis, rather than pain felt at the level of the pelvis, vagina or vulva, although clearly this is more commonly both. Vaginismus describes the sign elicited on attempting examination, of resistance – as demonstrated by thigh adductor muscle spasm and pelvic floor muscle spasm. This can be accompanied

by comments by the patient of distaste for the examination – 'What a horrible job you have doctor!' They may be disengaged from the process or very tearful, upset, fearful and hypervigilant. Vaginismus may occur not only with sex but also during tampon use and pessary insertion, and the woman often presents to the HCP with inability to have a cervical smear taken. The Internet has encouraged self-diagnosis, and many women are encouraged to believe that buying sex aids or dilators will help them retrain their muscles. Yet this frequently does not deal with the underlying problem that can be physical and psychological or a combination of both.

Non-Coital Pain Disorders

Non-coital pain disorders cause significant distress in younger women particularly, often because of the impact on sexual functioning. These include vulval pain syndromes, chronic bladder pain and pelvic pain. They may be psychogenic in origin or organic disease with poorly understood aetiologies and poor diagnostic criteria. This often results in delayed diagnosis with a consequent protracted impact on functioning. It is imperative that women with any chronic disease, particularly urogenital, are asked about the effect on their sexual life. Often it is a source of embarrassment and shame and will not be revealed unless specifically enquired after. Sexual well-being is a combination of general well-being, quality of life and relationship satisfaction and is frequently a good reflection of overall quality of life.

Non-Consummation

These are an isolated group with a combination of all or none of the above or may include male factors. Presentation may be late or delayed, frequently with time pressure of fertility or end of a relationship at stake. Treatment can be also long and protracted, requiring a multifaceted approach.

Phases of Life

Sexuality develops throughout childhood. Many theories of child development have had models of sexual maturation superimposed during the twentieth century. Commonly the belief that sexual dysfunction is symptomatic of adverse childhood experiences leading to disorders of maturation and personality, with the normal phases of child sexual development disturbed as a reflection of abnormal child–parent relationships, damaging the model for future intimate relationships, has led to referral for long-term psychoanalysis or psychotherapy. Yet this may not be a suitable intervention for many and understanding the sequence of events in the 'here and now' may be just as effective for most.

Puberty and Adolescence

Adolescence is a time of massive hormonal upheaval, physical changes, peer group pressure and evolving self-realization. Education with respect to genital function, menstrual cycles, sexual behaviour, contraception and functional relationships evolves with both underlying family attitudes and exposure to the Internet. Early sexual experiences and relationships can colour all future sexual life, but if there is an element of robust support and self-belief, these can be all part of the normal 'pushing of boundaries' and exploration inherent in a healthy adolescence. Yet the freedoms of these years can also expose the vulnerable young person to damaging behaviours acted out through a sense of sexual freedom. Non-judgemental guidance and easy access to contraceptive services can do much to diminish the long-term effects of this period in life.

The self-harming behaviour of young women can present in many ways. The teenager who has multiple sexual partners with little protection against infection or pregnancy may have a different life story thus far compared to the young person who requests labial reduction or, more extremely, 'closes' herself with self-administered sutures having been sexually active before an arranged marriage. Yet all have roots in self, parental/cultural and peer expectations and their ability to control their own destiny. Power and gender relationships may play a large role in sexual feelings. Although celibacy may be promoted in many cultures as a method of self- and population control, in practice for many this is not part of exploration this phase represents. The cultural setting for these restrictions can have lasting sequelae.

Reproductive Lifetime

Sexual function is inextricably linked with reproductive function despite the ability to control fertility and infection in the modern age. This chapter does not have the scope to cover all areas in any depth, but those commonly encountered in healthcare settings are mentioned for discussion.

Contraception, Sexually Transmitted Infection and Termination of Pregnancy

In many countries, contraceptive provision or gynaecologist review can be the window of opportunity for sexual health intervention. Prevention of both sexually transmitted infections (STIs) and pregnancy are inherent in healthy sexual practices. Access to safe abortion services is not available to all, but it is recognized as key to male and female reproductive and sexual health. Control over the consequences of sexual activity prevents long-term psychological sequelae as well as physical. Our contribution to damage as HCPs can be significant. The poor choices of a long-term hormonal contraception that significantly alters a woman's mood and bleeding can end relationships – often with a woman feeling she can no longer provide what she perceives her partner to need.

The nurse told me my body was all wrong. She couldn't find my cervix. Then after searching around for half an hour she said I had an erosion. I thought I had leprosy of the vagina. That bits were going to start dropping out!

A woman presenting to a gynaecology clinic with persistent vaginal discharge and superficial dyspareunia that had been investigated with numerous negative STI checks.

Thoughtless comments about, for instance, the position or appearance of the cervix can embed powerful fantasies that create significant psychosexual symptomatology. Symptoms associated with sex create disproportionate fear and elaborate explanations for them. Powerful defences are set up to protect the psyche. Loss of libido and sensation and an increase in pain perception are common pathways of sexual disturbance. Understanding these causes may be therapeutic.

My mother persuaded me that having an abortion was the right thing. I was in such a panic, I just wanted to get it over with. Now that I have had a miscarriage, I think of all those dead babies inside me.

A woman presenting with secondary anorgasmia.

The 'womb as a tomb' in both miscarriage and termination of pregnancy is a significant inhibitor and can have a late impact on sexual functioning. The perpetuation of distorted thinking will depend on the ability of the individual and HCP to recognize this.

Infertility

Sexual function in couples with subfertility or infertility is of such significance that most fertility clinics do and should employ counsellors, often persons with experience in psychosexual work. It is not uncommon to encounter couples who are not having penetrative intercourse, either consciously or not. The demands of performing to specific menstrual cycle dates and maintaining celibacy at other times take their toll on many couples. Sex becomes goal orientated and spontaneity disappears. The financial, physical and psychological impact of fertility treatment alters the relationship between the couple and for some raise questions regarding their motivation and wishes at odds with previous desires. Even if there was not a psychosexual problem before, it is easy to envisage how they may develop.

Pregnancy and Pelvic Floor Disorders

Pelvic floor disorders are common amongst all women. One in four adult women will have life-altering incontinence, and 30% of parous women will have up to a grade 2 cystocoele. These may have an impact on sexual functioning. The impact of childbirth, body mass index and daily activities including lifting and engagement in sport all affect acclimatization to bodily changes.

Pregnancy and childbirth herald major changes for a couple, embarking on a different role in society with their first child. Their primary position as partner and lover changes to include mother/parent. For some, pregnancy increases orgasmic potential, theoretically via an increase in oxytocin receptors, but changes may be secondary to other psychological and behavioural effects such as bonding and protection of the child (which may also be negative). Childbirth itself will alter sexual health, but there is no good evidence to suggest that vaginal delivery decreases postnatal sexual health compared with caesarean section [6], despite claims to justify the increasing caesarean section rate. Episiotomy, however, does increase the persistence of superficial dyspareunia. In a large longitudinal study, women who breastfed their babies were significantly less interested in sex than those who bottle-fed their babies, irrespective of tiredness or depression, although this was not maintained long term [7]. It also revealed 7–13% of women expressed a need for help, but 25% had not sought it. Changes and dissatisfaction are common but many factors contribute to this. Mind and body doctoring is fundamental in these circumstances. Debriefing is commonly a feature of perineal clinics for postpartum injuries and, although not evidence based at present, should be incorporated as far as possible into routine postnatal care. Advice regarding sexual function is also reassuring for the pregnant and postnatal, even if they feel it is the 'last thing on their mind'. Great care should be taken when deciding on operative intervention in those with dyspareunia, particularly if they plan to have more children and are oestrogen deficient. Topical oestrogen cream can safely be used in breastfeeding women and can 'reintroduce' the woman to her healing vulva and vagina.

We can't think of it as a nice place anymore. It is red and raw and feels like a bucket.

A new mother tearfully complaining of painful sex after a traumatic instrumental delivery.

Women presenting with pelvic floor dysfunction may describe themselves as too big/too loose or alternatively too small, or complain that sex is painful. After surgical intervention, perceptions may be of a scarred or small vagina, with consequential dissatisfaction. Although the 'vagina with teeth' was used as a metaphor in psychosexual medicine, the advent of meshes has introduced a vagina capable of causing 'hispareunia' (painful intercourse for the man). It was often assumed that restoration of normal anatomy would improve sexual function, but many urogynaecological studies have shown this to be simplistic.

The doctor didn't even have to touch me to see how disgusting I was.

Presenting with a 'loose vagina' according to her partner, this well-presented woman requested a second prolapse operation. Her abusive relationship was then addressed once the examination revealed her feelings about herself.

I can't feel anything anymore. We have made love every day of our 40 year marriage. He is very disappointed.

A patient who had been treated for overactive bladder symptoms successfully and attributed this sexual dysfunction to the treatment, but her husband had retired and requested sex twice daily. She was not able to say this to him in words.

Menopause

Am I not too old for that?
Isn't that to be expected at my age?

There have been many studies exploring sexual activity and dysfunction in perimenopausal and ageing women. Overall there is a reduction in activity with age, but this correlates with partner status – both those without partners and those whose partners have sexual problems. Studies suggest that approximately half of women over 50 will be sexually active if in relationships with a decline over the decades, although there may be some cultural variations in this [8]. Some evidence suggests cessation of activity is more likely to be linked to the male partner [9]. A reduction or cessation is often linked to general health status of either partner rather than age itself [10]. A study of Australian menopausal women aged between 45 and 55 years showed increased rates of FSD from 42 to 88% from the early to late menopause [11], but addition of a sexual distress measurement scale reduced this significantly to approximately one-third [12]. Other work from this group seems to indicate that sexual responsivity is related to ageing, but libido, frequency of intercourse and dyspareunia are associated with oestrogen deficiency.

Simple measures such as topical oestrogen, non-hormonal vaginal remoisturizers and lubricants can improve the physical sequelae of hormone deficiency and tissue ageing. Consideration of treatment (surgical and/or conservative) for those with symptomatic pelvic floor dysfunction or correction of other bothersome problems may improve sexual functioning. These therapies are complemented by a psychosexual approach.

Gynaecological Cancers

As medical interventions improve the treatment successes from cancer, the study of survivorship becomes more important. Aside from the physical effects of surgery, chemotherapy and radiation therapy, the impact of a cancer diagnosis on the patient and her carer is enormous (see Chapter 20). The role of sex in the relationship and the impact of menopause, fertility and physical changes are reflected in the presenting symptoms – postcoital bleeding, pain, etc. Guilt at survival, association with sex itself and sex being unimportant compared with life belie the importance of this basic component of a healthy, satisfying life. Understanding the individual feelings as experienced by the patient and partner is paramount. Encouraging frank discussion about the impact of treatment allows administration of support and other interventions.

I felt all the doctors who had examined me, operated on me and put things inside me were there in the room with me and my husband. I couldn't do it. I feel so sorry for him.

A resentful woman with arousal disorder after successful treatment with chemo-radiation for endometrial cancer.

The Silent Patient: Psychosexual Disorders and Men

As much as we like to try to focus our attention on women, their partners play a large role in women's obstetric and gynaecological issues. There may be a belief that men are less complex than women, but this undermines the man who is equally complex in his sexual response. Male partners rarely attend consultations with their wives/partners, but they are frequently 'in the room' with us. How often are we told that a woman needs her lax vagina tightening as sex doesn't 'feel' as it used to or non-consummators that need assistance in widening a vagina to 'let their partner in'? In this brief section, it is hoped that the silent partner is given a voice to assist women better with sexual dysfunction.

Subfertility Services

Subfertility clinics are probably the most overt presentation of the male partner. The healthcare professional concentrates 90% of clinic efforts on investigation into women and, almost as an afterthought, turns attention to semen analysis. In addition to looking at test results, it is essential to ask a couple about sex. Approximately 40% of couples with subfertility will have sexual difficulties, and many will find this increases with length of time trying or increasing interventions.

Every time I go to have sex with my husband, I think about the doctor examining me and our love life has become about failure rather than pleasure.

A female patient when asked about frequency of sexual intercourse in the fertility clinic.

It is important to consider not only the psychosexual dysfunction issues such as premature ejaculation, erectile dysfunction, retarded ejaculation and anorgasmia in men, but also the rarer physical anomalies such as hypospadias and neurological inability to ejaculate. All of these have been encountered in fertility clinics where an incomplete sexual history has been taken and their female partners have gone through numerous invasive procedures and treatments completely unnecessarily.

> 'Doctor,' embarrassed shuffle of feet and red face, 'I feel that I should tell you that when I come . . . . well, it comes out of the bottom of my cock just before my ball sack. I've tried to tell people but no one has listened before. Can you help us?'

A male partner in a couple who had had multiple failed cycles of IVF.

The psychological impact of azoospermia and oligospermia should not be underestimated and, whilst fertility specialists might notice the impact during treatment in a more protective partner, there are few support services for men.

> My husband couldn't come here today, I've dropped him off in the woods before the hospital. He's so distraught I'm worried about his welfare today. He's taken the sperm test result really bad, doctor.

A female partner of a man with azoospermia (no sperm seen on his semen sample).

Childbirth

There is a strong focus on the trauma of childbirth affecting women, but men may present with secondary sexual dysfunction following childbirth. Rather than feel that this is rarely seen, the obstetrician and gynaecologist should try to offer support to male partners in debriefing and explore their feelings in relation to the experience. There are currently no official support networks for partners of women in maternity services.

> The way I see it, doc, is that I'm here to protect her as her husband but not only did I fail in the maternity ward, I keep seeing it again all day and when I'm trying to sleep, and now I can't help her because I'm in pieces- it's all my fault.

A man with erectile dysfunction since a traumatic delivery.

Following Surgery

It is encouraged to give women as much information as possible during diagnostic and therapeutic pathways, but we must consider that the genitalia that we are trying to restore to normal anatomy are used by our women for their own and partners' sexual pleasure.

The significant proportion of women that are seen in gynaecology outpatients with pelvic floor symptoms have reduced, if not ceased, sexual function (often since they have been examined by healthcare professionals who have 'pathologized' their physical findings). How often are their hushed comments about things not being normal or sex difficult with their husbands ignored? If their phantasies (fantasies with physical manifestation) are transferred to their partners, sexual dysfunction can occur both pre-operatively and post-op.

Healthcare professionals are taught that patients recall just 20% of their consultations, so we give them peer-reviewed leaflets considered useful on their surgery, often not assessed by patients.

> I looked at those pictures and whenever we tried to make love, all I could think about was what was at the top of her vagina now?' Pause with widened eyes. 'A huge black hole that might eat me up . . . and I lost my erection.'

A male patient with erectile dysfunction after his wife's vaginal hysterectomy.

A vital area to consider is when women with vaginismus are 'treated' with dilators or surgery, they are frequently discharged after their therapeutic intervention, so we have little personal feedback on efficacy. Sadly, these patients are often seen in psychosexual clinics with their partners who can also develop secondary erectile dysfunction or premature ejaculation. There is little evidence to support widespread use of these interventions currently. The silent patient can in fact be communicating a great deal.

Sexual Dysfunction and Treatment in Men

Premature Ejaculation

The medical definition of premature ejaculation (PE) is under three minutes from penetration to ejaculation. This is a source of surprise to a number of men who are led to believe that this should be longer. Many couples have an enjoyable sex life even with a diagnosis of PE. Therefore treatment is not necessary unless it is distressing for men and/or their partners.

Whilst it is important to consider the cause of this fully (e.g. commitment issues/ambiguity about starting a family), there are many treatments that men may source before visiting anyone. Masters and Johnson pioneered the 'stop/start technique' where men are encouraged to stop stimulation for thirty seconds as their excitement builds and then restart. There is also the squeeze technique where the man or partner withdraws and squeezes the glans penis until the desire to ejaculate is suppressed.

I'm done just as she is getting started. We turn away from each other and I can hear her crying but she refuses to talk to me.

A couple with PE undergoing fertility treatment.

There are many sprays, lubricants and condoms with local anaesthetic marketed to reduce sensation and also some mechanical devices such as 'Prolong' which appear to be effective in some men. More recently, there has been the launch of dapoxetine, a selective serotonin reuptake inhibitor (SSRI) for PE. To date, this seems to cause nausea and sleepiness in many patients and so has limited efficacy. Men who take an SSRI with a phosphodiesterase inhibitor (e.g., Viagra) might find some benefit, and there are some successes with mindfulness and yoga in some patients. There is very little published data on behavioural therapies.

Retarded Ejaculation

Whilst there is a plethora of products for women on the market for anorgasmia, there is little available for men in this situation. This presents one of the more problematic sexual issues in men, in part because it is derided in society as being an advantage, rather than disadvantage, to female partners. Often these men can ejaculate on their own or with digital or oral stimulation from partners. This poses an issue for spontaneous conception and the difficulty that it presents may well be one of the causes.

Retarded ejaculation management is patient specific, but encouraging penetration at the 'point of no return' may help. Desensitizing treatments on the glans penis and/or vibratory devices may also help.

Erectile Dysfunction

Whilst 10% of men are said to suffer from erectile dysfunction (ED), this only represents the proportion who present to their primary care doctor for assistance. The Massachusetts male ageing study demonstrated rates of up to 40% in men in their forties and increasing with age up to 70% in the seventies [13]. Additionally increasing rates are seen in diabetic men

(over 51%) and ED is now seen as a strong indicator of cardiac disease [14]. Men with ED (particularly gradual onset) must be screened for cardiovascular disease.

Treatment depends on the cause – a psychosexual pathology should be diagnosed only by exclusion with screening for cardiovascular disease and diabetes with lipids and fasting blood glucose. Additionally an androgen profile should be checked to exclude low testosterone or panhypopituitarism. Men with psychosexual dysfunction often retain their morning erections and ability to masturbate, but men with physical causes find that they lose all ability to penetrate as the erection becomes gradually less firm.

I keep thinking when I'm with her that I am useless and it (sic-the erection) goes. It's fine when I'm on my own. I love this girl but why should she stay with me when I can't satisfy her?

A male patient with anxiety-related ED.

Men with diabetes are eligible for prescription phosphodiesterase inhibitors, but it should be remembered that they have a higher incidence of microvascular disease and may have limited response. Men with microvascular disease should be encouraged to purchase a pump to improve blood flow to the penis and use this daily. However they should be warned that the pump produces a cold, blue erection that often points down.

The pump is not the most romantic thing but it's given us back what we thought we might never regain-big grin to partner.

A male diabetic patient with ED.

An important patient group to remember are those men who are survivors of prostatic carcinoma. Sadly, many are affected by nerve degeneration secondary to radiotherapy or surgical damage. Whilst it is important to give patients a realistic idea of the risk of ED, it is also important to encourage them to have regular erections to keep their penis exercised. Retrograde ejaculation is common in this group and in those who have had surgery for benign prostatic hypertrophy. Many of these men also find benefit from a penile vacuum pump, and this should be used regularly, post surgery to limit progression of microvascular disease.

Since he had surgery and lost this little piece of him, he feels like a different man to me and the spark of our relationship has gone. I have to keep reminding myself that we should be grateful that he is still with us.

A partner of a man with ED post nerve-sparing prostate surgery.

Summary

Male sexual dysfunction impinges on gynaecological practice both directly and indirectly. It is vitally important to take a sexual history in all areas of our work and refer to a psychosexual service if problems are too complex to be managed locally.

Management of Psychosexual Disorders

There are many approaches to the diagnosis and treatment of psychogenic sexual disorders. This should include the establishment of the absence or impact of organic disease on sexual functioning despite a more dominant psychological effect. Differing disciplines will have varying emphasis of focus on aspects of behavioural control – early experiences, world vision, quality of relationship, impact of ongoing sense of self-worth, etc. However, treating a patient as the 'expert' in their condition, despite lacking the insight and perspective to understand the impact of these factors, will facilitate the therapeutic relationship between the healthcare professional and the patient to achieve these ends.

The key tenets of the psychosexual approach are:

Listen to the patients 'story' and view of their problem/s

Observe the effect of the patient and their presentation on the doctor and seek to understand the patient's body language

Feel the effect of the doctor's comments/questions and interventions on the patient (especially examination)

Think about the feelings generated during the consultation and/ or examination

Interpret the observations and reflect on their revelations of the sexual issues

Using these components of a consultation with reflection of the most revealing features can open an understanding of the issues and allow resolution.

A simple approach to asking about sexual problems will facilitate greater diagnosis.

- Are you in a sexual relationship?
- Do you have any difficulties?
- Are they a problem for you?
- Do you have pain during sex?

Putting the problems into context by trying to understand when the problem started (lifelong or acquired), whether there are trigger factors, and if it is situational is more helpful than a sexual biography.

The language used by health professionals is very different from that of patients and assuming that the meaning of words used without seeking clarification is likely to limit understanding of the patient's complaints. Basic language and euphemisms can allow misinterpretation and often prove difficult with patients whose native language is different from that of the health professional. This works both ways. Never assume we understand what the patient means! Let her explain the meaning in her own words and feelings. Use the words the patient uses. 'The patient is the expert.' The doctor often needs to assume a position of ignorance to interpret the patient's symptoms and feelings. This is difficult when we are trained to be the expert and ask closed questions to streamline care down preplanned pathways. All circumstances and individuals are unique, particularly with respect to sexual difficulties. Just as expectations and frequency of intercourse are individual to a particular woman or couple, so are the difficulties that ensue.

The key component of a psychosexual consultation may be the examination, when the patient's vulnerabilities can be exposed. The 'moment of truth' can be a therapeutic event in itself if used appropriately rather than an opportunity to reassure and exclude physical causes. The body can express feelings that the patient cannot. Observing body language and behaviour can unlock fantasies, fears and defences [15].

Summary

It is important to routinely ask about sexual activity. Possible physical factors should be assessed, but the psychological impact must be addressed. Symptoms should be acknowledged even if they seem outside of the doctor's expertise. Treat the physical factors *in addition to*, rather than instead of, the psychological as sex is the ultimate biopsychosocial event.

Key Points

- The natural progression of a child learning to be independent involves dealing with pain, fear, guilt, shame, anxiety and conflict. Difficulty with expressing these feelings may readily be acted out in sexual relationships and result in long-standing problems.

- It is imperative that women with any chronic disease, particularly urogenital, are asked about the effect on their sexual life.
- There is no good evidence to suggest that vaginal delivery decreases postnatal sexual health compared with caesarean delivery, despite claims to justify the increasing caesarean delivery rate.
- The needs and complex sexual response of the male partner should be addressed. He is often the 'silent' patient in the psychosexual consultation.
- Increasing rates of erectile dysfunction (ED) are seen in diabetic men, and ED is now seen as a strong indicator of cardiac disease. Men with ED (particularly gradual onset) must be screened for cardiovascular disease.

References

1. Field N, Mercer CH, Sonnenberg P, et al. Associations between Health and Sexual Lifestyles in Britain: Findings from the third National Survey of Sexual Attitudes and Lifestyles (Natsal-3). *Lancet.* 2013;**382**(9907):1830–44.

2. Hayes RD, Dennerstein L. The Impact of Aging on Sexual Function and Sexual Dysfunction in Women: A Review of Population-Based Studies. *J Sex Med.* 2005;**2**:317–30.

3. Bachmann GA, Leiblum SR, Grill J. Brief sexual inquiry in gynecologic practice. *Obstet Gynecol.* 1989; **73**(3 Pt 1): 425–7.

4. American Psychiatric Association (2013) *DSM-5: Diagnostic and Statistical Manual for Mental Disorders.* 5th edition. American Psychiatric Press, USA.

5. American Psychiatric Association (1984) *DSM-IV: Diagnostic and Statistical Manual for Mental Disorders.* 4th edition. American Psychiatric Press, USA.

6. De Souza A, Dwyer PL, Charity M, Thomas E, Ferreira CH, Schierlitz L. The effects of mode delivery on postpartum sexual function: a prospective study. *BJOG.* 2015;**122**(10):1410–8.

7. Glazener CM. Sexual function after childbirth: women's experiences, persistent morbidity and lack of professional recognition. *Br J Obstet Gynaecol.* 1997;**104**(3):330–5.

8. Nicolosi A, Laumann EO, Glasser DB, et al. Global Study of Sexual Attitudes and Behaviors Investigators' Group. Sexual behavior and sexual dysfunctions after age 40: The global study of sexual attitudes and behaviors.*Urology.* 2004;**64**(5): 991–7.

9. Beckman N, Waern M, Gustafson D, Skoog I. Secular trends in self reported sexual activity and satisfaction in Swedish 70 year olds: Cross sectional survey of four populations, 1971–2001. *BMJ.* 2008;**337**:a279.

10. Lindau ST, Schumm LP, Laumann EO, et al. A Study of Sexuality and Health among Older Adults in the United States Stacy. *N Engl J Med.* 2007; **357**:762–74. DOI: 10.1056/NEJMoa067423.

11. Dennerstein L, Randolph J, Taffe J, Dudley E, Burger H. Hormones, mood, sexuality and the menopausal transition. *Fertil Steril.* 2002;**77**(Supp4): S42–8.

12. Hayes RD, Dennerstein L, Bennett CM. Fairley CK What is the 'true' prevalence of female sexual dysfunctions and does the way we assess these conditions have an impact? *J Sex Med.* 2008;**5**(4): 777–87.

13. Feldman HA, Goldstein I, Hatzichristou DG, et al. Impotence and its medical and psychosocial correlates: Results of the Massachusetts Male Aging Study. *J Urol.* 1994;**151**:54–61.

14. McCabe MP, Sharlip ID, Lewis R, et al. Segraves RT Risk Factors for Sexual Dysfunction Among Women and Men: A Consensus Statement from the Fourth International Consultation on Sexual Medicine 2015. *J Sex Med.* 2016;**13**(2):153–67.

15. Smith A. The skills of psychosexual medicine. In *Psychosexual Medicine* Ed. H Montford, R Skrine 2001 Oxford University Press.

Chapter 23

Psychosocial Aspects of Fertility Control

Jonathan Schaffir

Introduction

The decision of when to start a family, or how to space children within a family, is inherently colored by social and psychological factors. Unlike biological events in a woman's life such as puberty or menopause, family planning is largely under a woman's control, and her decisions are shaped by other life events. Issues such as psychological maturity, dynamics of the partner relationship, demands of work and career, and financial readiness may all contribute to a woman's decision to put off pregnancy when she is sexually active. To do so, she has at her disposal a wide array of contraceptives, including behavioral (abstinence or natural family planning), pharmacological (oral, implantable or injectable contraceptives), and surgical choices (sterilization). Decisions regarding method of pregnancy prevention are dependent on which of these methods is most suitable to her lifestyle and mindset.

In fact, in no other aspect of medicine is the prescription of pharmaceuticals or medical procedures so closely tied to psychosocial as opposed to biological factors. Unlike the medications dispensed for illness, or surgeries intended to rectify a disorder, interventions for family planning are largely elective and the best course of treatment is decided not by the health care provider but by the patient. In this respect, family planning is more subject to the psychological and social attributes of the patient than most other aspects of medical practice, or even gynecological practice.

The goal of this chapter is to provide an overview of how psychosocial issues play a role when birth control is used and which choices of contraceptive method are made. It will also examine how particular methods, namely, hormonal contraceptives, may influence psychological and sexual function. Abortion, which is a possible sequela of failed contraceptive efforts, will also be examined for its effect on mental health. By examining the interplay between contraceptive techniques and the psyche, the reader should gain a better understanding of how best to counsel women about the effects they may anticipate when choosing a birth control method.

Psychosocial Influences on the Use of Contraception

In order for birth control to be used effectively and consistently, there are four conditions that must be met. In addition to the existence of techniques that are reliable and medically efficacious, there must be motivation for use, education as to what is available and how the techniques are used, and access to these techniques. It is these latter three conditions that are most subject to psychological, social and cultural influences.

Age and phase of life are key sociodemographic variables that influence contraceptive use. The needs of a sexually active teenager for whom pregnancy might be unwanted or socially stigmatizing are clearly different than those of a woman in her mid-reproductive years looking to space children, or a woman in later life who has completed all intention of childbearing. In fact, age is directly related to contraceptive utilization, which increases linearly with age [1]. Between ages 40 and 44, 75% of women use contraception, though 8.6% remain at risk of unintended pregnancy. Many of these women incorrectly believe that they no longer require contraception due to a perceived lack of fertility.

At the younger end of the age spectrum, adolescents have a unique set of barriers that interfere with their engagement in using contraception [2, 3]. Adolescence is defined by psychological maturity that is markedly behind the level of physical maturity. Consequently, adolescents may follow a pattern of cognitive thought that makes them unable to appreciate the long-term consequences of current acts,

199

coupled with a developmental tendency toward risk-taking behavior. As a result, they may deny or minimize the risks of pregnancy and fail to properly employ any contraception. In addition, they may lack education about contraceptive options, and not have a family or peer environment that is supportive of contraceptive use. Finally, adolescents may not have access to effective contraception, whether as a result of lack of guaranteed confidentiality and perceived adverse repercussions to asking about access, or as a result of being unable to financially or geographically access contraceptive services at this young age.

Socioeconomic status is itself a correlate of contraceptive use. Women who come from backgrounds of lower economic class are less likely to use effective contraception, due to a variety of factors including lack of education, distrust of medical providers, poor access to care and provider bias [4]. Improving coverage for contraceptive methods and access to medical care could dramatically affect the reproductive health of poorer populations, and public health studies suggest that women who live in areas where universal coverage is available have lower rates of unintended pregnancy and abortion.

There are many other cultural issues that also affect the use of contraception. For some, religion is a driving influence [5]. Some religions such as Catholicism expressly forbid sexual intercourse for purposes other than procreation, and contraception is considered intrinsically wrong. In some cases, the restrictions on contraceptive use are related to a cultural paternalism that puts the desires of the male member of the couple ahead of those of the woman. In such cases, women may not be allowed to choose whether to use contraception, or they may not be given access to pharmaceutical contraceptives or information about them. Such cultural viewpoints may cause significant conflicts and ethical dilemmas when women from a repressive culture present for care in a community with more liberal attitudes [6].

Issues Related to Choice of Contraceptive

Psychosocial factors not only influence the decision of whether to prevent pregnancy but also play a role in deciding on the type of contraception. Beyond the obvious considerations of medical safety and the avoidance of methods that would be contraindicated or apt to exacerbate existing medical conditions, most women have a variety of both pharmaceutical and nonpharmaceutical options available to them. High efficacy is often a concern, but even this issue may be influenced by psychological factors. For example, a single woman with limited resources for whom pregnancy would be psychologically traumatic might seek a more effective contraceptive method than a woman in an established relationship for whom pregnancy would not present such a burden.

Even those seeking highly effective forms of contraception have many options. Hormonal and intrauterine contraceptives are the most effective in preventing pregnancy, with failure rates with ideal use of less than 1%. Actual failure rates, however, are often higher due to issues surrounding compliance, with typical use failure rates anywhere from 9% for oral contraceptives that require daily use to 6% for injectable contraceptives requiring recurrent visits to a health care provider. For methods such as implants and intrauterine devices that do not rely on patient behaviors for compliance, typical use rates are much closer to perfect use rates [7]. One reason that so many hormonal contraceptives are available is to offer choices for women who may have difficulty meeting the demands of use, often for psychosocial reasons. For example, the use of a daily oral medication may be difficult for a woman with an inconsistent daily schedule or complex lifestyle. For such women, using a medication taken weekly or monthly, or a device inserted long term, may be preferable. In fact, convenience and ease of use are more important than other medical issues in the choice of contraception [8].

Choice of contraception may also be influenced by the degree to which use is affected by sexual behavior and functioning. Hormonal and intrauterine contraceptives have the advantages of not requiring administration with each act of intercourse and not relying on partner involvement to maintain efficacy. Barrier methods such as the diaphragm or condom, on the other hand, may be perceived as being more of a hindrance to spontaneous sexual behavior because they require application with each act of coitus. Condoms may also be avoided by individuals who perceive them as interfering with sexual pleasure [9]. On the other hand, condoms are the recommended method for couples in whom one or both partners are not monogamous, in order to serve the added purpose of preventing sexually transmitted disease.

Effects of Mental Health on Contraceptive Choice

Choice of contraceptive method may also be influenced by baseline mental health. In women with symptoms of depression or anxiety, the capacity for misuse or discontinuation of contraceptives (in particular oral contraceptives and condoms) may be greater, due to related issues such as decreased motivation, diminished desire for self-care, excessive worry and poor assessment of risk and planning. Such factors would make more reliable forms of contraception particularly desirable for this population [10].

Choices of women with underlying mental health issues, however, do not consistently reflect this goal. Young women who screen positive at baseline for depressive symptoms are less likely to choose effective or long-term contraceptives [11], and more likely to choose oral contraceptives that require daily dosing over long-acting reversible contraceptives such as implants and intrauterine devices [12]. Additionally, women who report increased depression symptoms or high stress are less likely to use contraception consistently and are at higher risk of user-related contraceptive failure [13].

Several theories have been put forth to explain these differences. Women with depression or high stress symptoms may lack the diligence or coping mechanisms necessary to use a daily prescription such as oral contraceptives. Depression and stress may have negative effects on cognitive processes and decision-making regarding contraception and sexual behavior. Furthermore, women with psychological symptoms may fear that hormonal contraception may have side effects that will negatively impact their baseline psychological functioning, which deters them from using more effective contraception. This latter concept, which may be expressed by women without a history of mental health issues as well, may reflect a misconception that requires further explication.

Effects of Hormonal Contraception on Psychological Function

Concerns about adverse effects of contraception on women's mental health stem from research done shortly after the introduction of oral contraceptives over 40 years ago. Some of these large cohort studies demonstrated significantly detrimental effects of oral

contraceptives, including 30% increase in depression diagnosis, increased risk of divorce, increased rate of suicide attempts, and an increased rate of death from accidents or violence [14]. Studies done in this era, however, may not reflect the risks present in modern times. Doses of estrogen and progestins in early versions of oral contraceptives were much higher than those in today's formulations. Furthermore, the social stigma associated with use of hormonal contraception, particularly in young and unmarried women, has faded with time.

Despite newer formulations with lower doses and changes in the characteristics of women who are prescribed hormonal contraception, there remains a perception that adverse psychological effects persist. Among women who discontinue oral contraceptive use due to adverse side effects, up to 33% report that emotional side effects prompted discontinuation [15], and among those who experience adverse changes in mood, a majority may stop using the pill within six months [16]. Even before initiating hormonal contraception, women fear that it will induce negative psychological effects, with 20% reporting an expectation of changes in mood [17].

The actual incidence of adverse effects on mood in women who choose hormonal contraception is far less than women may anticipate. Large observational cohort studies that compare women using various forms of contraception demonstrate either lower depression scores among hormonal contraception users compared with nonusers [18] or no difference in depression diagnosis or depression scores [19, 20]. Because these studies are observational, they are subject to biases that likely affect the results. Women who use hormonal contraception are likely to be healthier, which may affect psychological well-being. Also, hormonal contraception is likely to provide beneficial side effects such as decreased menstrual pain and bleeding that may affect mood scores. Additionally, the small number of women who do experience adverse effects may be offset by an equal or greater number who experience improved mood on hormonal contraceptives, leading to an apparent lack of difference in mean mood scores between groups [16]. Nonetheless, it is likely to be a small minority of hormonal contraceptive users who experience adverse mood effects.

The effects of oral contraceptives on the menstrual cycle may be salutary for many women. Compared to nonusers, women who use oral contraceptives experience less variability in affect across the menstrual cycle, such that they are less prone to the changes in affect that often occur with progression through the luteal phase of the menstrual cycle [21]. Pill formulations that contain a constant dose of hormone throughout the cycle (monophasic) have a greater stabilizing effect on mood than triphasic formulations that vary the amount of hormone through the cycle. Furthermore, adverse mood symptoms and somatic symptoms are more pronounced during the pill-free interval of the cycle, when exogenous hormone is not administered [22]. These findings suggest that women who experience distressing psychological effects of the menstrual cycle may benefit from hormonal contraceptive use.

Indeed, oral contraceptives have been offered as a treatment for women with premenstrual dysphoric disorder (PMDD). By suppressing ovulation and eliminating variability in hormonal concentrations over the menstrual cycle, oral contraceptives may improve bothersome mood changes that affect these women in the luteal phase. A randomized placebo-controlled trial of a levonorgestrel-containing oral contraceptive in women diagnosed with PMDD failed to show any significant difference in depressive scores between cases and controls at the conclusion of the trial [23]. However, the effect may depend on the type of progestin used in the pill. A review of trials using oral contraceptives formulated with drospirenone, a progestin with specific antimineralocorticoid properties, describes improvements in psychological symptoms in these women as well as improved productivity and relationships relative to women treated with placebo [24]. These studies suggest that there may be a unique property of drospirenone that improves mood in women with menstrual dysphoria.

The progestin component of combined oral contraceptives may determine some of the effect on mood. In women with no history of premenstrual emotional symptoms using oral contraceptives, those whose formulation had higher progesterone to estrogen ratios were more likely to have negative mood effects [21]. The effect may also be dependent on the type of progestin rather than the dose. Two randomized trials have demonstrated worse psychological side effects for users of an oral contraceptive containing levonorgestrel than for users of an alternative oral contraceptive whose progestin had fewer androgenic properties [25, 26].

If indeed the progestin component may be the hormonal component that determines psychological side effects of combined contraceptives, then one may suspect that progestin-only contraception would be likely to have such effects. The contraceptives currently available in the United States that contain progestin only include the progestin-only pill, the depot medroxyprogesterone injection (DMPA), the etonogestrel subdermal implant, and the levonorgestrel-containing intrauterine device. Unfortunately there are few controlled studies that examine these methods. In the only randomized controlled trial that compared progestin-only pills with combined oral contraceptives, there was a lower incidence of depression in the progestin-only group [27]. However, the trial was done using a pill containing levonorgestrel, rather than norethindrone, which is the only progestin currently approved as a progestin-only contraceptive pill in the United States.

DMPA might be expected to have greater effects than oral progestin-only pills, since it contains a higher overall dosage which raises serum progesterone levels and suppresses ovulation to a greater extent than oral preparations. Studies of DMPA, however, are overall reassuring, with most users demonstrating no significant adverse mood effects, and less than 5% experiencing clinically significant worsening depression [28]. When compared with nonusers, DMPA users do demonstrate increased depression scores over time, with differences noted after three years of use [29].

Although there are no direct comparisons of progestin subdermal implants with other forms of hormonal contraception, the side effects of such methods have been reported in association with efficacy trials. Among women using Norplant, an earlier version of subdermal progestin that used six rods containing levonorgestrel, there was a 10.6% rate of mood complaints, though only 1.8% discontinued the medication due to these effects [30]. For the newer etonogestrel implant currently on the market, prospective trials demonstrate a 7.3% rate of reporting depression after two years, with 2.4% citing this as a reason for discontinuation [31]. Overall, it seems that adverse mood effects of hormonal contraception are similar between users of combined oral contraceptives and progestin-only contraceptives, with less than 10% experiencing clinically significant issues in both groups.

Characteristics of Women Experiencing Adverse Mood Effects

If indeed a small minority of women experience mood effects on hormonal contraception severe enough to prompt discontinuation, then these women are at increased risk for poor compliance and unintended pregnancy. It would be helpful to identify what characteristics might predispose women to such effects so they may be properly counseled about their options before starting a hormonal contraceptive method.

Unfortunately, there is little information that is useful in predicting which women are likely to experience mood effects from hormonal contraception. A comparison of users who experienced mood and sexual side effects with those who did not found that neither age nor education was predictive, though women who experienced adverse mood effects were more likely to be unmarried and either Caucasian or South Asian [32]. Some other studies have suggested that women with an underlying mood disorder, notably depression, are more likely to develop negative mood changes on hormonal contraception [33, 34]. However, a literature review of existing studies that examine contraception in women with underlying depression has determined that there is no clear association between the use of hormonal contraceptives and deterioration of mood in women with preexisting depressive symptoms [35]. A history of major depression should not be a contraindication to the prescription of hormonal contraceptives.

In fact, the characteristic that is most predictive for developing adverse mood symptoms on hormonal contraception is the previous experience of such an effect. This suggests that there may be an underlying but yet unexplained aspect of physiological makeup that predisposes certain women to such effects. Several studies have examined this subset of women to identify explanations for this phenomenon. Some of the explanations given by these researchers suggest that these women may have changes in functioning of specific regions of the brain [36], differences in prenatal testosterone exposure [37], or differences in the structure of androgen receptors [38]. Additional research is needed to further elucidate exactly what predisposes this small minority of women to negative mood changes with exposure to hormonal contraception.

Sexual Side Effects of Hormonal Contraception

Sexual side effects of hormonal contraception are another concern that may lead susceptible women to discontinue an otherwise effective contraceptive method. Although some women may anticipate a negative impact of hormonal contraception on sexual functioning, the incidence is small. Most women who use hormonal contraceptives experience no change in sexual function scores, and as many as one-fifth report improvement [39]. Sexual function is influenced by many factors independent of the biological effects of contraception, and the women who experience improved sexual function may feel freed of the anxiety and fear of unwanted pregnancy, and have improvement in somatic symptoms such as menstrual bleeding and pain that may interfere with their sexual behavior.

Nevertheless, sexual side effects (most notably decreases in sexual desire) are consistently noted in 3–10% of women using hormonal contraception [40], a figure that mirrors the rates for mood effects. Despite similar rates of prevalence, there is not necessarily a correlation between the two. In studies measuring sexual effects as well as mood, sexual desire is suppressed in subsets of women whose mood is unaffected by the use of contraception [41, 42, 27].

The explanation often given for the decrease in sexual desire in some women using hormonal contraception is the effect on testosterone. Testosterone has been implicated as the primary hormonal influence on sexual desire in both men and women, with androgen deprivation leading to decreased sexual desire, and androgen replenishment restoring normal libido in surgically menopausal women with hypoactive sexual desire [43]. Exogenous estrogen, such as that found in combined oral contraceptives, is associated with decreased levels of biologically active testosterone, due to the increased production of sex-hormone binding globulin which binds circulating testosterone. Despite this effect, there is no consistent association between androgen levels and sexual desire in hormonal contraceptive users, and supplemental androgen is not helpful in reversing the diminished sexual desire that some oral contraceptive users experience [44]. Furthermore, prospective studies demonstrate that reductions in free testosterone associated with different estrogen doses do not affect enjoyment of sexual activity [45].

Since the changes that occur in sexual function in a minority of oral contraceptive users do not appear to be related to estrogen's effect on free testosterone, some have proposed that they may be a function of the progestin component. Comparisons of different progestational agents, however, fail to demonstrate a difference in sexual function scores [46]. Some evidence points to a difference in serotonin genotype between women with and without contraceptive-related sexual dysfunction [47]. The exact mechanism remains to be elucidated, and for now the small incidence of decreased sexual function in hormonal contraceptive users is generally viewed as an idiosyncratic and poorly predicted reaction.

Psychological Consequences of Sterilization

For women who are certain that they no longer want to have children, sterilization is a highly effective and permanent method of contraception. The procedure eliminates the need for worry and anxiety about unintended pregnancy, and is not dependent on patient compliance for its efficacy. As such, it might be expected to have positive psychological effects on those women who experience stress related to fear of pregnancy, and would be free of any potential hormonal influences on mood.

In fact, the psychological sequelae of this procedure generally range from neutral to positive. Many studies demonstrate a beneficial effect on sexual functioning, with reports of improvement in sexual satisfaction, sexual desire, and coital frequency. Sexual spontaneity and satisfaction are often improved due to decreased anxiety about the possibility of pregnancy [48]. Greater satisfaction with relationships has also been reported. For women who have preexisting psychiatric disease, sterilization demonstrates no significant effect on the course of illness and, in some women, was associated with reduced psychiatric morbidity at six months [49].

One potential negative outcome that women who undergo sterilization may experience is regret. Unlike other forms of birth control, sterilization is irreversible, and a woman who later decides that she is interested in childbearing may feel sad or angry about her previous decision to have her tubes occluded. The single risk factor that is most consistently associated with regret is age. Overall rates of regret following sterilization range from 2% to 6%, but among women younger than age 30 the risk rises to 20% at 14 years [50]. Studies of women younger than age 25 demonstrate even higher rates, with relative risk of regret being 3.5–8.6 the rate of women over 30. Other potential risk factors for regret include marital discord, changes in marital status following sterilization, death of a child, underlying psychological disease and inadequate counseling [51]. Interestingly, nulliparity is not a risk factor for regret, perhaps because those women who feel so strongly about completely avoiding pregnancy are highly motivated to obtain sterilization [49].

Mental Health Issues Related to Abortion

Although family planning methods allow most women to conceive and have children according to their desires and conveniences, a substantial number of pregnancies occur that are unintended and unplanned. Whether due to non-compliance with intended methods of contraception or due to lack of education and access to effective birth control, about half of pregnancies in the United States are unintended. Of these, four in ten are terminated in abortion. By the age of 45, it is estimated that three out of ten women will have had an elective abortion [52]. Given the frequency of this experience, it is worthwhile to review the psychological issues associated with voluntary termination of pregnancy.

Debate about the psychological effects of abortion has circulated for almost 30 years, as public health advocates and policy makers have sought to determine whether detrimental effects of induced abortion exist, and if such effects should be considered in efforts to control or limit abortion services [53]. Studies have appeared in peer-reviewed journals that identify adverse effects of induced abortion on women's mental health, and testimony citing such research has been given in political forums to support laws that would restrict abortion. A review attempting to quantify the adverse effects cited in such research estimates that women who have undergone abortion experience an 81% increased risk of mental health problems [54]. Such problems include increases in anxiety, depression, alcohol abuse, and suicidal behaviors, with 10% of the increased incidence attributable to abortion.

In an effort to create a balanced and strictly analytical review of the evidence on psychological effects of abortion, the American Psychological Association established a task force to review the subject, who published their findings in 2008 [55]. In their analysis of 50 papers published between 1990 and 2007, the authors conclude that for women undergoing legal first-trimester abortion, the relative risks of mental health problems are no greater than the risks among women who deliver an unplanned pregnancy. Although they did find a higher incidence of violence-related deaths among women who had an abortion, the correlation demonstrated the higher risk for violence in the lives of women who have abortions and the importance of controlling for such exposure in studies of mental health and pregnancy outcomes.

Several factors account for the differences in the conclusions drawn in these reviews based on similar sets of data. The research literature examining psychological effects of abortion includes studies of varying methodological strength, and it is vital that those who analyze such data identify the quality of the study on which conclusions are based [56]. Since underlying mental health issues are a strong risk factor for negative mental health outcomes, the measurements and definitions of preexisting mental health are extremely important but lacking in many studies. Furthermore, many studies use completed pregnancy as a comparison group, rather than completed pregnancy strictly among women with unintended pregnancy. Since many disadvantages such as low socioeconomic status, lack of education and violence put women at risk for unintended pregnancy, these factors are likely to be confounders in surveys of women having abortions. Rather than comparing women who have had abortions with those who completed pregnancies, a more suitable comparison group might be those who sought abortion but were denied the opportunity to have one. In such comparisons, those who received abortion have similar or lower levels of depression and anxiety than women denied an abortion [57].

Although carefully performed reviews conclude that women in general having abortions do not have a greater risk of mental health issues than women completing an unplanned pregnancy, many women do experience psychological sequelae to some degree. Sadness, grief, and feelings of loss are common following the elective termination of pregnancy. However, only a minority of women experience lasting sadness or regret sufficient to trigger mental health difficulties [58]. Risk factors for such problems include intendedness of the pregnancy, ambivalence about the decision, lack of social support and preexisting mental health disorders. The situation may also be different for women who terminate a wanted pregnancy late in pregnancy due to a fetal abnormality; these women experience psychological trauma similar to women who miscarry a wanted pregnancy or experience a stillbirth [55]. Being able to predict which women have a higher risk of mental health problems following induced abortion may help abortion providers to anticipate their needs for additional counseling.

Conclusions

Women today have more options than ever of methods to effectively delay or avoid pregnancy. Because she does not have to base decisions strictly on medical or biological suitability, each woman is able to choose contraception that is appropriate for her lifestyle. Although many of these choices are hormonal and have the potential to interact with biological factors, overall side effects are few and impact on psychological health is positive. For most women, the ability to enjoy sex free of concerns about unwanted pregnancy results in improved psychological well-being.

For any pharmaceutical or surgical option, however, there are minorities of women who do experience adverse effects. For some interventions, such as sterilization and abortion, there are identifiable risk factors that may alert the clinician to those at risk for developing mental health effects. For many pharmaceutical options, such as oral or injectable hormonal contraceptives, depressed mood and decreased sexual desire are idiosyncratic reactions that occur infrequently and are less predictable. For these issues, additional research is necessary to determine the characteristics that may identify a woman as being susceptible to such effects. Nevertheless, most women and their providers may rest assured that contraception is safe and unlikely to adversely affect the user's mental health.

Key Points

- Family planning is more subject to the psychological and social attributes of the patient than most other aspects of medical practice, or even gynecological practice.

- Psychosocial factors not only influence the decision of whether to prevent pregnancy but also play a role in deciding on the type of contraception.

- Psychosocial influences on the use of contraception include age and phase of life, socioeconomic status, culture and religion.

- Women cite convenience and ease of use as more important than other medical issues in the choice of contraception.

- Women who experience distressing psychological effects of the menstrual cycle may benefit from hormonal contraceptive use. There may be a unique property of drospirenone that improves mood in women with menstrual dysphoria.

- There is little information useful in predicting which women are likely to experience mood effects from hormonal contraception.

- Sexual side effects (most notably decreases in sexual desire) are consistently noted in 3–10% of women using hormonal contraception. These effects do not appear to be related to estrogen's effect on free testosterone.

- The single risk factor that is most consistently associated with regret after sterilization is age. Among women younger than age 30 the risk of regret rises to 20% at 14 years.

- Most studies of the effects of induced abortion on women's mental health are confounded by methodological limitations. Although carefully performed reviews conclude that women having abortions do not have a greater risk of mental health issues than women completing an unplanned pregnancy, many women do experience psychological sequelae to some degree.

References

1. Jones J, Mosher W, Daniels K. Current contraceptive use in the United States, 2006–2010, and changes in patterns of use since 1995. *National Health Statistics Reports* 2012; **60**: 1–25.

2. Hofmann AD. Contraception in adolescence: A review; 1. Psychosocial aspects. *Bulletin of the World Health Organization* 1984; **62**: 151–62.

3. Lagana L. Psychosocial correlates of contraceptive practices during late adolescence. *Adolescence* 1999; **34**: 463–82.

4. Dehlendorf C, Rodriguez MI, Levy K, Borrero S, Steinauer J. Disparities in family planning. *American Journal of Obstetrics and Gynecology* 2010; **202**: 214–20.

5. Kellogg Spadt S, Rosenbaum TY, Dweck A, Millheiser L, Pillai-Friedman S, Krychman M. Sexual health and religion: A primer for the sexual health clinician. *Journal of Sexual Medicine* 2014; **11**: 1606–19.

6. Rademakers J, Mouthaan I, de Neef M. Diversity in sexual health: Problems and dilemmas. *European Journal of Contraception and Reproductive Health Care* 2005; **10**: 207–11.

7. Trussell J. Contraceptive failure in the United States. *Contraception* 2011; **83**: 397–404.

8. Egarter C, Tirri BF, Bitzer J, Kaminskyy V, Oddens BJ, Prilepskaya V, et al. Women's perceptions and reasons for choosing the pill, patch, or ring in the CHOICE study: A cross-sectional survey of contraceptive method selection after counseling. *BMC Women's Health* 2013; **13**: 9.

9. Paterno MT, Jordan ET. A review of factors associated with unprotected sex among adult women in the United States. *JOGNN* 2012; **41**: 258–74.

10. Hall KS, Steinberg JR, Cwiak CA, Allen RH, Marcus SM. Contraception and mental health: A commentary on the evidence and principles for practice. *American Journal of Obstetrics and Gynecology* 2015; **212**: 740–6.

11. Garbers S, Correa N, Tobier N, Blust S, Chiasson MA. Association between symptoms of depression and contraceptive method choices among low-income women at urban reproductive health centers. *Maternal and Child Health Journal* 2010; **14**: 102–9.

12. Hall KS, Moreau C, Trussell J, Barber J. Role of young women's depression and stress symptoms in their weekly use and nonuse of contraceptive methods. *Journal of Adolescent Health* 2013; **53**: 241–8.

13. Hall KS, Moreau C, Trussell J, Barber J. Young women's consistency of contraceptive use – does depression or stress matter? *Contraception* 2013; **88**: 641–9.

14. Robinson SA, Dowell M, Pedulla D, McCauley L. Do the emotional side-effects of hormonal contraceptives come from pharmacologic or psychological mechanisms? *Medical Hypotheses* 2004; **63**: 268–73.

15. Sanders SA, Graham CA, Bass JL, Bancroft J. A prospective study of the effects of oral contraceptives on sexuality and well-being and their relationship to discontinuation. *Contraception* 2001; **64**: 51–8.

16. Westhoff CL, Heartwell S, Edwards S, Zieman M, Stuart G, Cwiak C, Davis A, Robilotto T, Cushman L, Kalmuss D. Oral contraceptive discontinuation: Do side effects matter? *American Journal of Obstetrics and Gynecology* 2007; **196**: 412.e1–e7.

17. Wimberly YH, Cotton S, Wanchick AM, Succop PA, Rosenthal SL. Attitudes and experiences with levonorgestrel 100 mcg/ ethinyl estradiol 20 mcg among women during a 3-month trial. *Contraception* 2002; **65**: 403–6.

18. Keyes KM, Cheslack-Postava K, Westhoff C, Heim CM, Haloossim M, Walsh K, Koenen K. Association of hormonal contraceptive use with reduced levels of depressive symptoms: A national study of sexually active women in the United States. *American Journal of Epidemiology* 2013; **178**: 1378–88.

19. Duke JM, Sibbritt DW, Young AF. Is there an association between the use of oral contraception and depressive symptoms in young Australian women? *Contraception* 2007; **75**: 27–31.

20. Toffol E, Heikinheimo O, Koponen P, Luoto R, Partonen T. Hormonal contraception and mental health: Results of a population-based study. *Human Reproduction* 2011; **26**: 3085–93.

21. Oinonen KA, Mazmanian D. To what extent do oral contraceptives influence mood and affect? *Journal of Affective Disorders* 2002; **70**: 229–40.

22. Sundstom Poromaa I, Segebladh B. Adverse mood symptoms with oral contraceptives. *Acta Obstetricia et Gynecologica Scandinavica* 2012; **91**: 420–7.

23. Halbreich U, Freeman EW, Rapkin AJ, Cohen LS, Grubb GS, Bergeron R, et al. Continuous oral levonorgestrel/ethinyl estradiol for treating premenstrual dysphoric disorder. *Contraception* 2012; **85**: 19–27.

24. Lopez LM, Kaptein AA, Helmerhorst FM. Oral contraceptives containing drospirenone for premenstrual syndrome. *Cochrane Database of Systematic Reviews* 2012, Issue 2. Art No: CD006586.

25. Shahnazi M, Khalili AF, Kochaksaraei FR, Jafarabadi MA, Banoi KG, Nahaee J, Payan SB. A comparison of second and third generations combined oral contraceptive pills' effect on mood. *Iranian Red Crescent Medical Journal* 2014; **16**: e13628.

26. Kelly S, Davies E, Fearns S, McKinnon C, Carter R, Gerlinger C, Smithers A. Effects of oral contraceptives containing ethinyl estradiol with either drospirenone or levonorgestrel on various parameters associated with well-being in healthy women. *Clinical Drug Investigation* 2010; **30**: 325–36.

27. Graham CA, Ramos R, Bancroft J, Maglaya C, Farley TMM. The effects of steroidal contraceptives on the well-being and sexuality of women: A double-blind, placebo-controlled, two-centre study of combined and progestogen-only methods. *Contraception* 1995; **52**: 363–9.

28. Westhoff C, Truman C, Kalmuss D, Cushman LO, Davidson A, Rulin M, Heartwell S. Depressive symptoms and Depo-Provera. *Contraception* 1998; **57**: 237–40.

29. Civic D, Scholes D, Ichikawa L, LaCroix AZ, Yoshida CK, Ott SM, Barlow WE. Depressive symptoms in users and non-users of depot medroxyprogesterone acetate. *Contraception* 2000; **61**: 385–90.

30. Sivin I, Mishell DR Jr, Darney P, Wan L, Christ M. Levonorgestrel capsule implants in the United States: A 5-year study. *Obstetrics & Gynecology* 1998; **92**: 337–44.

31. Funk S, Miller MM, Mishell DR Jr, Archer DF, Poindexter A, Schmidt J, Zampaglione E, Implanon US Study Group. Safety and efficacy of Implanon, a single-rodimplantable contraceptive containing etonogestrel. *Contraception* 2005; **71**: 319–26.

32. Wiebe ER, Brotto LA, MacKay J. Characteristics of women who experience mood and sexual side effects with use of hormonal contraception. *Journal of Obstetrics and Gynaecology of Canada* 2011; **33**: 1234–40.

33. Joffe H, Cohen LS, Harlow BL. Impact of oral contraceptive pill use on premenstrual mood: Predictors of improvement and deterioration. *American Journal of Obstetrics and Gynecology* 2003; **189**: 1523–30.

34. Segebladh B, Borgstrom A, Odlind V, Bixo M, Sundstrom-Poromaa I. Prevalence of psychiatric disorders and premenstrual dysphoric symptoms in patients with experience of adverse mood during treatment with combined oral contraceptives. *Contraception* 2009; **79**: 50–5.

35. Bottcher B, Radenbach K, Wildt L, Hinney B. Hormonal contraception and depression: A survey of the present state of knowledge. *Archives of Gynecology and Obstetrics* 2012; **286**: 231–6.

36. Gingnell M, Engman J, Frick A, Moby L, Wikstrom J, Fredrikson M, Sundstrom-Poromaa I. Oral contraceptive use changes brain activity and mood in women with previous negative affect on the pill – a double-blinded, placebo-controlled randomized trial of a levonorgestrel-containing combined oral contraceptive. *Psychoneuroendocrinology* 2013; **38**: 1133–44.

37. Oinonen KA. Putting a finger on potential predictors of oral contraceptive side effects: 2D:4D and middle-phalangeal hair. *Psychoneuroendocrinology* 2009; **34**: 713–26.

38. Elaut E, Buysse A, De Sutter P, De Cuypere G, Gerris J, Deschepper E, T'Sjoen G. Relation of androgen receptor sensitivity and mood to sexual desire in hormonal contraception users. *Contraception* 2012; **85**: 470–9.

39. Pastor Z, Holla K, Chmel R. The influence of combined oral contraceptives on female sexual desire: A systematic review. *European Journal of Contraception and Reproductive Health Care* 2013; **18**: 27–43.

40. Burrows LJ, Basha M, Goldstein AT. The effects of hormonal contraceptives on female sexuality: A review. *Journal of Sexual Medicine* 2012; **9**: 2213–23.

41. Leeton J, McMaster R, Worsley A. The effects on sexual response and mood after sterilization of women taking long-term oral contraception: Results of a double-blind cross-over study. *Australia and New Zealand Journal of Obstetrics and Gynaecology* 1978; **18**: 194–7.

42. Graham CA, Sherwin BB. The relationship between mood and sexuality in women using an oral contraceptive as a treatment for premenstrual symptoms. *Psychoneuroendocrinology* 1993; **18**: 273–81.

43. Bolour S, Braunstein G. Testosterone therapy in women: A review. *International Journal of Impotence Research* 2005; **17**: 399–408.

44. Schaffir J. Hormonal contraception and sexual desire: A critical review. *Journal of Sex & Marital Therapy* 2006; **32**: 305–14.

45. Graham CA, Bancroft J, Doll HA, Greco T, Tanner A. Does oral contraceptive-induced reduction in free testosterone adversely affect the sexuality or mood of women? *Psychoneuroendocrinology* 2007; **32**: 246–55.

46. Wallwiener M, Wallwiener LM, Seeger H, Muck AO, Bitzer J, Wallwiener CW. Effects of sex hormones in oral contraceptives on the female sexual function score: A study in German female medical students. *Contraception* 2009; **82**: 155–9.

47. Bishop JR, Ellingrod VL, Akroush M, Moline J. The association of serotonin transporter genotypes and selective serotonin reuptake inhibitor (SSRI)-associated sexual side effects: Possible relationship to oral contraceptives. *Human Psychopharmacology* 2009; **24**: 207–15.

48. Baill IC, Cullins VE, Pati S. Counseling issues in tubal sterilization. *American Family Physician* 2003; **67**: 1287–94.

49. Smith EM, Friedrich E, Pribor EF. Psychosocial consequences of sterilization: A review of the literature and preliminary findings. *Comprehensive Psychiatry* 1994; **35**: 157–63.

50. Curtis KM, Mohllajee AP, Peterson HB. Regret following female sterilization at a young age: A systematic review. *Contraception* 2006; **73**: 205–10.

51. Chi I-C, Jones DB. Incidence, risk factors, and prevention of poststerilization regret in women: An updated international review from an epidemiological perspective. *Obstetrical and Gynecological Survey* 1994; **49**: 722–32.

52. Guttmacher Institute Fact Sheet: Induced Abortion in the United States. www.guttmacher.org/fact-sheet/induced-abortion-united-states. Accessed 11 April 2017.

53. Major B, Appelbaum M, Beckman L, Dutton MA, Russo NF, West C. Abortion and mental health: Evaluating the evidence. *American Psychologist* 2009; **64**: 863–90.

54. Coleman PK. Abortion and mental health: Quantitative synthesis and analysis of research published 1995–2009. *British Journal of Psychiatry* 2011; **199**: 180–6.

55. American Psychological Association Task Force on Mental Health and Abortion. Report of the task force on mental health and abortion. Washington, DC: 2008. www.apa.org/pi/wpo/mental-health-abortion-report.pdf. Accessed 23 March 2017.

56. Steinberg JR, Russo NF. Evaluating research on abortion and mental health. *Contraception* 2009; **80**: 500–3.

57. Foster DG, Steinberg JR, Roberts SCM, Neuhaus J, Biggs MA. A comparison of depression and anxiety symptom trajectories between women who had an abortion and women denied one. *Psychological Medicine* 2015; **45**: 2073–82.

58. Cameron S. Induced abortion and psychological sequelae. *Best Practice & Research Clinical Obstetrics and Gynaecology* 2010; **24**: 657–65.

Chapter 24

Legal and Ethical Factors in Sexual and Reproductive Health

Bernard M. Dickens and Rebecca J. Cook

Introduction

Law and ethics are closely intertwined in the area of human sexuality and reproduction [1], but the law's inherent conservatism has an ambivalent expression. The law has tended to view indulgence of individuals' sexuality outside marriage through the lens of sin [2], introducing and accommodating condemnation, such as punishment and illegitimate status (bastardy) in the public sector and disadvantage, such as dismissal from employment or school in the private sector for immoral behavior. In contrast, however, many legal systems still allow men immunity from rape laws when forcing themselves on their resistant wives, even by violence. Men's self-restraint is then a requirement of personal ethics (microethics), although public ethics (macroethics) have inspired some judges and legislatures to reform permissive laws to condemn domestic sexual violence.

Sexuality

Consent

Whether individuals should succumb to their sexual urges outside marriage can be a source of considerable tension, anxiety, and guilt, aggravated by legal and ethical constraints and sexual indulgence between married partners is not free from ethical concerns of mutual respect. Similarly, whether partners have freely consented can be a source of anxiety and self-recrimination on ethical and legal grounds. Sexual relations with underage partners, of either sex, can be an obvious legal concern, but modern attention includes relations with elderly voluntary partners affected by degrees of dementia, such as when perhaps Viagra-aided men find same-age companions [3].

Touching without consent is generally addressed in law relating to assault. Consent to ordinary touching is often implied by conduct, such as when entering a crowded train or sports arena. Sexual touching is more intimate, and sexual assault is usually more heavily punishable than common assault because it affects not only individuals' bodily integrity but also their emotional well-being, dignity, and sense of security. Many legal systems set ages of consent before which adolescents' consent to sexual touching or intercourse is legally invalid, rendering the acts offences. Sexually precocious adolescents may be considered delinquents for consensual relationships, but are increasingly regarded less as offenders than as offended against, by partners and, for instance, by parents' lack of due care. Further, if a sexual partner is less than three years or so older than the other who is underage, this may be seen as misguided sexual curiosity rather than a serious offence. Adolescent girls may be induced to restraint, however, by being made apprehensive of unwed pregnancy if it carries a social stigma.

Sex and Gender

By whatever means sexuality is expressed, it concerns the contrast between sex, which is determined by biology, and gender, which is a product of social and cultural perception. The English language often obscures this difference, where 'gender' may be a polite euphemism when to speak of 'sex' would appear crude, provocative, or in poor taste. In the romance languages, notably French, Spanish, and Italian, the masculine is introduced by 'le,' 'el,' and 'il,' and the feminine by 'la.' In French, for instance, the kitchen, where women work, is 'la cuisine,' and the roof, a workplace outside the home, is 'le toit.' The spoon, a kitchen implement, is 'la cuillere,' while the knife, which could be a work tool, is 'le couteau.' Accordingly, because nursing is a female-gendered occupation, a 'male nurse' may be distinguished from a 'nurse,' and a male midwife is more exceptional.

The relevance of this to reproductive and sexual health is that some individuals experience dissonance between their biological sex and their social gender, the feminine person confined in a masculine body or vice versa. Gender dysphoria is a medical condition amenable to a variety of treatments, including surgeries often misdescribed as 'sex change' or 'sexual reassignment' operations that change social gender. This opens up a variety of 'sexualities' beyond male and female, including lesbian, gay, bisexual, transsexual or transgender, and intersex, without stigmatization for sexual deviance. Legal systems may be slow, however, to accommodate the psychological, emotional, and mental health needs of individuals whose sex differs from the gender they feel they possess.

Legal conservatism that identifies transgendered individuals by reference only to their biological sex determined at birth creates tensions in such areas as gender identification, for instance, on vehicle drivers' licenses and passports, but more significantly bars participation in social and sports activities and has profound lifelong effects in denial of rights to marry where, as is common, same-sex marriage is prohibited. Legal requirements that individuals who consider themselves female, wear makeup and women's attire and identify with women should use men's washrooms when in public places, because of their biology, and that masculine looking individuals in mens' clothing should similarly enter women's washrooms, is not just disruptive of public order, but a source of humiliation, distress, and social dysfunction. The ethical principle of justice should prevail, as a matter of human rights, over legal constructions of traditional law to permit individuals to present themselves in public as of the gender to which they feel they belong, even if different from their biological classification [4].

Sexual Violence

Many, if not all, individuals are susceptible to sexual violence, but widespread international experience shows the overwhelming majority of victims to be female. This is so in all settings, including victims' own homes, and across all social classes, but most visible instances tend to identify females in disadvantaged circumstances, such as of social disorder or displacement. Sexual assaults cover a wide spectrum, from unwanted fondling of an erogenous zone or frottage, such as deliberately rubbing against another's clothed body for sexual gratification, for instance, in crowds or crowded public conveyances,

to violent rape. Milder assaults may be a distasteful nuisance or embarrassment, but even these can be a source of distress, disgust and depression, in showing one's vulnerability, exploitability, and defenselessness, inducing fear of being in public places. Greater sexual outrages are liable to be traumatic, liable to trigger post-traumatic stress disorders.

The criminal nature of these assaults is self-evident, but legal processes of detection and prosecution may inadvertently be aggravating factors in victims' psychological anguish, sometimes related to social stigmatization they suffer through publicity in their communities. Forensic examinations of rape victims, for instance, may be afforded priority over attending to their medical and psychological needs. Internal examinations into body cavities may be conducted without sensitivity to recover assailants' tissues, sometimes described by victims as 'the second rape,' and victims may be required to remain in soiled clothing and underclothes and not wash. Insufficient priority may be given to training medical forensic personnel in accommodating victims' physical and psychological needs in order to enhance their recovery and rehabilitation [5]. Similarly, domestic violence victims' economic and psychological dependency on their assailants may require that their counselling review their social options, including counselling with, or of, their abusive partners or family members [6].

Judicial proceedings against criminal suspects may require victims to confront them, present detailed testimony of what they recall occurred and of their active and/or passive responses, including to whom they chose to complain and why, and be subject to possibly hostile cross-examination, such as denying the occurrence or suggesting their consent, and at times to judicial skepticism. Mature complainants may endure this with composure, such as when forewarned and prepared by experienced prosecuting counsel, but court procedures and personnel can be intimidating. Some legal systems, such as in North America including Mexico, have pioneered courses in judicial gender sensitivity training, such as to limit publicity of victims' identities, but this may have an impact, if at all, quite late in the process of law enforcement.

It is not uncommon for police officers, including of senior rank, to be unresponsive to complaints and evidence of sexual assault, especially of a domestic origin, reflecting a social culture of denial or normalization, but equally indifferent to evidence even of a gross nature such as of a violent gang rape. In such cases, they may require complainants or those accompanying them such as parents to provide more detailed information of the assailants, for instance, of their descriptions, clothing, and identities, than the circumstances allowed victims to record. They may also make prejudicial assessments of victims' social status and sexual virtue. Official passivity, hostility, and skepticism deny victims the opportunity to feel that the wrongs they have suffered, and that they themselves as members of their communities, matter, inducing unresolved feelings of frustration, helplessness and despair.

Some victims seek relief through suicide. The contributions that fair legal processes, by police forces, legal professionals, and court personnel including judges, can make to individuals' sense of well-being, and of being valued, have been addressed in the psychological literature [7]. Unfortunately, such literature is rarely included in legal or judicial training.

Sexually Transmitted Infections

Many legal systems have provisions for the protection of public health that include compulsory reporting to public health agencies of diagnoses of sexually transmitted infections (STIs). Mandatory reporting may be anonymous regarding diagnosed patients' identities, serving only statistical and demographic purposes of infection control, but where personal identities are reportable, for instance, to allow contact-tracing, legal and ethical issues of medical confidentiality arise. The terms 'confidentiality' and 'privacy' are often applied synonymously, but for legal and ethical purposes they are distinguishable. The distinction is drawn that confidentiality protects professional relationships, such as between doctor and patient, lawyer and client, priest and confessant, while privacy protects and may regulate use of information or data itself that may have implications for the individuals from whom it is derived and others, such as their family members [8]. Accordingly, mandatory reports of STIs may result in public health officers informing contacts of infected persons that they have been exposed to infection without disclosing the identities of the possible source of infection. This may result in an individual being suspected of being the source, correctly or mistakenly.

In some communities infection with STIs is accepted as a common lifestyle risk, but in others

knowledge of individuals' infection is stigmatizing, humiliating, and disempowering to them. Infected persons may lose employment, educational, social, and other opportunities. Disclosure may even expose them to violence and death, such as in so-called honor killings of women believed to have brought shame and dishonor on their families. In recent decades, since the appearance of HIV infection, HIV-positive women have been sterilized without their informed consent, ostracized from their communities and families, and obstructed or marginalized in access to health services, particularly in pregnancy and childbirth, which is liable to expose attendants to their body fluids.

Failure to disclose HIV positivity to prospective sexual partners has been a source of criminal conviction, dating to when HIV transmission was presumed to lead to the acquired immunodeficiency syndrome (AIDS) and rapid death. Where modern treatment is available, however, AIDS is no longer regarded as a lethal infection but as a chronic infection with which treated individuals can live prolonged lives. Nevertheless, even when a condom is used and a person's viral load is low, so that the risk of transmitting HIV infection is low, nondisclosure of HIV positivity often remains open to prosecution, with a possibility, if not likelihood, of conviction for aggravated sexual assault [9]. This possible liability is to provide strong assurance that individuals will not be deceived into unprotected sexual relations with HIV-infected partners.

Fertility

Fertility Control

The World Health Organization published a comprehensive legal and human rights overview of sexual health in 2015 [10]. Its report notes that discrimination and inequality can impair enjoyment of sexual health, and recognizes that human sexuality includes many different behaviors and expressions, observing that accommodation of this diversity contributes to individuals' overall sense of well-being and health. The report covers a wider area than the concept of reproductive health. This was defined at the UN International Conference on Population and Development, held in Cairo in 1994, and adopted at the UN International Conference on Women held in Beijing in 1995. The full definition reads:

Reproductive health is a state of complete physical, mental and social well-being and not merely the absence of disease or infirmity, in all matters relating to the reproductive system and to its functions and processes. Reproductive health therefore implies that people are able to have a satisfying and safe sex life and that they have the capability to reproduce and the freedom to decide if, when and how often to do so. Implicit in this last condition are the rights of men and women to be informed and to have access to safe, effective, affordable and acceptable methods of family planning of their choice, as well as other methods of their choice for regulation of fertility which are not against the law, and the right of access to appropriate healthcare services that will enable women to go safely through pregnancy and childbirth and provide couples with the best chance of having a healthy infant [11].

The claim that individuals have the ethical right and should have 'the freedom to decide if, when and how often' to have children through 'methods of family planning of their choice' refers to methods of contraception and contraceptive sterilization. The Beijing Declaration rejected abortion as a method of family planning, including this only among 'other methods ... for regulation of fertility which are not against the law.' Because some family planning associations may also provide abortion services for failure of contraceptive means, however, to limit resort to unsafe abortion, opponents of family planning identify such associations as abortion providers. A leading opponent of barrier, chemical, and other artificial means of human reproductive self-determination is the Roman Catholic Church, which has international influence. This may well be entering an era of change over the coming years.

Due to the historical European origins of international law and institutions, the Roman Catholic Church, through the Holy See, is the only religious denomination to have status in the United Nations Organization, and representation at UN conferences. Seeing pregnancy and childbirth as gifts of divine grace or blessing that it is impertinent for humans to frustrate or contrive for themselves, and human sexual intercourse outside lawful marriage for the purpose of procreation as sinful, officers of the church, having forsworn marriage and a 'satisfying and safe sex life' for themselves, rejected the definition and very concept of reproductive health. They sought alliances with delegates from the most conservative Islamic countries to preserve the illicit, and,

where possible, illegal character of family planning means, including in their view abortion, except perhaps for 'natural' family planning [12].

From the earliest times, which some date back before the original Hippocratic Oath's resistance to abortion, artificial means of fertility control have attracted religious and conservative condemnation, which conservative forces strove to maintain in Beijing. This aggravates emotional distress, turmoil, and tension for adherents to religious faiths regarding receipt, and delivery, of a wide spectrum of reproductive health services, beginning with chemical or barrier methods of contraception. The emotional struggle is not new, however, since humans have sought, and often successfully used, contraceptive means for millennia, as recorded in ancient texts of herbal medicine [13]. The tradition of herbal contraception and abortion has persisted, as women's special knowledge, for centuries, although suppressed in medieval Europe when possessors of this knowledge suffered religiously inspired death for witchcraft.

Religious discipline once operated principally by threat of divine and temporal retribution but, with the decline of legal sanctions for breach, now exerts force psychologically through guilt. Those reared in religious or conservative cultures may feel discomfort, distress, and remorse in their resort to contraception, contraceptive sterilization, or abortion, and in delivering many, if not all, reproductive health services. As healthcare professionals, they may seek to pursue specialties as little related as they can be to such services, but may violate terms of legal contracts with patients or of employment if they refuse services within their specialty associated indirectly with reproductive healthcare. Psychiatrists treating patients seeking relief from sadness following termination of pregnancy, for instance, on the end of a relationship, dermatologists treating sexually active patients for syphilitic scarring, and public health officers regulating location of massage parlors and striptease clubs they recognize may be bases of prostitution must use their professional skills and experience nonjudgmentally, unless perhaps legislation affords them exemption on grounds of conscience.

Conscientious Objection

Ethical respect for conscience would entitle physicians to participate as well as object to participate, for instance, in abortion procedures [14]. At present, however, legislation and judicially interpreted customary law have addressed only conscientious objection. Claims of conscientious objection have risen particularly with liberalization of restrictive abortion laws but are also involved regarding contraception and sterilization, including by nurses, midwives, and, for instance, pharmacists who refuse to fill contraception prescriptions. The right of conscientious objection allows healthcare practitioners the comfort of reconciling their personal beliefs with their professional practice. The burden falls, however, on patients eligible for care who face frustration and the negative, possibly humiliating judgment of those to whom they turn for care, perhaps when they lack practicable alternatives. Apart from being confronted by professionals' apparent moral condemnation, patients' knowledge that, without prior notice, the practitioners to whom they turn, often for time-sensitive care, may deny them indicated care without recourse, introduces uncertainty and apprehension into what they require and seek as a supportive professional relationship of patient dependency and trust.

An expansion of denial of lawful services occurs not only when those more remote from service delivery, such as health facility administrators, nursing attendants responsible to serve meals and provide routine comfort for bed-ridden hospitalized patients, and ambulance attendants, invoke conscientious objection in order to withhold services, but also when physicians, pharmacists, and others claim that contraceptive products are abortifacients. A further expansion occurs when objection is taken not only to participation in procedures but also to being complicit in their performance. This claim is under development in the United States, but, if it progresses, is likely to be presented elsewhere with support of international religious organizations. The claim is that it is as wrong even incidentally to permit another person's sin as to commit that sin oneself [15].

Ethics committees of professional associations in medicine, law, and other disciplines, and courts of law, are setting limits to procedures to which conscientious objection can be claimed, and requiring those who invoke conscience to refer patients, in a timely fashion, to comparable practitioners who do not object. It has similarly been proposed that medical professional associations might serve both patients and their members by becoming sources of referral to non-objecting practitioners [16]. There is also close

to universal agreement that conscientious objection cannot be invoked when a patient's life or continuing health is at grave risk, including by suicide. For instance, the Roman Catholic Church accepts the philosophical concept of double effect, accepting the incidental effect of a deliberate act that would be sinful to achieve as its primary purpose [17]. Terminating a life-endangering pregnancy would be seen as an unavoidable incident of a legitimate purpose, in the same way as removing a man's cancerous testicles, leaving him sterile, would not be seen as a sterilization procedure but legitimate cancer treatment.

Abortion

The human practice of abortion is as old as understanding of the cause and symptoms of pregnancy, as historical herbal medicine shows, but access to lawful services remains strongly contested, both for and against. International experience is that countries with the most restrictive laws have relatively high rates of abortion-related maternal mortality and morbidity, showing that laws affect the safety, rather than the incidence, of the practice, while countries with effective birth control access and education have low rates of unwanted pregnancy [18]. Rates of unlawful and therefore clandestine abortion are calculable only by estimates based on maternal deaths and hospital admissions, since safely conducted procedures go unrecognized and are not publicized, and definitional uncertainty remains in law between abortion and menstrual regulation or extraction procedures.

Unwanted pregnancy is commonly a source of anxiety, particularly where counselling is not reliably confidential and termination options may be unlawful. Decisions both to terminate and continue pregnancies, unplanned and planned, can be sources of regret [19], but opponents of abortion have claimed that a 'post-abortion stress syndrome' exists and is pathological, requiring strong emphasis in counselling [20]. This condition is not part of routine professional counselling beyond advising clients that they will live with the consequence of their choices. In contrast, the authoritative Diagnostic and Statistical Manual of Mental Disorders, now DSM-5, includes postpartum depression and psychosis, with diagnostic symptoms of a major depressive disorder with postpartum onset [21]. This has a history of legal recognition, for instance, by reducing the crime committed when women, within 12 months of delivery, kill their newborn children, from murder to infanticide, with lesser punishment.

Opponents of liberal abortion law reform are conscious that much of the institutional organization is mobilized by religious hierarchies in which women are underrepresented, absent or excluded. Members of the Roman Catholic hierarchy, for instance, are unaffected in their personal lives by their doctrines' effects on women's lives, because they have neither wives, daughters nor granddaughters. To overcome the charge of being unsympathetic to women, abortion opponents, many of whom are women, adopt the strategy of advocating 'women-protective' legal restrictions, among which banning sex-selection abortions, presumed to target female fetuses, may have appeal, and make prohibition of abortion rather than its acceptance legally 'normal,' as it was throughout most of the past two and more centuries [22].

Infertility

Medically Assisted Reproduction (MAR)

The standard of care of their patients that health service professionals are required to maintain is determined as a matter of law, but courts usually defer to the professions themselves, unless exceptionally the professions set standards or endorse practices that courts find to be against public interest or protection. In March 2015, the Psychology and Counselling Guideline Development Group of the European Society of Human Reproduction and Embryology published guidance for clinic staff members that courts may accept as evidence of what is required in routine care [23]. It should be remembered, however, that guidelines guide but do not necessarily govern practice, so that in particular cases practitioners may be able to justify to courts' satisfaction why they departed from professional guidance.

Intense emotions are frequently aroused by infertility, such as the frustration and despair of those failing to achieve much-wanted pregnancy, and the hopes that clinic staff share with them that this cycle of treatment will succeed. The law, however, takes an unromantic, even materialistic approach to the process involved in MAR. For instance, leading courts facing new issues raised by MAR regard gametes and embryos as a species of legal property [24]. When in 2000 the Constitutional Chamber of the Supreme Court of Justice of Costa Rica invoked violation of the right to life of embryos liable to remain untransferred to women's bodies in order to ban in vitro fertilization (IVF), the Inter-American Court of Human Rights required removal of the ban, since it violated infertile couples' human and legal rights, among others, to privacy and to private and family life in their quest to have children. The Court observed that embryo loss and wastage are as legally tolerable in IVF as in natural reproduction, because the Court-appointed expert scientific witness testified that, of every ten embryos naturally generated in humans, no more than two or three survive natural selection to be born as persons. The Court reviewed European and additional international jurisprudence to conclude that:

> the historic and systematic interpretation of precedents that exist in the Inter-American system confirms that it is not admissible to grant the status of person to the embryo. [25]

The new reproductive technologies require the law to be flexible, and willing to reconsider its conventional attitudes, lest it may become an obstacle to necessary or desirable scientific progress for the public benefit [26]. The progress in social attitudes to MAR in many economically developed countries follows the trajectory observed a half-century ago regarding artificial insemination:

> Any change in custom or practice in this emotionally-charged area has always elicited a response from established custom and law of horrified negation at first; then negation without horror; then slow and gradual curiosity, study, evaluation, and finally a very slow but steady acceptance. [27]

Gametes, Embryos, and Parenthood

The World Health Organization characterizes infertility as a disease [28]. In the same way that blood transfusion and organ donation have been developed to treat disease, gamete and embryo donation has come, where legally permitted, to treat infertility disease. Comparable issues of legal ownership, possession, and control of gametes and embryos in transit between donors and recipients arise, but a key difference concerns determination of parenthood when a child is born of these transactions [29]. Laws in most countries, with United States' exceptionalism, prohibit commercial payments, but even where allowed, custody of children at birth or afterward is usually determined not by private agreements among adults but according to Article 3(1) of the UN

Convention on the Rights of the Child, which provides that:

> In all actions concerning children, whether undertaken by public or private social welfare institutions, courts of law, administrative authorities or legislative bodies, the best interests of the child shall be a primary consideration.

Laws historically have been based on tenacious presumptions, such as that a child born to a married woman during the marriage or within 300 days of its end, by death or divorce, is her husband's, to avoid the stigma of illegitimacy (bastardy), unless he denies this and another man claims paternity, and that a woman is the legal mother of a child she gestates and delivers. Such presumptions are now disrupted by legal accommodation of gamete and embryo donation, and surrogate motherhood. The law's intention to provide the psychological comfort of legal certainty of parenthood presents the discomfort of ethical adjustment or opposition, since religions and cultures rarely evolve at the speed of which legal reform is capable [30]. Legal recognition, for instance, of same-sex marriage and parenthood, often by the medicalization of reproduction through MAR or surrogacy, permits the biological impossibility of a child both of whose legal parents are of the same sex as each other [31]. Conservative cultures and individuals tend to find such legal developments stressful and destabilizing.

Surrogate Motherhood

First evident through the tumultuous *Baby M* child custody trials in New Jersey late in the 1980s [32], when a surrogate mother recovered the child, her genetic daughter, from the genetic father and his wife to whom she had surrendered the child at birth, surrogate motherhood is now legally accommodated and regularized in many countries to achieve participants' intentions, namely, that women who gestate children for others, usually through IVF and embryo transfer, are not their legal mothers, and commissioning parents, often but not always genetically related to the children surrendered to them, are their legal parents [33]. The much publicized *Baby M* trial resulted in a judicial order of joint custody between the mutually reproachful and hostile genetic mother and father, described by an authority on children's laws as 'indisputably the logical, reasoned, and straightforward result of existing legal concepts of parenthood, adoption, baby-selling and the like' but

also as 'surely the worst result possible' [34]. The experience served early notice of the need for psychological assessment and counselling of participants in such arrangements. Failure of assessment and counselling resulting in emotional trauma for adult participants, which may affect resulting children, may constitute legal negligence.

Adding to the cultural and often socioeconomic gap that often divides those who offer surrogate motherhood services to strangers from those who engage them are geographical divisions, when would-be parents cross national borders for services. This phenomenon affects many, if not all, forms of MAR, most contentiously to obtain services unlawful in individuals' countries of residence [35], but has potential for mutual exploitation regarding surrogacy, where women may be hired for low-cost services or hold newborns for ransom to increase payments. So-called reproductive tourism is an aspect of 'medical tourism,' [36] but the description 'tourism' is ethically objectionable. The term associates seeking care abroad with the indulgence of spare time and money for leisure and curiosity, but trivializes and demeans the intense emotions usually invested in seeking medical care in general and parenthood in particular.

Surrogate pregnancies are usually initiated by IVF and embryo transfer, and travel for these purposes may expose individuals to differences between cultures and religions, and differences within them. In Islamic countries, for instance, some allow sperm and embryo donation, while others, giving more weight to the authenticity of parental, particularly paternal, genetic lineage, do not [37]. How births are registered can also differ, some birth registration systems holding the gestational women the mothers, while others that consider the sources of sperm to be the fathers consider the sources of the ova the mothers. When neither of the commissioning parents supplied gametes, systems may leave open registration of parentage, which makes a case in favor of more comprehensive legislation. France, for instance, which has an outright ban on surrogacy and has denied recognition to children so born, refusing immigration to children born outside the country to French nationals who participated in surrogacy transactions, now has judicial rulings, including from the European Court of Human Rights, requiring recognition and issuing of documents recognizing the children's French nationality [38].

This illustrates how laws on sexual and reproductive rights and health are under continuous evolution through the interaction of legislation and court judgments. It also illustrates how practitioners and analysts of this field must remain vigilant to observe legal developments under various influences.

Key Points

- Legal requirements that identify transgendered individuals by reference only to their biological sex determined at birth disrupt public order and constitute a source of humiliation, distress, and social dysfunction.
- In cases of sexual assault, the legal processes of detection and prosecution may inadvertently be aggravating factors in victims' psychological anguish.
- In some communities knowledge of individuals' sexually transmitted infection is stigmatizing, humiliating, and disempowering to them.
- Health professionals must use their professional skills and experience nonjudgmentally when dealing with matters relating to fertility control. This includes not only gynecologists but also psychiatrists, dermatologists, public health officers, nurses, midwives, pharmacists and other professionals.
- The new reproductive technologies require the law to be flexible, and willing to reconsider its conventional attitudes, to facilitate scientific progress.
- Historical presumptions pertaining to parenthood are now disrupted by the accommodation of gamete and embryo donation, surrogate motherhood, and same-sex marriage in contemporary law. Conservative cultures and individuals tend to find such legal developments stressful and destabilizing.
- Surrogate motherhood may expose individuals to differences between and within cultures, religions, and legal systems. Practitioners and analysts of reproductive medicine must remain conversant with rapidly changing laws in their field.

References

1. Cook R, Dickens B, Fathalla M. *Reproductive Health and Human Rights: Integrating Medicine, Ethics and Law*. Oxford, Oxford University Press, 2003.

2. Ferriter D. *Occasions of Sin; Sex & Society in Modern Ireland*. London, Profile Books, 2009.

3. Alzheimer's Society (England and Wales) Factsheet 514 LP: Sex and Dementia (PDF) 2013.

4. Knop K (ed.) *Gender and Human Rights*. Oxford, Oxford University Press, 2004.

5. US Department of Justice. Office of Violence against Women. *A National Protocol for Sexual Assault Medical Forensic Examinations. Adults/Adolescents*. 2nd edn. April 2013. NCJ 2281 19. www.ncjrs.gov/pdf files 1/ovw/241903. pdf. Accessed 23 March 2017.

6. World Health Organization. *Responding to Intimate Partner Violence and Sexual Violence Against Women*. WHO clinical and policy guidelines Geneva, WHO, 2013.

7. Thibaut J, Walker L. *Procedural Justice: A Psychological Analysis*. Hillsdale, NJ, Lawrence Erlbaum Associates, 1975; Lind EA, Tyler TR. *The Social Psychology of Procedural Justice*. New York, Plenum Press, 1988.

8. Laurie GT. Challenging medical-legal norms: The role of autonomy, confidentiality, and privacy in protecting individual, and familial group rights in genetic information. *J Legal Medicine* 2001; 22: 1–54.

9. See the full discussion in the Supreme Court of Canada in the case *R. v. Mabior*, [2012] 2 Supreme Court Reports 584.

10. World Health Organization. *Sexual Health, Human Rights and the Law*. Geneva, WHO, 2015.

11. UN Department of Public Information. Platform for Action and Beijing Declaration. Fourth World Conference on Women, Beijing, China, 4–15 September 1995. New York, UN, 1995, para. 94.

12. Fehring RJ, Kurz W. Anthropological differences between contraception and natural family planning. In: Koterski JW, ed. *Life and Learning X: Proceedings of the Tenth University Faculty for Life Conference, June 2000*, Washington, DC, University Faculty for Life. 2002; 237–64.

13. See De Materia Medica by the Greek physician, pharmacologist and botanist Pedanius Discorides, born c. AD 40.

14. Dickens BM. The right to conscience. In: Cook RJ, Erdman JN, Dickens BM (eds) *Abortion Law in Transnational Perspective: Cases and Controversies*. Philadelphia, University of Pennsylvania Press. 2014; 210–38.

15. Nejaime D, Siegel RB. Conscience wars: Complicity-based conscience claims in religion and politics. *Yale Law J.* 2015; 124: 2516–91.

16. Lynch HF. *Conflicts of Conscience in Health Care: An Institutional Compromise.* Boston, Massachusetts Institute of Technology Press. 2008; FIGO [International Federation of Gynecology and Obstetrics]. Committee for the Study of Ethical Aspects of Human Reproduction, *Ethical Issues in Obstetrics and Gynecology* London, FIGO, 2015.

17. Boyle JM. Toward understanding the principle of double effect. *Ethics* 1980; 90: 527–38. See also FIGO [International Federation of Gynecology and Obstetrics]. Committee for the Study of Ethical Aspects of Human Reproduction, *Ethical Issues in Obstetrics and Gynecology*, London, FIGO, 2015.

18. Sedgh G, Singh S, Shah IH, Ahman E, Henshaw SK, Bankole E. Induced abortion: Incidence and trends worldwide from 1995 to 2008. *Lancet* 2012; 379 (9816): 625–32.

19. Appleton SF. Reproduction and regret. *Yale J Law and Feminism* 2011; 23: 255–333.

20. Vandewalker I. Abortion and informed consent: How biased counseling laws mandate violations of medical ethics. *Michigan J Gender and the Law* 2012; 19: 1–70.

21. American Psychiatric Association. *Diagnostic and Statistical Manual of Mental Disorders.* 5th edn. Arlington, VA, American Psychiatric Publishing. 2013: 186–7.

22. Yahalom TR. Strange bedfellows: The destigmatization of anti-abortion reform. *Columbia J of Gender and Law* 2015; 30(2): 529–48; Siegel RB. The right's reasons: Constitutional conflict and the spread of women-protective antiabortion argument, *Duke Law J* 2008; 57: 101–49.

23. European Society of Human Reproduction and Embryology (ESHRE). *Routine Psychosocial Care in Infertility and Medically Assisted Reproduction – A Guide for Fertility Staff.* ESHRE; March 2015, www .eshre.eu/Guidelines-and-Legal/Guidelines/Psychosoc ial-care-guideline.aspx. Accessed 23 March 2017.

24. Dickens B, Cook R. The Legal Status of In Vitro Embryos. *Int J Gynecol Obstet* 2010; 111: 91–4.

25. Artavia Murillo et al. ("In Vitro Fertilization") v. Costa Rica Judgment of November 28, 2012 (Inter-American Court of Human Rights), para. 223.

26. Cook RJ, Dickens BM. Reproductive health and the law. In: Ferguson PR, Laurie GT, eds. *Inspiring*

a Medico-Legal Revolution: Essays in Honour of Sheila McLean. Farnham, Surrey and Burlington, VT, Ashgate. 2015; 3–23.

27. Kleegman SJ, Kaufman SA. *Infertility in Women.* Philadelphia, PA Davis, 1966; 178.

28. World Health Organization. The International Committee for Monitoring Assisted Reproductive Technology (ICMART) and the World Health Organization (WHO) Revised glossary on ART terminology. *Human Reproduction* 2009; 24: 2683–7, at 2686.

29. Meyer DD. Parenthood in a time of transition: Tensions between legal, biological and social conceptions of parenthood. *Amer J Comparative Law* 2006; 54: 125–44.

30. Schenker JG, ed. *Ethical Dilemmas in Assisted Reproductive Technologies* Berlin/Boston, De Gruyter, 2011.

31. Norrie KMcK. Parenthood and artificial human reproduction: The dangers of inappropriate medicalisation. In Ferguson PR, Laurie GT, eds. See 26 above; 37–52.

32. In the Matter of Baby M, 1988, 537 Atlantic Reporter 2d 1227 (New Jersey Supreme Court), reversing in part 1987, 525 Atlantic Reporter 2d 1128 (New Jersey Superior Court).

33. Cook R, Sclater SD, Kaganas F, eds. *Surrogate Motherhood: International Perspectives.* Oxford, Hart Publishing, 2003.

34. Bezanson RP. Solomon would weep: A comment on In the Matter of Baby M and the limits of judicial authority. *Law, Medicine and Ethics* 1988; 16: 126–30 at 126.

35. Hodges JR, Turner L, Kimball AM, eds. *Risks and Challenges in Medical Tourism: Understanding the Global Market for Health Services.* Santa Barbara, CA, Praeger, 2012; Cohen IG. Circumvention tourism. Cornell Law Rev. 2012; 97: 1309–98.

36. Bookman MZ, Bookman KR. *Medical Tourism in Developing Countries.* New York, Palgrave Macmillan. 2007.

37. Behjati-Ardakani Z, Karoubi MT, Milanifar AR, Masrouri R, Okhandi MM. Embryo donation in Iranian legal system: A Critical Review. *J Reprod Infertil* 2015; 16: 130–7.

38. Sotto P. Surrogate children get legal recognition in France. *Time* magazine. July 3, 2015.

Chapter

25

The Psychobiology of Birth

Amali Lokugamage, Theresa Bourne and Alison Barrett

The long-term implications for birth and the early postnatal period on maternal, fetal and neonatal health are evidenced within the literature [1–25]. Normal labour and birth can bring about psychobiological changes that promote physical and emotional health which is limited not only to the fetus/neonate and mother but also to the family unit and society. The understanding of some of the elements underlying these psychobiological perspectives of birth allows health professionals to embed these factors and values within their care.

Section 1 – The Women

Understanding the biophysical processes in labour is an important aspect of maintaining 'normality', even when the processes may be disturbed by medical events. An example would include an understanding of the mechanics of the birth and how more upright, forward positions (including kneeling) assist the birth process. This allows pelvic joints to increase in mobility creating wider pelvic diameters and enabling gravity to assist the pelvic floor and the fetus to negotiate the intra-pelvic turns necessary for effective birth. In addition upright positions have been reported to stimulate the release of oxytocin and cervical prostaglandins [17]. It has been proposed that encouraging women to mobilize and adopt upright positions in labour would be of value in reducing later interventions. This has been demonstrated to improve birth outcomes with reduced duration of first stage, less epidurals and fewer instrumental and caesarean births [26]. It clearly is also associated with a sense of increased maternal control.

Oxytocin

There is a divergent and conflicting relationship between oxytocin and adrenalin (which produces the fight, flight or frozen response) [27] so the underlying factors that increase stress and fear in the labour ward

can have implications for labour and breastfeeding. Uvnäs Moberg emphasizes the importance of enabling the normal birth process which amplifies the oxytocin response, and the higher oxytocin levels are associated with positive emotions [17, 28].

This corroborates the social neurobiological theory that oxytocin encourages calmness, trust, generosity, compassion and social cohesion through the neurobiology of maternal and pair bonding, thus also, conversely, providing insights into the origins of human anxiety and violence[25].

The use of synthetic or exogenous oxytocin in nulliparous labour has continued to grow in recent years with an associated increase in epidurals, instrumental and caesarean births and their related complications [29]. Bugg et al. [30] note no differences between the use and non-use of oxytocin in either the type of delivery or Apgar score; the only apparent difference was an average increase of two hours in the duration of labour in those receiving synthetic oxytocin. They consider that maternal, rather than medical, decision making should be the deciding factor in use.

However, in a period of healthcare rationalization the judicious use of oxytocin should also be considered, and proactive attention to other factors that may inhibit or enhance labour would be beneficial. These may include mobility and positioning, continuity of caregiver, touch, the prevention of ketone formation (eating and drinking) and reducing adrenaline in the early first stage of labour [31].

The use of oxytocin for the augmentation of labour can increase the risk of uterine hyperstimulation and associated problems. The literature also suggests that exogenous oxytocin, whether for delivery of the baby or placenta, can influence the mother's postdelivery production of natural oxytocin. In addition, although exogenous oxytocin is an effective uterotonic drug, its delivery is usually continuous (rather than pulsatile), its effect is short-lived and it may fail to cross the blood–brain barrier, providing the necessary physiological changes required in maternal and fetal adaption [32]. Oxytocin is also involved in the release of prostaglandins, endorphins, cortisol and other hormones, all of which have interrelated functions and effects in labour and the puerperium [33].

There is a growing knowledge around the effects of endogenous oxytocin. Many of the effects are short term, but it is also linked with the initiation of many biophysical and chemical responses that are of a longer duration [34]. It is recognized as a neurotransmitter that is important not only for labour and breastfeeding but also for its influence on a wide range of social behaviours including mother–infant interactions [35].

Apart from its role in contracting the uterus, the management of third stage and the let-down reflex, oxytocin has an essential role in maternal and neonatal neuroplasticity around birth. This hormone has a strong role in maternal/neonatal smell, interactions and the formation of social bonds [4]. Disturbances may have implications for social imprinting, stress management for later life and parenting [36].

It should be noted though that this mood-altering hormone can mediate against depression, it may itself be affected by drugs prescribed for depression [27]. Thus there may be interaction between antidepressant use in the third trimester and postpartum haemorrhage, but evidence at present is inconclusive [37].

Fear and Pain

Women have long feared the pain of labour and the consequences (see Chapter 34, Tokophobia). Indeed fear is linked with an increased risk of elective caesarean not only among nulliparous women but also for a growing number of women in subsequent pregnancies [38]. In the pressured health service an elective caesarean may appear a satisfactory resolution to a previous traumatic event. Nevertheless Ryding et al. [38] point out that there are often linked mental health issues and unresolved concerns with a previous birth. These unresolved issues may manifest themselves in alteration of physiological effects. In providing an automatic elective caesarean on request for such women, we negate the very processes important in the release of natural oxytocin during late pregnancy and labour with the linked health and social benefits for the development of the neonate, child and adult. Also negated by elective caesarean section is the effect of the pelvic curve and head compression on the baby's adaptation to neonatal life [4].

Fear of childbirth has been associated with emergency caesarean, prolonged labour, dystocia and poor experiences for mothers. Ryding et al. [38] suggest that appropriate referral for discussion and behavioural therapies rather than 'avoiding' the issue may yield more positive outcomes and better coping strategies; the research of Rouhe et al. [39] would support this. It is important to consider social, media and cultural aspects of fear in relation to labour and birth as well as previous experience.

Pain sensations of labour are important elements in birth. Pain sensation releases endorphins and other hormones in the mother which pass to the baby in labour and if the mother does not experience some degree of pain sensation the opportunity for fetal transfer of endorphins is reduced or eliminated. As labour develops, cortisol and the hormones adrenaline and noradrenaline begin to rise. Later in labour these are beneficial to the fetus in that they have opposite effects on the central nervous system and sympathetic and parasympathetic nervous system of the fetus compared to the adult, diverting blood from fetal extremities to the brain, which is neuroprotective [40]. Moreover, cortisol activates the central nervous system, promotes lung maturity and transition to extra-uterine life as well as promotes increased maternal behaviours following birth [4]. Forgoing the 'stress' of labour thus may have significant long-term consequences [40]. To what extent this is fact versus conjecture remains to be elucidated.

For example, in non-randomized studies, the neonates of mothers who had epidurals and/or systemic opioids during labour (compared to the neonates of mothers who had none) exhibited reduced breast-seeking and breastfeeding behaviours [4, 41]. These neonates were less likely to breastfeed within 150 minutes of birth and tended to cry more, whereas 90–100% of neonates not exposed to these medications exhibited all six measured positive breastfeeding behaviours. Epidurals have also been associated with the persistence of the occipito-posterior malposition of the fetus which is directly linked to more interventions and operative delivery [42].

Parents may be all too aware of the 'risk' of pain but not the rationale. At present, phrasing in discussions may be about the removal of pain rather than the increase of pain tolerance. Health professionals can discuss choices, including non-pharmacological approaches that may improve pain tolerance and support the maternal and neonatal physiological changes at these times. In order to do so, they need to be conversant with these techniques as much as the pharmacological methods.

Labour-mediated changes in the stress hormones adrenaline and cortisol have important effects in labour. Adrenaline aids the expulsive efforts of the contraction and cortisol potentially aids oxytocin in crossing the blood/brain and placental barriers and initiating further biophysical/chemical responses in mother and fetus [4]. In early labour adrenaline may have an inhibitory effect and strategies to lower stress such as labouring at home and the provision of continuity of carer may impact on birth outcomes such as reducing the incidence of labour dystocia [31]. These have certainly been factors shown to improve such outcomes; the evidence that these are mediated through the endocrine mechanisms is less clear, though theoretically plausible.

Infection

Sepsis remains a concern of every health professional. In maternity care, invading bacteria can cause postpartum sepsis, an especially feared complication of childbirth before the era of antibiotics but still a leading cause of maternal mortality today. In the past, measures to eradicate sepsis included baths, enemas, shaving, sterile prep and drapes as well as the zealous use of antibiotics.

While judicious use of antibiotics has obvious benefits, an evolving understanding of the human microbiome has led to growing concern about the long-term consequences of their injudicious use. Through indiscriminate use of drugs and practices that alter the maternal microbiome not only may we be creating drug resistant bacteria we may also be eliminating or curtailing the seeding of healthy bacteria within the fetus and neonate [43]. Links with non-communicable disease and conditions are becoming stronger and no longer can we ignore the importance of addressing this issue [44].

Stress in pregnancy, antibiotics and the mode of delivery all influence the microbiome (uterine and vaginal) available for the fetus and this 'seeding' [43, 45].

It is likely that commensal maternal vaginal flora, seeded into the neonatal gut flora during a vaginal birth, may play an important part in the development of the neonate's immunity. Gut microbiota influence gut neurochemistry which in turn may impact on central nervous function.

Therefore healthy gut microbiota may be important factors in some psychological as well as physical conditions of the offspring, some of which may impact on subsequent societal health [43, 45]. Where possible the aim for a vaginal birth will reduce long-term health risks; however, early skin-to-skin and long-term breastfeeding may help mediate against some of this [46, 47]. Nonetheless, most forms of medical intervention are likely to decrease the establishment of breastfeeding and mother-baby attachment [46, 48].

Complications at Birth

In a study of a Danish cohort of 4,269 consecutive live male births, investigators found that birth complications in combination with early child rejection can predispose to violent crime [49, 50]. There are associations with early life stress and low adult plasma concentrations of oxytocin. The findings illustrate the critical importance of integrating biological with social measures to fully understand how violence develops and also suggest that prenatal, perinatal and early postnatal healthcare interventions could influence predisposition to violent behaviour later in life.

When complications occur and there is a need for intervention, how does the health professional enable normal birth processes? Parental involvement in decisions and control is often associated with increased birth satisfaction but often, where obstetric complications occur, it is difficult to facilitate this process [51]. In 2013 in a UK report on the quality of care in England [52], one of the most common concerns during labour was inadequate care and advice. Women also raised concerns about delayed and conflicting advice. The report also highlighted that health professionals spoke to women in a 'disrespectful, patronising and condescending manner', resulting in women feeling anxious, being demeaned and not listened to [52, p.11]. This has improved in the 2015 report [53] but still 25% of mothers do not always feel fully involved in the decision making process and 30% felt post delivery they were not always treated with kindness and respect.

Shared decision making and strategies to support this in the antenatal period are important elements in enabling and empowering the woman during the birth period. This is also seen as essential for women who have had a previous caesarean section [53].

In a high-risk situation, however, this may be more challenging. Consideration of how control might remain with the woman when complications occur should be an important aspect of care. This may be achieved by improving and preserving aspects of normality, for example

- encouraging mobility and differing labouring positions despite the necessary medicalized elements of the birth
- where an instrumental delivery is necessary bringing the head to the introitus and encouraging her to deliver her child
- maintaining communication, dignity and compassion where a caesarean is required
- encouraging skin to skin contact as soon as maternal/neonatal condition permit.

Where complications have occurred it is essential to consider future births and the impact this birth may have on future pregnancies and delivery. Opportunities should be available to discuss issues arising and clear documentation should be available to support decision making and support in the future.

Breastfeeding

Birth is only the beginning of a journey and the biopsychosocial approach encompasses the postnatal care. No aspect of postnatal care is more significant to the long-term health of and child than breastfeeding. Breastfeeding is linked with reduced incidence of premenopausal breast cancer, ovarian cancer, retained gestational weight gain, type 2 diabetes, myocardial infarction and metabolic syndrome for the mother, and for the child a reduction in diabetes; obesity; recurrent ear infections; leukaemia; diarrhoea and hospitalization for lower respiratory tract infections [15].

Breastfeeding and active bonding protect against children's internalizing behaviour problems [54]. This leads to the dovetailing of the Early Years Agenda into the arguments of how important this foundation of psychobiology is to human development and likely represents a biosocial and holistic effect of physiological, nutritive and maternal–infant bonding benefits.

The Early Years Agenda and the economic gains to society from avoiding maladaptive neurodevelopment attributable to the of lack of parental bonding and emotional investment to childrearing have been adopted in a UK cross–political party manifesto called 1001 Critical Days: The Importance of the Conception to Age Two Period [55]. An All-Party Parliamentary Group also published a further report

in 2014 called 'Building Better Britons'[56], recommending the creation of a maternity system which optimizes normal birth, breast feeding and maternal bonding amongst other interventions in early childhood which are more cost effective than behavioural interventions delivered after this stage.

Section 2 – The Health Professional

Care around birth is constantly evolving and has an impact on its culture. There are potential tensions between women, their families, their caregivers and society itself; all create changes that direct how women perceive birth. Birthing is not purely a biomedical event. It is a biopsychosocial experience for mother and baby providing the link with either optimum or less than optimum physiological and emotional well-being for mother and baby. It is not meaningfully defined for many women in terms of 'morbidity and mortality outcomes' but in quality of the experience overall. If a woman has complications, some of these terms may have more relevance to her. Nevertheless it is not just the life/death moments that remain indelible but memories linked to the event and care provided which may cause long-term psychosocial pathology [57].

The psychosocial elements of birth are difficult to measure. Empowerment is one such aspect and is explored in some epidemiological studies, but other factors are explored through documentaries such as 'Orgasmic Birth' [58].

Dissociating short-term from long-term outcomes around birth within epidemiological studies also alienates the medical from social models of birth. Since midwives and obstetricians generally restrict their care to pregnancy, birth and early postnatal period, the longitudinal perspective on the mode of childbirth and its impact on the family – and therefore society as a whole – is lost. Zander, a GP with a rich experience in home birth and long-term care of families, observed differences between women giving birth at home and in hospital [22–24]. He noticed that the memories around birth were vivid and were associated with sharp recall, an important consideration in our care and the long-term mental well-being of women.

Ogden et al. [22–24] noted that whether or not birth actually occurred at home or in the hospital, women who chose home birth as an option were more likely to rate the experience as positive as opposed to the hospital-based mothers who tended to recall negative events. They also identified how women who gave birth in the hospital were more likely to cite the achievement of others (the doctor or midwife) than themselves in their own birth.

Fear, Litigation and the 'Blame Game'

When outcomes are potentially poor and risk is high, health professionals fear they may be implicated. This tends to generate the fear of litigation and drives defensive or risk-averse practice. The driving forces may be professional accountability and altruism, but the health professionals' concerns may include professional survival and impact on their family and the impact both financially and psychologically from threats to their career. Self and professional protection relies on the shift of blame and the 'blame' game which may impede professional and care relationships. Additionally, decisions 'offered' to women may be couched to limit perceived 'safe' choices[59].

Moreover, the focus of obstetricians' care is where there is a need for crisis management rather when the normal physiology is working. This creates a skewed view of birth, where the body is perceived as infirm and reliant on the need for intervention. Care shifts from supporting the normal physiological process to monitoring and visiting 'just in case' of a problem arising. Additionally, where medical intervention is needed there is a tendency to take over, rather than support, the normal physiological processes. This may be so as much for midwives where resources and culture limit the possibility for promoting normality [60].

Furthermore, clinical negligence schemes for hospitals require staff to complete increasingly larger amounts of contemporaneous documentation whilst caring for a woman in labour. Although vital in reviewing care, this inevitably detracts from the time a professional has to give emotional support to a woman in labour and enable self-driven decision making. Continuous emotional and physical support improves the physiology and outcomes of labour, but this may be hindered as the focus shifts to paperwork [61]. Perversely, the drive to appraise risk may actually be increasing it, by limiting the capacity to enable physiological birth and exacerbating the risk of requiring an intervention.

Stress

Work-related critical incidents may also induce post-traumatic stress symptoms or even post-traumatic stress disorder, anxiety and depression[62]. This can negatively affect healthcare practitioners' behaviours towards patients. It also affects the choices and care they provide as well as practitioner confidence in themselves, women and others. Moral distress is not uncommon and is found in all health professionals[63]. It occurs when the professional wishes to follow one course of action but is unable to because of organizational, cultural or resource constraints. It is associated with lowered compassion, burnout and employment mobility.

Interpersonal neurobiology recognizes that the carer impacts on the maternal neural plasticity and programming in the short term as much as the maternal care impacts on the long-term neonatal psychological development. Stress and fear can be transmitted and cause changes in the maternal neurobiology as much as compassionate care and confidence [9]. Conversely, stress and anxiety from the women and their families can impact on the professional reactions, decision making and health [18].

As discussed previously, the hormone oxytocin counterbalances fear, promoting positive emotions not only for labouring women and the neonate but also for their caregivers[17]. The environment of physiological birth may stimulate a higher oxytocin secretion within all who are present. Touch is one such mechanism that increases oxytocin in others and ourselves. Neuroeconomic research points to oxytocin nasal sprays helping humans to overcome their natural aversion to uncertainty with regard to the behaviour of others [64].

Stress may impact negatively on the production of cerebral oxytocin in the individual. Could this affect how practitioners care and offer choices? Conversely, oxytocin could mediate against high levels of stress [27]. It may be pertinent to consider ways to increase oxytocin activity in practitioners, strengthening the relationship between professional and woman as well as the practitioner's inner resources.

Section 3 – The Institution

Institutional ideologies such as obsession with economic targets, protocols, rigidly applied evidence-based medicine, medico-legal fear, lack of understanding of human rights in childbirth and high levels of burnout in staff are important in creating an atmosphere that makes birth hard or easy. *The Lancet*'s 2014 Midwifery Series [65] highlights that the industrial mechanistic model of maternity services may lack the insight to deliver compassion whether through lack of training, modelling in practice, internal and external pressures or a culture where staff as well as women are treated without respect or value [66]. Market forces where value is monetary rather than personal can result in a dehumanised approach to care where staff are considered units of provision as women are assets as long as they take no more time than that allotted.

Youngson [67] highlights how this approach may be flawed as compassion and holistic care leads to better health outcomes and therefore lower costs to the service[68]. Indeed higher empathy within health professionals in the delivery of care may reduce hospital admissions [69]. In maternity, continuous care by the same caregiver has an impact on maternity outcomes and costs [70, 71].

In addition, Youngson clearly demonstrates that healthcare worker burnout through working in dehumanized industrialized healthcare conditions leads to lack of compassion towards patients [67, 72]. Poor communication and attitudes, including lack of respect, are major areas of complaints within the NHS and professional bodies [73]. So there is direct impact on the woman's health from the psychological status of the care giver, which is influenced by working conditions.

There is a long history regarding the balance of female power versus patriarchal systems and particularly in childbirth [74]. Recent surveys in both the United Kingdom and the United States emphasize the need for practitioners to aim towards a healthcare system that supports women in their choices, offering respect and autonomy[75].

Summary

This chapter has articulated some of the important psychobiological factors in the modern maternity system. We have discussed the meaning of becoming a 'mother', the influence of the 'care providers' and the pressures exerted by the institution. The psychobiological dimensions of these three areas should influence future maternity system planning for the health of individuals as well as the health of society.

Key Points

- Birthing is not purely a biomedical event; it is a biopsychosocial experience for the family, and is not meaningfully defined for many women in terms of 'morbidity and mortality outcomes' but in quality of the experience overall.
- Endogenous oxytocin secretion is associated with a sense of maternal control, reduced duration of first stage, less epidurals and fewer operative deliveries. It also influences a wide range of social behaviours including mother–infant interactions. Disturbances of peri-partum endogenous oxytocin secretion can have implications for parenting, social imprinting and stress management in later life.
- Labour pain stimulates the release of maternal endorphins, cortisol and catecholamines which cross the placenta, activate the fetal central nervous system, promote fetal lung maturity and promote neonatal breast-seeking and breastfeeding behaviours. This means that forgoing the 'stress' of labour (e.g. through a planned caesarean birth) may have significant long-term consequences.
- Commensal maternal vaginal flora seeded into the neonatal gut flora during a vaginal birth may play an important role in the psychological and physical well-being of the offspring.
- Even in high-risk situations calling for medical intervention, it is often possible to preserve some aspects of 'normality' in childbirth.
- Breastfeeding protects the offspring from a range of medical and social problems in childhood and adult life.
- Obstetric and midwifery practice should support the normal physiological processes of labour. Perversely, obsessive risk appraisal and risk aversion may create hazard, by reducing the likelihood of physiological birth and increasing the chances of an avoidable medical intervention.
- Maternity institutions should nurture an organizational culture that promotes compassionate care, respect for rights, high staff morale and flexible application of evidence-supported care.

References

1. Bird JA, Spencer JA, Mould T, Symonds ME. Endocrine and metabolic adaptation following caesarean section or vaginal delivery. *Arch Dis Child Fetal Neonatal Ed* 1996; 74(2):F132–F134.

2. Vogl SE, Worda C, Egarter C, Bieglmayer C, Szekeres T, Huber J et al. Mode of delivery is associated with

maternal and fetal endocrine stress response. *BJOG* 2006; **113**(4):441–445.

3. Franzoi M, Simioni P, Luni S, Zerbinati P, Girolami A, Zanardo V. Effect of delivery modalities on the physiologic inhibition system of coagulation of the neonate. *Thromb Res* 2002; **105**(1):15–18.

4. Olaz-Fernandez I, Marin Gabriel M, Gil-Sanchez A, Garcia-Segura L, Arevalo M. Neuroendocrinology of childbirth and mother-child attachment: The basis of etiopathogenic model of perinatal neurobiological disorders. *Frontiers in Neuroendocrinology* 2014; **35**(4):459–472.

5. Otamiri G, Berg G, Ledin T, Leijon I, Lagercrantz H. Delayed neurological adaptation in infants delivered by elective cesarean section and the relation to catecholamine levels. *Early Hum Dev* 1991; **26**(1):51–60.

6. Scheller JM, Nelson KB. Does cesarean delivery prevent cerebral palsy or other neurologic problems of childhood? *Obstet Gynecol* 1994; **83**(4):624–630.

7. Sedeghat N. The effect of mode of delivery and anaesthesia on neonatal blood pressure. *Obs Anaes Dig* 2008; **28**:225–226.

8. Tahirovic H, Toromanovic A, Grbic S, Bogdanovic G, Fatusic Z, Gnat D. Maternal and neonatal urinary iodine excretion and neonatal TSH in relation to use of antiseptic during caesarean section in an iodine sufficient area. *J Pediatr Endocrinol Metab* 2009; **22**(12):1145–1149.

9. Louise Cozolina. *The Neuroscience of Human Relationships: Attachment and the Developing Social Brain* (2nd edn.) New York: WW Norton & Company; 2014.

10. Kim P, Feldman R, Mayes LC, Eicher V, Thompson N, Leckman JF, et al. Breastfeeding, brain activation to own infant cry, and maternal sensitivity. *J Child Psychol Psychiatry* 2011; **52**(8):907–915.

11. Nissen E, Lilja G, Widstrom AM, UvnäsMoberg K. Elevation of oxytocin levels early postpartum in women. *Acta Obstet Gynecol Scand* 1995; **74**(7):530–533.

12. Nissen E, UvnäsMoberg K, Svensson K, Stock S, Widstrom AM, Winberg J. Different patterns of oxytocin, prolactin but not cortisol release during breastfeeding in women delivered by caesarean section or by the vaginal route. *Early Hum Dev* 1996; **45**(1–2):103–118.

13. Smith LJ. Impact of birthing practices on the breastfeeding dyad. *J Midwifery Women's Health* 2007; **52**(6):621–630.

14. Stein DJ, Vythilingum B. Love and attachment: The psychobiology of social bonding. *CNS Spectr* 2009; **14**(5):239–242.

15. Stuebe A. The risks of not breastfeeding for mothers and infants. *Rev Obstet Gynecol* 2009; **2**(4):222–231.

16. Swain JE, Tasgin E, Mayes LC, Feldman R, Constable RT, Leckman JF. Maternal brain response to own baby-cry is affected by cesarean section delivery. *J Child Psychol Psychiatry* 2008; **49**(10):1042–1052.

17. UvnäsMoberg K. *The Hormone of Closeness: The Role of Oxytocin in Relationships*. London: Pinter and Martin; 2013.

18. Porges S. *The Polyvagal Theory: Neurophysiological Foundations of Emotions, Attachment, Communication and Self-regulation*. New York: WW Norton & Company; 2011.

19. Zeki S. The neurobiology of love. *FEBS Lett* 2007; **581**(14):2575–2579.

20. Downe S. *Normal Childbirth: Evidence and Debate*. (2nd edn.) Edinburgh: Churchill Livingstone Elsevier; 2008.

21. Lokugamage A. *The Heart in the Womb: An Exploration of the Roots of Love and Social Cohesion*. London: Docamali Ltd; 2011. ISBN: 9780956966704.

22. Ogden J, Shaw A, Zander L. Part1. Woman's memories of homebirth 3–5 years on. *British Journal of Midwifery* 1997; **5**(4):208–211.

23. Ogden J, Shaw A, Zander L. Part 2. Deciding on a homebirth: Help and hindrance. *British Journal of Midwifery* 1997; **5**(4):212–215.

24. Ogden J, Shaw A, Zander L. Part 3. A decision with a lasting effect. *British Journal of Midwifery* 1997; **5**(4):216–218.

25. Pedersen CA. Biological aspects of social bonding and the roots of human violence. *Ann N Y Acad Sci* 2004; **1036**:106–127.

26. Lawrence A, Lewis L, Hofmeyer G, Styles C. Maternal positions and mobility during first stage of labour (Review) *The Cochrane Library* 2013; Issue 10.

27. UvnäsMoberg K, Petersson M. Oxytocin, a mediator of anti-stress, well-being, social interaction, growth and healing. *Z. Psychosom. Med. Psychother.* 2005; **51**:57–80.

28. Moberg, Kerstin Uvnas. *Oxytocin: The Biological Guide to Motherhood*. Hale Publishing, 2015, ISBN-13: 978-1939847423.

29. Buchanan S, Patterson J, Roberts C, Morris J, Ford J. Trends and morbidity associated with oxytocin use in labour in nulliparas at term. *Australian and New Zealand Journal of Obstetrics and Gynaecology* 2012; **52**:173–178.

30. Bugg G, Siddiqui F, Thornton J. Oxytocin versus no treatment or delayed treatment for slow progress in the first stage of spontaneous labour (Review) *The Cochrane Library* 2013; Issue 6.

Section 4 Obstetrics and Maternal Health

31. Karacam Z, Walsh D, Bugg G. Evolving understanding and treatment of labour dystocia. *European Journal of Obstetrics and Gynaecology and Reproductive Biology* 2014; **182**:123–127.

32. Bell A, Erickson E, Carter S. Beyond Birth; The role of natural and synthetic oxytocin in the transition to motherhood. *Journal of Midwifery and Women's Health* 2014; **59**(1):35–42.

33. Gerhardt S. *Why love matters: How affection shapes a baby's brain* (2nd edn.) London: Routledge; 2015.

34. Ishak W, Kahloon M, Fakhry H. Oxytocin role in enhancing well-being: A literature review. *J. Affect. Disord.* 2011; **130**:1–9.

35. Shen H. Neuroscience: The hard science of oxytocin. *Nature* 2015; **522**:410–412.

36. Feldman R. The adaptive human parental brain: Implications for children's social development. *Trends in Neurosciences* 2015; **38**(6):387–399.

37. Bruning A, Heller H, Kieviet N, Bakker P, de Groot C, Dolman K, Honig A. Antidepressants during pregnancy and postpartum haemorrhage: A systematic review. *European Journal of Obstetrics & Gynaecology and Reproductive Biology* 2015; **189**:38–37.

38. Ryding E, Lukasse M, Van Parys A, Wangel A, Karro H, Kristjansdottir H, Schroll A, Schei B and on behalf of the Bidens Group. Fear of Childbirth and risk of Cesarean Delivery: A cohort study in six European Countries. *Birth* 2015; **42**(1):48–55.

39. Rouhe H, Salamela-Aro K, Toivanen R, Tokola M, Halmesmaki E, Saisto T. Obstetric outcome after intervention for severe fear of childbirth in nulliparous – randomised trial. *BJOG* 2013; **120**(1):75–84.

40. Hyde M, Mostyn A, Modi N, Kemp P. The health implications of birth by caesarean section. *Biological Reviews* 2012; **87**(1):229–243.

41. Ransjo-Arvidson AB, Matthiesen AS, Lilja G, Nissen E, Widstrom AM, UvnäsMoberg K. Maternal analgesia during labor disturbs new born behavior: Effects on breastfeeding, temperature, and crying. *Birth* 2001; **28**(1):5–12.

42. Lieberman E, Davidson K, Lee-Parritz A, Shearer E. Changes in fetal position during labor and their association with epidural analgesia. *Obstet Gynecol* 2005; **105**(5 Pt 1):974–982.

43. Dietert R, Dietert J. The Microbiome and sustainable healthcare. *Healthcare* 2015; **3**:100–129; doi:10.3390/healthcare 3010100.

44. Dietert RR. Natural Childbirth and Breastfeeding as Preventive Measures of Immune-Microbiome Dysbiosis and Misregulated Inflammation. *J Anc Dis Prev Rem* 2013; **1**:103.

45. Jasarevic E, Howerton CL, Howard CD, Bale TL. Alterations in the vaginal microbiome by maternal stress are associated with metabolic reprogramming of the offspring gut and brain. *Endocrinology* 2015; **156**(9):3265–3276.

46. Forster DA, McLachlan HL. Breastfeeding initiation and birth setting practices: A review of the literature. *J Midwifery Women's Health* 2007; **52**(3):273–280.

47. Nissen E, UvnäsMoberg K, Svensson K, Stock S, Widstrom AM, Winberg J. Different patterns of oxytocin, prolactin but not cortisol release during breastfeeding in women delivered by caesarean section or by the vaginal route. *Early Hum Dev* 1996; **45**(1–2):103–118.

48. Smith LJ. Impact of birthing practices on the breastfeeding dyad. *J Midwifery Women's Health* 2007; **52**(6):621–630.

49. Raine A, Brennan P, Mednick SA. Birth complications combined with early maternal rejection at age 1 year predispose to violent crime at age 18 years. *Arch Gen Psychiatry* 1994; **51**(12):984–988.

50. Raine A, Brennan P, Mednick SA. Interaction between birth complications and early maternal rejection in predisposing individuals to adult violence: Specificity to serious, early-onset violence. *Am J Psychiatry* 1997; **154**(9):1265–1271.

51. Fair C, Morrison T. The relationship between prenatal control, expectations, experienced control and birth satisfaction among primiparous women. *Midwifery* 2012; **28**(1):39–44.

52. Care QualityCommission. *National findings from the 2013 survey of women's experience of maternity care.* 2013. www.nhssurveys.org/Filestore/MAT13/MAT13_maternity_report_for_publication.pdf.

53. Nilson C, Lundgren I, Smith V, Vehvilainen-Julkunen K, Nicoletti J, Devane D, Bernloehr A, van Limbeek E, Lalor J, Begley C. Women-centred interventions to increase vaginal birth after caesarean section (VBAC): A systematic review. *Midwifery* 2015; **31**(7):657–663.

54. Liu J, Leung P, Yang A. Breastfeeding and active bonding protects against children's internalizing behavior problems. *Nutrients* 2014; **6**(1):76–89.

55. Leadsom A, Field F, Burstow P, Lucas C. 'The 1001 Critical Days: The Importance of the Conception to Age Two Period'. London: A Cross Party Manifesto; 2013.

56. All Party Parliamentary Group forConception to Age 2: First 1001 Days. *Building Great Britons*. London; WAVE Trust and Parent Infant Partnership UK (PIPUK) February 2015; Available at www.wavetrust.org/sites/default/files/reports/Building_Great_Britons_Report-APPG_Conception_to_Age_2-Wednesday_25th_February_2015.pdf. Accessed 23 March 2017.

226

57. Fenech G, Thompson G. Tormented by ghosts from the past: A meta-synthesis to explore the psychosocial implications of a traumatic birth on maternal well-being. *Midwifery* 2014; **30**(2):185–193.

58. Cundiff J. Orgasmic birth; The best kept secret. *Journal of Midwifery and Women's Health*. 2010; **55**(3):49.

59. Powell R, Walker S, Barrett A, Informed Consent to breech birth in New Zealand. *New Zealand Medical Journal* 2015; **128**(1418):6599.

60. Scamell M. The swan effect in midwifery talk and practice: A tension between normality and the language of risk. *Sociology of Health and Illness* 2011; **33**(7):987–1001.

61. de Boer J, Lok A, Van't VE, Duivenvoorden HJ, Bakker AB, Smit BJ. Work-related critical incidents in hospital-based health care providers and the risk of post-traumatic stress symptoms, anxiety, and depression: A meta-analysis. *Soc Sci Med* 2011; **73**(2):316–326.

62. Hodnett ED, Gates S, Hofmeyr GJ, Sakala C. Continuous support for women during childbirth. *Cochrane Database Syst Rev* 2013; 7:CD003766.

63. Whitehead P, Herbertson R, Hamric A, Epstein E, Fisher J. Moral distress among healthcare professionals: Report of an institution-wide survey. *Journal of Nursing Scholarship* 2015; **47**(2):117–125.

64. Kosfeld M. Trust in the brain. Neurobiological determinants of human social behaviour. *EMBO Rep* 2007; 8 Spec No:S44–S47.

65. The Lancet. Achieving respectful care for women and babies. *The Lancet* 2015; **385**(9976):1366.

66. Freedman LP, Kruk ME. Disrespect and abuse of women in childbirth: Challenging the global quality and accountability agendas. *The Lancet* 2014; **384**(9948):42–44.

67. Youngson R. *TIME to CARE: How to Love Your Patients and Your Job*. Raglan: Rebelheart Publishers; 2012.

68. Dahlin CM, Kelley JM, Jackson VA, Temel JS. Early palliative care for lung cancer: Improving quality of life and increasing survival. *Int J Palliat Nurs* 2010; **16**(9):420–423.

69. Del CS, Louis DZ, Maio V, Wang X, Rossi G, Hojat M, et al. The relationship between physician empathy and disease complications: An empirical study of primary care physicians and their diabetic patients in Parma, Italy. *Acad Med* 2012; **87**(9):1243–1249.

70. Hodnett ED, Gates S, Hofmeyr GJ, Sakala C. Continuous support for women during childbirth. *Cochrane Database Syst Rev* 2013; 7: CD003766.

71. Tracy SK, Hartz DL, Tracy MB, Allen J, Forti A, Hall B, et al. Caseload midwifery care versus standard maternity care for women of any risk: M@NGO, a randomised controlled trial. *The Lancet* 2013; **382**(9906):1723–1732.

72. Orton P, Orton C, Pereira GD. Depersonalised doctors: A cross-sectional study of 564 doctors, 760 consultations and 1876 patient reports in UK general practice. *BMJ Open* 2012; **2**:e000274.

73. Haxby E. Thinking differently about complaints in the NHS. *Future Hospital Journal* 2014; **1**(2):103–7.

74. Ehrenreich B, English D. *Witches, midwives, and nurses a history of women healers.* (2nd edn.) New York City: Feminist Press at the City University of New York; 2010.

75. Lowe N. Dignity in Childbirth. *Journal of Obstetric Gynecological and Neonatal Nursing* 2014; **43**(2): 137–138.

227

Chapter

26

Assessment of Psychosocial Health during the Perinatal Period

Julie Jomeen

Introduction

The concept of psychosocial health is now considered more broadly as a state of mental, emotional, social and spiritual well-being. Such an approach recognizes mental state as resulting from life experiences and adaptive processes; hence, psychosocial assessment is specifically linked to the psychological and social experiences of individuals and families in relation to life processes. The importance of the relationship between psychosocial processes and health has been increasingly recognized. Psychological aspects of childbirth and perinatal mental illness (PMI) rose to prominence in the United Kingdom following the 2004 Confidential Enquiry in Maternal and Child Health [1] when for the first time PMI was demonstrated to be the largest cause of maternal deaths. However, the effective assessment of psychosocial health is of growing concern to policy makers and practitioners more globally. Clinical guidelines in the United States, Canada, Scotland and Australia [2] recommend assessment of women at risk of perinatal mental health problems (PMHP). Australia, particularly, has introduced psychosocial assessment alongside routine physical care in a maternity context, in recognition of the impact of psychosocial problems on maternal and child outcomes [3]. Recent evidence has highlighted the burden in economic terms of a failure to identify and manage women with PMI, citing a cost to UK society of about £8.1 billion for each one-year cohort of births [4]. This chapter will highlight why healthcare practitioners need to understand and consider psychosocial health. It will identify psychosocial risk factors and consider their relationship with PMI. It will consider the usefulness of key measures that have been developed to undertake that assessment, acknowledging some of the challenges inherent in those processes for health professionals, women and their families.

The Importance of Psychosocial Health in a Maternity Context

It is now well acknowledged that social and emotional health problems in the perinatal period can lead to poor outcomes for women, their infants and families [5, 6]. Women who are vulnerable to or develop perinatal mental health problems (PMHP) do benefit from treatment interventions [7]. Antenatal assessment for mental health issues and risk factors facilitates appropriate liaison with relevant professionals, timely discussion regarding treatment, support options and the development of management plans for the perinatal period, with the ultimate aim of reducing the negative impact on both mother and child [8]. It is suggested that a history of previous postpartum depression (PPD) and psychosocial factors are the most significant precursors of antenatal depression (AND) and PPD [8], highlighting the value of assessing both those elements within the perinatal context.

Previous or Current Mental Health Problems

PMHP are not uncommon and can have serious consequences. In high-income countries, 10% of pregnant women and 13% of mothers of infants have significant PMHP, depression and anxiety being the most common [9]. If 700,000 women give birth each year, as in England, approximately 70,000 women will be affected antenatally and 91,000 postpartum, with rates much higher in resource-constrained countries [9]. Whilst the focus within the literature is on depression, historically on PPD and more recently on AND, PMI is actually a spectrum of conditions, varying in severity from adjustment disorders and distress, through mild to moderate depressive illness and anxiety states, severe depressive illness and post-traumatic stress disorder, to chronic serious mental illness and post-partum psychosis.

PMHP affect women from across the population and can have a significant impact upon the healthy functioning of the woman and her long-term mental health, obstetric outcomes, her partner, the quality of family relationships, as well as on the well-being of the fetus and a child's development in the short and the long terms. The burden of PMI in individual, societal and economic terms must not be underestimated. Perinatal care provides a clear opportunity for professionals who come into contact with women to make a positive impact on adverse obstetric and mental health outcomes related to PMI [10]. This, however, requires awareness and understanding of common mental health problems, as well as the confidence to make enquiries of women about their mental health status. This is an area that has been traditionally identified as problematic for midwives [11, 12], health visitors [13, 14] and general practitioners [15] as well as health professionals generally [16]. It is essential that practitioners effectively assess and recognize PMI risk to underpin appropriate and proactive referral and care decisions, which assure the necessary support that women and their families need.

Public attention on PMI internationally followed the 2004 UK Confidential Enquiries in Maternal and Child Health report. For the first time, deaths from PMI were identified as the overall leading cause of maternal mortality (1998–2001) [1]. This report lucidly highlighted PMI as an issue requiring greater attention, catapulting PMI onto the maternity public health agenda. Subsequent reports [17, 18] have continued to evidence PMI as a significant cause of death and highlight, unlike other conditions, no decrease in suicide rates in perinatal women.

PMI is a potentially preventable cause of perinatal mortality. Recommendations from the UK confidential enquiries into maternal deaths [1, 17, 18] stress that assessment through questioning about mental health should be routine in antenatal clinics, backed up by effective communication between services and professionals to optimize care pathways.

Identifying and Assessing Women's Psychological Status

Individual women will demonstrate wide variation in their emotional status, from a minor transient experience, 'baby blues' to severe mental illness (SMI), such as puerperal psychosis. Whilst the range and type of PMI might vary, they form part of a continuum, which can present right across the perinatal period. Practitioners will see women with existing mental health disorder who become pregnant, as well as women who develop PMHP when they have previously been well. The existing evidence base makes a distinction between those two groups of women and the associated differing approach to assessment, that is 'prediction' of the risk of developing a mental health disorder and attempts to 'detect' onset of a distress/depression/anxiety episode in previously non-depressed women. A number of countries have developed approaches to assessing psychological health, and the literature shows a wide variability of screening tools [8]. In practice these screening tools are often more focussed on depression and more latterly anxiety, rather than a wider spectrum of PMHP, linked to the prevalence of depression (and anxiety) in this population.

The Whooley Questions (Modified PHQ-2)

In the United Kingdom the National Institute for Health and Care Excellence (NICE) guidelines for antenatal and postpartum mental health [19] give all healthcare professionals working with pregnant and postpartum women a clearly defined remit for prediction of the current disorder and detection of risk factors. The original guidance, issued in 2007 [20], focussed on the detection of depression using the Whooley questions (see Box 26.1). The 2014 guidelines have responded to the increasing evidence base around perinatal anxiety and additionally sought to address assessment of the range and prevalence of anxiety disorders (including generalized anxiety disorder, obsessive-compulsive disorder, panic disorder, phobias, post-traumatic stress disorder and social anxiety disorder). The significance of anxiety is its independent predictive nature for deleterious infant/child outcomes with evidence indicating links to long-term behavioural/emotional problems in the child [8].

If a health condition is serious, prevalent, under-detected and treatable, as in the case of most PMHP, and if an acceptable assessment procedure of known accuracy is available, then assessment can be an effective measure in principle. Ultimately, however, a worthwhile screening process must result in a clinical benefit for those screened, that is, a reduction in mortality/morbidity associated with the condition

---

BOX 26.1 Prediction and Detection Questions [19]

Prediction Questions

At the woman's first contact with services during pregnancy and the postpartum period, healthcare professionals (including midwives, obstetricians, health visitors and GPs), should ask about:

1. Past or present severe mental illness, including schizophrenia, bipolar disorder, psychosis in the postpartum period and severe depression.
2. Previous treatment by a psychiatrist/specialist mental health team, including inpatient care.
3. Family history of perinatal mental illness.

Detection Questions (Whooley Questions: PHQ-2)

At the woman's first contact with primary care, booking visit and postpartum (usually at 4 to 6 weeks and 3 to 4 months), healthcare professionals (including midwives, obstetricians, health visitors and GPs) should ask two questions to identify possible depression.

1. During the past month, have you often been bothered by feeling down, depressed or hopeless?
2. During the past month, have you often been bothered by having little interest or pleasure in doing things?

Also consider using the 2-item Generalized Anxiety Disorder scale (GAD-2):

1. Over the last 2 weeks, how often have you been bothered by feeling nervous, anxious or on edge?
2. Over the last 2 weeks, how often have you been bothered by not being able to stop or control worrying?

If a woman responds positively to either of the depression questions, is at risk of developing a mental health problem or there is clinical concern, consider using the Edinburgh Postnatal Depression Scale (EPDS) or the Patient Health Questionnaire (PHQ-9) as part of a full assessment or referring the woman to her GP or to a mental health professional.

If a woman scores 3 or more on the GAD-2, consider using the GAD-7 for further assessment or referring the woman to her GP or to a mental health professional.

If a woman scores less than 3 on the GAD-2 scale, but you are still concerned she may have an anxiety disorder, ask the following question:

1. Do you find yourself avoiding places or activities and does this cause you problems?

If she responds positively, consider using the GAD-7 scale for further assessment or referring the woman to her GP or to a mental health professional.

---

[21]. Measures therefore need to be accurate in their assessment.

The Whooley questions (Patient Health Questionnaire: PHQ-2) as in NICE [19], have been used with the perinatal population. Two recent studies have sought to validate these questions in both the antenatal and postpartum context and suggest that the approach has excellent properties for 'ruling out' depression in perinatal women (a negative predictive value of 100%). This could be valuable for busy health practitioners, and has led to the recommendation of its use as a pre-screening tool for depression [22, 23]. In some studies, however, it has been found to yield high false-positive rates [24]. Such results suggest the requirement to follow the pre-screening with another measure and ultimately a diagnostic interview. Darwin et al. [2], however, found the Whooley questions 'missed' half the possible cases identified using the EPDS (EPDS threshold ≥ 10) as the comparator. The authors suggest that this is a result of under-disclosure by women, the outcome of which is that depression symptoms are under-identified in practice [2].

The Edinburgh Postpartum Depression Scale

The EPDS has been the most consistently used measure for identifying risk of antenatal and postpartum depression in a global context [21]. It is a self-rated, 10-item instrument consisting of 10 statements relating to symptoms of depression (depressed mood, anhedonia) in the previous seven days, offering one of four possible responses for each statement (on a scale of 0–3). The EPDS deliberately excludes somatic symptoms, often seen as symptoms of a mental health disorder that would overlap with the physical and/or social changes that occur in the perinatal context, such as changing sleep patterns. Responses are summed to yield a maximum score. Item number 10 addresses thoughts of suicidal ideation. The most commonly applied cut-off score indicating possible depression (i.e. a positive screening result) is 13 points or over [21]. A synthesis of more than 40 studies using the EPDS suggested an optimum cut-off point of 12 for major depression and 10 for major/minor depression combined. The EPDS has been found to be variable in terms of sensitivity and specificity and will inevitably yield both false positives and false negatives. The EPDS has been validated for antenatal use; there are many non-English translations [21]. Its brevity and generally acceptable performance mean the EPDS is widely used.

Whilst often taken as the 'gold standard', issues have been raised in relation to the claimed unidimensional nature of the EPDS. Psychometric testing has demonstrated embedded items within the EPDS, both antenatal and postpartum, that assess anxiety rather than depression. This may have some use in a clinical context but, if being used to identify depression in isolation, that it may also be measuring anxiety has implications for cut-off scores [25]. Authors have recommended differing thresholds for antenatal and postpartum use of the EPDS [26], which may help to account for raised anxiety in the antenatal period, but these have not been internationally validated with any consistency or evaluation. The use of the EPDS as a multidimensional measure has now been posited by several authors [25–27], yet the evidence base to date has not translated into practice. Overall a good assessment measure should reflect both reliability and validity, and the UK National Screening Committee have expressed concerns about widespread implementation of the EPDS as a screening tool [28]. Therefore, as with any 'screening' tool, the EPDS should complement, rather than replace, clinical judgement, especially when we consider that the positive predictive value of the English-language version of the EPDS in the general postpartum population (the probability that a positive screening result is correct) has been estimated at between 50 and 60%, leaving a large margin for error.

Other Assessment Measures for Depression and Anxiety

A measure often utilized more in research than clinical practice and less widely validated than the EPDS, the Postpartum Depression Screening Scale (PDSS), appears to perform similarly in terms of sensitivity and specificity as a screening instrument for perinatal depression [21]. The PDSS comprises seven domains: sleeping and eating disturbances; anxiety and insecurity; emotional ability; cognitive impairment; loss of self; guilt and shame; thoughts of self-harm. The measure is self-rated and scores range from 35 to 135. A cut-off of 60 or over is deemed significant symptomology of depression, and 80 or over is considered a positive screen for major depression.

Another measure, which addresses the domains of depression and anxiety and hence might be considered of greater utility in a perinatal context, is the Hospital Anxiety Depression Scale (HADS). This measure was indeed recommended in the 2007 NICE guidelines [20] as a second line measure of assessment. However, its validity in a childbearing population has been questioned [29], and it is no longer a recommended second-line assessment measure within the current UK guidelines [19].

Other tools originally developed for generic depression screening have been used in perinatal populations. These include the Beck Depression Inventory and Zung Self-Rating Depression Scale [21] as well as the General Health Questionnaire (GHQ-12). Though again such measures have not been without critique, questions have been raised about scoring methods, appropriate threshold and factorial stability [30]. A recent study has sought to validate a modified GHQ-12 (GHQ-12-WB or GHQ-12-Wellbeing), which demonstrates relatively good psychometric properties in a postpartum group, particularly when reduced to eight questions [30]. Though this measure requires further testing, the concept of measuring and screening for psychological well-being rather than psychological morbidity in perinatal populations is gaining some ground [10]. The well-being perspective may offer a compelling framework to encompass and exemplify the holistic nature of pregnancy and new motherhood, one which can involve a multifaceted and evolving continuum ranging from a positive to a negative sense of well-being, which is inherently normal [30].

Translation into Clinical Practice

The above tools beyond the EPDS have generally failed to translate into clinical practice, in part due to their failure to perform as effectively in childbearing populations, making tools designed specifically for pregnancy and postpartum more attractive.

Worthy of consideration is that whilst short self-report measures are undoubtedly attractive for use in clinical practice due to their ease of use and potential cut-off scores and which may help facilitate practitioner judgements [31], such measures are not without their problems. They are not diagnostic in nature and a score on a screening tool only serves to highlight possible or probable PMI. While tools might be useful in underpinning mood assessment, they should not be considered a replacement for clinical diagnostic skills and expertise. King [24], for example, suggests that the use of the PHQ-2 runs the inherent risk of de-skilling midwives who, with appropriate training, are capable of identifying and managing women with mild to moderate distress. However, they can have significant utility when used sensitively and considerately as part of a broader assessment and decision-making [32].

Identifying Risk Factors

National reports and academic literature highlight the difficulties with identifying risk for PMI, as well as managing the risk appropriately. Risk factors are best described as vulnerability, adverse factors or characteristics that are present in a woman's life and hence put them at greater risk of developing PMI [28]. Risk factors, as independent causal variables, are not necessarily recommended to predict AND or PND [19, 20] because there is no inevitable cause-and-effect relationship. Presence of risk factors may well, however, increase an individual's vulnerability, particularly if the individual is subject to 'a cluster of these adverse factors' [28, p.55, 33]. Psychosocial assessment aims to place PMI assessment in the context of a woman's life circumstances, providing a holistic, integrated, woman-centred approach to mental health status. The administration of a standardized screening tool when coupled with discussing women's life situation may also make screening more acceptable and support disclosure [34]. Identifying psychosocial risk factors can support healthcare professionals to sketch out profiles of vulnerable women, profiles which can then be considered when assessing a woman's needs across the perinatal period.

> **BOX 26.2** Potential Risk Factors for PMI [1, 17, 18]
>
> Previous psychiatric disorder
> Family history of serious mental ill-health
> Social disadvantage and isolation
> Poverty
> Minority ethnic group
> Asylum seekers and refugees
> Late bookers and non-attenders
> Domestic violence
> Substance misuse
> Known to child protection services
> Employment status
> Physical ill health
> Life events
> Lack of support

Evidence accrued over several decades now recognizes some fairly consistent risk factors for PMI (see Box 26.2).

Indeed, these risk factors, whilst framed slightly differently, are reflected in the UK NICE guidelines [19] (see Box 26.3). Whilst these are not recommended as a risk predictor checklist per se, the guidance states that they should be included in the assessment and diagnosis of a suspected PMHP.

An Australian study of over 40,000 women by BeyondBlue also confirmed the importance of the above risk factors [33]. That the risk factors suggested have been found to be fairly globally consistent should furnish practitioner confidence in the consideration of these as part of the assessment of women's perinatal psychosocial status. Australia has been one country where there has been an explicit move to assessing psychosocial risk factors, which includes depression screening as one part [33].

Assessing Psychosocial Health

A number of measures have been developed in attempts to effectively assess multidimensional factors thought to influence PMH, rather than measure PMH status at a particular point in time. A recent review by Johnson et al. [33] sought to critically evaluate those measures assessing PMH risk (Box 26.4).

Johnson et al. [33] concluded that none of the above instruments met all of the requirements of psychometric properties defined within the review. Whilst the Antenatal Risk Questionnaire (ANRQ) and the Australian Routine Psychosocial Assessment (ARPA) had large sample sizes, the former reported low positive predictive values or failed to provide information regarding their clinical performance. Other measures had insufficient sample sizes, such as the Antenatal Psychosocial Health Assessment (ALPHA), Camberwell Assessment of Needs – Mother (CAN-M) and Contextual Assessment of Maternity Experience (CAME). The ANRQ fulfilled the requirements of the review analysis more comprehensively than the other instruments examined, based on the defined rating criteria, so it will be explored briefly next.

Antenatal Risk Questionnaire

The Antenatal Risk Questionnaire (ANRQ) was developed by Austin et al. [35] in consultation with midwives and mental health care professionals working in a large maternity hospital. It consists of 12 items which were selected from the original 23 Pregnancy Risk Questionnaire (PRQ). This tool assesses psychosocial risk domains: emotional support from subject's own mother in childhood, past history of depressed mood, mental illness and treatment received, perceived level of support available following the birth of the baby, partner emotional support, life stresses in the previous 12 months, personality style (anxious or perfectionistic traits) and history of abuse (emotional, physical and sexual). It is scored with a possible maximum score of 62 and minimum score of 5. It was rated against a diagnostic interview and performed acceptably at the most clinically relevant cut-off of 23 (sensitivity 0.62, specificity 0.64, the PPV was 0.30 [low]; the NPV was 0.87). While the acceptability of the ANRQ was high amongst both pregnant women and midwives [35], the performance of the tool in terms of effective identification is relatively weak, and the non-provision of demographic information within the study to determine normative data leads the review authors to state that the ANRQ is not recommended [33].

While it might be desirable to recommend a tool for clinical practice, for all the reasons previously discussed, it is important that clinicians are made aware of their limitations. It is probably reflective of the relatively new nature of this type of assessment in a maternity context that the efficacy of such assessment tools in improving women's clinical outcomes is currently unsupported by the evidence [21].

Acceptability and Effectiveness of Psychosocial Assessment

To have any effect on morbidity, an assessment process must be acceptable to the target population, as well as among health professionals conducting the procedure. In the case of PMI, as defined in international guidance, reasonable evidence now shows that most women and health professionals find the process tolerable [21], though this is not a universal finding [2]. Some women are not comfortable with such screening, finding the process intrusive and potentially stigmatizing, resulting in a failure to answer questions honestly [2]. Noteworthy is that stigma appears to be more pervasive in the case of cultural diversity. Jarrett [36] highlighted that midwives, in some cases, demonstrated discriminating attitudes and formed illness perceptions based on cultural stereotypes rather than on professional knowledge.

In general, most studies highlight a positive change towards a shared responsibility for the assessment and management of PMHP. Many healthcare professionals acknowledge that caring for women with PMHP is part of their professional role [3, 12, 14, 15, 37]. Confidence and knowledge are overwhelmingly the most influential factors in determining professional attitudes. Jones et al. [37] highlight that willingness to provide care links to a practitioner's own perceived confidence and competence. The need for specialist PMH services where pregnant and postpartum women can be referred via rapid access pathways is emphasized in all the confidential enquiry reports as something that must support any psychosocial assessment process.

Training offers the most effective way to enhance practitioners' awareness of their role in PMH care and to support a change in practice [21]. Skilful conduct of psychosocial assessment is essential to underpin a consistent standard of care and an acceptable experience for women [21]. Continued research is clearly necessary to determine the best models of conducting psychosocial assessment, but training of health professionals is likely to be the key element.

The context in which screening is conducted also appears relevant, with busy clinic settings not providing the optimal environment. A lack of adequate time and suitable care settings are systemic issues affecting midwives' experiences of providing care [24, 36]. Women in turn find screening more acceptable if they feel their health professional is engaged and empathetic; they expressed preferences for verbal feedback and discussion rather than a simple report of a test score [21], all of which is inevitably related to the time available, creating challenges for how this might be addressed.

Conclusion

The intensification of national policies and guidelines signal a drive and commitment from several governments to ensure that healthcare professionals address the issue of PMI, with countries introducing guidance

to support identification of vulnerable women. Whilst internationally different approaches to psychosocial assessment are used, there is a general acknowledgement that unless identification forms an integral part of a resourced infrastructure, with clear pathways that can offer diagnostic assessment, effective and available treatment options and support, then 'screening' is not beneficial or, worse, may cause greater potential harm [38].

Accruing evidence highlights the support women and their families living with PMI require. Training of health professionals in the recognition of clinical symptoms and the conduct of psychosocial assessment is also key in that regard [21]. Identification strategies, using appropriate measures as part of that assessment, when delivered by healthcare professionals equipped with the knowledge and skills, can deliver effective outcomes for women and their families.

Key Points

- Perinatal mental illness is a spectrum of conditions, varying in severity from adjustment disorders and distress, through mild to moderate depressive illness and anxiety states, severe depressive illness and post-traumatic stress disorder, to chronic serious mental illness and postpartum psychosis.
- It can have a significant impact upon the healthy functioning of the woman and her long-term mental health, obstetric outcomes, her partner, the quality of family relationships, as well as on the well-being of the fetus and a child's development in the short and the long terms.
- A worthwhile screening process must result in a clinical benefit for those screened.
- Tools that are available for assessing risk of perinatal mental health problems in a clinical or research setting include the Whooley Questions, Edinburgh Postpartum Depression Scale (EPDS), the Postpartum Depression Screening Scale (PDSS), the Beck Depression Inventory and Zung Self-Rating Depression Scale, the General Health Questionnaire (GHQ-12) and a modified GHQ-12 (Wellbeing). These tools are not without their critique, are non-diagnostic and should complement, rather than replace, clinical judgement.

- Tools for antenatal psychosocial assessment include the Antenatal Risk Questionnaire (ANRQ), Antenatal Psychosocial Health Assessment (ALPHA), Australian Routine Psychosocial Assessment (ARPA), Camberwell Assessment of Needs – Mothers (CAN – M) and Contextual Assessment of Maternity Experience (CAME). None of these currently meet all requisite psychometric criteria to be confident of their widespread introduction into practice, and continued research is necessary.
- Psychosocial assessment is acceptable to most, but not all, women and health professionals, but skilful conduct of psychosocial assessment is essential to underpin a consistent standard of care and an acceptable experience for women.
- Lack of adequate time, suitable care settings and robust referral and treatment infrastructure are issues that require attention at a systemic level.
- The training of health professionals and infrastructure for the referral of women are essential for successful implementation of psychosocial assessment.

References

1. Confidential Enquiry into Maternal and Child Health. *Why mothers die (2000–2002)*. London, RCOG. 2004.

2. Darwin Z, McGowan L, Edozien LC. Antenatal mental health referrals: Review of local clinical practice and pregnant women's experiences in England. *Midwifery* 2015; **31**(3): e17–22.

3. Rollans M, Schmied V, Kemp L, Meade T. 'We just ask some questions . . .' the process of antenatal psychosocial assessment by midwives. *Midwifery* 2013; **29**: 935–42.

4. Bauer A, Parsonage M, Knapp M, et al. *The costs of perinatal mental health problems*. London, London School of Economics and Political Science. 2014.

5. Murray L, Cooper P, Hipwell A. Mental health of parents caring for infants. *Archives of Women's Mental Health* 2003; **6**: s71–77.

6. Speranza AM, Ammaniti M, Trentini C. An overview of maternal depression, infant reactions and intervention programmes. *Clinical Neuropsychology* 2006; **3**(1): 57–68.

7. Fontein-Kuipers YJ, Nieuwenhuijze MJ, Ausems M, et al. Antenatal interventions to reduce maternal distress: A systematic review and meta-analysis of randomised trials. *British Journal of Obstetrics and Gynaecology* 2014; **121**: 389–97.

8. Paschetta E, Berrisford G, Coccia F, et al. Perinatal psychiatric disorders: An overview. *American Journal of Obstetrics and Gynecology* 2014; **210**(6): 501–509.e6.

9. Fisher J, de Mello M, Patel V, et al. Prevalence and determinants of common perinatal mental disorders in women in low- and lower-middle-income countries: A systematic review. *Bulletin of the World Health Organization* 2010; **90**: 139–49H. Available from www.who.int/bulletin/volumes/90/2/11–091850/en/.

10. Alderdice F, McNeill J, Lynn F. A systematic review of systematic reviews of interventions to improve maternal mental health and well-being. *Midwifery* 2013; **29**(4): 389–99.

11. Jomeen J, Glover LF, Davis S. Midwives' illness perceptions of antenatal depression, *British Journal of Midwifery* 2009; **17**(5): 296–303.

12. Hauck T, Kelly G, Dragovic M, et al. Australian midwives' knowledge, attitude and perceived learning needs around perinatal mental health. *Midwifery* 2015; **31**(1): 247–55.

13. Morrell CJ, Slade P, Warner R, et al. Clinical effectiveness of health visitor training in psychologically informed approaches for depression in postnatal women: Pragmatic cluster randomised trial in primary care. *British Medical Journal* 2009; **338**: a3045. Available from: www.bmj.com/content/bmj/338/bmj.a3045.full.pdf.

14. Jomeen J, Glover L, Jones C, et al. Assessing women's perinatal psychological health: Exploring the experiences of Health Visitors. *Journal of Reproductive and Infant Psychology* 2013; **31**: 479–89.

15. Centre for Mental Health. *Falling through the gaps*. London, Centre for Mental Health. 2015.

16. NSPCC. *Prevention in mind. All babies count: Spotlight on perinatal mental health*. 2013. www.nspcc.org.uk/Inform/resourcesforprofessionals/underones/spotlight-mental-health-landing_wda96578.html. (Accessed 25 September 2015.)

17. Confidential Enquiry into Maternal and Child Health. *Saving mothers' lives: Reviewing maternal deaths to make motherhood safer (2003–2005)*. London, RCOG. 2007.

18. Centre for Maternal and Child Enquiries. Saving mothers' lives: Reviewing maternal deaths 2006–2008. *British Journal of Obstetrics and Gynaecology* 2011; **118** (Suppl. 1): 1–203.

19. National Institute for Health and Care Excellence. *Antenatal and postnatal mental health: Clinical*

management and service guidance. London, Department of Health. 2014.

20. National Institute for Health and Clinical Excellence. *Antenatal and postnatal mental health: Clinical management and service guidance.* London, Department of Health. 2007.

21. Milgrom J, Gemmill A. Screening for perinatal depression. *Best Practice Research Clinical Obstetrics and Gynaecology* 2014; **28**: 13–23.

22. Mann R, Adamson J, Gilbody SM. Diagnostic accuracy of case-finding questions to identify perinatal depression. *Canadian Medical Association Journal* 2012; **184**: E424.

23. Mann R, Gilbody S. Validity of two case-finding questions to detect postnatal depression: A review of diagnostic test accuracy. *Journal of Affective Disorders* 2011; **133**: 388–97.

24. King L, Pestell S, Farrar S, et al. Screening for antenatal psychological distress. *British Journal of Midwifery* 2012; **20**: 396–401.

25. Jomeen J, Martin CR. Confirmation of an occluded anxiety component within the Edinburgh Postnatal Depression Scale (EPDS) during early pregnancy. *Journal of Reproducive and Infant Psychology* 2005; **23**: 143–54.

26. Matthey S, Fisher J, Rowe H. Using the Edinburgh Postnatal Depression Scale to screen for anxiety disorders: Conceptual and methodological considerations. *Journal of Affective Disorders* 2013; **146**: 224–30.

27. Reichenheim ME, Moraes C, Oliveira A, Lobato G. Revisiting the dimensional structure of the Edinburgh Postnatal Depression Scale (EPDS): Empirical evidence for a general factor. *BMC Medical Research Methodology* 2011; **11**: 93.

28. Raynor M, England C. *Psychology for midwives: Pregnancy, childbirth and puerperium.* Maidenhead, Open University Press. 2010.

29. Jomeen J, Martin CR. Is the Hospital Anxiety and Depression Scale (HADS) a reliable screening tool in early pregnancy? *Psychology and Health* 2004; **19**(6): 787–800.

30. Spiteri CM, Jomeen J, Martin CR. Reimagining the General Health Questionnaire as a measure of emotional wellbeing: A study of postpartum women in Malta. *Women and Birth* 2013; **26**(4): e105–11.

31. Alderdice F, Ayers S, Darwin Z, et al. Measuring psychological health in the perinatal period: Workshop consensus statement, 19 March 2013. *Journal of Reproductive and Infant Psychology.* 2013 November; **31**: 431–8.

32. Jomeen J. Women's psychological status in pregnancy and childbirth–measuring or understanding? *Journal of Reproductive and Infant Psychology* 2012; **30**: 337–40.

33. Johnson M, Schmied V, Lupton SJ, et al. Measuring Women's Perinatal Mental Health Risk. *Archives of Women's Mental Health* 2012; **15**: 375–86.

34. Brealey SD, Hewitt C, Green JM, et al. Screening for postnatal depression: Is it acceptable to women and healthcare professionals? A systematic review and meta-synthesis. *Journal of Reproductive and Infant Psychology* 2010; **28**: 328–44.

35. Austin M-P, Colton J, Priest S, et al. The Antenatal Risk Questionnaire (ANRQ): Acceptability and use for psychosocial risk assessment in the maternity setting. *Women and Birth* 2010; **26**: 17–25.

36. Jarrett P. Attitudes of student midwives caring for women with perinatal mental health problems. *British Journal of Midwifery* 2014; **22**(10): 718–24.

37. Jones CJ, Creedy DK, Gamble JA. Australian midwives' attitudes towards care for women with emotional distress. *Midwifery* 2012; **28**(2): 216–21.

38. Jomeen J, Martin CR. Developing specialist perinatal mental health services. *Practising Midwife* 2014; **17**(3): 18–21.

Chapter 27

Biopsychosocial Factors in Prenatal Screening and Diagnosis for Fetal Anomaly

Louise D. Bryant

Introduction

Large numbers of pregnant women are offered prenatal testing in one form or another, for example, via screening programmes for Down syndrome that form part of routine antenatal care in most parts of the developed world. Screening tests are used to identify women at higher risk of having a baby affected by a particular condition. Women found to be at higher risk, for example, of having a 1 in 150 or greater chance of having an affected baby (a 'screen positive') will be offered invasive diagnostic tests. Invasive diagnostic tests, usually chorionic villus sampling (CVS) or amniocentesis, carry a risk of miscarriage of around 0.5–1%, and not all women opt for this further test [1]. If a diagnostic test identifies that the fetus is affected by a particular condition, women may then be offered a termination of pregnancy. Testing technologies are constantly being developed and as each new test is introduced into the clinic there is the potential for unintended psychological consequences for pregnant women. Prenatal testing for congenital conditions can cause women and their partners to examine their views and beliefs about disability, abortion, what it means to be a parent, and the role of technologies in selecting the type of people being born. For some women, these challenges can be unexpected and unwanted.

Of particular interest to those working within a biopsychosocial model of reproductive health is this potential for screening and diagnostic tests to generate anxiety in pregnant women. High levels of anxiety and stress in pregnancy are known to affect maternal-placental-fetal neuroendocrine activity and have been associated with an increased risk of preterm labour and preeclampsia [2]. While anxiety has been the main focus of research in this area, depressive symptoms in relation to prenatal testing have also been considered. Depression during pregnancy is associated with a range of negative effects including preterm birth that may be

due to increasing levels of hypothalamic-pituitary-adrenal axis and sympathetic nervous system hormones including cortisol [3]. Research suggests that depression experienced in early to mid-pregnancy appears to be most associated with an increased risk of adverse outcomes [3]. This is important when considering the impact of prenatal testing, as screening and diagnosis are almost exclusively conducted in the first half of the pregnancy. Understanding how and where psychological distress might manifest during the prenatal testing pathway is important in the provision of woman-centred antenatal care.

Prenatal Screening and Anxiety

There are three main systematic reviews that together provide a comprehensive assessment of anxiety in relation to screening for Down syndrome [4–6]. There is much less published evidence on the anxiety associated with screening for other conditions. Research in this area mainly addresses the question of whether there are differences in anxiety before and after screening for those women who choose to accept the tests. The most commonly used measure is the Spielberger State Trait Anxiety Index (STAI) [7]. The STAI is a self-report measure that assesses two aspects of anxiety. State anxiety relates to current feelings of tension, anxiety and nervousness being experienced 'right now', whereas trait anxiety relates to the relatively stable, generalized propensity to be tense, anxious and nervous. Of most interest when considering a response to screening tests is state anxiety measured on the S-Anxiety Scale. S-Anxiety scores can be between 20 and 80, with higher scores indicating higher levels of current anxiety. The STAI is one of the most widely used measures of general anxiety in both clinical and non-clinical populations and has good psychometric properties, although there has been limited validation in a pregnant population [8]. State anxiety norms for a general population set the mean S-Anxiety score at 36 for women aged between 19 and 39 [7]. Pregnant women scoring above 40 on the S-Anxiety are considered to be highly anxious [8].

There is evidence to suggest that for women electing to have prenatal screening, levels of state anxiety prior to undergoing screening range from normal levels to around 40 [4, 5]. An elevation of anxiety can be considered appropriate in this situation and may reflect an increased awareness of a potential threat to the fetus. For women who receive a screen negative result (a risk lower than the specified threshold) anxiety levels stay in the normal range or return to normal levels if they have been raised [4, 5]. The story for women who receive a screen positive result is markedly different. Green et al. reviewed 15 studies that assessed anxiety in women following a serum screen positive result and reported a significant rise in anxiety [4]. Qualitative research consistently reports feelings of shock, panic, distress and anxiety as well as sleep disturbance, loss of appetite and altered feelings towards the pregnancy. Five studies reported S-Anxiety scores in the range of 49–57, which is considered to be an acute anxiety response. The more recent review by Lou et al. [5] assessed three later studies and reported S-Anxiety scores of 42–44 for women who received a screen-positive result, which still reflects significantly high levels of anxiety. The limited research on maternal reactions to screening results for cystic fibrosis carrier screening shows that anxiety is also raised in screen-positive women compared to those who receive a negative result [4].

The evidence is reasonably good that S-Anxiety scores return to normal levels after a negative diagnostic test result [4, 5], suggesting that that while highly unpleasant, anxiety associated with a false screen positive does not result in long term, potentially harmful, maternal stress. Green et al. [4] suggested that for some women, residual anxiety can remain after a diagnostic test confirms the fetus is not affected [4]. Although the review by Lou et al. did not find evidence to support this in studies using the STAI [5], other research has identified residual concerns that may be picked up in different ways; this will be discussed in the next section on ultrasound screening. Of course, not all women choose to have an invasive diagnostic test following a positive screen. It might be expected that these women would continue to experience heightened levels of anxiety throughout the pregnancy, although there is very limited evidence in this area [4]. One study has suggested that women who choose not to have a diagnostic test may experience less anxiety after a positive screen than those women who opt for an invasive procedure [9]. This study did not use a validated measure of anxiety, and 'worry' was collected retrospectively, so no clear conclusions can be drawn.

Screening via Ultrasound and Anxiety

Ultrasound is unlike any other technology used in pregnancy and has transformed women's experiences of antenatal care. Scans provide an opportunity to confirm the reality of the pregnancy, 'meet the baby' and provide reassurance about its well-being [10]. Seeing the fetus can create an immediate emotional tie to a baby which, depending on the stage of pregnancy, cannot be felt or seen from the outside [11]. Parents often view the scans as something to look forward to – a social rather than medical event – and most scans are reassuring and pleasurable experiences [12]. Ultrasound images are often posted on social media and via mobile phones, are shared amongst friends and family, leading to what has been called the 'personification of the fetus' [13].

Ultrasound is also a multipurpose screening technology, for example, used to ascertain gestational age to input to the risk calculation for biochemical screening. Ultrasound is used directly as a screening tool to identify 'soft markers' that are associated with an increased risk of chromosomal and genetic conditions in the fetus. Soft markers are minor structural variants, for example, an increased nuchal translucency measurement, cysts in the fetal choroid plexus or an echogenic bowel. Soft markers do not constitute a defect in themselves but can be considered to raise the risk of a range of genetic and chromosomal conditions, especially if found in conjunction with other structural anomalies or advanced maternal age [14]. The mid-pregnancy scan can also diagnose a number of major structural abnormalities and detailed examinations are conducted of the fetal skeleton, skull, brain, spinal cord, face, abdomen, heart and kidneys.

For some women therefore, a keenly anticipated scan can become the opposite of the expected happy occasion [15]. Soft markers will be identified in around 5% of pregnancies [16] and in around a further 1–2% of cases major structural abnormalities will be found. It is recognized that many women are psychologically unprepared for an anomalous finding from a scan, even if cognitively they are aware of the potential for problems to be identified [10]. Good-quality, large studies on the psychological impact of soft marker identification are not available, but a number of studies demonstrate that potentially anomalous ultrasound findings can engender high levels of anxiety in pregnant women. Qualitative research shows that many women describe intense negative reactions to the identification of a soft marker, for example, shock, extreme anxiety and, especially where choroid plexus cysts in the fetal brain are identified, vivid imaginings of fetal deformity [17, 18].

Two studies have used the STAI to assess levels of anxiety after a soft marker has been identified. The first reported a mean S-Anxiety score of 40 (ranging between 31 and 53 depending on ethnic group) immediately after the scan [19]. The second study measured mean S-Anxiety scores during the week after the scan of 49, but reported that S-Anxiety levels returned to normal by 30 weeks' gestation after follow-up scans or a diagnostic test [20]. While it is reassuring that high levels of anxiety do subside, for some women this may be at the cost of unexpectedly undergoing an invasive test midway through their pregnancy. Two studies reported that a significant proportion of women with isolated fetal markers for chromosomal anomalies may request amniocentesis even when their objective risk level does not warrant it [17, 19]. An early qualitative study found that residual concerns raised by something having 'been seen' via ultrasound may remain unresolved until the baby is born [21]. Other studies suggest that there can be longer-term psychological consequences to soft marker identification, including an altered view of pregnancy, and a continued vulnerability to related anxieties in certain circumstances, for example, during childhood illness [22, 23].

Ultrasound Screening and Depression

There is very limited research in the area of depressive symptoms in relation to prenatal screening. One such study measured depression in women whose scan identified a soft marker and compared them with a group of pregnant women who had a history of psychiatric illness but no soft marker, and a control group with neither experience [24]. Using the Edinburgh Postnatal Depression Rating Scale (EPDS), which has been validated for use in pregnancy [25], the study reported significantly higher levels of depressive symptomatology in the soft marker group than in the control group. Around one-third of the soft marker group were above the EPDS threshold for major depression. No significant difference in EPDS scores between the soft marker group and those with a history of psychiatric disorder was found. The study concluded that clinically significant levels of depressive symptomatology may be associated with anomalous ultrasound findings; however, the researchers did not follow up participants to see if these symptoms resolved later on in pregnancy.

One other study suggests that the psychological impact of a false-positive ultrasound screening can persist after the birth of a healthy baby [26]. Women for whom a soft marker had been identified and a control group with no soft marker were assessed for depressive symptoms at three time points: in the third trimester of pregnancy, one week post-partum and two months post-partum. At each time point, both anxiety and depression were significantly greater in the soft marker group, with the differences increasing at two months post-partum. The study also identified a detrimental impact on early mother–infant interaction in the soft marker group, for example, lower maternal sensitivity to infant signals.

Impact on the Pregnancy and Developing Fetus

Many of the studies discussed previously cite the potentially negative associations between psychological distress in pregnancy and pregnancy outcomes as a reason for studying anxiety and depression in relation to prenatal testing. What is the evidence that these reactions are detrimental to the pregnancy or the developing fetus?

Research has shown that the process of waiting for and undergoing an invasive diagnostic procedure is associated with high levels of maternal anxiety as measured by the STAI [27]. This anxiety is related not only to fear of the procedure itself (risk of miscarriage, expectation of pain) but also to fear of an abnormal result [27]. Raised levels of anxiety are also therefore associated with the immediate period after the amniocentesis and while waiting for results [28]. Anxiety is such a predictable response to amniocentesis that it has been used as a clinical model to study the impact of maternal anxiety on the fetal environment. For example, research has found that maternal plasma cortisol is significantly correlated with amniotic fluid cortisol levels and that this relationship increases in strength as maternal anxiety levels increase [29, 30]. An assessment of routinely collected data on birth outcomes at three health centres in France identified that women who underwent amniocentesis appeared to be at greater risk of preterm birth and a low-birth-weight baby than did controls [31]. The authors hypothesized that maternal stress may be a mediating factor of these outcomes, although a small sample rendered findings 'imprecise'.

Other research has found no relationship between S-Anxiety as linked to amniocentesis and adverse birth outcomes. One study recorded increased levels of the enzyme 11 β-HSD2 (11 β-hydroxysteroid dehydrogenase type 2), which deactivates cortisol in the fetoplacental unit, and the authors suggest that when faced with a period of acute psychological stress, upregulation of 11 β-HSD2 acts to protect the fetus from exposure to excessive maternal cortisol [32]. The biological pathways between psychological variables such as anxiety and adverse pregnancy outcomes have not yet been established and are likely to be complex, for example, amniotic fluid cortisol levels are not directly predicted by anxiety [29, 30]. In conclusion, despite the significant body of research on the potential psychological consequences of prenatal testing, there is as yet no clear answer to the question of whether anxiety or depression engendered by prenatal testing directly increases the risk of a negative outcome for the pregnancy or fetus.

Non-invasive Prenatal Testing for Aneuploidy

Non-invasive prenatal testing (NIPT) for Down syndrome and other aneuploidies is one of the most important technological developments in the history of prenatal testing for congenital anomaly. NIPT uses cell-free DNA (cfDNA) circulating in the maternal bloodstream combined with DNA sequencing technologies to identify fetal anomalies by comparing the fetal genetic profile with that of the mother [33]. The so called 'fetal' cfDNA migrates into the maternal blood stream via the natural cell death of trophoblast cells shedding off the placental tissue. The three main 'selling points' of NIPT are that it is accurate – detection rates for Down syndrome of over 99% are reported [34]; that it is a safe maternal blood test with no risk of miscarriage; and that it can be carried out reliably from approximately ten weeks' gestation. NIPT can be delivered as a primary 'first-line'

screening test to a low-risk population or as a second-stage contingent test for women identified at higher risk, for example, via serum screening, the identification of ultrasound markers, or advanced maternal age. Currently in the United Kingdom only private health providers offer NIPT as a first-line screen, but in 2016 the UK National Screening Committee recommended an initial 'evaluative implementation' of NIPT in National Health Service (NHS) maternity services and roll out in the NHS is planned for 2018. Research demonstrates that the technology is mostly viewed by women as a positive advancement in prenatal care, particularly for those who may wish to obtain reassurance about their pregnancy but who would avoid a test with a risk of miscarriage [35]. One of the obvious advantages of NIPT in the biopsychosocial context is that the anxiety associated with the procedural element of invasive tests is removed [27]. However, to assess whether there may be any other psychological implications of NIPT, it is necessary to understand more about the test itself.

Despite the early promise of NIPT as a non-invasive diagnostic test for fetal aneuploidy, NIPT can be considered as an advanced screening test rather than a replacement for invasive procedures [33]. This is mainly because the cfDNA is placental in origin. Confined placental trisomy (where the placenta has chromosomal rearrangements not found in the fetus) is found in approximately 1% of pregnancies and is one source of false-positive NIPT results [33]. CfDNA relating to a deceased twin with aneuploidy can also remain in the maternal bloodstream for the duration of a pregnancy [33]. In rare but recorded cases, maternal chromosomal rearrangements or even a maternal malignancy can also be the source of trisomy in cfDNA [34]. For all these reasons, a positive NIPT result needs to be confirmed via CVS or amniocentesis. When NIPT is used as a screening test in a low-risk population, there is a screen positive rate of around 0.1–1% [40]. Although much rarer, false-negative results have also been reported [33].

To date there has been very little research on women's psychological responses to this new technology. A Japanese study compared levels of 'non-specific' psychological distress (depression and anxiety symptoms) in women who underwent NIPT for advanced maternal age and a matched control group of pregnant women who did not undergo NIPT [36]. The women who underwent NIPT recorded higher levels of distress than did controls, but higher levels of anxiety would be expected in women who already knew they were at increased risk [37]. As part of a large British evaluation of NIPT for trisomies 13, 18, and 21, women who were offered NIPT following identification of being at higher risk of an aneuploidy following combined screening completed the STAI after the NIPT blood draw but before the results were given (Time 1) and then one month after their results (Time 2) (28). At Time 1, women in the highest risk group (> 1:150) were unsurprisingly more likely to be anxious than those in the medium risk group (> 1: 1000). Those in the highest risk group who opted for a diagnostic test (as well as NIPT as part of the study) had higher levels of anxiety than those who opted for NIPT only. At Time 2, anxiety levels had dropped for most, but some women who had received a negative NIPT result still had raised anxiety. In this study there was no measurement of anxiety taken after a positive NIPT result but before diagnostic test results (between Times 1 and 2) so it is unknown what impact a positive or inconclusive finding had on these women's anxiety. However, we know already that a positive screening result can induce high levels of anxiety in women, so we might anticipate very high levels in response to a screen-positive NIPT result.

An analysis of media reporting of NIPT shows that the test is sometimes misrepresented as an equivalent to invasive procedures with a focus on high detection rates, and that women may have incorrect or incomplete knowledge and expectations of its capabilities [39]. Therefore a positive NIPT result may be misunderstood as a 99% (or 100%) chance that the fetus is affected. Even in a high-risk population (3% prevalence of Down syndrome) the proportion of 'test-positive' babies who have Down syndrome (the positive predictive value [PPV]) is around 90% [40], meaning that up to one in ten women with a NIPT screen positive in this scenario will be found to have an unaffected fetus [41]. PPV is therefore an important statistic to communicate to women when counselling prior to screening and in the event of a positive NIPT result [34].

NIPT also has the potential to extend the waiting period from the point in time where the increased risk is raised until a final diagnosis. This is especially the case where NIPT is used as a secondary screening test and some women who are identified as being at high risk in the initial screening will need two further tests before they receive their final result [28]. In a small number of cases (varying between 1% and 12% depending on the reporting study) NIPT will result in an inclusive result requiring a redraw; around a third of redraws will fail for the second time [34]. It might be appropriate for some women to be offered the option of an invasive test instead of a redraw in order not to extend the waiting period, especially those in the higher risk group or women for whom second trimester termination is not an option [42]. In the case of uninterpretable NIPT results that are thought to be due to confined placental trisomy, second-trimester amniocentesis rather than first-trimester CVS is recommended, as CVS also samples placental tissue rather than actual fetal material [34].This will happen in very few cases, but for those women, the intervening extended period of raised anxiety may counteract any original psychological benefit of NIPT [43].

As yet, there is no research on the potential for residual anxiety in those women who have received a false-positive NIPT result. There is evidence that some women continue to have lingering concerns after a false-positive screening result and even after a negative NIPT result [28], and so it is likely that this may also be the case after a false-positive NIPT result, especially as by this point the woman may have been identified twice as being at higher risk. It has been recommended that false-positive NIPT results due to confined placental mosaicism are followed up via ultrasound because of an increased risk of placental insufficiency or intrauterine growth restriction [34]. In this situation, women will remain in a raised risk category and, while they will be small in number, it is important that they receive appropriate support throughout their pregnancies.

Summary

There are some clear conclusions about psychological responses to prenatal testing that can be drawn from the existing literature despite the limitations of the evidence base. Firstly, a positive screening result from either biochemical testing or via ultrasound is frequently accompanied by high levels of anxiety, which in some women reaches clinically significant levels. These high levels of anxiety subside after a reassuring diagnostic result but, for some women, residual worries appear to remain even if these are not clinically significant. Secondly, having NIPT or an invasive test is often associated with high levels of anxiety related to both the procedure (in the case of amniocentesis or CVS) and to fear of an abnormal result. A reassuring NIPT result or diagnostic test is associated with a reduction of anxiety to normal levels in most cases. Health professionals involved with the delivery of prenatal testing services can help ameliorate anxiety to some extent by providing accurate and up-to-date information in a timely fashion [44]. Research on depression as related to prenatal testing is much more limited and no clear conclusions can be drawn. Some research suggests that an experience of a screen positive or ultrasound marker may lead to higher rates of depressive symptomatology and that this may impact on maternal–infant interactions once the baby is born. More research on this is required, particularly in relation to false-positive NIPT results. There is no clear evidence that anxiety or depression relating specifically to prenatal testing experience has a detrimental effect on fetal development or pregnancy outcome, although studies show that anxiety in women undergoing amniocentesis is associated with raised stress markers in the fetal environment.

As technologies change it is important to continually revisit the potential for unintended psychological consequences of prenatal tests particularly in relation to non-invasive prenatal tests using cell-free DNA. There has been a move away from this more psychologically focussed research to topics of informed choice and decision making and, while this is important, there is a danger that we neglect some of the basic biopsychosocial questions around prenatal testing that are yet to be adequately answered.

Key Points

- Understanding how and where psychological distress might manifest during the prenatal testing pathway is important in the provision of woman-centred antenatal care.
- For women who receive a screen-negative result, anxiety levels return to normal levels after screening if they have been raised.
- For those with a screen-positive result, research consistently reports feelings of shock, panic, distress and anxiety as well as sleep disturbance, loss of appetite and altered feelings towards the pregnancy. Following a negative diagnosis, anxiety levels usually return to normal suggesting that a false screen-positive does not result in potentially harmful long-term maternal stress.

- Many women are psychologically unprepared for an anomalous finding from an ultrasound scan, even if cognitively they are aware of the potential for problems to be identified.
- There can be longer-term psychological consequences to soft marker identification, including an altered view of pregnancy, and a continued vulnerability to related anxieties in certain circumstances, for example, during childhood illness.
- The biological pathways between psychological variables such as anxiety and adverse pregnancy outcomes have not yet been established.
- So far, there has been very little research on women's psychological responses to non-invasive prenatal testing (NIPT).
- An advantage of NIPT in the biopsychosocial context is that the anxiety associated with the procedural element of invasive tests is removed.
- Media and commercial representation of NIPT as being almost equivalent to a diagnostic test is misleading and may lead to heightened anxiety in some women receiving a screen-positive result.

References

1. Tabor A, Alfirevic Z. Update on procedure-related risks for prenatal diagnosis techniques. *Fetal Diagnosis and Therapy*. 2009;**27**(1):1–7.

2. Edozien LC. Beyond biology: the biopsychosocial model and its application in obstetrics and gynaecology. *BJOG: An International Journal of Obstetrics & Gynaecology*. 2015;**122**(7):900–3. doi: 10.1111/1471-0528.13328.

3. Szegda K, Markenson G, Bertone-Johnson ER, Chasan-Taber L. Depression during pregnancy: a risk factor for adverse neonatal outcomes? A critical review of the literature. *The Journal of Maternal-Fetal & Neonatal Medicine*. 2014;**27**(9):960–7.

4. Green JM, Hewison J, Bekker HL, Bryant LD, Cuckle HS. Psychosocial aspects of genetic screening of pregnant women and newborns: a systematic review. *Health Technology Assessment*. 2004;**8**(33).

5. Lou S, Mikkelsen L, Hvidman L, Petersen OB, Nielsen CP. Does screening for Down's syndrome cause anxiety in pregnant women? a systematic review. *Acta Obstet Gynecol Scand*. 2015;**94**(1):15–27.

6. Harris JM, Franck L, Michie S. Assessing the psychological effects of prenatal screening tests for maternal and foetal conditions: a systematic review.

Journal of Reproductive and Infant Psychology. 2012;**30**(3):222–46.

7. Spielberger C. *Manual for the State-Trait Anxiety Inventory. STAI (Form Y). ('Self-Evaluation Questionnaire').* Palo Alto, CA: Consulting Psychologists Press; 1983.

8. Grant K-A, McMahon C, Austin M-P. Maternal anxiety during the transition to parenthood: a prospective study. *J Affect Disord.* 2008;**108**(1–2):101–11.

9. Kobelka C, Mattman A, Langlois S. An evaluation of the decision-making process regarding amniocentesis following a screen-positive maternal serum screen result. *Prenatal Diagnosis.* 2009;**29**(5):514–9.

10. Garcia J, Bricker L, Henderson J, Martin M-A, Mugford M, Nielson J, et al. Women's views of pregnancy ultrasound: a systematic review. *Birth.* 2002;**29**(4):225–50.

11. Alhusen JL. A literature update on maternal-fetal attachment. *Journal of Obstetric, Gynecologic, & Neonatal Nursing.* 2008;**37**(3):315–28.

12. Åhman A, Runestam K, Sarkadi A. Did I really want to know this? pregnant women's reaction to detection of a soft marker during ultrasound screening. *Patient Education and Counseling.* 2010;**81**(1):87–93.

13. Zechmeister I. Fetal images: the power of visual technology in antenatal care and the Implications for women's reproductive freedom. *Health Care Analysis.* 2001;**9**:387–400.

14. Breathnach F, Malone F. Ultrasound screening for fetal abnormalities and aneuploidies in first and second trimesters. In: Rodeck CH, Whittle M, editors. *Fetal Medicine: Basic Science and Clinical Practice.* Second ed. London: Elsevier; 2009. pp. 265–71.

15. Larsson A-K, Svalenius EC, Maršál K, Ekelin M, Nyberg P, Dykes A-K. Parents' worried state of mind when fetal ultrasound shows an unexpected finding a comparative study. *J Ultrasound Med.* 2009;**28**(12):1663–70.

16. Åhman A, Axelsson O, Maras G, Rubertsson C, Sarkadi A, Lindgren P. Ultrasonographic fetal soft markers in a low-risk population: prevalence, association with trisomies and invasive tests. *Acta Obstet Gynecol Scand.* 2014;**93**(4):367–73.

17. Cristofalo E, Dipietro J, Costigan K, Nelson P, Crino J. Women's response to fetal choroid plexus cysts detected by prenatal ultrasound. *Journal of Perinatology.* 2006;**26**(4):215–23.

18. Larsson A-K, Crang-Svalenius E, Dykes A-K. Information for better or for worse: interviews with parents when their foetus was found to have choroid plexus cysts at a routine second trimester ultrasound.

Journal of Psychosomatic Obstetrics & Gynecology. 2009; **30**(1):48–57. doi: 10.1080/01674820802621775.

19. Lee MJ, Roman AS, Lusskin S, Chen D, Dulay A, Funai EF, et al. Maternal anxiety and ultrasound markers for aneuploidy in a multiethnic population. *Prenatal Diagnosis.* 2007;**27**(1):40–5.

20. Watson MS, Hall S, Langford K, Marteau TM. Psychological impact of the detection of soft markers on routine ultrasound scanning: A pilot study investigating the modifying role of information. *Prenatal Diagnosis.* 2002;**22**(7):569–75.

21. Baillie C, Smith J, Hewison J, Mason G. Ultrasound screening for chromosomal abnormality: women's reactions to false positive results. *British Journal of Health Psychology.* 2000;**5**:377–94.

22. Carolan M, Hodnett E. Discovery of soft markers on fetal ultrasound: maternal implications. *Midwifery.* 2009;**25**(6):654–64.

23. Croton JA. The long-term maternal sequelae to false positive soft marker screens in prenatal ultrasound screening [Ph.D.]. Leeds: University of Leeds (United Kingdom); 2006.

24. Hippman C, Oberlander TF, Honer WG, Misri S, Austin JC. Depression during pregnancy: the potential impact of increased risk for fetal aneuploidy on maternal mood. *Clinical Genetics.* 2009;**75**(1):30–6.

25. Cox JL, Holden JM, Sagovsky R. Detection of postnatal depression. Development of the 10-item Edinburgh Postnatal Depression Scale. *The British Journal of Psychiatry.* 1987;**150**(6):782–6.

26. Viaux-Savelon S, Dommergues M, Rosenblum O, Bodeau N, Aidane E, Philippon O, et al. Prenatal ultrasound screening: false positive soft markers may alter maternal representations and mother-infant interaction. *PloS one.* 2012;**7**(1):e30935.

27. Košec V, Nakić Radoš S, Gall V. Development and validation of the prenatal diagnostic procedures anxiety scale. *Prenatal diagnosis.* 2014;**34**(8):770–7.

28. Lewis C, Hill M, Chitty LS. Women's experiences and preferences for service delivery of non-invasive prenatal testing for aneuploidy in a public health setting: A mixed methods study. *PLoS One.* 2016;**11**(4):e0153147. doi: 10.1371/journal.pone.0153147.

29. Sarkar P, Bergman K, O'Connor T, Glover V. Maternal antenatal anxiety and amniotic fluid cortisol and testosterone: possible implications for foetal programming. *J Neuroendocrinol.* 2008;**20**(4):489–96.

30. Glover V, Bergman K, Sarkar P, O'Connor TG. Association between maternal and amniotic fluid cortisol is moderated by maternal anxiety. *Psychoneuroendocrinology.* 2009;**34**(3):430–5.

31. Garrouste C, Le J, Maurin E. The choice of detecting Down syndrome: does money matter? *Health Economics*. 2011;**20**(9):1073–89.

32. Ghaemmaghami P, Dainese SM, La Marca R, Zimmermann R, Ehlert U. The association between the acute psychobiological stress response in second trimester pregnant women, amniotic fluid glucocorticoids, and neonatal birth outcome. *Dev Psychobiol*. 2014;**56**(4):734–47.

33. Gregg AR, Van den Veyver IB, Gross SJ, Madankumar R, Rink BD, Norton ME. Noninvasive prenatal screening by next-generation sequencing. *Annual review of genomics and human genetics*. 2014;**15**:327–47.

34. Cuckle H, Benn P, Pergament E. Cell-free DNA screening for fetal aneuploidy as a clinical service. *Clinical biochemistry*. 2015;**48**(15):932–41. doi: 10.1016/j.clinbiochem.2015.02.011.

35. Lewis C, Hill M, Silcock C, Daley R, Chitty L. Non-invasive prenatal testing for trisomy 21: A cross-sectional survey of service users' views and likely uptake. *BJOG: An International Journal of Obstetrics & Gynaecology*. 2014;**121**(5):582–94. doi: 10.1111/1471-0528.12579.

36. Suzumori N, Ebara T, Kumagai K, Goto S, Yamada Y, Kamijima M, et al. Non-specific psychological distress in women undergoing noninvasive prenatal testing because of advanced maternal age. *Prenatal diagnosis*. 2014;**34**(11):1055–60.

37. Grinshpun-Cohen J, Miron-Shatz T, Ries-Levavi L, Pras E. Factors that affect the decision to undergo amniocentesis in women with normal Down syndrome screening results: it is all about the age. *Health Expectations*. (ePub). 2015;**18**(6):2306–17. doi: 10.1111/hex.12200.

38. Hill M, Wright D, Daley R, Lewis C, McKay F, Mason S, et al. Evaluation of non-invasive prenatal testing (NIPT) for aneuploidy in an NHS setting: a reliable accurate prenatal non-invasive diagnosis (RAPID) protocol. *BMC pregnancy and childbirth*. 2014;**14**(1):229.

39. Lewis C, Choudhury M, Chitty LS. 'Hope for safe prenatal gene tests'. A content analysis of how the UK press media are reporting advances in non-invasive prenatal testing. *Prenatal Diagnosis*. 2015;**35**(5):420–7. doi: 10.1002/pd.4488.

40. Taylor-Phillips, S, Freeman K, Geppert J, Agbebiyi A, Uthman OA, Madan J, Clarke A, Quenby S, Clarke A. Accuracy of non-invasive prenatal testing using cell-free DNA for detection of Down, Edwards and Patau syndromes: a systematic review and meta-analysis. *BMJ open*. 2016;**6**(1):e010002.

41. Hewison J. Psychological aspects of individualized choice and reproductive autonomy in prenatal screening. *Bioethics*. 2015;**29**(1):9–18.

42. Jafri H, Ahmed S, Ahmed M, Hewison J, Raashid Y, Sheridan E. Islam and termination of pregnancy for genetic conditions in Pakistan: Implications for Pakistani health care providers. *Prenatal diagnosis*. 2012;**32**(12):1218–20.

43. Newson AJ. Ethical aspects arising from non-invasive fetal diagnosis. *Seminars in Fetal and Neonatal Medicine*. 2008;**13**(2):103–8.

44. Bryant L, Ahmed S, Hewison J. Conveying information about screening. In: Rodeck C, Whittle M, editors. *Fetal Medicine: Basic Science and Clinical Practice*. Second ed. Edinburgh: Elsevier; 2009. p. 225.

Chapter 28

The Maternal–Fetal Relationship
Conceptualization, Measurement and Application in Practice

Zoe Darwin and Judi Walsh

Introduction and Overview

Pregnancy and the transition to parenthood involve great psychological adaptation. Part of this adaptation is the development of the woman's relationship with her unborn child – the maternal–fetal relationship (MFR) – which manifests in a woman's thoughts, feelings, attitudes and behaviours towards her developing baby. Routine psychosocial assessment increasingly features in maternity care, and it has been argued that this could be expanded to include antenatal assessment of MFR to target interventions towards those judged to have 'suboptimal' MFR, to improve health-related behaviours and optimize parenting and the child's social and emotional development. There is, however, inconsistency in how MFR has been conceptualized, raising questions about what 'suboptimal' MFR might look like, and a lack of evidence on its associated risks, and amenability to intervention. To consider the implications of MFR for health professionals and clinical practice we outline what is meant by MFR, how it may be measured, what MFR influences and is influenced by, and why and when MFR may be measured.

What Is MFR?

Pregnancy is a time of physiological, emotional and psychological adaptation and adjustment [1] for both mothers and fathers. Early work exploring the transition to parenthood suggested that mothers need to achieve several psychological tasks during pregnancy, which include developing a maternal identity (e.g. [2]), differentiation of the self from the fetus, and developing an emotional relationship with the fetus [3]. Cranley [4] conceptualized this maternal–fetal relationship (MFR) as maternal 'attachment' in 1981, and there has since been a steadily increasing body of research which has grown to include the adaptation experienced by fathers [5].

The terminology used to describe this phenomenon has been the subject of debate in recent years because in developmental psychology, 'attachment' is a term used to describe a system which exists, from an evolutionary standpoint, to keep the child safe by promoting proximity-seeking and care-eliciting behaviours on the part of the child (although adults too can be attached and can seek care from others). The counterpart to attachment, the 'caregiving system', exists to promote the provision of care to others when they are distressed [6]. In this developmental sense, the child is 'attached' to the caregiver, but the caregiver is not 'attached' to the child. Thus, the relationships that parents form with their children before birth, often called 'bonding', are likely to be about parental attitudes, projections, cognitions and emotional responses to the pregnancy and developing fetus [7], not about seeking care from that fetus. For this reason, some scholars have argued that using 'attachment' in this context is a misnomer (e.g. [8, 9]), but the term 'attachment' to describe the antenatal relationship has become increasingly accepted.

There appears to be a reasonable consensus in the literature that whatever terminology we use, the construct under investigation is similar, centering around behaviours, thoughts, feelings and actions that demonstrate care and commitment to the developing child [8]. But even here there are differences. Definitions have variously emphasized different parental thoughts about and behaviours towards the fetus: love for [10], affiliation and interaction with [4], and protection of [11]. Most scholars have seen the construct as multidimensional (e.g. [4, 10]), but some have conceptualized it as unidimensional (e.g. [12]). There has been discussion too, of whether the concept includes feelings about the pregnancy in addition to feelings about the fetus (e.g. [4]), or whether these things are separate (e.g. [10]). These different conceptualizations have led to the development of different measures.

Measuring MFR

Over 30 years of published literature exists on the measurement of MFR. Measurement research has been dominated by verbal self-report tools where women are asked to rate various manifestations of the relationship, e.g. behaviours, feelings, attitudes and thoughts including talking to the baby, talking about the baby, feeling love for the baby, physical preparation and picturing the developing baby. Three main self-report measures are currently in use. A comprehensive review by Van den Bergh and Simons [8] summarizes these measures, their psychometric properties and how they link with theoretical understanding and description of the phenomenon. The measures are the Maternal-Fetal Attachment Scale (MFAS, [4]), the Maternal Antenatal Attachment Scale (MAAS, [10]) and the Prenatal Attachment Inventory (PAI, [12]). The measures vary in conceptualization, but all are scored on one or more continuous scales with higher scores being viewed as indicative of higher levels of MFR, and considered more favourable.

The MFAS focusses on 'the extent to which pregnant women engage in behaviours that represent an affiliation and interaction with their unborn child' ([4], p. 262). Reflecting concerns that the MFAS placed too great an emphasis on the motherhood role and pregnancy state, the MAAS was developed to focus on feelings and behaviours towards the fetus, scored in terms of the *quality* of attachment (e.g. closeness, pleasure in interaction, tenderness towards the fetus) and *intensity* of preoccupation (time spent thinking about the fetus). In contrast, the PAI focusses on the 'unique affectionate relationship', and on thoughts and feelings rather than behaviours. Measures of the paternal–fetal relationship also exist, and these have largely been adapted from measures developed for use in mothers, for example the Paternal Fetal Attachment Scale modified from the MFAS [13], and the Paternal Antenatal Attachment Scale, modified from the MAAS [10].

The various self-report measures each contain approximately 20 items and have been criticized for lacking application to clinical settings due to length and language requirements (e.g. [14]). Overall, reliability of the 'total' attachment scales in these measures tends to be fairly high, but there are often problems with sub-scales and factor structures, which might reflect differences and difficulties in conceptualizing the component parts of the concept [8]. In response to concerns about length and language requirements, researchers in the Netherlands developed the Pictorial Representation of Attachment Measure (PRAM) [15] to offer a brief, non-verbal tool which can be self-completed or talked through with the researcher or practitioner requesting the assessment. Completion requires the respondent to indicate on a visual diagram where they would place the baby in their life at this moment, with shorter distances between the baby and self thought to indicate greater interpersonal closeness and a higher level of MFR. The tool's authors report convergent validity in mothers and fathers using the MAAS and propose that the PRAM might have an application as a screening tool to identify 'suboptimal' MFR, but highlight the need to first conduct further research [14].

We lack clinical cut-offs for the measures described previously and they are instead generally used to compare higher and lower scores. Another approach to measurement is to focus on women's working models (i.e. representations) rather than their feelings of affection and commitment. This is usually done via a structured interview that generates a narrative, which is subsequently coded and scored. Examples include the Pregnancy Interview-Revised [16], the Working Model of the Child Interview [17] and the Interview of Maternal Representations during Pregnancy-Revised Version [18]. Scoring of structured interviews tends to be used to classify women as having different types or 'styles', an approach more comparable with assessing attachment through interviews, and one that may better lend itself to providing an indication of clinical concern, as compared with the MFR measures described previously. Although structured interviews are comprehensive and informative, they are resource-intensive: interviews are long (typically an hour) and the resulting tapes need to be coded by someone with appropriate training. As such, research using these structured interviews has been limited to relatively small sample sizes and the approach would be unsuitable for universal assessment or routine use in clinical settings.

There are several implicit assumptions around measurement that warrant further consideration.

First, measurement assumes that individuals are aware of the manifestations of MFR and able to quantify them. Second, measurement is assumed to be an inert process, but it is likely that there is some degree of measurement reactivity; whereby the process of measurement influences the thing being measured. Third, assessing MFR is a potentially emotive area where social desirability is likely to be a challenge for measurement, and women may be unwilling to disclose their 'true' feelings, particularly in a clinical context. There is also the potential for assessment to itself be a source of anxiety or feelings of guilt and inadequacy around parenting [19]. As argued by Walsh and colleagues, research is needed to explore whether discussion of MFR is meaningful or acceptable to pregnant women, what such discussions should reflect, and how such discussions should take place ([20]). We also need to take into account cultural factors: representations of the baby and self as parent are likely to differ across cultures. Most of the current research is dominated by a western concept and western measures of MFR which may not be applicable in other cultures. Further research is needed here.

Antecedents, Correlates and Consequences of MFR

Overall, demographic factors such as age, marital status, income, parity, education and ethnicity do not appear to considerably impact MFR [21]. Evidence exists linking MFR with other variables in pregnancy, most notably pregnancy-specific contextual factors, social support and physical and psychological health. Some of these variables have commonly been treated as 'predictors' of MFR and others as being dependent on MFR (i.e. considered 'outcomes'). Much of the work examining MFR in pregnancy is cross-sectional, and it is difficult to disentangle temporal relationships between constructs; such relationships should instead be considered associations. Although there is a great deal of research which examines these associations, research synthesis demonstrates that findings are often inconsistent [8, 21–23]. Next, we overview some of the factors found to be associated with MFR, but with the caution in mind that the challenge now is to build models which look at the complexity of how these factors interact with each other, rather than looking at predictors in isolation [8, 20, 24–26].

Factors Associated with MFR

Pregnancy-Specific Contextual Factors

The findings linking obstetric factors and MFR are inconsistent, and meta-analyses show trivial to low effect sizes overall [21]. There is little research on pregnancy planning, but research synthesis shows a small effect size on MFR [21]. Further clarity is needed distinguishing between attitudes and behaviours, and examining elements such as the extent to which the pregnancy was planned, intended, timed and wanted [27].

Many studies do not find an association between mode of conception and MFR (e.g. see [28] for a review), but recent research has found that mothers conceiving through assisted reproductive technology (ART) form more intense relationships with the fetus than mothers conceiving spontaneously once age has been taken into account [29]. Parents conceiving through ART may have experiences which are coupled with some form of perinatal loss such as miscarriage, but also loss around conception and parenthood. There may therefore exist parallels between parents whose pregnancies follow ART and/or perinatal loss, as parents may perceive their pregnancies as high risk even where they are considered obstetrically 'normal' (e.g. [30]) (see also chapter 14)).

Studies do not always find significant differences in terms of MFR between mothers with and without a history of pregnancy loss (e.g. [31]), although some find differences in particular scales, like 'differentiation of self from fetus' [32]. Although some studies have not found a difference between high-risk and obstetrically 'normal' pregnancies in terms of MFR (e.g. [33]), some have found lower levels in those hospitalized for high risk of preterm delivery [34], and others have found that amongst those hospitalized for pregnancy complications, positive coping strategies mediate between maternal appraisals of risk and MFR [35]. In future research, further attention needs to be given to the relationship between coping and MFR in pregnancies that are perceived to be high risk.

Social Support and Relationships

Women who are satisfied with their social supports have been consistently found to report higher levels of MFR. There is evidence in fathers of a strong association between the strength of the partner relationship and indicators of the parental–fetal relationship [13].

Challenges exist in disentangling these factors. Attitudes towards pregnancy and intendedness of pregnancy are associated with social support and relationship with partner (e.g. [36]). In addition, indicators of psychological health are consistently found to be highly correlated with the quality of the partner relationship and with social support [37], an observation that is found across populations and settings. Bouchard's research [24] was amongst the first to examine moderating effects in predicting the parental–fetal relationship for mothers and fathers, and found that, for mothers, relationship with partner was associated with MFR, but only for those with low levels of neuroticism or less optimal attachment with their own parents. For fathers, relationship quality interacted with high levels of parental attachment, but not neuroticism, to predict parental–fetal relationship. Recent research by Maas et al. [38] tested a model which comprised parental (personality and attachment), contextual (partner support and perceived stress) and expected child (temperament) characteristics, and which found MFR to be multiply determined, with parental characteristics explaining most variance. These recent research findings highlight that we need to consider unique combinations of risk and protective factors in considering pathways to MFR.

Physical and Psychological Health

MFR is related to health behaviours in pregnancy including balance of rest and exercise, safety measures, nutrition, avoiding harmful substances, obtaining healthcare and obtaining information [26]. Research has been dominated by primarily Caucasian middle-class samples, but recent studies suggest that these health behaviours are linked with MFR in low-income African-American families, and that these health behaviours mediate the link between MFR and later neonatal outcome [39]. However, some research shows that high levels of MFR can be associated with assurances of fetal well-being, and thus a less strict adherence to healthy behaviours [40]. Another consideration, particularly given suggestions that MFR should be targeted in order to improve health behaviours (e.g. [8]), is that associations between MFR and health behaviours may reflect a third variable that itself should be targeted by intervention. One possible candidate is 'stress' including causes (such as social deprivation and life events) and symptoms (such as depression and anxiety), which have been associated with both MFR and health behaviours [26].

Findings are especially inconsistent when examining the relationship between psychological health and MFR and although most work finds that MFR is higher in those with lower psychological distress (e.g. [41]), some studies do not find an association (e.g. [1]). Again, we find complex mediating and moderating pathways between factors. Walsh et al. [42] tested a model which found mental health to be a strong predictor of MFR, alongside care-giving style to partner, which itself mediated the link between attachment and MFR. In contrast, Diniz et al. [43] did not find a link between depression and MFR in their sample of Brazilian adolescents, but they did find emotional support to be a key variable associated with MFR.

Links between MFR and Postnatal Factors

Alongside considering how factors interact with each other, longitudinal work is needed to better understand the possible effects of MFR. Researchers suggest that 'it seems intuitively likely that the feelings parents have during pregnancy about their baby are likely to be associated with later parental and infant behaviour' ([7], p. 221). MFR measures in pregnancy have been found to be associated with more optimal child outcomes, and with better psychological health in the postnatal period [44]. There is emerging evidence that MFR is linked with parenting and child–parent relationship outcomes, but this work is in its infancy and there is a wide range of factors which impact the relationship. Parenting is a constellation of behaviours, emotions and cognitions [45], and we find inconsistent and modest findings between MFR and indicators of parenting, parental representations and parent–child interaction. Siddiqui and Hägglöf [46] found a link between MFR as measured by the PAI and postnatal involvement in interaction but not responsiveness in interaction. Condon et al. [47] found continuity between prenatal paternal attachment and postnatal parental 'attachment' measures (thoughts and connections with the baby), but with strong effects from relationship quality and mental health, whilst Müller [12] found only a modest correlation between MFR and postnatal attachment. Thun-Hohenstein et al. [48] did not find any significant relationship between maternal antenatal representations and parenting competence in interaction with infants of 12 weeks. They did find significant associations between antenatal representations and regulatory ability in the mothers, and interaction behaviour on the part of the infant. In conclusion, it appears that there are some links between antenatal representations of the child, or connections with the child, and some postnatal outcomes, but we need more research to explicate these complex links and mechanisms more fully.

It is often suggested that antenatal attachment can predict later attachment on behalf of the child. Secure infant attachment, most often measured through the 'gold standard' of the 'Strange Situation' [49], is associated with better functioning in many areas, including emotional, social and cognitive development [49], and so if we could find an indicator before birth, we might be able to target intervention. Some studies have found an association between working models of the child in pregnancy and later attachment security (e.g. [50]), but we currently have no strong evidence that MFR as measured by self-report on the part of the mother is linked with more secure attachment in infancy for children.

Why Measure MFR?

Many studies which examine associations between MFR and other perinatal factors conclude that if MFR in the antenatal period is associated with well-being and positive health practices in pregnancy, and more optimal outcomes for children and parents post birth, then intervening in the maternal–fetal relationship or representations thereof might have positive outcomes throughout this period, and might be a useful place to start. It has been proposed that problems with MFR may be targeted by interventions spanning several areas, including understanding and managing reactions to antenatal screening and perinatal loss, promoting parents' antenatal health behaviours (and subsequent birth and infant health outcomes), and the parent–infant relationship (and subsequent child's development) [8].

What constitutes a pathological maternal–fetal relationship remains 'almost entirely unexplored' ([51], p.10). MFR is most often scored on a continuum, and we have few indications of scores or cut-offs which would indicate a clinical difficulty (either at the 'low' end or the 'high' end). Thus, it remains that, in the clinical environment, difficulties should be clinically determined rather than relying on scores on a screening instrument. In addition, we do not well enough understand the long-term outcomes of 'problematic' levels of MFR, or for whom they

might pose a risk. We also find that some subscales of MFR are more commonly linked with difficulty or adjustment than others. Much of the research seems to suggest that when using the MAAS measure, the *quality* sub-scale is linked with functioning, especially psychological well-being, whereas associations with *intensity* subscale are much less clear and need further attention in research, although some suggest this scale is linked more strongly with external factors [52]. There is little evidence that low levels are linked with major difficulties in any arena or to provide justification for intervention. Of course, this is not to say that there may not be times where it might be useful to use measures of MFR in conjunction with, or to aid, clinical decision making, or indeed to provide a starting point for clinical interview. Research by Condon [53] suggests that there are cases of deliberate harm towards the fetus in terms of active or passive abuse. Pollock and Percy [54] investigated a high-risk sample of pregnant women. They used Condon's alternative categorical scoring method which combines scores on the *quality* and *intensity* dimensions to form four styles: negative disinterested, negative preoccupied, positive disinterested and positive preoccupied. Pollock and Percy found that all but two of the 40 mothers had a 'negative' antenatal attachment style and those with a negatively preoccupied MFR pattern (low levels of quality and high levels of intensity) were more likely to report irritation with the fetus. These mothers were also more likely to report an urge to harm the fetus, although this did not reach statistical significance and actual levels of abuse were not measured. This research shows that high scores, particularly on the *intensity* scale, might not always be optimal, and Laxton-Kane and Slade [25] suggest that we might devote future research to investigating 'styles' of MFR, rather than 'levels'.

Another approach may be to offer intervention on the basis of possible risk factors or characteristics, rather than individual assessment of MFR. This is the current approach for 'attachment-based interventions' which aims to support the parent in being available, responsive and sensitive to the child's needs and generally target groups considered 'at-risk' of insecure attachment based on certain characteristics, for example being homeless, a care leaver, or a young parent. Possible groups that may be targeted by intervention could include those who have experienced perinatal loss, those with high-risk pregnancies, those experiencing psychological distress, those with attachment difficulties in their family of origin and those whose health behaviours increase the risk of poor pregnancy and infant outcomes. These different areas of need would require different interventions and would differ in their mechanisms and intended outcomes, although some women may fall into multiple groups. Even if eligibility were not based on individual assessment of MFR, we may still want to measure MFR in order to understand how the intervention works (or fails to work) and capture change following an intervention – thus accurate assessment and indicators of clinically significant change are still needed and currently lacking.

When to Measure MFR

The timing at which measurement could and should be undertaken depends on its purpose. Early intervention requires early assessment. Maternity care in high-income countries has moved towards increasingly detailed antenatal psychosocial assessment in order to shape care pathways according to identified need. In the United Kingdom, psychosocial assessment is undertaken at the booking visit (the first formal antenatal appointment) and includes assessment of mental health, social support, involvement of social care and other services, residential status and health behaviours (including substance use and smoking). Targets (UK) now exist for the booking visit to be conducted by 10–12 weeks' gestation [55].

The need for early intervention must be balanced with the accuracy of results. MFR tools lack validation in early pregnancy as measurement of MFR has focussed on later pregnancy, although exceptions exist (e.g. [42]). This in part reflects the timing of the events that contribute to the development of the mother–child relationship, including the significance of quickening, with fetal movements generally being felt from around the middle of pregnancy (18–20 weeks in primigravida and 15–17 weeks in multigravida). Peppers and Knapp [56] described nine contributory events in MFR development, the first five of which happen before the birth: planning, confirming and accepting the pregnancy; feeling the fetus (fetal movements); accepting the fetus as an individual; giving birth; seeing the baby; touching the baby and giving care to the baby. With the introduction of ultrasound scanning, seeing the fetus has become an additional event that contributes to the relationship's development [57], and one which routinely first takes place before fetal movements have been felt unless a woman has attended for antenatal care relatively late. The occurrence and timing of events and associated trajectory of MFR development may thus vary with changes in clinical practice. In addition, it should be noted that not all of these events apply to all women or in all pregnancies, and events may vary with contextual factors such as intendedness of pregnancy and gestation at which pregnancy is confirmed, yet this remains under-researched.

It has been argued that the existing measures can be adapted for use in early pregnancy by simply omitting those items that apply only to the later stages (e.g. those concerning fetal movements) or using weighted means [8]. It is possible, however, that the situation is more complex than different items being relevant at different time points, and concepts in the trajectory of MFR development may not be suited to measurement in early pregnancy.

Alongside concerns around the accuracy of early measurement and its ability to identify women who may benefit from intervention, little is known about how these factors may vary with maternal characteristics, for example in women where there is a perceived or actual risk to the viability of the pregnancy. There is evidence of 'emotional cushioning' following perinatal loss whereby women's MFR in a subsequent pregnancy may be delayed as a self-protective mechanism [58]. Women who are informed about prenatal serum screening in pregnancy, compared with those who are not informed, delay MFR until testing is complete [59]. This process of the holding back of emotions has been described as 'the tentative pregnancy' [58]. Similar processes may be observed in women whose conception follows ART and women whose pregnancies are considered obstetrically high risk. Critically, it remains unknown whether the outcomes for these mothers and their children are different to those where a pregnancy does not follow perinatal loss and is not considered high risk.

Using tools in early pregnancy that lack validation for this specific time period has the potential to unnecessarily burden women and healthcare systems by overidentifying women whose MFR may progress in such a way that it is no longer considered 'suboptimal' at a later point in the pregnancy. It may therefore be that repeated assessment would be needed before determining concerns about a woman's MFR. In addition, trajectories may differ between individuals and between pregnancies in the same individual without being problematic. MFR is more likely to be higher in first-time pregnancies, and the limited research on measurement across all three trimesters indicates that levels of MFR rise after the first trimester and remain relatively stable over the second to third trimesters [10, 42]. Further work is needed to better understand these processes.

Trajectories of MFR development may also vary between mothers and fathers; measurement (and any intervention) may therefore be appropriate at different stages in fathers. Specifically, ultrasound scans have been identified as a key event in the development of the paternal–fetal relationship [57] and therefore may provide an opportunity for assessment and, where appropriate, intervention targeting the parental–fetal relationship and health behaviour change.

Implications for Healthcare Professionals

The argument for antenatal assessment of MFR in order to target interventions makes several assumptions that need to be questioned: that 'suboptimal' MFR exists, that MFR can be accurately measured (i.e. that individuals are conscious/aware of the manifestations and able to quantify them), that women will disclose in a clinical context and that women (and health professionals) would find it acceptable to target interventions on the basis of assessment.

There is currently insufficient evidence to support 'screening' for potential 'suboptimal' MFR in clinical practice. In addition, there exist some considerations that echo concerns raised in relation to antenatal mental health assessment more generally; specifically, that it is unethical to introduce assessment without appropriate management, and that we need to be mindful of over-pathologizing women [60]. In terms of identifying 'risk' or pathological concerns, rather than considering the introduction of a self-report measure to quantify levels of MFR, it may be fruitful to identify certain indicators that may be considered 'red flags', for example denial or concealing of the pregnancy, not engaging with antenatal care or thoughts of harming the baby (an item on the MAAS). Existing measures of MFR such as the PRAM may currently be more appropriately used as a communication device to discuss the context of a woman's pregnancy, and offer an enabling environment in which to voice her views and any concerns

that could be revisited throughout maternity care [61]. Here too is an opportunity to involve fathers and partners in discussions which may help to support them and promote their engagement, an aspiration identified in policy (e.g. [62]).

Summary
MFR-based screening may be appropriate only when we better understand what is being measured, how to facilitate MFR, and what the potential outcomes might be. Further research is needed before we are in a position to harness the potential of MFR for clinical application. This includes a need for greater conceptual clarity, greater understanding of the development and impact of MFR in the perinatal period and beyond, and how it may vary across cultures. Applied research is also needed to develop and test interventions in a clinical setting, with embedded consideration of resource implications and other factors influencing implementation. This is not to say that MFR is not a useful, valid or important concept. An understanding of what is known about MFR can aid professionals in their support of parents and in decision making. Similarly, an understanding of what we still need to know will help drive research and practice to provide appropriate, acceptable and timely support and care.

Key Points

- The terminology used to describe the relationship between a mother (or father) and the unborn child has been the subject of debate, but most authors agree that it centres around the parent's behaviours, thoughts, feelings and actions that demonstrate care and commitment to the developing child.
- There is a link between maternal–fetal relationship (MFR) and health behaviours in pregnancy including balance of rest and exercise, safety measures, nutrition, avoiding harmful substances, obtaining health care and obtaining information. There is also emerging evidence that MFR is linked with some indices of postnatal parenting and child–parent relationship outcomes, but currently there is no strong evidence that MFR as measured by self-report on the part of the mother is linked with attachment security in children.

- Women who are satisfied with their social supports have been consistently found to report higher levels of MFR, and there is evidence in fathers of an association between the strength of the partner relationship and indicators of the parental–fetal relationship.
- Research is needed to explore whether discussion of MFR is meaningful or acceptable to pregnant women, what such discussions should reflect, and how such discussions should take place.
- The most commonly used tools for measuring MFR are the Maternal-Fetal Attachment Scale (MFAS), the Maternal Antenatal Attachment Scale (MAAS) and the Prenatal Attachment Inventory (PAI), all of which are verbal self-report measures.
- Most current research is dominated by concepts and measures of MFR developed in western contexts which may not be applicable in some cultures.
- It may be advisable for future research to explore 'styles' in addition to 'levels' of MFR.
- Ideally, women at risk of adverse outcomes should be identified in early pregnancy to receive timely support, but MFR tools generally lack validation in very early pregnancy.
- We do not yet well enough understand the long-term outcomes of 'problematic' levels of MFR.
- There is currently insufficient evidence to support 'screening' for potential 'suboptimal' MFR in clinical practice, and research is needed to explore the application of MFR assessment as a communication device or aid to clinical decision making.

References

1. Hart, R. and C.A. McMahon, Mood state and psychological adjustment to pregnancy. *Archives of Women's Mental Health*, 2006. **9**(6): 329–337.

2. Rubin, R., Maternal tasks in pregnancy. *Maternal-Child Nursing Journal*, 1975. **4**(3): 143–153.

3. Valentine, D.P., The experience of pregnancy: A developmental process. *Family Relations*, 1982. **31**(2): 243–248.

4. Cranley, M.S., Development of a tool for the measurement of maternal attachment during pregnancy. *Nursing Research*, 1981. **30**(5): 281–284.

5. Condon, J.T., The parental-foetal relationship: A comparison of male and female expectant parents. *Journal of Psychosomatic Obstetrics and Gynecology*, 1985. **4**: 271–284.

6. Bowlby, J., *Attachment and loss. Volume 1: Attachment.* 2nd edition. 1982. New York: Basic Books.

7. Redshaw, M. and C. Martin, Babies, 'bonding' and ideas about parental 'attachment'. *Journal of Reproductive and Infant Psychology*, 2013. **31**(3): 219–221.

8. Van den Bergh, B. and A. Simons, A review of scales to measure the mother-foetus relationship. *Journal of Reproductive and Infant Psychology*, 2009. **27**(2): 114–126.

9. Walsh, J., Definitions matter: If maternal-fetal relationships are not attachment, what are they? *Archives of Women's Mental Health*, 2010. **13**(5): 449–451.

10. Condon, J.T., The assessment of antenatal emotional attachment – Development of a questionnaire instrument. *British Journal of Medical Psychology*, 1993. **66**(2): 167–183.

11. Sandbrook, S.P. and E.N. Adamson-Macedo, Maternal-fetal attachment: Searching for a new definition. *Neuroendocrinology Letters*, 2004. **25**: 169–182.

12. Müller, M.E., Development of the prenatal attachment inventory. *Western Journal of Nursing Research*, 1993. **15**(2): 199–215.

13. Weaver, R.H. and M.S. Cranley, An exploration of paternal-fetal attachment behavior. *Nursing Research*, 1983. **32**(2): 68–72.

14. van Bakel, H.J.A., et al., Pictorial representation of attachment: Measuring the parent–fetus relationship in expectant mothers and fathers. *BMC Pregnancy and Childbirth*, 2013. **13**: 138–147.

15. van Bakel, H.J.A., C.M.J.M. Vreeswijk, and A.J.B.M. Maas, Verbal and pictorial representations of the antenatal mother-foetus relationship. Proceedings of the 29th Society for Reproductive and Infant Psychology Conference, *University of Newcastle. (Abstract). Journal of Reproductive and Infant Psychology*, 2009. **27**(3): 323.

16. Slade, A., et al., *The parent development interview-revised: Unpublished protocol.* 2004, New York: The City University of New York.

17. Zeanah, C.H., et al., Mothers' representations of their infants are concordant with infant attachment classifications. *Developmental Issues in Psychiatry and Psychology*, 1994. **1**: 1–14.

18. Ammaniti, M. and R. Tambelli, *Prenatal self-report questionnaires, scales and interviews., in Parenthood and mental health. A bridge between infant and adult*

psychiatry, S. Tyano, et al., Editors. 2010, Oxford: Wiley-Blackwell.

19. Jomeen, J., *Choice and control in contemporary childbirth: Understanding through Women's Experiences*. 2010, London: Radcliffe.

20. Walsh, J., et al., Maternal–fetal relationships and psychological health: Emerging research directions. *Journal of Reproductive and Infant Psychology*, 2013. **31**(5): 490–499.

21. Yarcheski, A., et al., A meta-analytic study of predictors of maternal-fetal attachment. *International Journal of Nursing Studies*, 2009. **46**(5): 708–715.

22. Alhusen, J.L., A literature update on maternal-fetal attachment. *JOGNN-Journal of Obstetric Gynecologic and Neonatal Nursing*, 2008. **37**(3): 315–328.

23. Cannella, B.L., Maternal-fetal attachment: An integrative review. *Journal of Advanced Nursing*, 2005. **50**(1): 60–68.

24. Bouchard, G., The role of psychosocial variables in prenatal attachment: An examination of moderational effects. *Journal of Reproductive and Infant Psychology*, 2011. **29**(3): 197–207.

25. Laxton-Kane, M. and P. Slade, The role of maternal prenatal attachment in a woman's experience of pregnancy and implications for the process of care. *Journal of Reproductive and Infant Psychology*, 2002. **20**(4): 253–266.

26. Lindgren, K., Relationships among maternal-fetal attachment, prenatal depression, and health practices in pregnancy. *Research in Nursing & Health*, 2001. **24**(3): 203–217.

27. Klerman, V.T., The intendedness of pregnancy: A concept in transition. *Maternal and Child Health Journal*, 2000. **4**(3): 155–162.

28. Hammarberg, K., J. Fisher, and K. Wynter, Psychological and social aspects of pregnancy, childbirth and early parenting after assisted conception: A systematic review. *Human Reproduction Update*, 2008. **14**(5): 395–414.

29. McMahon, C.A., et al., Age at first birth, mode of conception and psychological wellbeing in pregnancy: Findings from the parental age and transition to parenthood Australia (PATPA) study. *Human Reproduction*, 2011. **26**(6): 1389–1398.

30. McMahon, C.A., et al., 'Don't count your chickens': a comparative study of the experience of pregnancy after IVF conception. *Journal of Reproductive and Infant Psychology*, 1999. **17**(4): 345–356.

31. Tsartsara, E. and M.P. Johnson, The impact of miscarriage on women's pregnancy-specific anxiety and feelings of prenatal maternal–fetal attachment during the course of a subsequent pregnancy: an exploratory follow-up study. *Journal of Psychosomatic Obstetrics & Gynecology*, 2006. **27**(3): 173–182.

32. Mehran, P., et al., History of perinatal loss and maternal–fetal attachment behaviors. *Women and Birth*, 2013. **26**(3): 185–189.

33. Kemp, V.H. and C.K. Page, Maternal prenatal attachment in normal and high-risk pregnancies. *Journal of Obstetric, Gynecologic, & Neonatal Nursing*, 1987. **16**(3): 179–184.

34. Pisoni, C., et al., Risk and protective factors in maternal–fetal attachment development. *Early Human Development*, 2014. **90**: S45–S46.

35. White, O., et al., Maternal appraisals of risk, coping and prenatal attachment among women hospitalised with pregnancy complications. *Journal of Reproductive and Infant Psychology*, 2008. **26**(2): 74–85.

36. Kroelinger, C.D. and K.S. Oths, Partner support and pregnancy wantedness. *Birth*, 2000. **27**(2): 112–119.

37. Pilkington, P.D., et al., Modifiable partner factors associated with perinatal depression and anxiety: A systematic review and meta-analysis. *Journal of Affective Disorders*, 2015. **178**: 165–80.

38. Maas, A.J.B., et al., Determinants of maternal fetal attachment in women from a community-based sample. *Journal of Reproductive and Infant Psychology*, 2014. **32**(1): 5–24.

39. Alhusen, J.L., et al., The influence of maternal–fetal attachment and health practices on neonatal outcomes in low-income, urban women. *Research in Nursing & Health*, 2012. **35**(2): 112–120.

40. Ross, E., Maternal–fetal attachment and engagement with antenatal advice. *British Journal of Midwifery*, 2012. **20**(8): 566–575.

41. McFarland, J., et al., Major depressive disorder during pregnancy and emotional attachment to the fetus. *Archives of Women's Mental Health*, 2011. **14**(5): 425–434.

42. Walsh, J., E.G. Hepper, and B.J. Marshall, Investigating attachment, caregiving, and mental health: a model of maternal-fetal relationships. *BMC Pregnancy and Childbirth*, 2014. **14**(383).

43. Diniz, E., S.H. Koller, and B.L. Volling, Social support and maternal depression from pregnancy to postpartum: the association with positive maternal behaviours among Brazilian adolescent mothers. *Early Child Development and Care*, 2014. **185**(7): 1053–1066.

44. Alhusen, J.L., M.J. Hayat, and D. Gross, A longitudinal study of maternal attachment and infant developmental outcomes. *Archives of Women's Mental Health*, 2013. **16**(6): 521–529.

45. Jones, J.D., J. Cassidy, and P.R. Shaver, Parents' self-reported attachment styles a review of links with

parenting behaviors, emotions, and cognitions. *Personality and Social Psychology Review*, 2014. **19**(1): 44–76.

46. Siddiqui, A. and B. Hägglöf, Does maternal prenatal attachment predict postnatal mother-infant interaction? *Early Human Development*, 2000. **59**(1): 13–25.

47. Condon, J.T., et al., A longitudinal study of father-to-infant attachment: antecedents and correlates. *Journal of Reproductive and Infant Psychology*, 2013. **31**(1): 15–30.

48. Thun-Hohenstein, L., et al., Antenatal mental representations about the child and mother–infant interaction at three months post partum. *European Child & Adolescent Psychiatry*, 2008. **17**(1): 9–19.

49. Ainsworth, M.D.S., et al., *Patterns of attachment: A psychological study of the strange situation*. 1978, London: Lawrence Erlbaum.

50. Crawford, A. and D. Benoit, Caregivers' disrupted representations of the unborn child predict later infant–caregiver disorganized attachment and disrupted interactions. *Infant Mental Health Journal*, 2009. **30**(2): 124–144.

51. Condon, J.T., Women's mental health: a 'wish-list' for the DSM V. *Archives of Women's Mental Health*, 2010. **13**(1): 5–10.

52. Condon, J.T. and C. Corkindale, The correlates of antenatal attachment in pregnant women. *British Journal of Medical Psychology*, 1997. **70**: 359–372.

53. Condon, J.T., The spectrum of fetal abuse in pregnant women. *Journal of Nervous Mental Disorders*, 1986. **174**(9): 509–516.

54. Pollock, P.H. and A. Percy, Maternal antenatal attachment style and potential fetal abuse. *Child Abuse & Neglect*, 1999. **23**(12): 1345–1357.

55. National Collaborating Centre for Women's and Children's Health, *Antenatal care: Routine care for the healthy pregnant woman*. 2008, London: RCOG Press.

56. Peppers, L.G. and R.J. Knapp, *Motherhood and mourning: Perinatal death*. 1980, New York: Praeger Publishers.

57. Ekelin, M., E. Crang-Svalenius, and A. Dykes, A qualitative study of mothers' and fathers' experiences of routine ultrasound examination in Sweden. *Midwifery*, 2004. **20**: 335–344.

58. Côté-Arsenault, D. and K. Donato, Emotional cushioning in pregnancy after perinatal loss. *Journal of Reproductive and Infant Psychology*, 2011. **29**(1): 81–92.

59. Rowe, H., J. Fisher, and J. Quinlivan, Women who are well informed about prenatal genetic screening delay emotional attachment to their fetus. *Journal of Psychosomatic Obstetrics and Gynecology*, 2009. **30**(1): 34–41.

60. Austin, M.-P., Marcé International Society position statement on psychosocial assessment and depression screening in perinatal women. *Best Practice & Research Clinical Obstetrics & Gynaecology*, 2014. **28**(1): 179–187.

61. Darwin, Z., L. McGowan, and L.C. Edozien, Measuring the maternal-fetal relationship (MFR) in early pregnancy. Proceedings of the 30th Society for Reproductive and Infant Psychology Conference, University of Leuven. (Abstract). *Journal of Reproductive & Infant Psychology*, 2010. **28**: e1–e19.

62. Department of Health, *Health child programme: Pregnancy and the first five years of life*. 2009, London: Department of Health.

Chapter 29

Reproductive Health Care for Women with Psychosocial Issues

Mary Hepburn

Introduction

Many different psychosocial issues affect women and their reproductive health. These constitute an ill-defined group, and different issues and problems are included with terminology. The UK National Institute for Health and Care Excellence (NICE) published its guideline for management of women with "complex social factors" [1]. The term "special needs" is sometimes used but is nonspecific, means different things to different people in different situations, and is disliked by many of those to whom it is applied. It is used in reference to women with social or psychosocial issues but is also used in reference to women with medical or physical problems. In the context of women's reproductive health it is commonly the former. Women with psychosocial factors, complex social factors, or special needs often have a combination of issues. A common underlying factor is poverty and/or inequality which is often the cause of their problems but, if not the cause, will exacerbate other problems. It is now recognized that socially disadvantaged women and women with psychosocial problems need multidisciplinary health and social care [1]. However, while the problems may dictate or influence obstetric or medical management and making it more complex, the main challenge is more commonly to provide services that women will want and be able to use and that incorporate effective collaboration between the services involved.

Poverty, social exclusion and inequality adversely affect health. Women with problems caused by or exacerbated by socioeconomic deprivation have poorer outcomes of pregnancy with increased rates of mortality and morbidity for both mothers and babies. In addition to the general adverse effects of inequality there can be specific effects. So, for example, use of alcohol and/or other drugs can lead to blood-borne virus infection, liver damage, cardiac valvular damage or thromboembolic disease;

prostitution can lead to sexually transmitted infection, and violence or abuse which in any setting can result in physical injuries, mental illness, and use of alcohol or other drugs. Treatment of these problems can in turn have adverse effects and for example drugs used to treat blood borne viruses, mental illness, and drug use can also cause ill-health in the neonate. The adverse health effects of social problems are often long term and extend into adulthood; poor social outcomes are also more common, with short- and long-term consequences. Women with psychosocial problems therefore have potentially high-risk pregnancies. The combination of high-risk pregnancy and failure to engage with health and other services is a dangerous one.

It has long been recognized that poverty and inequality adversely affect health. However, traditionally there was clear separation between the medical conditions caused by or associated with poverty and the coexisting social problems with responsibility similarly demarcated. While for many years the links and consequent benefits of an integrated approach have been recognized at an individual or individual service level, formal professional and strategic recognition of the need for multidisciplinary care is a relatively recent phenomenon.

Engagement with Services

As well as the impact of poverty on health, the effect of poverty on service use has been recognized, and it has been widely reported that poverty and inequality are associated with less effective engagement with services. Consequently those with greatest need often receive the least adequate care, a phenomenon described in the Black Report in 1982 as the "Inverse Care Law" [2]. Nevertheless, the reasons for poor engagement with services and late or non-attendance for antenatal care by socially disadvantaged pregnant women were – and still often are – widely reported to lie with service users rather than service providers. Poor compliance has been variously blamed on lack of motivation (and in the case of pregnant women as predictive of inadequate parenting) and on the lifestyles associated with poverty and inequality, especially use of alcohol and other drugs. The possibility that the problem might lie with the design and delivery of services was resisted. The behavioral and lifestyle issues that compromise engagement were also seen as outwith the responsibility of all but the specific specialist health and social services such as addiction services. Moreover, recognition that interventions that would improve social circumstances, stabilize lifestyle, and indirectly improve health could be an important part of medical management – or at least of relevance to medical management – was also discounted. Lifestyle issues and failure to engage with services were traditionally viewed as matters of individual choice and the remedies therefore a matter of individual responsibility.

Reasons for Nonengagement

Nonattendance is more marked for non-urgent and preventive care and in reproductive healthcare this includes contraception and family planning services and also antenatal care. While their lifestyles may make it difficult to attend for screening or preventive care and while they may view such care as less important, most women, regardless of their backgrounds or problems, do think it is important to attend for antenatal care. If asked why they do not attend for antenatal care, women may be reluctant to be frank with professionals perceived as having authority and power especially if they are concerned about child custody. The Glasgow Women's Reproductive Health Service (WRHS), a community-based multidisciplinary service for women with "special needs," was developed over five years from a pilot community clinic in 1985 to a citywide service in 1990 [3]. Women attended with a range of problems including use of alcohol and other drugs, mental illness, learning disability, HIV infection, homelessness, young maternal age, and asylum seeking or refugee status. Women said they did not attend traditional antenatal services for various reasons including administrative problems (e.g., non-registration with a general practitioner), geographic location of hospital clinics relative to where they lived, feeling uncomfortable in hospital settings perceived as unfriendly, and other competing demands on their time. The new service

was developed in close collaboration with the target population with a central hospital-based clinic and a network of five community clinics in districts identified as appropriate by the women. Booking gestations quickly fell to the same level as the rest of the hospital and in the early years of the service a majority of the women attended as self referrals. Formal evaluation of women's views of the WRHS was carried out among women who used drugs [4]. Their views of the service were extremely positive, and their priorities were firstly non-judgmental staff attitudes, secondly staff who were knowledgeable about their problems, and thirdly good clinical care. These findings have been confirmed in subsequent studies by other services. However, while asking women what they want is an obvious – and necessary – requirement when developing services, the reality is rather more complicated. Over the subsequent decade an increasing proportion of women booked with the service attended the hospital clinic even when there was a geographically more convenient community clinic and, when women were asked why they did so, they said they preferred to attend the hospital! It appears that they initially opted to attend the community clinics in familiar settings and with familiar community staff participating, but when they found similar staff and staff attitudes in the hospital clinic they actually preferred to attend the hospital. It can be difficult for women to make choices from theoretical options, and it may be necessary for them to try the options before making a decision. Moreover, what they want may not be what they need and the challenge is to develop services that address both aspects, provide the best compromise and that women are willing and able to use. It is also essential that all services working with vulnerable, marginalized women should regularly review women's views and their service requirements and be willing and able to make any necessary changes.

Staff Attitudes and Service Requirements

While it has long been recognized that the socially disadvantaged in general (and socially disadvantaged women in particular) use services less effectively, recognition that this is a problem of services per se came much later, and even later came the recognition that addressing this is the responsibility of service providers. The NICE guideline makes the point but sadly does not reflect general acceptance of all that this implies. A major obstacle has been and remains the attitude – in society in general as well as among service providers – that disadvantaged people are in some way responsible for their circumstances and problems, that these problems are due to 'lifestyle choices,' and that such women do not need or deserve special care. While women with medical conditions are viewed as meriting specialized care, socially disadvantaged women, women with psychosocial problems or 'lifestyle'-related problems have traditionally been expected to access care within mainstream services. They have often been viewed as less motivated and less worthy parents and as being responsible for the health and social problems experienced by their children; they and their families are in effect punished for being disadvantaged. In recent years there has been progress (both before and after publication of the NICE guidelines) with the recognition of the need for and development of specialized services for pregnant women with a variety of problems. These include, especially use of alcohol or other drugs, but also other issues such as mental illness, HIV infection, young maternal age, homelessness as well as development of specialized services for women who are asylum seekers or refugees or members of black and minority ethnic groups. Some of these groups of women need specific healthcare, such as women with HIV infection and women with mental illness. However, while socially disadvantaged and/or marginalized women are now recognized as needing specialized services, this is often viewed in terms of additional psychosocial support and, although many of these women are overrepresented among maternal deaths and their children have higher rates of mortality and morbidity, they and their pregnancies are often not regarded as obstetrically 'high risk.' Poverty per se increases mortality and morbidity for mothers and babies, and many of these 'special needs' are associated with additional increased risk. The severity of poverty and inequality varies geographically, and so the actual level of medical and obstetric risk will also vary accordingly. Service requirements will therefore also vary. The finding that marginalized women in Glasgow actually preferred to attend the hospital was fortuitous since it coincided with changes in the cohort of women, especially among women using alcohol and other drugs where the average age and length of drug use had both steadily increased with simultaneously increased

morbidity and adverse pregnancy outcomes. Consequently, while most of the women had always been obstetrically high risk and therefore requiring medically led maternity care, at the time the service was established many could still receive much of their care in the community. Latterly, most of the women required regular monitoring only available if they attended the hospital. The Glasgow service and experience gained in its construction informed service development for various categories of vulnerable women in a number of other centers nationally and internationally with similarly successful outcomes. Some of these services were similar in design to the Glasgow model, but other successful models of service provision have also evolved, in particular the liaison midwife model. This is especially useful in areas where numbers of women with significant special needs are too small to justify a separate specialized service and the liaison midwife provides an effective link between mainstream maternity services and other agencies involved in the women's care. In some areas, marginalized women receive midwifery-led care in the community, similarly popular with the women and appropriate for those who do not have complex healthcare needs. As discussed, many of the health problems are poverty related and the overall health of the cohort of marginalized women will to some extent be a reflection of local levels of poverty and inequality. Clinical need must be a priority in service design and ways found to combine that with women's wishes. However, it is important to understand women's wishes. In Glasgow it initially appeared that women wanted a community-based service but they subsequently opted for the hospital-based equivalent. From discussions with the women it became clear that their priority was not for community-based care but for care from non-judgmental knowledgeable staff.

Attitudes to Different Problems

While a nonjudgmental approach to care should apply to all types of problem, experience in Glasgow and elsewhere has demonstrated that this is not the case and that attitudes both societal and professional are also influenced by the type of problem and the way it is perceived. There is also confusion between a nonjudgmental and a collusive approach. For example problems perceived to be under individual control such as use of alcohol and other drugs are often viewed as being the result of individual choice, while others such as learning disability are seen as outwith the control of the individual who is therefore regarded as an 'innocent victim.' Blame and individual responsibility (and consequently fitness to be a parent and rights to child custody) are often viewed accordingly but often without logical basis. So, women who use alcohol or drugs may be incapable of adequately caring for their children, but their parenting skills may be greatly improved by effective treatment for their problem. On the other hand, while some 'innocent' women with learning disability may also be unable to care for their children, there may be less scope for improvement and their difficulties may not be amenable to any medical or social interventions. As well as differences in attitudes to different types of 'special needs,' there are also differences in attitudes to effects on the neonate of maternal medication for 'real' maternal conditions such as diabetes, epilepsy, or mental illness as opposed to 'self-inflicted' conditions such as use of alcohol or other drugs. So, while neonatal effects of treatment for maternal diabetes, epilepsy, and mental illness are viewed as unfortunate but not the women's responsibility, effects on the neonate of methadone therapy for women dependent on opiates (included in the WHO list of essential medicines) are often seen as the woman's 'fault' and in some countries (including the United Kingdom both historically and currently) are inappropriately viewed as evidence of maternal antenatal child abuse.

Staff Attitudes and Training

Ideally all healthcare workers would have nonjudgmental attitudes but in practice this cannot be guaranteed. An appropriately nonjudgmental (but non-collusive) approach is essential for the care of all women but especially for women with psychosocial problems; however, this is not a substitute for clinical knowledge, and skills and women should always receive care appropriate to their needs. Training in identification and management of the problems encountered among marginalized women is not yet included in generic postgraduate training for most healthcare workers. To ensure all healthcare staff acquire appropriate clinical knowledge and expertise for caring for those who use alcohol and other drugs, a working group of the UK Academy of Postgraduate Medical Colleges developed a core curriculum to be adopted by all the medical colleges and corresponding postgraduate bodies for healthcare professionals. This

was a challenging project, but implementation, since it requires the existence within these bodies of trainers with the relevant knowledge and skills, poses an even greater challenge! This remains a work in progress.

Antenatal Education and Provision of Information for Women

Education and provision of information is an important part of service provision. This must reflect the women's circumstances in every respect. For example the information about feeding the baby and the way in which it is delivered will be different for women from countries and cultures where breastfeeding is common and culturally accepted and those for whom this is not the case. So, among disadvantaged white Scottish women (with low breastfeeding rates) it is important to explore reasons why they are reluctant to breastfeed. These include having never observed others breastfeeding, involvement in prostitution and consequently viewing breasts only as sexual organs, embarrassment, and lack of self-confidence and self-worth, all often exacerbated by experience of violence or abuse. Moreover they may be not be persuaded to breastfeed by factors that influence middle-class women; the information that breastfeeding could help them regain their pre-pregnancy figure is usually considered irrelevant, while in the Glasgow service the knowledge that breastfed babies have a lower risk of cot death has proved to be a powerful motivator. Among women who use drugs, knowledge that breastfeeding will reduce the risk of the baby requiring pharmacological treatment for drug withdrawals has also contributed to a rise in breastfeeding rates among these women. For babies of socially disadvantaged women with increased rates of low birth weight and prematurity, breastfeeding will be especially advantageous. On the other hand discussions with asylum-seeking women from sub-Saharan Africa are more likely to involve exploring ways to destigmatize artificial feeding necessitated by maternal HIV infection. It is therefore essential to adopt a culturally sensitive and appropriate approach and to begin education and preparation as early as possible.

A History of Violence and Trauma

A common issue for many women with psychosocial problems is a history of trauma or abuse, sometimes the cause of their problems and sometimes exacerbating them. Recognition of the existence and significance of this link came later in the United Kingdom than in many other countries, but even when it was recognized it was viewed as outwith the remit of healthcare workers and that to ask women about it would be intrusive and potentially offensive. In 1988 the introduction of routine inquiry about violence and abuse including domestic abuse into maternity care in the WRHS was met with considerable professional hostility. However, while women may not choose to disclose such a history, it is now clear that they want to be asked and routine inquiry is now an established and required part of the maternity booking history in the United Kingdom and many other countries (see Chapter 8). Use of alcohol or other drugs is recognized as being a coping mechanism for women who are experiencing violence or abuse or a means of suppressing the memory of abuse. In turn both can be closely linked with mental illness. Despite these associations, use of alcohol and other drugs is still frequently viewed as a matter of individual choice. A history of abuse can also influence other choices including, as discussed, the decision on whether to breastfeed.

Early Intervention and Postpartum Contraception

Early engagement with services is important from both a medical and social perspective. Early commencement of education and planning is also essential as already noted in the context of breastfeeding. Discussion about fertility control and planning of future pregnancies should also be introduced as early as possible. Traditionally this is considered to be part of postnatal care, but for vulnerable women and women with special needs this is too late. Ideally the issue should be addressed before they become pregnant but this rarely happens and for women already pregnant the subject should be raised at or shortly after their first attendance. This allows sufficient time for women to learn about their options, think about them, and make a decision so that appropriate effective contraception can be initiated prior to postnatal discharge. For women who are successful in getting custody of their children it is important to ensure they do not jeopardize this success by unintentionally becoming pregnant again too soon. For women who are less fortunate and do not get custody of their children it is equally important to avoid an early unplanned pregnancy with a high risk of

repeated similar outcomes. Given their difficulties in attending for family planning and contraception these are women for whom long-acting reversible contraception (LARC) will be particularly indicated. The contraceptive implant is especially useful since it is easy to train staff to fit it. A disadvantage is the risk of irregular bleeding, sometimes heavy and/or prolonged, which is more common if the implant is fitted in the early postpartum period. This is a common reason for requests to have the implant removed early, but this can be mitigated to some extent if women are made aware of the possibility and if they are given effective management should it arise. This is less of a problem with the levonorgestrel intrauterine system (IUS) which is in many ways a preferable method and is also effective for women on enzyme-inducing medication including some antiretroviral HIV medication and some antiepileptic drugs. Fitting the IUS is, however, rather more complex and is mainly carried out by medical staff who are less likely to be available to do so. In Glasgow attempts to arrange to have the IUS inserted at ceasaren section were only occasionally successful. There is also often misplaced anxiety about transvaginal fitting of an IUS or IUCD in the immediate postpartum period, although it is simple and safe. The main risk is of expulsion but experience in Glasgow showed this was not significantly higher than with insertion at other times. However, if trained staff are not available and the woman is discharged with a review appointment, this is often missed and the woman may end up without any contraception. In Glasgow in the mid-1990s, introduction of antenatal discussion and routine offer to initiate LARC prior to postnatal discharge coincided with an approximately 50% reduction in the number of pregnancies among women using drugs. While a direct causal relationship cannot be proved, this was clearly a factor in the reduction. Formal studies elsewhere have now confirmed that this practice is cost effective and associated with higher implementation of contraception and reduction in subsequent early unplanned pregnancy [5, 6]. It has now been recognized as beneficial by FIGO, and in the near future the institutionalization of immediate postpartum IUD services will be evaluated in a clinical trial in a number of countries [7].

Prevention, Not Crisis Intervention

Early attendance for antenatal care and early discussions about medical and social management are vitally important for women with psychosocial problems. However, no matter how early in pregnancy women attend, it is too late for optimum outcomes, and no matter how early in pregnancy discussion is initiated about future reproductive plans, a valuable pre-pregnancy planning opportunity has been missed. In such circumstances damage limitation is the best that can be achieved. The importance of pre-pregnancy care and planning of pregnancies is well recognized for women with 'medical' problems especially diabetes and to a lesser extent epilepsy, but there is inadequate recognition of its importance for women with problems with a significant social component. In Glasgow, various forms of pre-pregnancy care for vulnerable women were established even before the citywide service was established, but its role as a routine part of specialist care was not recognized: women and/or their partners were referred only if they requested help or advice and it relied mainly on taking the service to the women. Referrals to a clinic for men and women with HIV infection initially came exclusively from the service caring for men with hemophilia but subsequently came also from general HIV services. WRHS provided reproductive healthcare including reproductive planning for women attending addiction services, residential and nonresidential. Among professionals dealing with problems such as mental illness and learning disability, there was less recognition of this service need. Many women with psychosocial problems or complex social factors are already in contact with some type of service, health or social, statutory or voluntary, but despite awareness of potential medical and/or social problems during or after pregnancy, the question of reproductive health and planning of pregnancies is rarely raised since this is not seen as their responsibility. This is disappointing and inexcusable. While, as noted, the need for and importance of reproductive planning is recognized (to varying degrees) for strictly medical problems such as diabetes or epilepsy, integrated reproductive healthcare and planning is not routinely included in the management of women with socially related problems, for example, use of alcohol or other drugs, or medical problems with a strong social component, for example, mental illness. Such women are often simply regarded as unsuitable to be parents, but discussion regarding their wishes and plans is often not undertaken and effective appropriate contraception is not provided. When they become pregnant without definitive planning, they are regarded as irresponsible.

Reproductive Choices

While women with social problems who become pregnant are often regarded as irresponsible and their adverse outcomes of pregnancy as evidence of poor motivation, it is important to recognize that women with socially related problems will have the same desire to have children as their non-disadvantaged peers. They will also aspire to have healthy babies that they are able to parent adequately.

Reducing the Risk

Across the whole social spectrum, many pregnancies are unplanned. However, while pregnancies among socially disadvantaged women are often unplanned, they are not necessarily unintended or unwelcome. Nevertheless, if a pregnancy is ill-timed the adverse medical and social outcomes may be more severe. The need for pre-pregnancy services in the management of women with pre-existing medical conditions such as diabetes, epilepsy, and heart disease is well established based on recognition that such conditions are associated with increased maternal and perinatal mortality and morbidity. The impact on medical and social outcomes of socioeconomic deprivation and social problems caused by or exacerbated by deprivation can be at least as severe as that due to maternal medical problems, but there is not the same recognition that these women need specialized pre-pregnancy care. This is particularly disappointing since many such women are already in contact with medical and/or social services affording an ideal opportunity to engage with them, discuss their reproductive plans, and provide them with the necessary services to enable them to control and protect their fertility so that any pregnancies they may have are planned and timed for optimal medical and social outcomes. The chances of having good medical and social outcomes will be increased by careful planning and timing of pregnancies. This will not, however, guarantee good outcomes. For some women the time will never be right and such women often have insight into this reality: nevertheless it is important not to prejudge the issue and to work with such women toward a positive goal recognizing that any pre-conceptual health and social input will be worthwhile and will improve the outcome of any pregnancy that occurs.

Service Delivery

Women with high-risk pregnancies need obstetrically led care embedded in maternity services. Thus, for example, women with diabetes receive obstetrically led antenatal care provided by a multidisciplinary team within a maternity setting. Similarly, women with high-risk pregnancies as a consequence of social problems should receive obstetrically led multidisciplinary care embedded in maternity services as described in the UK Maternal Mortality Report. Outwith pregnancy, however, reproductive healthcare, while vitally important, does not have such a central role and can be opportunistically delivered within other services attended by the women. For example, women attending addiction services, psychiatric and mental health services, women in residential care or engaged with services dealing with learning disability, homelessness, violence and/or abuse, women who are seeking asylum, and many other vulnerable women involved with a variety of agencies are readily accessible and would benefit from reproductive healthcare and planning. It should be pointed out that in such settings reproductive healthcare and support and advice with reproductive planning should also be routinely provided for vulnerable, socially disadvantaged men and/or couples.

Promoting Uptake of Services

Where such care is provided for vulnerable women it is often provided as an optional opt-in service that women must choose to have. However, even if such women are routinely offered the option of pre-pregnancy counseling and care, they may not know what is on offer or be aware of the potential benefits. Consequently, women may decline the offer, perceiving it as irrelevant to them. Moreover, while many services used by vulnerable women provide some types of healthcare or at least a basic health check as part of their routine initial assessment, they also often regard pre-pregnancy care or indeed reproductive healthcare in general as a specialist service to be targeted at selected women either on request or when perceived to be necessary. Raising of awareness is therefore necessary among service providers as well as service users; many services and agencies working with disadvantaged, socially marginalized, or vulnerable women are ideally placed to routinely provide pre-pregnancy care to all women who enter the service. Such pre-pregnancy care should include information and advice about pregnancy planning together with screening for sexually transmitted infections, cervical cytology, and provision of effective contraception (commonly LARC) to enable optimal timing of pregnancies. It should be provided in parallel with review of all medical and social problems that could affect pregnancies to ensure appropriate management and minimize their impact. As discussed, men in such settings should also be routinely provided with sexual healthcare and information and advice about reproductive planning.

Summary

The potential adverse effects on pregnancy of social problems and inequality should be more widely recognized. However, it is equally important to recognize the benefits of working together with relevant medical and social agencies in partnership with women with psychosocial problems, complex social factors, or special needs to help them to protect and control their fertility to ensure that any pregnancies they have are intended with optimal timing for good medical and social outcomes. During pregnancy, such women should also be provided with multidisciplinary care that is appropriate to their needs. All those working with such women in whatever capacity should have the appropriate attitudes, knowledge, and skills, and professional training should reflect this need. Experience confirms that women welcome such help and will use appropriate services appropriately provided.

Key Points

- Poverty and inequality increase morbidity and mortality for mothers and babies: the same principles should apply in provision of maternity care for all women with high-risk pregnancies, whether due to social or medical factors.
- Socially disadvantaged women and women with psychosocial problems need multidisciplinary health and social care.
  The main challenge is to provide services that women will want and be able to use and that incorporate effective collaboration between the services involved.
- Staff attitudes and service design issues constitute barriers to the uptake of mainstream maternity and reproductive health services by socially disadvantaged women and women with major psychosocial issues.

- An appropriately nonjudgmental but non-collusive approach is essential for care of women with psychosocial problems.
- As applies to women with medical disorders such as diabetes, pre-pregnancy care, early attendance for pre- or antenatal care, and early discussions about medical and social management are important for women with psychosocial problems.
- Services working with vulnerable, marginalized women should regularly review women's views and their service requirements and be willing and able to make any necessary changes.

References

1. NICE. Pregnancy and Complex Social Factors: A Model for Service Provision for Pregnant Women with Complex Social Factors. (2010). NICE Clinical Guideline 110. www.nice.org.uk/guidance/cg110. Accessed on 25 March 2017.

2. Townsend P, Davidson N. (1982) *Inequalities in Health: The Black Report*. Harmondsworth: Penguin.

3. Hepburn M. (1997) Horses for Courses: Developing Services for Women with Special Needs. *British Journal of Midwifery* Vol **5**, No 8: 482–484.

4. Hepburn M, Elliott L. (1997) A Community Obstetric Service for Women with Special Needs. *British Journal of Midwifery* Vol **5**, No 8: 485–488.

5. Gariepy A M, Duffy J Y, Xu X. (2015) Cost Effectiveness of Immediate Compared with Delayed Postpartum Etonogestrel Implant Insertion. *Obstetrics and Gynecology* Vol **126**, No 1: 47–55.

6. Levi E E, Stuart G S, Zerden M L, Garrett J M, Bryant A G. (2015) Intrauterine Device Placement During Cesarean Section and Continued Use 6 Months Postpartum: A Randomised Controlled Trial. *Obstetrics and Gynecology* Vol **126**, No 1: 5–11.

7. International Federation of Gynecology and Obstetrics (FIGO). *FIGO Project for 'Institutionalising Post-Partum IUD Services and Increasing Access to Information and Education on Contraception and Safe Abortion Services'* (PPIUD Project) www.figo.org/ppiud-project. Accessed on 25 March 2017.

Chapter 30

Maternal Psychosocial Distress

Leroy C. Edozien

Introduction

National guidelines in the United Kingdom, the United States, Canada and Australia recommend psychosocial screening as part of routine comprehensive maternity care [1–4]. This is because maternal psychosocial 'stress'* is associated with adverse obstetric outcomes such as preterm labour, fetal growth restriction and long-term problems in the offspring. Doctors, midwives and other professionals face challenges in implementing these recommendations. The knowledge of most front-line clinicians on principles and concepts pertaining to 'stress' is limited. Often the literature is more confusing than helpful, as definitions and understandings of 'stress' vary from author to author. There are no universally accepted and/or adopted tools for implementing the recommendations on psychosocial screening. Consequently, 'stress' during pregnancy is frequently undetected by doctors and midwives, and cases of anxiety and depression are missed. Where psychosocial 'stress' is detected, there usually is no certainty regarding how it should be managed. Evidence of the efficacy of various interventions is sparse, and resources for delivering these interventions are often not available. Preventative, rather than curative, interventions are needed, but interventions such as stress alleviation programmes and social support have produced mixed results. This may be due to complex interactions between biological and other factors, and a better understanding of the underlying mechanisms is required. This chapter provides a basic, empirical description of the pertinent definitions and concepts. It also describes a simple self-management approach that doctors and midwives could apply in the antenatal clinic.

Definitions and Concepts

'Stress' originates from engineering: it is the force that is applied to an object, and it produces an impact ('strain') on the object. The concept of 'stress' was embedded in the medical lexicon by the endocrinologist Hans Selye, who defined it as the nonspecific response of the body to any demand, this response accounting for the wear and tear of the body [5]. Eighty years after Selye gave his own definition, no definition of 'stress' has established itself as the universal standard. One critic summarized the situation in the literature as follows:

> We found that the control term 'stress' may be a cause one minute and an effect the next. Conflation of cause and effect occurred surprisingly frequently, even though they are self-evidently opposites. Stress may on the one hand be a stimulus, on the other a response.... This uncertainty of meaning is rife in the stress research literature. Sometimes stress is an interaction, sometimes a transaction. For some purposes it is a verb, for others a noun; and stress may be all or any of these things within one 'scientific' paper. [6]

The paradigm adopted in this chapter is as follows. An event, activity, experience or other stimulus that potentially or actually threatens the physiological and/or psychological status of a pregnant woman is termed a stressor. Psychosocial stressors include nonphysical events and experiences such as bereavement, financial insecurity and social isolation but could also be physical, such as poor housing and noise. The stressor may be acute (e.g. sudden death of a close relative) or chronic (a difficult relationship with partner).

The stressor elicits a response by the woman. This response has physiological and psychological components. In acute situations, the physiological response is that described as 'fight or flight', a term coined by the physiologist Walter Cannon [7]. In this response the sympathetic nervous system is triggered, with release of epinephrine and norepinephrine (adrenaline and noradrenaline) manifesting as increased pulse rate, perspiration and dry mouth. This arousal response is an adaptive mechanism; it facilitates survival, and is triggered before cognitive capacities are engaged. The reflex initial response is regulated by the limbic system of the brain (see Chapter 6), and further appraisal of the stressor engages higher centres, resulting in a psychological response. The psychologist Richard Lazarus famously proposed the theory of cognitive appraisal: in response to the stressor, a person makes a primary appraisal (the stressor is interpreted as positive, dangerous or irrelevant) and a secondary appraisal (an assessment of whether one's resources are sufficient or insufficient to deal with the stressor) [8].

The term 'eustress' is applied when a stressor is interpreted as positive and responded to accordingly. In this situation the stressor facilitates good outcomes by heightening attention and vigour. If the stressor is interpreted negatively and there is the perception that the stressor exceeds one's resources for dealing with it, the term 'distress' applies. Perceived control is the belief that one has control over a stressor. A feeling of lack of control exacerbates the negative response to a stressor.

The stressor can be reduced or eliminated by means of a behavioural response ('behavioural control') or the application of mental processes ('cognitive control'). Individuals vary in the extent to which they have a sense of control of various elements in their lives and also in the extent to which they feel in need of control. Those who feel that they have practically no control are in a state of resignation or learned helplessness. This is a maladaptive state and can lead to physical and/or psychological morbidity. Those who excessively feel in need of control may have difficulties in coping with challenging situations that call for flexibility.

Behavioural responses may blunt the physiological and psychological impact of the stressor if they are health-promoting (e.g. dietary adjustments and exercise) or may exacerbate it, as happens with the use of smoking, alcoholism and bulimia as coping mechanisms.

Coping strategies are the behaviours, thoughts and emotions employed in adjustment to a stressor or stressors. In some cases these are counterproductive (maladaptive coping). Active coping strategies confront the stressor and seek to diminish its impact (strain). Avoidant strategies, on the other hand, seek to bypass the stressor, e.g. by denial, sleeping, drinking. This usually signals capitulation

and is maladaptive (i.e. does not enhance the prospects of survival). Some strategies focus on problem-solving, others on optimizing emotions and enhancing the sense of control. Coping strategies that can be promoted in the management of maternal psychosocial distress include antenatal education (aiming to enhance perceived control), venting (outward expression of thoughts and feelings in a supportive environment), exercise, relaxation and social support.

It is essential for well-being that physiological and psychological responses to stressor stimuli should be commensurate with the threat posed by the stressor and that the response should be switched off when the threat has been controlled or eliminated. In maladaptive states these do not happen.

The concept of allostasis provides a framework with potential to distinguish between normal adaptors to stressor stimuli and maladaptors [9]. Allostasis is defined as 'maintaining stability through change'. Clinicians are familiar with the concept of homeostasis, the mechanism by which critical systems in the body (such as temperature and blood pH) are maintained within a narrow range of operation, with various processes restoring the system to a set point after any disturbance. Hormones and catecholamines produced as part of the response to stressor act to restore stability, and then the hormonal response is turned off. However, when there is a chronic elevation or dysregulation of these neuroendocrine mediators of response to stressor, the 'set point' for stability changes (allostasis) and an allostatic load subsequently develops. Allostatic load is the wear and tear that the body experiences due to frequent exposure to stress hormones, repeated cycles of allostasis and the inefficient turning-on or shutting off of responses to stressors. It manifests clinically in a variety of ways, such as hypertension and obesity. Further alterations of the set point may result in allostatic overload, that is actual disease states. Allostatic load reflects more than chronic exposure to stressors; it encompasses other factors such as genes, early development and lifestyle choices (diet, smoking, alcohol use, exercise) which influence the 'stress' response system. Although the terminology of allostasis has not been welcomed by all and it has been criticized for being 'little more than a re-labelling exercise'[10], the underlying concept that the cumulative effects of sustained distress (load, with whichever adjective applied) is injurious to long-term health is generally accepted.

Biomarkers of allostatic load provide a measure of the cumulative effects of exposure to stressors and the associated behavioural responses. They include hormonal indices such as serum dehydroepiandrosterone sulphate (DHEA-S, a hypothalamo-pituitary axis antagonist); inflammatory markers such as C-reactive protein, albumin and interleukin-6; and indices of cardiovascular and metabolic risk such as systolic and diastolic blood pressure, glycosylated haemoglobin, serum HDL and total cholesterol and waist-hip ratio (WHR). Stressor-induced elevation of cortisol and activation of the sympathetic nervous system lead to sustained elevations in glucose and insulin resistance, which manifest as increased WHR and elevated glycosylated haemoglobin. Cholesterol and HDL cholesterol are measures of metabolic imbalance.

Maternal Psychosocial Distress and Its Impact on Mother and Baby

Given the challenges of definition and measurement, the paucity of robust data on the prevalence of maternal psychosocial distress is not a surprise. In a maternity experiences survey of Canadian women, almost one-fifth (17.1%) of women reported experiencing three or more stressful life events in the 12 months prior to the birth of their baby [11]. A wide range of events and experiences could make a pregnant woman distressed [12]. These include a difficult relationship with her partner, family or friends, socioeconomic deprivation, work-related stressors, immigration issues and adverse life events. She may also be troubled by pregnancy-related concerns such as fears for the health of her baby, fear of childbirth and insecurities about parenthood. These are legitimate concerns and do not equate to disease conditions. If not controlled, however, exposure to psychosocial stressors and the negative perception of these stressors could cause anxiety during pregnancy. Anxiety in pregnancy has a direct relationship with a negative perception of stressors and with socioeconomic deprivation but an inverse relationship with social support and self-esteem.

Studies (including meta-analyses) of the association between 'psychosocial stress' and perinatal outcome are not helpful if (as happens) they fail to distinguish between a mother's exposure to stressor(s) and her experience of psychosocial distress.

Maternal psychosocial distress is associated with increased risk of preterm delivery (see Chapter 33),

BOX 30.1 Reported Effects of Maternal Psychosocial Distress on the Child's Development Compiled from the Literature

Lower 12-month mental development scores

Attention problems

Negative temperament

Sleep problems

Behavioural/emotional problems

Autism

Attention deficit/hyperactivity disorder (ADHD) symptoms

Poor executive function

Decreased grey matter density

Greater impulsivity in adolescence

Reduced telomere length (associated with reduced lifespan)

Schizophrenia

hypertensive disorder in pregnancy, intrauterine growth restriction and neurodevelopmental disorders including attention deficit hyperactivity disorder and impaired cognitive development in the offspring [13–16] – see Box 30.1. Also, it influences the offspring's future behaviour as a mother. The effect of maternal psychosocial distress on the baby is illustrated by a study of 116 women and their full-term infants in which the infants' responses (cortisol levels and behavioural response) to painful heel-stick blood draw were evaluated 24 hours after birth [17]. Maternal plasma cortisol and report of stress, anxiety and depression were assessed at 15, 19, 25, 31 and 36+ weeks' gestational age. The infants who had exposure to elevated concentrations of maternal cortisol during the late second and third trimesters had larger cortisol responses to the prick. The infants of mothers with elevated levels of cortisol early in pregnancy as well as maternal psychosocial distress throughout gestation tended to show a slower rate of behavioural recovery from the pain of the heel-stick blood draw. These associations could not be explained by mode of delivery, prenatal medical history, socioeconomic status or child race, sex or birth order. This implies that in utero exposure to maternal psychosocial distress detrimentally affects the baby's future response to stressors.

By What Mechanism Does Maternal Distress Exert Its Putative Effects on the Offspring?

The mechanisms by which maternal psychosocial distress contributes to these outcomes for mother and baby are diverse and by no means easy to study. Results from animal models may not necessarily be transferable to humans, and long-term longitudinal studies on humans are difficult to design and conduct. Measurement of distress and its effects remains constrained by the challenge of defining and characterizing 'stress', the non-uniform methods of assessing hormonal and psychological indices, and the uncertainty regarding the window (gestational age) at which maternal distress has its optimal effect on the baby.

It is generally agreed that activation of the hypothalamic-pituitary-adrenal axis in both the mother and the baby occurs. The authors of a systematic review report that only a small number of studies showed significant associations between maternal prenatal cortisol concentrations and child outcomes, but the majority of these studies showed that maternal cortisol is related to adverse child outcomes (more health problems, lower cognitive/motor development, more psychological/behavioural problems and higher child cortisol concentrations) [18]. Factors other than cortisol are involved. Maternal psychosocial distress is also associated with increased production of oxytocin and inflammatory markers such as cytokines [19]. One study showed that intrusive thoughts and emotional distress regarding the fetus were associated with reduced volume of fetoplacental blood flow in the third trimester, which suggests that a decrease in fetoplacental blood flow is a possible pathway between maternal distress and reduced fetal growth [20]. It has also been found that maternal anxiety is associated with increased uterine artery resistance index, but this finding does not persist after adjusting for alcohol and nicotine use [21, 22].

Epigenetic mechanisms (see Chapter 3) have also been implicated [23].

Assessing Maternal Distress: Screening and Detection

To achieve timely recognition of pregnant women who may need psychosocial support and to offer them effective care, it would be helpful to have robust means of screening and detection. Various psychological and psychosocial tools have been used for this purpose (see Chapter 26). A systematic review identified 43 different psychometric instruments to assess maternal psychosocial distress [24].

Psychological instruments elicit symptoms indicative or predictive of psychological distress. Psychosocial screening tools assess issues such as substance abuse, life stresses, psychiatric history and family violence. The obvious limitation of these approaches is that they tend to address one dimension of what is clearly a multidimensional phenomenon. They take no account of the biological dimension, whereas biology may be just as important as stressor appraisal and coping strategies in determining whether a disease condition develops as a consequence of exposure to stressors. Also these approaches do not specifically address 'wear and tear'. A further limitation is that they mostly assess the situation at the time of pregnancy, whereas the potential impact of maternal distress may have been determined by factors originating well before pregnancy. Unfortunately, composite measures that take account of all three domains – biological, psychological and social – are yet to be developed.

Responding to Maternal Distress: Interventions

Drawing conclusions from studies of interventions to alleviate maternal psychosocial distress is difficult because of the methodological issues. Some studies evaluate preventative interventions; others evaluate therapeutic interventions. Some recruited a general population; others focussed on at-risk women. Some interventions were multicomponent; others were single. There are also ethnic and geographical variations and, critically, differences in definition, identification and measurement of maternal distress. The issues targeted by the interventions varied from 'stress' to anxiety, depression and psychosis.

A systematic review and meta-analysis showed that antenatal therapeutic interventions for women who have or are at risk of maternal distress are effective [25]. These interventions include acupuncture, mindfulness and a self-help support workbook with telephone support. Music has been shown to be beneficial to pregnant women and newborns [26].

Studies of computer- or web-based interventions have given mixed results [27]. Induced maternal relaxation during the 32nd week of pregnancy has been shown to cause changes in fetal neurobehaviour including increased fetal heart rate variability [28].

To an extent, it is arguable that even the best-designed studies will have limited applicability in the management of an individual woman. This is because the response to stressor stimuli is marked by individuality. Management of maternal psychosocial distress should be tailored to the needs and circumstances of the particular woman, albeit using tools known to be safe and effective. The paradigm of psychosocial distress adopted in this chapter places emphasis on coping mechanisms. To target interventions appropriately we have to ask, why do some pregnant women cope relatively well with stressors but others do not? When better tools are developed for identifying those likely to have a maladaptive response to stressors, then preventive interventions can be targeted more appropriately. Meanwhile care providers should focus on guiding the woman to strengthen her coping mechanisms and build resilience.

Resilience is the ability to mobilize one's resources, internal and external, and adapt to the challenges of a stressor, thereby facilitating achievement of a desirable ('positive') outcome. This outcome includes not only overcoming the stressor but also emerging as a stronger person. The resources include personal coping strategies and social support. Maternity services should assist distressed women to develop the relationship skills, cognitive skills and strategies required for resilience. To do this, doctors and midwives have to gain the trust of distressed women. They also need to have the relevant training and education so that they possess a working knowledge of the concepts discussed in this chapter, develop skills in woman-centred interviewing of distressed women and have both the temperament and the technical proficiency to support and monitor the women as appropriate.

The UK mental health charity, Mind devised a model for building resilience which comprises three elements: well-being ('positive' activities and managing emotions), social capital (relationships) and coping skills. This model was applied to maternity settings in the Mind resilience-building programme. In a mixed-methods evaluation of the programme 71.8% of 108 pregnant women and new mothers reported an improvement in well-being, and 79.1% of pregnant women showed an increase in their combined score across well-being, problem solving

and setting goals, and social support [29]. Qualitative evaluation indicated that engagement in positive activities, building social connections and learning coping strategies enhanced the resilience of women in urban and rural settings [30].

Cognitive behavioural therapy [31] and mindfulness-based cognitive therapy [32] are promising non-pharmacological approaches to the management of anxiety in pregnancy.

In a challenging economic climate, maternity units and service commissioners may not have the resources to deliver a comprehensive and intensive model of care similar to the Mind resilience building programme. Sign-posting women to external services that deliver psychological therapies is useful only if there is ready access to such services, as waiting times may be of such length that delivery of baby is imminent by the time treatment is commenced. Despite these challenges, the professional obligation to address the concerns of distressed women should not be abandoned. Obstetric and midwifery services are capable of delivering brief psychological interventions in-house. One way of doing this is by guided self-help, an abbreviated form of cognitive therapy. The woman is supported to commence a journey of behavioural activation and cognitive restructuring.

Behavioural activation aims to reduce maladaptive behaviours, such as social withdrawal and excessive sleeping, and increase engagement in reinforcing behaviours, such as spending time with family and engagement in other social or relaxation activities. The underlying principle is that helping people to change what they do is the key to changing how they feel [33]. Activities that are routine, pleasurable or necessary to the woman (and, in other contexts, men) are identified, and she is helped to construct a diary of activities and goals. Diary sheets for doing this are freely available on the Internet [34].

Cognitive restructuring involves identification of unhelpful thoughts, evaluation of the evidence for and against these thoughts and substitution of these thoughts with more positive and evidence-based alternatives. Worksheets for conducting this exercise are also freely available on the Internet [35].

A schema for delivering guided self-help is outlined in Box 30.2. Some women may have severe anxiety or comorbid depression requiring psychiatric assessment and treatment. For them guided self-help is inappropriate, and they should be seen by a psychiatrist (see Chapter 35).

BOX 30.2 Suggested Schema for Delivering Guided Self-Help to Psychosocially Distressed Pregnant Women

Establish rapport

Identify physical symptoms and signs of distress: lethargy, somnolence, sweating, palpitations, tachycardia.

Identify cognitive factors: negative thoughts, fears, lack of concentration

Identify behaviours consistent with distress: withdrawal from social activities; other avoidance behaviours

Define the underlying problem: what/when/where/with whom?

Assess lifestyle: sleep, diet, exercise, relaxation

Assess the impact, including risk of harm to/from self and others (including baby)

Collaboratively set specific, measurable and realistic goals

Introduce behavioural activation and/or cognitive restructuring

Arrange face-to-face or telephone follow-up.

Monitor and document obstetric and psychological outcomes

Conclusion

Obstetricians and midwives should possess a working knowledge of principles and concepts pertaining to maternal psychosocial distress. The term 'stress' is in common usage but neither clinicians nor academicians have a uniform understanding of what this means. It has variously been construed as a potentially threatening stimulus, the response to such stimulus or a negative response to the stimulus. The term 'maternal psychosocial distress' should be used when a pregnant woman has the perception that the challenge posed by psychosocial stressors in her life exceed her internal (coping) and external (social support) resources for dealing with it. Doctors and midwives should assess women for psychosocial distress not only at the booking visit but also in each trimester of pregnancy. For most women simple, non-pharmacological interventions would be alleviative, but some will require more intense psychological therapies or psychiatric treatment.

Key Points

- There is no universally agreed definition of the term 'stress'.
- The ability to respond to a stressor is important for survival and for optimizing performance, and humans have physiological and psychological mechanisms for responding positively.
- When these mechanisms are substituted with maladaptive behavioural responses such as smoking and eating disorder, a vicious circle develops.

- Chronic elevation or dysregulation of neuroendocrine modulators of the response, including failure to switch off the hormonal response, predisposes the woman (or man) to metabolic, cardiovascular and inflammatory pathologies; and programmes the baby for similar pathologies in adulthood.
- Assessment for maternal psychosocial distress should be part of routine pregnancy care.
- Guided self-help can be effective in building resilience and is deliverable in the setting of an antenatal clinic.

Note

* Inverted commas applied in view of the nebulous nature of this term.

References

1. American College of Obstetricians and Gynecologists Committee on Health Care for Undeserved Women. ACOG Committee Opinion No. 343: Psychosocial risk factors: Perinatal screening and intervention. *Obstet Gynecol* 2006;**108**(2):469–77.

2. National Institute for Health and Care Excellence. Antenatal and Postnatal Mental Health: Clinical Management and Service Guidance. NICE Clinical Guideline 192. London: NICE. 2014.

3. Australian Health Ministers' Advisory Council. Clinical Practice Guidelines: Antenatal Care – Module 1. Canberra: Australian Government Department of

Health and Ageing. 2012. www.health.gov.au/antenatal. Accessed 26 March 2017.

4. Society of Obstetricians and Gynaecologists of Canada (SOGC). Healthy beginnings: Guidelines for care during pregnancy and childbirth. Policy statement. December 1998.

4b. Health Canada. *Family-centred maternity and newborn care: National guidelines*. 4th edition. Ottawa, Canada: Minister of Public Works and Government Services. 2000.

5. Szabo S, Tache Y, Somogyi A. The legacy of Hans Selye and the origins of stress research: A retrospective 75 years after his landmark brief 'letter' to the editor# of Nature. *Stress* 2012;**15**(5):472–8. doi: 10.3109/ 10253890.2012.710919.

6. Patmore A. *The truth about stress*. London: Atlantic Books 2006, p42.

7. Brown TM, Fee E. Walter Bradford Cannon: Pioneer physiologist of human emotions. *Am J Public Health* 2002;**92**(10):1594–5.

8. Lazarus RS, Folkman S. *Stress, Appraisal, and Coping*. New York: Springer Publishing Company 1984.

9. McEwen BS. Stress: Homeostasis, Rheostasis, Allostasis and Allostatic Load. In Fink G (ed.), *Stress Science: Neuroendocrinology*. Elsevier, 2010.

10. Day TA. Defining stress as a prelude to mapping its neurocircuitry: No help from allostasis. *Prog Neuropsychopharmacol Biol Psychiatry* 2005;**29**(8): 1195–200.

11. Public Health Agency of Canada. What Mothers Say: The Canadian Maternity Experiences Survey. 2009 Available at www.phac-aspc.gc.ca/rhs-ssg/ survey-enquete/mes-eem-eng.php. Accessed 26 March 2017.

12. Dunkel Schetter C, Niles AN, Guardino CM, Khaled M, Kramer MS. Demographic, medical, and psychosocial predictors of pregnancy anxiety. *Paediatr Perinat Epidemiol* 2016;**30**(5):421–9. doi: 10.1111/ ppe.12300.

13. Cardwell MS. Stress: Pregnancy considerations. *Obstet Gynecol Surv* 2013;**68**(2):119–29. doi: 10.1097/ OGX.0b013e31827f2481.

14. Glover V. Maternal depression, anxiety and stress during pregnancy and child outcome; What needs to be done. *Best Pract Res Clin Obstet Gynaecol* 2014;**28** (1):25–35. doi: 10.1016/j.bpobgyn.2013.08.017.

15. Davis EP, Sandman CA. Prenatal psychobiological predictors of anxiety risk in preadolescent children. *Psychoneuroendocrinology* 2012;**37**(8):1224–33. doi: 10.1016/j.psyneuen.2011.12.016.

16. Brunton PJ. Effects of maternal exposure to social stress during pregnancy: Consequences for mother and offspring. *Reproduction* 2013;**146**(5):R175–89. doi: 10.1530/REP-13-0258.

17. Davis EP, Glynn LM, Waffarn F, Sandman CA. Prenatal maternal stress programs infant stress regulation. *J Child Psychol Psychiatry* 2011;**52**(2): 119–29. doi: 10.1111/j.1469-7610.2010.02314.x.

18. Zijlmans MA, Riksen-Walraven JM, de Weerth C. Associations between maternal prenatal cortisol concentrations and child outcomes: A systematic review. *Neurosci Biobehav Rev* 2015;**53**:1–24. doi: 10.1016/j.neubiorev.2015.02.015.

19. Coussons-Read ME, Okun ML, Nettles CD. Psychosocial stress increases inflammatory markers and alters cytokine production across pregnancy. *Brain Behav Immun* 2007;**21**(3):343–50.

20. Helbig A, Kaasen A, Malt UF, Haugen G. Does antenatal maternal psychological distress affect placental circulation in the third trimester? *PLoS One* 2013;**8**(2):e57071. doi: 10.1371/journal. pone.0057071.

21. Teixeira JM, Fisk NM, Glover V. Association between maternal anxiety in pregnancy and increased uterine artery resistance index: Cohort based study. *BMJ* 1999;**318**(7177):153–7.

22. Vythilingum B, Geerts L, Fincham D, Roos A, Faure S, Jonkers J, Stein DJ. Association between antenatal distress and uterine artery pulsatility index. *Arch Womens Ment Health* 2010;**13**(4):359–64. doi: 10.1007/ s00737-010-0144-8.

23. Palma-Gudiel H, Córdova-Palomera A, Eixarch E, Deuschle M, Fañanás L. Maternal psychosocial stress during pregnancy alters the epigenetic signature of the glucocorticoid receptor gene promoter in their offspring: A meta-analysis. *Epigenetics* 2015;**10** (10):893–902. doi: 10.1080/15592294.2015.1088630.

24. Nast I, Bolten M, Meinlschmidt G, Hellhammer DH. How to measure prenatal stress? A systematic review of psychometric instruments to assess psychosocial stress during pregnancy. *Paediatr Perinat Epidemiol* 2013;**27** (4):313–22. doi: 10.1111/ppe.12051.

25. Fontein-Kuipers YJ, Nieuwenhuijze MJ, Ausems M, Budé L, de Vries R. Antenatal interventions to reduce maternal distress: a systematic review and meta-analysis of randomised trials. *BJOG* 2014;**121**(4): 389–97. doi: 10.1111/1471-0528.12500.

26. Ashford MT, Olander EK, Ayers S. Computer- or web-based interventions for perinatal mental health: A systematic review. *J Affect Disord* 2016;**197**:134–46. doi: 10.1016/j.jad.2016.02.057.

27. Hollins Martin CJ. A narrative literature review of the therapeutic effects of music upon childbearing women and neonates. *Complement Ther Clin Pract* 2014;**20**(4): 262–7. doi: 10.1016/j.ctcp.2014.07.011.

28. DiPietro JA, Costigan KA, Nelson P, Gurewitsch ED, Laudenslager ML. Fetal responses to induced maternal relaxation during pregnancy. *Biol Psychol* 2008;**77**(1):11–19. doi: 10.1016/j.biopsycho.2007.08.008.

29. Steen M, Robinson M, Robertson S, Raine G. Pre and post survey findings from the Mind 'Building resilience programme for better mental health: Pregnant women and new mothers'. *Evidence Based Midwifery* 2015;**13**(3): 92–9.

30. Steen M. The perfect mum doesn't exist but a good enough mum does: Building resilience for better maternal mental health. *Australian Nursing & Midwifery journal* 2016;**24**(1):39.

31. Green SM, Haber E, Frey BN, McCabe RE. Cognitive-behavioral group treatment for perinatal anxiety: A pilot study. *Arch Women's Ment Health* 2015;**18**(4): 631–8. doi: 10.1007/s00737-015-0498-z.

32. Goodman JH, Guarino A, Chenausky K, Klein L, Prager J, Petersen R, Forget A, Freeman M. CALM pregnancy: Results of a pilot study of mindfulness-based cognitive therapy for perinatal anxiety. *Arch Women's Ment Health* 2014;**17**(5): 373–87. doi: 10.1007/s00737-013-0402-7.

33. Martell C, Dimidjian S, Herman-Dunn R. *Behavioral Activation for Depression: A Clinician's Guide.* Guilford Press 2013 ISBN-10: 1462510175 ISBN-13: 978-1462510177.

34. Psychology Tools. Behavioural Activation http://psychologytools.com/behavioral-activation-self-help.html. Accessed 26 March 2017. www.talkplus.org.uk/downloads_folder/Behavioural_Activation.pdf. Accessed 26 March 2017.

35. Psychology Tools. Cognitive Restructuring. http://psychologytools.com/technique-cognitive-restructuring.html. Accessed 26 March 2017.

The Effects of Stress on Pregnancy: A Not-So-Evident Association Revisited

Denise Defey

Introduction

As a practising clinical psychologist working both in maternity hospitals and private specialized consultation, as well as training medical doctors, midwifes, nurses, psychologists and community workers in perinatal psychology for almost 40 years, I have been progressively impressed by the burden laid on prospective mothers by the issue of stress in pregnancy.

I have seen mothers overwhelmed by guilty feelings over a perinatal loss or a newborn with a birth defect, thinking it has all been their fault and a result of the stressful situations they underwent during pregnancy. I have often worked clinically with mothers undergoing grief processes during pregnancy, struggling between their intense subjective need to mourn their lost loved one, on the one hand, and, on the other hand, the consistent pressure from their environment (both lay and professional) not to think or cry in order to avoid damaging their unborn child.

I remember once, walking along a hospital corridor, hearing a young pregnant woman coming out of the first prenatal consultation, who was telling her partner that the doctor had emphasized (prescribed?) she had to feel happy from that moment on till the last day of pregnancy, or otherwise she would damage her fetus.

I can even recall a colleague whose husband committed suicide in the time they were expecting their first child. This pregnancy ended in a premature delivery and later neonatal death, which was commented on by the psychologists around her as a positive event, because of the ill fate of that child, whose mind had been so early impregnated by the loss of its father.

As young psychologists, a colleague and I were impressed by so much pressure. Assuming we had plenty to learn about such a relevant issue we set out to read as much as we could on the subject. We were quite puzzled to discover that 50 different variables were used to measure stress in the first hundred papers on stress in pregnancy that we found. These variables ranged from laboratory tests assessing well-known indicators of stress to intangible indicators such as the number of prenatal control consultations (which, obviously, could be determined by other issues such as geographical/cultural/financial obstacles or poor quality/ inaccessibility/ hostility/cultural inadequacy, etc. of prenatal care offered). Midway stood cigarette smoking, assumed to be an indicator of stress, an assumption oblivious to the fact that smoking may be more connected to chronic addictive behavior, or even relaxing moments, for example, after lunch or sex.

As the years and decades passed after those times of early professional practice, issues have become worse. The Internet has become extensively used for dissemination of poorly grounded 'scientific' information, and such information pertaining to stress during pregnancy is abundant on the World Wide Web. Insecurity of every pregnant woman, social paradigms about 'good motherhood,' and consumerism of technology and 'science' have also done their part. In today's world it is almost impossible for pregnant women living in modern (especially urban) Western societies to be free from the pressure stemming from the naturalization of the 'evidence' of negative effects of stress during pregnancy. These effects are assumed to have an impact on their child not only as a fetus but also as an infant, a school child, an adolescent, even an adult.

This chapter is the written version of a lecture delivered in the 2016 International Meeting of ISPOG (International Society of Psychosomatic Obstetrics and Gynaecology). It is written not only

This chapter is based on a lecture delivered at the triennial congress of the International Society of Psychosomatic Obstetrics and Gynaecology (ISPOG) held in Malaga, Spain, May 2016.

because the editors of this book were interested in the ideas presented but also because a vast number of young and not-so-young professionals attending the meeting approached me to declare heartily that they shared these ideas but had never dared to speak it out because they thought that this stemmed purely from their ignorance on the subject and they simply had to read and learn more on it.

Therefore, the following considerations are written not only in respect to scientific evidence but also in the hope that they will help to give voice to many who would like to challenge the ever-prevailing burden on mothers and families of the naturalization and generalization of deleterious effect of stress during pregnancy. It is also written, of course, in the hope to help relieve some of the additional burden pregnant women have to undergo when their life stresses and strains coincide in time with their pregnancies.

Is Stress Everywhere . . . or Nowhere?

As suggested above, stress is not a variable but a construct, that is, an abstraction created to bring together elements which share common characteristics but are quite diverse from one another.

'Stress' is often taken as an univocal concept and habitually associated to its ill-effects on health, quality of life, and so on. However, a deeper understanding of the concept leads, for instance, to the appreciation of the differences between eustress and distress.

*Eus*tress is the arousal produced by exciting positive events such as a first date, the wedding day, or delivering a lecture to a large audience. It has, no doubt, a biological counterpart, and it is followed by fatigue, even exhaustion. But it is the zest of life that much of makes the difference between a meaningful, rich, exciting life and a dull, repetitive existence.

*Dis*tress, on the other hand, is what is habitually identified as 'stress': tension, alert, and a disquieting subjective reaction of alert, which may respond to real peril, imagined situations or, simply, a chronic reaction to all situations, be they demanding or not.

Both eustress and distress are part of life itself and are part of the tools that we use to deal with everyday events. There is even an ethical side to this discussion, which has led many to question the WHO definition of health as 'complete well-being.' Many people, both lay and academic, question this passive view of health which implies some kind of 'social autism,' that is, the incapacity to be sympathetic and suffer over another being's suffering.

In the field of motherhood and maternal care, there can also be found many contradictions on the issue of the ill- or beneficial effects of stress during pregnancy. Those who advocate that prospective mothers should avoid stress are the same who label as 'neglect' and irresponsibility the behavior of those women who conduct their pregnancy in a 'relaxed' way, without much concern for medical care, prenatal diagnosis, or preventive actions to protect their pregnancy.

It can be misleading in clinical assessment to equate stress to poor pregnancy outcome in a univocal direction, as many pathological conditions (some personal, some social, or both) strongly determine a lifestyle exempt from stress: severe depression, demoralization, learned helplessness, a-motivational syndrome after intense cannabis consumption, and so on. The most extreme example for this is 'nude life,' a concept devised by Walter Benjamin to describe the lives of those whose existence is irrelevant to others and who live and die in solitude and neglect.

There can be no doubt that, when pregnant, these women are not affected by stress, but there can be no doubt either that this lack of stress is lack of stamina, 'moral famine,' and bonding deprivation. All these conditions severely affect pregnancy care and, later, care of and bonding to the offspring.

Stress during Pregnancy and Women's Liberation

The idea that stress has negative effects on pregnancy subtly advocates a passive stance in life which, in the case of women, can be thought of as the persistence of nineteenth-century ideas of the ideal woman as static, always 'in wait of' (the ideal husband, financial provision from others, offspring, etc.).

This, on the one hand, is in rampant contradiction with ideas prevalent in Western urbanized settings, where women are expected to lead an active life, pursue their own self-fulfillment, have a choice about motherhood, and so on. Apparently, once they become pregnant and decide to carry on with their pregnancy, the surrounding overt and subtle messages conveyed to them change radically, and they are expected to be calm and relaxed, ready to accomplish with bed rest and the interruption of their professional or personal aims for the sake of 'his Majesty, the baby,' as Freud would put it.

This contradiction is even more radical when recommendations and burdening messages about the effect of stress on pregnancy are delivered by female doctors, midwives, nurses, and the like, who often lead very stressful lives themselves and are not able to take proper care of their own pregnancies or infants. Quite surprisingly, their own experience of pregnancy under stress very rarely makes them more sympathetic to their patients' life situation.

Stress Mediators and Compensating Mechanisms

The interminable production of papers on the ill effects of stress on pregnancy is in no way equaled by the replication or further development of pioneering research showing protective mechanisms and mediators when stress affects pregnancy.

As early as 1973, Ando et al. [2] conducted their well-known study on pregnant women living around the Osaka airport in Japan, where the thundering noise of airplane takeoff haunts them and their fetuses every minute, every hour, every day. Assessing newborns who had undergone this indisputable, continuing stressful situation during pregnancy, they found that, in the case of mothers who had moved into the area five months after conception, the fetuses were severely affected. However, in the cases in which mothers had been living there along the nine months of pregnancy, fetuses were not different in any way to fetuses whose mothers had had no stressful stimuli during pregnancy. This brings along the ever-important conclusion that fetuses may *adapt* to stress and therefore avoid its deleterious consequences.

Not only by biological involuntary mechanism can stress be neutralized. In a less well-known study [24], pregnant rats were exposed to severe stress during pregnancy, forcing them to undergo periodical electric shocks. After delivery, their newborns were quite affected, which was very clear in contrast to the control group of pregnant rats with an uneventful pregnancy. Affected newborns were separated in two groups for maternal postnatal care; one half was given to mothers who had had a normal pregnancy and the other half to mothers who had suffered severe stress during pregnancy. The first half, cared for in a similar way as their healthy counterparts, showed no postnatal improvement. However, mothers who had suffered stressful pregnancies were able to compensate for the damage this had had on their offspring by means of extraordinary maternal care. In a short time, their offspring were equally healthy and as well developed as their unaffected counterparts.

Prominent studies on resilience have shown how, even in the presence of the most extreme stressful conditions, humans can not only survive but also thrive. These studies are seldom (if ever) mentioned in the innumerable conference presentations or literature reviews in papers published on the issue of stress during pregnancy. Furthermore, master degree and doctoral students are very seldom (if ever) stimulated to pursue these pioneering, ground-breaking studies.

The adaptive behavior of the mother rats with their affected offspring can well be included in the concept of 'coping mechanisms,' which mediate the effect of stress in any circumstance, obviously including pregnancy. The search for orientation and support from an experienced, soothing other (be it a relative, professional, doula, and the like) is a resource often used successfully by women to cope with normal or extraordinary stress during pregnancy. Unfortunately, more cultivated pregnant women turn to a coping mechanism which is often ineffective, if not counterproductive: the search for information, especially by means of the Internet which will more often than not confirm their fears about the damage they are producing on their fetuses by being so anxious about their pregnancy.

Stress: Voluntary or Involuntary?

In the previously mentioned anecdote where the young woman was 'prescribed happiness,' the underlying message is that undergoing stressful situations in life can be a voluntary event which can be avoided by means of equally voluntary actions or attitudes.

In fact, although pregnancy often brings along hypersensitivity, most studies focus on real stressful events during pregnancy, such as unexpected loss of loved ones, war, meteorological ill-events, forced migration, dwelling difficulties, and so on. Stress is part of every person's life, and it has been assessed that 78% of women undergo some kind of stress during pregnancy [18].

Of late, many studies have tried to shed light on the overlooked issue of maltreatment during pregnancy, now considered to increase at that time of life and probably be one of the reasons for lack of prenatal care, when husbands do not allow another man to touch their wives or healthcare personnel to see the effects of abuse on their wives'/partners' bodies.

It is quite astonishing to find the stark contradiction between the relevance assigned to the assumed ill-effect of stress on pregnancy, on the one hand and, on the other, the lack of perception of those who advocate this concerning the stressful effect on pregnant women produced by dissemination and clinical use of their ideas. A very clear example of this can be seen when hypertensive women are hospitalized to produce 'bodily and mental rest' and then they have to passively undergo the everyday stress of hearing their doctors (in university hospitals, also students) expose them to the discussion among them during the daily round about the risks that endanger them and their fetuses.

Highly or Poorly 'Mentalized' Stressful Experiences

In the situation aforementioned, hypertensive women are trapped in a situation in which they are not expected to interact with doctors, who often use terms that cause them confusing and disquieting concerns, such as 'fetal distress' or 'neonatal depression.' Since they are not expected to talk to doctors during the professional exchange of ideas at the clinical round, they do not have the opportunity to handle their fears and anxiety in what has been termed a 'mentalized' way [12], that is, being able to use their upper cognitive functions which help discriminate between fantasy and reality, thus developing adaptive behavior and soothing subjective reactions.

This issue of mentalized versus non-mentalized stress is seldom taken into account, despite being of utmost importance. While the person is paralyzed and bound to his/her primitive animal reaction, the reaction is the well-known fight/flight duet, with its corresponding neurobiological counterpart. However, when upper mental functions can be put into action, stress can turn into challenge that may lead to mental upper functions and adaptive reactions.

Some persons, who are termed 'psychosomatic' or 'psychosomatically vulnerable' patients, are doomed to respond to life stress, be it minor or dramatic, with bodily reactions which endanger their health, even their life. When stress is mentioned in connection with pregnancy, it is this model which is borne in mind. However, many women are highly mentalized and react in a different, more protective way to stress situations they have to face in their daily lives, including the time they are pregnant.

The association between stress and pregnancy is habitually regarded as a causal, one-to-one relation, but in fact studies show only a relative, not absolute, increase in likelihood of harm to mother or baby. In these studies, many women have not been affected by the stressful situation analyzed. These women in whom stress has not harmed the fetus or affected the course of pregnancy are not studied as to their differential characteristics and qualities (such as mentalization) which may have protected them from the ill-effect of stress during pregnancy.

An example of this can be that of a young woman who was told during the second trimester of her first pregnancy that her fetus was so severely malformed that it was doomed to die shortly after birth. She recalled her grandmother had weighed 500g at birth and, with no intensive neonatal care or anything similar at the time, she was set aside to die while personnel attended on her mother. They involuntarily laid her on a heat source and she survived. Therefore, her fetus could also survive, an idea that soothed her and allowed her to carry on her pregnancy without being overwhelmed by anguish and anticipated grief. (In fact, though finally death took place, her infant lived much longer than expected, in which time she provided him with tender loving care.)

Stress: Severe or Minor; Acute or Chronic

It is evident from observation, and also a conclusion that can be drawn from methodologically validated scientific literature, that daily troubles stemming from such normal situations as childrearing, work, even heavy traffic (i.e. minor stress) do not have an ill-effect on pregnancy. Otherwise, practically no newborn would be healthy and practically no pregnancy would have an uneventful course.

However, this is not always stated in scientific papers. In fact, they often measure stress through variables such as bereavement, which has stages evolving in time, which generate varying degrees and intensity of subjective suffering, that could be successively termed as major or minor, acute or stable.

Furthermore, dissemination of information termed as 'scientific' seldom specifies the quality of stress assessed; thus, a snow storm is presented as equally harmful as a severe traumatic event as the collapse of the Twin Towers (which, in fact, generated the premature birth of twice as many newborns as the usual number in New York in the next week).

Reliable, Consistent Evidence

The association which appears consistently in the literature in papers using reliable methodology is between an extraordinary traumatic event during the second or third trimester of pregnancy, and a highly increased risk of premature birth in the following week.

The other information that can be taken as reliable evidence is that, in hypertensive or diabetic pregnant women, stress (both acute and chronic, major or minor) may decompensate their chronic condition, thus favoring negative outcomes for both mother and fetus. These effects are not to be overlooked, since they include (in the case of hypertensive patients) placental abruption or vascular accidents eventually leading to maternal or fetal demise, and (in the case of diabetic patients) eventual malformations, should decompensation take place in the first trimester, or stillbirth, should it happen later.

Beyond this, the body of 'evidence' becomes contradictory, often methodologically weak and, as previously stated, often contaminated by confounding variables.

A meta-analysis published in the ISPOG *Journal of Psychosomatic Obstetrics and Gynecology* [18] showed an association of less than 1% between stress and poor pregnancy outcome, which led the authors to the conclusion that maternal psychosocial stress has no clinical significance.

Methodological Issues

In line with those who have expressed concerns over methodological issues in this subject (e.g., [21]), the revision by Littleton et al. (2010) [18] dismissed as methodologically invalid almost four-fifths of the papers published.

In the first place, confounding variables are the rule. For example, during Nazi occupation the Dutch population was pushed to the limit of starvation during a very long time, which obviously led to extremely poor outcomes in the pregnancies taking place at the time. Though obviously stressing, the damage on the fetus produced by extreme lack of nutrients cannot be overseen. However, this historical fact is often taken as a paradigm when studying the ill-effects of stress during pregnancy on the children born at that time or shortly after.

Probably the confounding variables most frequently overlooked are those related to the extremely well-studied effects of early mother–infant bonding as well as later family relations and rearing practices on infant and child well-being and health, both mental and bodily. Thus, stressful events taking place during pregnancy are studied in connection to later problems such as poor school performance or psychopathology during adolescence, in which dismissing the weight of other variables is equivalent to denying the developments of Pediatrics and Child and Adolescent Psychology in the last century.

Stress studies are based on an underlying conception of cause-and-effect which can no longer be held as acceptable in modern epistemology (which acknowledges the complexity and multi-determined condition of events in nature, let alone human life and bondings).

As mentioned previously, a key flaw to reliability of studies is the choice of variables used by researchers to study the intangible group of events we call 'stress.' The description of the variables is often disregarded in published research, especially abstracts. Furthermore, researchers are free to choose whichever variable they consider suitable, no matter how poorly it reflects the construct (as the aforementioned case of studies measuring stress in pregnancy according to the number of prenatal care consultations attended) or how contaminated it is by confounding variables.

Another methodological flaw takes place in studies relying upon biological measures of elements which truly reflect a reaction to stress (such as cortisol or adrenaline), samples are often taken in situations where it is difficult to determine whether stress can be considered the cause of poor pregnancy outcome or it is the consequence of the unfortunate event itself. (A good example of this can be studies on the association between stress and early pregnancy loss using blood samples taken during hospitalization immediately after spontaneous abortion.)

Dealing with the Causes or the Effect?

In both lay and scientific publications, effects of stress on pregnancy are measured by means such as questionnaires, scales, and biological samples, which, in fact, take for granted that all the problem lies exclusively *within* the woman's body, mind, or both. Stressful work, family discord, and domestic violence, for instance, are considered as purely subjective processes affecting biological variables (e.g., catecholamines) which, in turn, affect fetal healthy development.

The dissemination and/or clinical use of this limited view has a burdensome effect on women, most especially if their child is eventually unhealthy or dies for whichever reason. Furthermore, this favors an attitude from both healthcare personnel and their family milieu to lay responsibility exclusively on mothers, thus unfairly overlooking the fact that the source of stress during pregnancy may actually stem from others, such as employers or violent partners. In the case of stress generated by illness or difficulties with the woman's other children, it is extraordinarily difficult for the pregnant woman to keep calm to protect the unborn child, while at the same time keep active to take care of the ill or problematic other child(ren).

The habitual approach of some doctors or midwives to stress during pregnancy (based upon paradoxically stressing the mother by 'prescribing' an unstressful course of events during pregnancy) seems inadequate and unfair, even potentially harmful. An approach attempting to help women and families solve the cause of stress seems more sensible, sensitive, and effective, as will be shown.

A good example of this is the habitual practice in some hospitals in Germany, where pregnant women needing bed rest are not confined to a hospital bed but granted eight-hour daily help in the household and childrearing chores while they remain at home in bed rest.

Pinard and the Social Roots of Poor Pregnancy Outcome

Adolphe Pinard (1844–1934), famous for the creation of the stethoscope which bears his name, created Puericulture, which is considered the root of what we know today as Perinatology, an interdisciplinary approach to the complex biopsychosocial events and structural issues which determine perinatal health and outcome, both for mothers and their offspring.

Observing working women and the course of events around them during pregnancy and the early times of their children, Pinard made pioneering observations on the influence of life and work conditions on pregnancy outcome, especially in all that concerns maternal nutrition and poor fetal growth.

Considering that premature birth and intrauterine restricted fetal growth are still today the main unresolved problems of Perinatal Medicine and the major causes of perinatal and infant death, as well as for negative consequences for health along the life span, these reflections coming from a wise, experienced clinican are contributions to be taken into account.

The Concept of Scenarios

The Ministry of Health of Uruguay (a country with a pioneering role in perinatal medicine and psychosocial obstetrics) has designed several healthcare programs for complex issues, such as drug abuse duringpregnancy, based upon the concept of 'scenarios.'

Stemming from the theories of complexity which are the landmark of modern social sciences and a community approach to healthcare, this concept attempts to go beyond the idea of 'clinical cases' to determine both diagnosis and treatment of whichever health problem affects the individual or the community. 'Scenarios' not only includes the biological or even the psychosocial variables at stake but takes, instead, a much wider stance to provide a scope of variables that determine ill-health and the possibilities of healthcare approaches to them.

Thus, in the aforementioned programs of the Uruguayan Ministry of Health for drug abuse during pregnancy, not only biological consequences on the fetus and maternal psychopathology and compliance to treatments proposed are taken into account, but also social class, dwelling conditions, partner drug abuse, attitude of her family and social milieu toward drug abuse, country legal regulations, family history, a history of child abuse, healthcare personnel attitude toward women, accessibility of drugs during pregnancy, and any other issue which has been shown in research (as have the former) to be risk or protective factors for the occurrence and persistence of drug abuse during pregnancy.

This concept of scenarios not only provides wider, deeper understanding of the problem to be dealt with but also protects the person bearing the problem (e.g., drug abuse, stress during pregnancy) from being held as the only source of and, therefore, solely responsible for the ill-effects of the problem. This concept also allows clinicians and researchers to profit from information stemming from both quantitative and qualitative research, as well as from both the medical and the psychosocial disciplines.

It goes without saying that the idea of *scenarios* can be applied to the problem of stress during pregnancy. In the vast majority of cases, stress arises not from the woman herself but from scenarios generated by involuntary events such as the loss of a loved one, severe illness in another child, work or dwelling conditions, and even tragedies beyond her personal or family life (such as the collapse of the Twin Towers).

The use of the concept of *scenarios* in the approach to stress during pregnancy not only helps to avoid aggravating stress by laying the burden of responsibility on the woman but, most importantly, allows us to understand the *causes* of stress, not just its *consequences*.

The Case for Intrauterine Growth Restriction

Intrauterine growth restriction (IUGR) is a leading cause for perinatal problems including perinatal death and health problems which go beyond infancy and childhood to reach adulthood and increase the risk for metabolic and cardiovascular disease during late adulthood.

IUGR has been shown to have a much higher prevalence in life conditions stemming from poverty, inadequate dwelling, poor educational status, straining work conditions and malnutrition or undernutrition. In Uruguay, for instance, the prevalence of IUGR in these unfavorable social conditions was 28% versus 9% in global country prevalence, according to reliable official information for 2014.

An approach based upon the concept of scenarios and providing relief from the causes instead of highlighting the consequences has managed to bring the prevalence in the affected population groups down to 9%. This program ("Uruguay Grows with You"), which has been designed to be one of the five national priority health programs, is based upon interdisciplinary intensive work in territory providing psychosocial interventions devised for the needs of each family. Basically working through home visits (42 is the mean) during a time span of nine months, the program approaches families which include pregnant women and/or children under 4 years of age. The aims are not only related to psychosocial variables but also biomedical issues, such as prevention of preterm birth, promotion of fetal and infant growth, and prevention of anemia in both mothers and their offspring. Psychosocial intervention is used as a *tool* to reach a wider, deeper, and more reliable situational diagnosis (scenario), as well as a means to generate a 'working alliance' with families that may lead them to receive effective healthcare and nutritional help during these determining periods of life. As mentioned previously, the outcome measures show not only better psychosocial conditions after the interventions but also remarkable changes in the prevalence of prematurity (19–9%), IUGR (28–9%), and anemia during pregnancy and the early years. [23]

Conclusions and Recommendations

The conclusions stemming from all the aforesaid are basically related to ethical concerns. The issue of stress during pregnancy and its consequences has been dealt with, both by the academic community and the 'scientific dissemination' press, in a way that we consider careless as to its effects on women and their families. Both lay and clinical use of this methodologically feeble information has disregarded the subjective effect on women, thus paradoxically filling their gestational time with unnecessary stress.

We advocate an active attitude from scientific societies and the academic world in general in protecting the public from what can be considered 'toxic' effect of inaccurate information. In the same trend, we consider there should be both stimulus to and dissemination of research showing protective and compensatory factors to protect pregnancy, fetuses, and infants from the stress their mothers have (mostly involuntarily) undergone during pregnancy.

Finally, we consider dissemination and teaching on this issue should include and emphasize not only these protective factors but also a perception of the effects of stress during pregnancy in a way that is not general and unspecific but with clear indication of condition, effects, time span of effects, and actions to be taken to prevent damage. The example for this kind of 'protective dissemination' would bear the following wording:

> Intense, acute stress may improve the chance of premature birth in the following week, therefore exposed pregnant women should have an extra prenatal consultation specifically aimed at assessing and responding to the risk of preterm labour.

It can be considered that these recommendations reflect the present-day concern over patient safety following a reliable and ethically valid approach.

Key Points

- The stress literature often fails to distinguish between eustress and distress.
- Doctors and midwives may inadvertently aggravate maternal stress by their approach to the management of this condition.
- While it is important to know the *consequences* of stress, it is also important to understand the *causes* of stress.
- The complex nature of the correlates of maternal stress means that the relationship between maternal stress and pregnancy outcomes cannot be framed as a simple cause–effect relationship.
- Due to methodological problems it is often difficult to draw robust conclusions from published research on maternal stress.
- The approach based on the concept of 'scenarios' (instead of clinical cases), employed successfully by the Uruguayan Ministry of Health in the care of women with complex biological and social needs, is an example of a holistic approach to managing maternal stress.

References

1. American College of Obstetrics and Gynecology. Committee on health care for underserved women psychosocial risk factors: Perinatal screening and intervention. *Obstet Gynecol* 2006, **108**: 469–477.

2. Ando Y, Hattori H. Statistical studies on the effects of intense noise during human fetal life. *Journal of Sound and Vibration* 1973, **27**(1): 101–110.

3. Auger N, Giraud J, Daniel M. The joint influence of area income, income inequality, and immigrant density on adverse birth outcomes: a population-based study. *BMC Public Health* 2009, **9**: 237–248.

4. Bacallao J, Peña M, Díaz A. Reducción de la desnutrición crónica en las bases bio-sociales para la promoción de la salud y el desarrollo. *Revista Panamericana de Salud Pública (Organización Panamericana de la Salud)* 2012, **32**(2): 145–150.

5. Ball S, Jacoby P, Zubrick S. Socio-economic status accounts for rapidly increasing geographic variation in the incidence of poor fetal growth. *Int. J. Environ. Res. Public Health* 2013, **10**: 2606–2620.

6. Cardwell M. Stress: pregnancy considerations. *Obstet Gynecol Survey* 2013, **68**(2): 119–129.

7. Coussons-Read ME, Okun ML, Schmitt MP, Giese S. Prenatal stress alters cytokine levels in a manner that may endanger human pregnancy. *Psychosomatic Medicine* 2005, **67**(4): 625–631.

8. Diego M, Jones T, Field T, Hernandez-Reif O, Schanberg S, Kuhn C, Gonzalez/Garcia A. Maternal psychosocial distress, maternal cortisol and fetal weight. *Psyhosomatic Medicine* 2006, **68**(5): 747/753.

9. Dötsch J. Perinatal programming: myths, facts and future of research. *Mollecular and Celullar Pediatrics* 2014, **1**: 2.

10. Dunkel-Schetter C. Psychological science on pregnancy stress processes, biopsychosocial models, and emerging research issues. *Annual Review of Psychology* 2011, **62**: 531–558.

11. Feldman P, Dunkel-Schetter C, Wadhwa P. Maternal social support predicts birth-weight and fetal growth in human pregnancy. *Psychosomatic Medicine* 2000, **62**: 715–725.

12. Fonagy P, Target M. *Psychoanalytic theories: Perspectives from developmental psychopathology.* Londres: Brunner-Routledge, 2004.

13. Glynn L, Wahdwa P, Sandman M, Dunkel Schetter C, Chicz-DeMet A. When stress happens matters: effects of earthquake timing on responsivity in pregnancy. *American Journal of Obstetrics & Gynecology* 2001, **184**(4): 637–642.

14. Grote N, Bridge J, Javin A, Melville J, Lyenger S, Katon W. A meta-analysis of depression during pregnancy and the risk of preterm birth, low birth weight and IUGR. *Arch General Psychiatry* 2010, **67**(10): 1012–1024.

15. Hobel C, Goldstein A, Barrett E. Psychosocial stress and pregnancy outcome. *Clin. Obstet. Gynecol* 2008, **51**: 333–348.

16. Kotliarenco M, Gómez E, Muñoz M, Aracena M. Características, efectividad y desafíos de la visita domiciliaria en programas de intervención temprana. *Rev. Salud Pública* 2010, **12**(2): 184–196.

17. Laplante D, Barr R, Brunt A, Gelbert du Fort G, Meaney M, Saucier J, Zelazo P, King S. Stress during pregnancy affects general intellectual and language functioning in human toddlers. *Pediatric Research* 2004, **56**: 400–410.

18. Littleton HL, Bye K, Buck K, Amacker A. Psychosocial stress during pregnancy and perinatal outcomes: a meta-analytic review. *Journal of Psychosomatic Obstetrics & Gynecology* 2010, **31**(4): 219–228.

19. Mulder E, de Medina P, Huizink A, Van den Bergh J, Buitelaar J, Visser G. Prenatal maternal stress: effects on pregnancy and the (unborn) child. *Early Hum Dev* 2002, **70**: 3–14.

20. Nakamura K, Sheps S, Arck PC. Stress and reproductive failure: past notions, present insights and

future directions. *Journal of assisted reproduction and genetics* 2008, **25**(2–3): 47–62.

21. Paarlberg M, Vingerhoets A, Passchier J, Dekker G, Van Geijn H. Psychosocial factors and pregnancy outcome: a review with emphasis on methodological issues. *Journal of Psychosomatic Research* 1995, **39**(5): 563–595.

22. Park M, Son M, Kim Y, Paek D. Social inequalities on birth outcomes in Korea, 1995–2008. *J Korean Med Sci* 2013, **28**: 25–35.

23. Presidencia de la República. Area de Políticas Territoriales. *Uruguay Crece Contigo: resultados alentadores*. Territorios Comunes. Edición Junio-Julio 2014: 4–5.

24. Pryce CR, Feldon J. Long-term neurobehavioural impact of the postnatal environment in rats: manipulations, effects and mediating mechanisms. *Neuroscience& Biobehavioral Reviews* 2003, **27**(1): 57–71.

25. Smith L, La Gasse L, Derauf C, Grant P, Rizman S, Arria Wahdwa P. Psychoneuroendocrine processes in human pregnancy influence fetal development and health. *Psychoneuroendocrinology* 2005, **30**(8): 724–743.

26. Wahdwa P, Sandman C, Porto M, Dunkel-Schetter C, Garite T. The association between prenatal stress and infant birth weight and gestational age at birth. *Am. J Obstet Gynecol* 1993, **169**(4): 858–865.

27. Woods S, Melville J, Yuqing G, Fan M, Gavin A. Psychosocial stress during pregnancy. *Am J Obstet Gynecol* 2010, **202**(1): 611–617.

28. Yehuda R, Mulherin-Engel S, Brand S, Seckel J, Markus S, Berkowitz G. Transgenerational effects of traumatic stress disorder in babies of mothers exposed to traumatic stress in the attack to the World Trade Center during pregnancy. *Journal of Clinical Endocrinology & Metabolism* 2013, **90**(7): 4115–4118.

Chapter 32

Biopsychosocial Approach to the Management of Drug and Alcohol Use in Pregnancy

Nancy A. Haug, Raquel A. Osorno, Melissa A. Yanovitch, and Dace S. Svikis

Use of alcohol, tobacco, and illicit drugs during pregnancy is associated with serious health complications for mothers and infants alike. Pregnant women with substance use disorders are less likely to seek or obtain consistent prenatal care throughout their pregnancies. This population is also at increased risk for infectious diseases such as HIV, hepatitis, and sexually transmitted infections, as well as co-occurring mental health conditions, including mood dysregulation, anxiety, eating disorders and trauma. The direct and indirect cost of prenatal substance use has major economic consequences for every society and remains a significant public health concern.

Pregnant women who use substances have unique biopsychosocial needs that warrant careful consideration in a socioeconomic and cultural context. Substance use during pregnancy falls along a severity continuum with regard to drug type and usage patterns (i.e., quantity, frequency, route of administration). Perinatal care providers have a unique opportunity to educate women, encourage cessation and reduction, prevent medical problems, and promote treatment when needed and available. A comprehensive care model facilitates access to care for women who may have limited resources and struggle with significant barriers to treatment. This chapter provides an overview of evidence-based research and best clinical practices for managing substance use and misuse in pregnant women with a focus on biological, psychological and sociocultural factors.

Screening, Brief Intervention, and Referral to Treatment (SBIRT)

Screening, Brief Intervention, and Referral to Treatment (SBIRT) is an evidence-based approach used to identify and address problematic substance use outside of traditional addiction treatment settings. SBIRT is used in emergency, community

health, and primary care settings in the United States [1], and is endorsed by several national organizations (e.g., American College of Obstetricians and Gynecologists [ACOG]) [2]. SBIRT for pregnant women typically includes routine screening for substance use as part of prenatal care, brief advice or intervention when use is detected, and referral to treatment when appropriate. SBIRT provides an armamentarium practitioners can use to educate and promote substance use cessation, which in turn is associated with better maternal and infant outcomes.

Screening

Early identification of prenatal substance use is vital so that potentially harmful effects on mother and fetus can be ameliorated. Universal (i.e., routine) screening is central to the basic SBIRT model. Since it detects the continuum of substance use, screening provides opportunity for education about the risks of use during pregnancy as well as prevention of progression to misuse. It also minimizes biases that come with screening only when drug use is suspected.

Screening in pregnancy brings unique challenges. In particular, the context in which screening occurs and how it is implemented can have a profound impact. Because drug use during pregnancy in many countries can have legal or social repercussions, women may deny substance use, seek care late in pregnancy, or avoid prenatal care entirely if they expect punitive measures to be taken against them [3]. Other barriers include shame, stigma, lack of family support, substance-using partners, lack of childcare and transportation. As a result, it is imperative that a nonjudgmental, respectful, supportive, and safe environment is provided to ensure that these women become engaged in treatment and obtain proper medical care.

Table 32.1 Prenatal screen for alcohol, tobacco, and substance use: 5Ps

1. Parents	Did any of your parents have a problem with alcohol or other drug use?
2. Peers	Do any of your friends have a problem with alcohol or other drug use?
3. Partner	Does your partner have a problem with alcohol or other drug use?
4. Past	In the past, have you had difficulties in your life due to alcohol or other drugs, including prescription medications?
5. Present	In the past month have you used alcohol, other drugs, or smoked cigarettes?

A single "yes" response suggests the need for further assessment.

For practical reasons, screening tools must be short and easy to administer. Increased stigma of using drugs during pregnancy raises concerns about underreporting. Several brief screening tools have been developed specifically for use with pregnant women, which demonstrate good reliability and validity for detection of prenatal substance use. These include the TWEAK [4], AUDIT-C [5], and the T-ACE [6] for alcohol, and the Perinatal Substance Abuse Screen (5Ps) [7] for other drugs (see Table 32.1), as well as the CRAFFT for young women under the age of 21 years [8]. Providers should inquire specifically about prescribed medications, over-the-counter medications, alcohol, tobacco, cannabis, and other illicit drugs (i.e., methamphetamine, cocaine, MDMA, opioids, inhalants, and benzodiazepines). If universal screening is impractical, research has identified risk factors that predict alcohol and substance use during pregnancy which include smoking cigarettes in the month before pregnancy, continuing to smoke during pregnancy, living with or having a partner who uses substances, presence of a psychiatric disorder, and history of physical or sexual trauma.

Urine drug testing can also confirm suspected or reported drug use in pregnant women. Urine drug tests should only be used with the women's consent and should not be relied on as the sole indication of drug use; routine drug testing is not highly sensitive for many prescription drugs and may produce false-positive and false-negative results. Imposing mandatory urine testing is impractical, expensive, and may

disproportionately impact minority groups, worsen negative legal consequences, and compromise access to health care [9].

Pregnant women, particularly those who report a history of injection drug use or who have injecting male partners, should be screened for blood–borne viruses: human immunodeficiency virus (HIV), hepatitis C virus (HCV) and hepatitis B virus (HBV). The World Health Organization (WHO) has published recommendations for prevention of mother-to-child transmission of HIV and postnatal care in HIV-positive women [10]. Although HCV cannot be treated during pregnancy, medical review and liver function tests should be conducted if the HCV antibody is positive. HBV vaccination of the infant can be performed to reduce vertical transmission from HBV-positive mothers.

Brief Intervention

When a pregnant or postpartum woman screens positive for alcohol, tobacco, or other drug use, the practitioner should proceed to brief intervention (BI) [11]. BI components may include practitioner advice, feedback and motivational interviewing. BI are typically short in duration (approximately 5–30 minutes) and rely upon the FRAMES model (Feedback, Responsibility, Advice, Menu of Options, Empathy, Self-Efficacy) to increase awareness and elicit behavior change [12]. Since having a healthy baby is often a prime motivation to reduce or cease drug use, BIs can be tailored to include information about substance use during pregnancy and benefits for the fetus of reducing or stopping substance use. Practitioner advice should be offered in a nonjudgmental way without using scare tactics, ideally in response to a women's concern about the pregnancy and request for information. Evidence of BI effectiveness in pregnant women is strongest for alcohol [13] but was also effective for other substances in a London sample of pregnant adolescent girls [14].

For smoking, a modified brief counseling program, the 5As, is recommended by ACOG and the National Cancer Institute. The "5As": Ask, Advise, Assess, Assist, and Arrange offer a practical, effective intervention with pregnant smokers and may motivate a quit attempt [15]. For those unwilling to set a quit goal, the 5Rs (i.e., Relevance, Risks, Rewards, Roadblocks, and Repetition) can be discussed. Training materials for the 5As are available, and computerized versions show moderate increases in motivation, self-efficacy, and intention to change among pregnant smokers [16].

The "SBIRT" smartphone application can also screen for alcohol, tobacco, and substance use, complete a BI, and make referrals to treatment based on motivational interviewing. The phone app contains a three-question screen and other established screening measures, which link to the stages of change (i.e., precontemplation, contemplation, preparation, action and maintenance). These can be helpful in determining a woman's readiness to reduce or quit alcohol, tobacco, or drugs, so that a tailored BI can be provided. Phone and computerized intervention strategies have the potential to save time, lower costs, and reduce the need for intensive staff and practitioner training. These technologies also offer anonymity and confidentiality to patients, yielding more self-disclosure and less socially desirable responding, particularly in regard to stigmatized behavior such as substance use [17].

Referral to Addiction Treatment

A complete history of medical conditions, obstetric health, psychiatric disorders, and family/social functioning should be obtained in order to determine the level of care and appropriate modality of addiction treatment. Detoxification may be indicated to resolve withdrawal symptoms and to stabilize patients prior to inpatient treatment.

Psychosocial and behavioral treatments for alcohol and substance use are effective when delivered in both inpatient and outpatient addiction treatment settings. These interventions typically include motivational interviewing, cognitive behavioral therapy, group and family therapies, and relapse prevention. Psychosocial treatment based on the therapeutic community model is common in many European countries. Psychosocial approaches specifically showing effectiveness for pregnant women are more limited. Nonetheless, contingency management approaches have demonstrated improved retention in drug treatment and access to prenatal services for pregnant women [18].

Comprehensive Care Model

Many pregnant women with substance use disorders require comprehensive and coordinated care to address the complex biopsychosocial factors they often face throughout pregnancy and postpartum.

Services should fit the needs of the patient, rather than adapting the patient's needs to the services offered by a particular agency; multidisciplinary coordination is necessary to counteract the historical separation of prenatal care and substance use treatment. The Advisory Council on the Misuse of Drugs (ACMD) recommends maternity services offered to substance using pregnant women be integrated with services that address both long-standing psychosocial concerns and those that emerge during the pregnancy. Services linked with obstetric care ideally include primary health care, social work for children and families, pediatrics, psychiatry, and pain and addiction medicine. Along with adherence to the comprehensive care model, the ACMD emphasizes the importance of providing comfortable, accessible services and including patients in any decision-making regarding their care [19].

There are many ways in which medical providers can facilitate access to substance use treatment. Direct linkage from obstetrical care to substance use outpatient services doubles the chance that patients will complete the referral. For high-risk women, the role of prenatal care providers does not stop with a referral or list of resources. Providers can initiate contact with the referral, escort patients to appointments, and then follow up after the scheduled appointment with a substance use specialist. When the obstetrical staff facilitate access to necessary resources, interorganizational linkages develop, which can help prevent patients from falling through the cracks between referrals. Agencies should develop treatment plans in conjunction with one another, and collaborate on tracking patients' progress throughout the course of pregnancy [20].

Comprehensive case management addresses social and environmental factors that may affect a pregnant woman's ability to engage in treatment, such as assistance with finances, linkages to legal and welfare services, safe housing options, education and job training and domestic violence services [20]. In particular, transportation can be a significant obstacle for patients who live in rural areas or have limited income. Lack of reliable transportation may increase the number of missed prenatal care appointments, as well as impact a patient's ability to engage in substance use treatment. Offering transportation services and attending to social barriers improve the probability that women remain in treatment and reduce post-treatment substance use [21].

Familial and work obligations are also associated with poor treatment retention. Onsite childcare and children's programming during treatment are an important aspect of comprehensive care. Residential treatment settings that allow children to stay with their mothers are associated with positive outcomes across various domains of psychosocial functioning. Unfortunately, many outpatient and residential programs do not offer childcare services, and children are usually not permitted to accompany mothers in addiction treatment settings [20].

Substance use, psychiatric illnesses, and psychosocial stressors are often associated with adverse childhood experiences within the family of origin or foster care system. Because women in treatment for substance use often lack positive models of parenting themselves, they may benefit from parenting classes. Parenting classes may mitigate the effects of a woman's substance use on her family and result in higher rates of abstinence when offered in conjunction with childcare and prenatal care. Providers can make referrals to parenting classes or incorporate these classes directly into treatment programming [22, 23].

Psychiatric Disorders

Research shows that women with substance use disorders are more likely than other women to have co-occurring mental disorders. Psychiatric symptoms, such as depression and anxiety, can be exacerbated by pregnancy and may have adverse effects on addiction treatment outcomes [20]. Women with co-occurring mental health diagnoses may benefit from pharmacological treatment, psychiatric services, diagnosis-specific care (e.g., nutrition counseling for women struggling with eating disorders), and/or children's mental health services. Some pregnant women may feel more comfortable engaging in treatment that offers support for such issues as intimate partner violence, sexual abuse and trauma [23]. High rates of current exposure to physical and emotional violence are found among pregnant women with substance use disorders. Trauma-focused interventions for women with co-occurring drug problems are empirically validated and widely adopted [24].

Cultural Competency

Cultural factors are closely related to women's participation in substance use treatment during pregnancy, as well as continued benefit from treatment after completion. Services for patients with disabilities should include translation services for the hearing impaired and provision of materials for the visually impaired. Interpreter services should be available when treatment is not offered in a patient's primary language. Culturally competent providers should be knowledgeable about a variety of ethnic and cultural backgrounds, and maintain a sense of openness about how these identities intersect with gender and substance use. Guidelines for culture-specific treatment considerations exist and are an important part of sensitive and respectful care [20].

The stigma of substance use for pregnant women may hinder treatment seeking. Due to societal attitudes and gender role expectations, women often experience feelings of shame and guilt, low self-esteem, decreased self-efficacy, and fear of negative consequences such as loss of child custody. Women who are of color, disabled, older, lesbian, and/or poor may experience additional challenges in many cultures. To counter stigma, providers should maintain a nonjudgmental, supportive, and respectful stance, alongside an understanding of women's issues and cultural differences.

Gender-specific programming significantly affects both short- and long-term outcomes in multiple areas of psychosocial functioning. In the first year after completing gender-specific treatment, studies have shown reduced utilization of mental health services, decreased aftercare treatment for substance use and lower rates of arrest [25].

Postpartum Maintenance

The effects of gender-specific programming extend beyond the course of treatment to aftercare. Women in gender-specific treatment are more likely to engage in continuing care than women in mixed-gender treatment. Even for women who achieve abstinence during pregnancy, postpartum relapse is common and necessitates continued care. In terms of postpartum relapse prevention, gender-specific relapse prevention groups yield better outcomes for women six months after treatment completion than mixed-gender groups [21, 26].

Maintaining postpartum abstinence, or substantively reducing use, is not only important to maternal and newborn health but can also make a difference with subsequent pregnancies. Women with substance use disorders are at risk for unplanned pregnancies.

Due to the dramatic effect substances can have on fetal health during the first trimester, interpartum interventions may offer an opportunity to intervene before pregnancy awareness or prior to the first prenatal visit. For example, CHOICES: A Program for Women about Choosing Health Behaviors is a BI that targets risky drinking and contraception for non-pregnant women of reproductive age as a public health strategy to prevent alcohol-exposed pregnancies [27].

Physiological Considerations

The following section focuses on biological and physiological considerations for practitioners who care for pregnant women, including maternal intoxication, withdrawal, fetal effects and breastfeeding. While the majority of female drug users consume multiple substances, this synopsis looks separately at each class of drugs. This provides an opportunity to highlight unique characteristics and sequelae associated with each substance during pregnancy and postpartum. Table 32.2 presents the effects of perinatal substance use, and Table 32.3 provides breastfeeding guidelines.

Alcohol. Of all substances, alcohol may be most dangerous to the developing fetus. No safe levels have been established for consumption in pregnancy. Once alcohol is imbibed, fetal alcohol levels approximately equal the mother's in about one to two hours. Because of fetal reuptake of amniotic fluids, the fetus remains exposed for extended periods of time [28].

Maternal alcohol intoxication is marked by the development of cerebellar-motor retardation, resulting in incoordination and unsteady gait, slurred speech, nystagmus, impairment in attention or memory, and more severely in stupor or loss of consciousness. Signs of withdrawal include tremens, autonomic reactivity, insomnia, nausea/vomiting, anxiety, psychomotor agitation and, in extreme cases, auditory, visual, or tactile hallucinations and grand mal seizures [29]. Management of alcohol withdrawal is imperative to the safety of mother and fetus. Peak withdrawal occurs 24 hours after the last alcoholic beverage is consumed and can be potentially fatal.

According to WHO, pregnant women with alcohol use disorders should be encouraged to stop alcohol use and, if necessary, referred immediately to a detoxification program under direct medical supervision. Detoxification from alcohol can be undertaken at any point during the pregnancy, though maximum benefits are achieved for both mother and fetus with

early intervention. Pharmacologic treatment of alcohol withdrawal in infants includes short-term administration of long-acting benzodiazepines. Medically supervised pharmacological withdrawal is not associated with any significant negative consequences to the fetus. In fact, the risks of continued alcohol use during pregnancy far outweigh the risks of undergoing medically supervised detoxification [11].

If breastfeeding is being considered, women should be educated about alcohol's effect on lactation. Following consumption, lactation is temporarily decreased due to inhibition of the milk ejection reflex. However, alcohol will pass into breast milk, and can be found in concentrations similar to those found in the mother's blood. Long-term effects of exposure to the infant are unknown, thus the WHO recommends waiting at least two hours following the consumption of one drink before breastfeeding. Women who drink more than one standard drink on an occasion should wait four to eight hours before breastfeeding [11].

Tobacco. Pregnancy is an important time to motivate women to stop smoking. Reduction of tobacco intake or abstinence from smoking provides benefits for mother and fetus, most notably higher birth weight and reduced risk of preterm birth. Fetal growth is most affected by maternal smoking during the second and third trimesters. Women who quit smoking in the first trimester have infants with growth parameters similar to those of non-smokers [30]. Financial incentives (e.g., gift certificate or voucher) have evidence for supporting pregnant women in quitting smoking, especially when provided intensively [31]. However, even with resources for clinic-wide implementation, two recent studies in Scotland and England underscore the difficulty in practical translation of financial incentives, with low rates of pregnant women signing on (i.e., 20% and 39%, respectively) and low quit rates, particularly among those from lower socioeconomic status [32, 33].

WHO recommendations for the management of tobacco use in pregnancy state that there is currently insufficient evidence to determine whether or not pharmacotherapy (i.e., nicotine replacement therapy [NRT], bupropion, varenicline) is effective or safe when used in pregnancy for smoking cessation [34]. Several national guidelines have recommended NRT in pregnancy under close medical supervision when psychosocial interventions fail. Higher doses of nicotine may be required to prevent withdrawal symptoms since nicotine is metabolized more rapidly during

Table 32.2 Effects of Perinatal Substance Use

Drug	Perinatal Complications	Neonatal Effects	Long-Term Effects
Nicotine	• Intrauterine growth restriction • Premature delivery • Placental abruption • Low birth weight	• Low birth weight • Breathing difficulties • SIDS • Increased mortality	• Asthma • Obesity • Type 2 diabetes • ADHD • Heart disease • Neurodevelopmental impairments
Alcohol	• Withdrawal, including delirium tremens if severe • Placental abruption • Preterm delivery • Fetal distress	• Small head size • Withdrawal, including seizures if severe	• Restricted growth • Abnormalities of heart, skeleton, and brain • Fetal alcohol spectrum disorders (FASD) • Fetal alcohol syndrome • Facial abnormalities including upper lip border, smooth philtrum, and short palpebral fissures
Cannabis	• Fetal growth restriction	• Small head size • Altered neurobehavioral performance	• Greater difficulty with visuospatial tasks, language, verbal reasoning, short-term memory, attention • Depression • Attentional difficulties
Cocaine	• Placental abruption • Early membrane rupture • Preterm delivery • Spontaneous abortion	• Low birth weight • Tremors, rapid breathing • Withdrawal	• Growth restriction • Neurodevelopmental impairments
Amphetamines	• Premature delivery • Preeclampsia • Eclampsia • Placental abruption • Pregnancy-induced hypertension	• Low birth weight • Fetal death • NAS	• Growth restriction • Cognitive impairments • Decreased arousal • Increased stress
Benzodiazepines	• Spontaneous abortion	• Withdrawal	• Cardiovascular abnormalities • Digestive tract abnormalities • Limb malformations • Oral cleft
Opioids	• Preterm delivery • Stillbirth	• Low birth weight • NAS, including seizures if severe	• Growth restriction • Behavioral and developmental delays

Adapted from SOGC Clinical Practice Guidelines [52].

pregnancy. Maternal tobacco withdrawal symptoms include irritability, frustration or anger, insomnia, depressed mood, increased appetite, anxiety and restlessness [29]. When NRTs are combined with a faster-acting form of nicotine (nicotine patch, in addition to nicotine inhaler, gum, or lozenge),

Table 32.3 Breastfeeding Guidelines for Pregnant Women with Substance Use Disorders

Drug	Breastfeeding Indicated?	Effects on Mother and Infant
Nicotine	Yes, following medical consult	• Effects unknown
Alcohol	Yes: 2 hours following one drink; 4–8 hours following multiple drinks	• Lactation decrease in mother • Infant effects unknown
Cannabis	No	• Effects unknown, but passes into breast milk in high quantities
Cocaine	No, if actively using Yes: 48 hours following consumption	• Infant intoxication and seizures
Amphetamine	No, if actively using Yes: 48 hours following consumption	• Inhibits prolactin release • Can reduce supply
Benzodiazepines	Short-acting: Yes, following medical consult Long-Acting: No	• Some incidents of suckling difficulties and sedation reported • Increased drowsiness in the mother raises risk that she will fall asleep and smother infant
Illicit Opioids	Yes: 24 hours after consumption	• Infant central nervous system depression • Infant death
Methadone	Yes	• No significant effects reported
Buprenorphine/Naloxone	Yes	• No significant effects reported
Slow-Release Morphine	Yes, following medical consult	• Infant central nervous system depression

smoking cessation rates increase [35]. Although NRTs eliminate additional toxins present in cigarette smoke and pregnant women should be encouraged to use them as a step toward smoking cessation, nicotine in any dose is ultimately unhealthy for the developing fetus.

If smoking is continued or resumed postpartum, the mother should be educated about risks to the child posed by breastfeeding. Nicotine and its metabolites can be found in breast milk, though at lower levels than those present in maternal saliva. Long-term effects of exposure to nicotine in breast milk are not known, but postpartum smoking should be discouraged even if not breastfeeding because secondhand smoke poses additional significant risks to the infant [36].

Cannabis. Cannabis sativa (marijuana) is the most commonly used illicit drug in pregnancy, with increasing prevalence in many parts of the world due to legalization, decriminalization and medicalization. In the mother, symptoms of cannabis intoxication include red eyes, increased appetite, dry mouth and slowed heart rate. Signs of withdrawal

include irritability, anger or aggression, nervousness, difficulty sleeping, decreased appetite, restlessness, depressed mood, tremors, sweating, fevers, chills, headache and abdominal pain [29].

Harmful effects of cannabis exposure in utero are more nuanced than those of other substances, and outcomes are often confounded by other substance use and psychosocial factors. Cannabinoids such as tetrahydrocannabinol (THC) may disrupt normal brain development and function. Smoking, the most common route of administration for THC, has negative implications for pregnancy and lactation. Cannabis passes easily into breast milk and can reach levels significantly higher than maternal serum levels. Though the effects of cannabis use on lactation are inconclusive, breastfeeding should be discouraged if the mother uses cannabis postpartum to eliminate risk of later neurodevelopmental impairments [37].

Cocaine. Cocaine is a plant-derived stimulant and local anesthetic with a short half-life. Cocaine intoxication in the mother is characterized by increased or decreased heart rate and blood pressure; dilated pupils; sweating or chills; nausea or vomiting;

psychomotor agitation or retardation; evidence of weight loss; muscular weakness, slowed breathing, chest pain, or cardiac arrhythmias, confusion, seizures, involuntary muscle movements or coma. Maternal withdrawal symptoms include fatigue, vivid nightmares, insomnia or hypersomnia, increased appetite and psychomotor retardation or agitation [29].

Women who use cocaine postpartum are advised not to breastfeed. Cocaine passes readily into the breast milk, potentially exposing the infant to significant amount of the drug. Though research in this area is limited, studies have documented that infants exposed to cocaine in this manner can suffer cocaine intoxication and seizures [38].

Amphetamine. Amphetamine-type substances (i.e., amphetamine, methamphetamine, MDMA) have increased in prevalence worldwide, particularly in North America, Europe, and Asia [39]. Methamphetamine is a potent, man-made stimulant drug with a half-life longer than cocaine's and additional mechanisms of action in the central nervous system. Providers should be aware of amphetamine properties to improve identification and referral to treatment. Short-term effects include increased wakefulness and energy, decreased appetite, increased sexual activity, and physiological complications such as arrhythmias, hypertension, seizures and hyperthermia. Chronic use often leads to depression, anxiety, confusion, insomnia, memory loss, weight loss, dental problems, violent behavior and psychosis [40]. In managing withdrawal from stimulants for pregnant women, psychopharmacological medications may be useful in addressing psychiatric symptoms but are not routinely required [11].

A specific withdrawal syndrome is not defined for amphetamine-exposed neonates, but a small percentage develop severe withdrawal symptoms, a condition known as neonatal abstinence syndrome (NAS), that require intervention. One study determined that approximately 49% of methamphetamine-exposed infants exhibited withdrawal symptoms within the first three days of life but only 4% required medication management [41]. Amphetamine is documented to pass into breast milk in varying quantities. The effects of breastfeeding following amphetamine include increased infant irritability, agitation and crying. Breastfeeding is discouraged for at least 48 hours following amphetamine use to reduce risk of infant exposure [42].

Benzodiazepines. Women may be prescribed benzodiazepines to treat symptoms of anxiety, sleep difficulties or hyperemesis gravidarum that present during pregnancy. Typical maternal withdrawal symptoms include irritability, sweating, tachycardia, hand tremor, increased anxiety, sleep difficulty and, more seriously, cognitive distortions, delirium and seizures [29]. Benzodiazepines should not be discontinued abruptly because withdrawal symptoms may present complications for mother and fetus. Longer-acting benzodiazepines should be used for tapering to limit withdrawal symptoms and risk of seizure [11].

Benzodiazepines enter breast milk in varying quantities depending on the exact substance and dosage. Research shows low incidence of adverse effects during breastfeeding while taking benzodiazepines, though some incidents of suckling difficulties or sedation have been reported in the infant [43].

Opioids. Prescription misuse of opioids is increasingly common, and drugs in this category include oxycodone, hydrocodone, codeine and morphine. Heroin is an illicit opioid that is injected intravenously, smoked or snorted. Signs of maternal opioid intoxication include constriction of the pupils, drowsiness, slurred speech, impaired attention or memory and loss of consciousness. Withdrawal symptoms in pregnant women include depressed mood, insomnia, fever, yawning, diarrhea, nausea or vomiting, muscle aches, runny nose or tearfulness, dilation of pupils, goose bumps and sweating [29].

Opioid use in pregnancy is associated with pre-term delivery, low birth weight, and still birth, and mothers are more likely to suffer from major depression, anxiety disorders, and chronic health conditions such as HIV, diabetes, renal disease and hypertension. Further, opioid-using patients are four times as likely to remain in the hospital five or more days post delivery and four times more likely to die before hospital discharge. On average, the cost of hospitalization of an opioid user is much higher non-opioid related hospitalizations.

Neonates exposed to opioids in utero may develop NAS between one and seven days after delivery, which can last one to two weeks. Symptoms of NAS span the autonomic, gastrointestinal and central nervous systems, and often require medical intervention. Doses of morphine or methadone are common pharmacologic treatments, but risks of administration must be weighed with severity of NAS symptoms [44].

Different opioids transfer into breast milk in varying amounts. While some opioids are frequently prescribed to mothers postpartum for pain management, others such as codeine and oxycodone have been shown to cause central nervous system depression or death in the infant.

Opioid Pharmacotherapy

Access to opioid pharmacotherapy depends on governmental restrictions as well as political, social and cultural factors. In some countries, methadone and/or buprenorphine maintenance treatment is unavailable or illegal. For example, all treatment for substance use disorders in the Russian Federation is abstinence-oriented and opioid substitution therapy is against the law. Other countries in Eastern Europe and Asia such as China and India have significant unmet treatment needs for opioid users [45].

Methadone. Methadone is an opioid agonist indicated for patients suffering from opioid use disorders. It is used worldwide to promote abstinence from illicit opioid substances and to improve treatment attendance and prenatal care utilization. Methadone is generally considered safer than illicit opioids for both mother and fetus because it reduces associated behaviors of illicit drug seeking such as sharing injection needles or trading drugs for sex. Most research demonstrates methadone efficacy at doses between 60 and 100 mg for pregnant women [46].

Methadone use in pregnancy increases likelihood of compliance with prenatal care and substance use treatment during pregnancy. Despite its benefits, methadone maintenance treatment in pregnancy is not without risks. The probability of methadone-exposed infants developing NAS is comparable to those of infants exposed to other opioids in utero regardless of the mother's methadone dose. Methadone-induced NAS is treated in the same manner as other opioid-induced NAS, usually with tapered morphine administration. However, methadone treatment during pregnancy is associated with fewer pregnancy complications, reduced illicit opioid use and better treatment outcomes for mother and fetus [46]. Breastfeeding is not contraindicated for mothers on methadone maintenance treatment because amounts found in breast milk are sufficiently small [47].

Slow-Release Morphine. Slow-release morphine is also known to effectively treat opioid use disorder during pregnancy. A comparative study of methadone and morphine maintenance in pregnant women indicated that infants born to the women in both groups had statistically similar birth weights that were within normal range, while newborns in both groups exhibited signs of NAS [48]. Since little research exists on the safety of breastfeeding while taking slow-release morphine, infants should be monitored for signs of central nervous system depression.

Buprenorphine/Naloxone. Buprenorphine is a partial opioid agonist that is an alternative to methadone for opioid use disorder treatment. An advantage of buprenorphine is that it can be dispensed in weekly or biweekly doses, unlike the daily distribution at a licensed clinic required by methadone. This results in a more convenient treatment option, especially for patients living in rural settings or those with limited access to transportation.

Buprenorphine's safety profile is generally considered better than methadone's because it is a partial agonist, reducing likelihood of overdose. Buprenorphine-exposed neonates also exhibit a lower incidence of NAS and have shorter hospital stays. However, patients treated with buprenorphine are statistically less likely to continue in treatment than those treated with methadone [49].

A more recent formulation of buprenorphine includes naloxone, an opioid antagonist. The addition of naloxone prevents overdose and discourages diversion, selling or giving the drug away instead of being taken as prescribed. Clinical judgment should be used when deciding to keep a woman on the combined formulation or switching to buprenorphine alone when pregnancy is confirmed. Breastfeeding while on buprenorphine is generally considered safe and should be encouraged [47, 49].

Pregnant women maintained on opioid replacement therapy generally require higher doses of pain medication during labor than women not taking opioid substitution. Opioid replacement therapy should not be discontinued during labor or cesarean section, but medication is typically divided into three or four doses over the course of the day to improve pain management and prevent withdrawal [50, 51].

Conclusion

Perinatal use of alcohol, tobacco and other drugs increases risk for adverse maternal and infant outcomes. Early detection is important, and obstetric care providers are in a unique position to provide education and brief intervention to women using drugs during pregnancy. When substance use is severe, providers can also refer such women to addiction treatment. To assist practitioners in such efforts, the WHO has published guidelines for the identification and management of substance use disorders during pregnancy [11]. Intended for a global audience of practitioners, including those from low- and middle-income countries, these guidelines highlight the importance of adapting recommendations to meet the needs of local health care systems. This is important, because while research has shown that pregnant women with substance use disorders are likely to benefit most from comprehensive, coordinated care, such programs do not exist in many parts of the world. Practitioners are encouraged to identify and address barriers, develop services, and form care plans within their socioeconomic and cultural context.

Key Points

- Pregnant women with substance use disorders are more likely than other women to have co-occurring mental disorders and/or current exposure to physical and emotional violence.
- Screening, Brief Intervention, and Referral to Treatment (SBIRT) for pregnant women typically includes routine screening for alcohol, tobacco, and other drug use as part of prenatal care; brief advice or intervention when use is detected; and referral to treatment when appropriate.
- Brief screening tools for use with pregnant women include the TWEAK, AUDIT-C, and the T-ACE for alcohol, the Perinatal Substance Abuse Screen (5Ps) for other drugs; and the CRAFFT for young women under the age of 21 years.
- Brief intervention components may include practitioner advice, feedback and motivational interviewing.
- Technology-based interventions have potential to save time, lower costs and reduce the need for intensive staff and practitioner training, while offering anonymity and confidentiality to patients.
- Evidence-based psychosocial and behavioral treatments for alcohol and other drug use during pregnancy include motivational interviewing, cognitive behavioral therapy, contingency management, group and family therapies, and relapse prevention.

- Services should fit the needs of the patient, rather than adapting the patient's needs to the services offered by a particular agency.
- Multidisciplinary care coordination is necessary to counteract the historical separation of prenatal care and substance use treatment.
- Pregnant women maintained on opioid replacement therapy generally require higher doses of pain medication during labor than women not taking opioid substitution. Opioid replacement therapy should not be discontinued during labor or cesarean section.
- Parenting classes may mitigate the effects of a woman's substance use on her family and result in higher rates of abstinence when offered in conjunction with childcare and prenatal care.
- Even for women who achieve abstinence during pregnancy, postpartum relapse is common and necessitates continued care.

References

1. Madras B, Compton W, Avula D, Stegbauer T, Stein J, Clark H. Screening, brief interventions, referral to treatment (SBIRT) for illicit drug and alcohol use at multiple healthcare sites: Comparison at intake and 6 months later. *Drug Alcohol Depend*. 2009;**99**:280–295.

2. O'Brien P. Performance measurement: A proposal to increase use of SBIRT and decrease alcohol consumption during pregnancy. *Matern. Child Health J.* 2014;**8**(1):1–9.

3. Howell EM, Heiser N, Harrington M. A review of recent findings on substance abuse treatment for pregnant women. *J Subst Abuse Treat*. 1999;**16**:195–219.

4. Russell M, Martier SS, Sokol RJ, Mudar P, Jacobson S, son J. Detecting risk drinking during pregnancy: A comparison of four screening questionnaires. *Am. J. Public Health* 1996;**86**:1435–1439.

5. Dawson D, Grant B, Stinson F, Zhou Y. Effectiveness of the derived Alcohol Use Disorder Identification Test (AUDIT-C) in screening for alcohol use disorders and risky drinking in the US general population. *Alcohol Clin Exp Res*. 2005:**29**(5): 844–854.

6. Sokol RJ, Martier SS, Ager JW. The T-ACE questions: Practical prenatal detection of risk-drinking. *Am J Obstet Gynecol*. 1989;**160**(4):863–868.

7. Watson E. The evolution and application of the 5 P'S behavioral risk screening tool. *The Source*. 2010;**20** (2):27–29.

8. Knight JR, Shrier LA, Bravender TD, Farrell M, Vander Bilt J, Shaffer HJ. A new brief screen for adolescent

substance abuse. *Arch Pediatr Adolesc Med.* 1999;**153**:591–596.

9. American Congress on Obstetricians and Gynecologists. Toolkit on state legislation. [cited 26 March 2017]. Available from: www.acog.org/-/media/Departments/Government-Relations-and-Outreach/NASToolkit.pdf.

10. World Health Organization. PMTCT Strategic Vision 2010–2015. Preventing mother-to-child transmission of HIV to reach the UNGASS and millennium development goals. 2010 [cited 26 March 2017]. Available from: http://whqlibdoc.who.int/publications/2010/9789241599030_eng.pdf.

11. World Health Organization. Guidelines for the identification and management of substance use and substance use disorders in pregnancy. 2014 [cited 26 March 2017]. Available from: http://apps.who.int/iris/bitstream/10665/107130/1/9789241548731_eng.pdf.

12. American Congress of Obstetricians and Gynecologists. Committee opinion number 423: motivational interviewing: A tool for behavior change. 2009 [cited 26 March 2017]. Available from: www.acog.org/-/media/Committee-Opinions/Committee-on-Health-Care-for-Underserved-Women/co423.pdf?dmc=1&ts=20150802T1346475239.

13. O'Connor MJ, Whaley SE. Brief intervention for alcohol use by pregnant women. *Am J Public Health.* 2007;**97**:252–258.

14. Whicher EV, Utku F, Schirmer G, Davis P, Abou-Saleh MT. Pilot project to evaluate the effectiveness and acceptability for single-session brief counseling for the prevention of substance misuse in pregnant adolescents. *Addict Disord Their Treat.* 2012;**11**:43–49.

15. Phelan S. Smoking cessation in pregnancy. *Obstet Gynecol Clin N Am.* 2014;**41**(2):255–266.

16. Ondersma SJ, Svikis DS, Lam PK, Connors-Burge C, Ledgerwood DM, Hopper JA. A randomized trial of computer-delivered brief intervention and low-intensity contingency management for smoking during pregnancy. *Nicotine Tob Res.* 2012;**3**:351–360.

17. Bull S. *Technology-Based Health Promotion.* Thousand Oaks, CA: Sage Publications; 2011.

18. Terplan M, Lui S. Psychosocial interventions for pregnant women in outpatient illicit drug treatment programs compared to other interventions. Cochrane Database Syst. Rev. 2007 [cited 26 March 2017]. Available from: www.cochrane.org/CD006037/ADDICTN_psychosocial-interventions-for-pregnant-women-in-outpatient-illicit-drug-treatment-programmes-compared-to-other-interventions.

19. Advisory Council on the Misuse of Drugs. Hidden harm – responding to the needs of children of problem drug users. Home Office. 2003 [Cited 26 March 2017] Available from: www.gov.uk/government/uploads/system/uploads/attachment_data/file/120620/hidden-harm-full.pdf.

20. Center for Substance Abuse Treatment. Substance abuse treatment: addressing the specific needs of women. Treatment Improvement Protocol (TIP) Series 51. 2009 [cited 26 March 2017]. Available from: https://store.samhsa.gov/shin/content/SMA13-4426/SMA13-4426.pdf.

21. Ashley OS, Marsden ME, Brady TM. Effectiveness of substance abuse treatment programming for women: A review. *Am J.Drug Alcohol Abuse.* 2003;**29**:19–53.

22. Gopman S. Prenatal and postpartum care of women with substance use disorders. *Obstet Gynecol Clin N Am.* 2014;**41**:213–228.

23. Milligan K, Niccols A, Sword W, Thabane L, et al. Maternal substance use and integrated treatment programs for women with substance abuse issues and their children: A meta-analysis. *Subst Abuse Treat Prev Policy.* 2010;**5**:21.

24. Haug NA, Duffy M, McCaul ME. Substance abuse treatment services for pregnant women. *Obstet Gynecol Clin N Am.* 2014;**41**:267–296.

25. Hser Y, Evans E, Huang D, Messina N. Long-term outcomes among drug-dependent mothers treated in women-only versus mixed-gender programs. *J Subst Abuse Treat.* 2011;**41**:115–123.

26. Claus RE, Orwin RG, Kissin W, et al. Does gender-specific substance abuse treatment for women promote continuity of care? *J Subst Abuse Treat.* 2007;**32**(1):27–39.

27. Project CHOICES Intervention Research Group. Reducing the risk of alcohol-exposed pregnancies: a study of a motivational intervention in community settings. Pediatrics. 2003;**111**:1131–1135.

28. Izquierdo LA, Yonke N. Fetal surveillance in late pregnancy and during labor. *Obstet. Gynecol Clin N Am.* 2014;**41**(2):307–315.

29. American Psychiatric Association. *Diagnostic and Statistical Manual of Mental Disorders*, Fifth Edition. Arlington, VA: American Psychiatric Association; 2013.

30. Prabhu N, Smith N, Campbell D, Craig LC, Seaton A, Helms PJ, et al. First trimester maternal tobacco smoking habits and fetal growth. *Thorax.* 2010;**65**:235–240.

31. Lumley J, Chamberlain C, Dowswell T, Oliver S, Oakley L, Watson L. Interventions for promoting smoking cessation during pregnancy. *Cochrane Database Syst. Rev.* 2009 [cited 26 March 2017] Available from: http://onlinelibrary.wiley.com/doi/10.1002/14651858.CD001055.pub3/full.

32. Radley A, Ballard P, Eadie D, MacAskill S, Donnelly L, Tappin D. Give it up for baby: Outcomes and factors influencing uptake of a pilot smoking cessation incentive scheme for pregnant women. *BMC Public Health.* 2013;**13**(343):1–13.

33. Ierfino D, Mantzari E, Hirst J, Jones T, Aveyard P, Marteau TM. Financial incentives for smoking cessation in pregnancy: A single-arm intervention study assessing cessation and gaming. *Addiction.* 2015;**110**:680–688.

34. World Health Organization. WHO recommendations for the prevention and management of tobacco use and second-hand smoke exposure in pregnancy. Geneva, 2013.

35. Brose LS, McEwen A, West R. Association between nicotine replacement therapy use in pregnancy and smoking cessation. *Drug Alcohol Depend.* 2013;**132**(3):660–664.

36. Jacob N, Golmard J-L, Berlin I. Relationships between nicotine and cotinine concentrations in maternal milk and saliva. *Acta Paediatrica.* 2015;**104**(8):1–7.

37. American Congress of Obstetricians and Gynecologists. Committee Opinion Number 637. Marijuana use during pregnancy and lactation. 2015 [cited 26 March 2017]. Available from: www.acog.org/Resources-And-Publications/Committee-Opinions/Committee-on-Obstetric-Practice/Marijuana-Use-During-Pregnancy-and-Lactation.

38. D'Apolito K. Breastfeeding and substance abuse. *Clin. Obstet. Gynecol.* 2013;**56**(1):202–211.

39. United Nations Office on Drugs and Crime. World drug report 2012. 2012. [cited 26 March 2017] Available from: www.unodc.org/documents/data-and-analysis/WDR2012/WDR_2012_web_small.pdf.

40. Committee on Health Care for Underserved Women. Committee opinion no. 479: Methamphetamine abuse in women of reproductive age. Am. Coll. Obstet. Gynecol. 2011. [cited 26 March 2017]. Available from: www.acog.org/-/media/Committee-Opinions/Committee-on-Health-Care-for-Underserved-Women/co479.pdf?dmc=1&ts=20150802T1602256805.

41. Smith LM, LaGasse LL, Derauf C, Grant P, Shah R, Arria A, et al. The infant development, environment, and lifestyle study: Effects of prenatal methamphetamine exposure, polydrug exposure, and poverty on intrauterine growth. *Pediatrics.* 2006;**118**(3):1149–1156.

42. Bartu A, Dusci LJ, Ilett KF. Transfer of methylamphetamine and amphetamine into breast milk following recreational use of methylamphetamine. *Br. J. Clin. Pharm.* 2009;**67**(4):455–459.

43. McElhatton PR. The effects of benzodiazepine use during pregnancy and lactation. *Reprod. Toxicol.* 1994;**8**(6):461–475.

44. Kocherlakota P. Neonatal Abstinence Syndrome. *Pediatrics.* 2014;**134**(2):e547–61.

45. World Health Organization. The methadone fix. Bull. World Health Organ. 2008 [cited 26 March 2017] Available from: www.who.int/bulletin/volumes/86/3/08-050308.pdf

46. Fullerton CA, Kim M, Thomas CP, Lyman DR, Montejano LB, Dougherty RH, et al. Medication-assisted treatment with methadone: Assessing the evidence. *Psychiatr. Serv.* 2014;**65**(2):146–157.

47. Gopman S. Prenatal and postpartum care of women with substance use disorders. *Obstet. Gynecol. Clin. N. Am.* 2014;**41**(2):213–228.

48. Fischer G, Jagsch R, Eder H, Gombas W, Etzersdorfer P, Schmidl-Mohl K, et al. Comparison of methadone and slow-release morphine maintenance in pregnant addicts. *Addiction.* 1999;**94**(2):231–239.

49. Mozurkewich EL, Rayburn WF. Buprenorphine and methadone for opioid addiction during pregnancy. *Obstet. Gynecol. Clin. N. Am.* 2014;**41**(2):241–253.

50. Committee on Health Care for Underserved Women and the American Society of Addiction Medicine. Committee opinion no. 524: opioid abuse, dependence, and addiction in pregnancy. Am. Coll. Obstet. Gynecol. 2012 (Reaffirmed 2016) [cited 26 March 2017]. Available from: www.acog.org/-/media/Committee-Opinions/Committee-on-Health-Care-for-Underserved-Women/co524.pdf?dmc=1&ts=20150802T1641540132.

51. Jones HE, Deppen K, Hudak ML, Leffert L, McClelland C, Sahin L, et al. Clinical care for opioid-using pregnant and postpartum women: The role of obstetric providers. *Am. J. Obstet. Gynecol.* 2014;**210**(4):302–310.

52. Wong, S, Ordean, A, Kahan, M. SOGC Clinical Practice Guidelines: Substance use in pregnancy: no. 256. *Int. J. Gynaecol. Obstet.* 2011;**114**(2):190–202.

Chapter

33

Biopsychosocial Factors in Preterm Labor and Delivery

Gabriel D. Shapiro, William D. Fraser, and Jean R. Séguin

Introduction

Preterm birth (PTB) is a significant and growing problem in contemporary obstetrics, leading to increased neonatal morbidity and mortality and entailing substantial social and economic costs. PTB is the leading cause of infant mortality in industrialized countries, accounting for 60% of perinatal mortality and about half of long-term neurologic morbidity [1]. PTB is defined by the World Health Organization as delivery before 37 completed weeks of gestation. In 2013, the rate of PTB was 11.4% of live births in the United States [2], where annual acute care costs for preterm infants are estimated at more than $26 billion [3]. Preterm infants are at increased risk of respiratory distress, jaundice, hypoglycemia, and neonatal death, as well as developmental delays and needs for special education. There is also mounting evidence linking PTB to health outcomes in adulthood. Additionally, PTB exacts an emotional and financial burden on parents, increasing maternal distress and depressive symptoms [3]. Of great concern is the fact that PTB has not shown the same reductions in recent decades as other adverse neonatal health indicators. Rates of PTB are actually increasing in many industrialized countries [4], though recent reductions have been seen in the United States [2].

PTB shows a biological complexity and phenotypic heterogeneity that make prediction and prevention especially difficult [4]. Preterm labor precedes about half of all PTBs, while preterm premature rupture of membranes and iatrogenic causes (indications for induced delivery such as severe preeclampsia) are each involved in roughly a quarter. Identified risk factors include previous preterm delivery, multiple gestation pregnancy, low pre-pregnancy body mass index or gestational weight gain, chorioamnionitis or other intrauterine infection, mechanical factors such as incompetent cervix and uterine malformations, and indications for early delivery [5]. While

many risk factors, particularly biological ones, are quite reliable in terms of their associations with PTB across different populations, they are not highly specific to PTB, and the ability to predict PTB from a risk factor profile remains poor. In fact, only about half of preterm deliveries are preceded by one of these known risk factors. In addition, PTB exhibits troubling disparities across racial groups and socioeconomic strata [2, 3]. Identification of novel risk factors and elucidation of the pathways linking risk factors to PTB are thus crucial research priorities.

While understanding of biological risk factors for PTB is more advanced than for psychosocial risk factors, a growing literature supports the role of psychosocial stress during pregnancy (PSP) in the etiology of preterm labor and birth [5]. Neuroendocrine, inflammatory, and maternal lifestyle and behavioral pathways are hypothesized to mediate the link between PSP and PTB [6–8]. However, there has been heterogeneity in findings regarding the role of various forms of PSP as a potential predictor of PTB. Therefore, this chapter will survey the published evidence on the association between PSP and PTB, and will highlight established and hypothesized physiologic pathways mediating this relationship. Beginning with an overview of different measures of PSP, we will describe the literature investigating their associations with PTB. We will then discuss the biological manifestations of PSP, the physiologic responses to chronic and acute stress, and the mechanisms hypothesized to mediate the link between PSP and PTB.

Psychosocial Stress during Pregnancy and Preterm Birth

Several types of PSP including stressful life events, perceived stress and pregnancy-related anxiety have been associated with PTB [8, 9]. There is also some understanding of the biological pathways underlying these links and how they vary across pregnancy, but it remains incomplete. Heterogeneity of exposure measurement and outcome definitions pose challenges to the determination of overall links. The following sections summarize existing knowledge on the measurement of PSP and on its association with PTB.

Measures of Psychosocial Stress during Pregnancy

Stress constitutes a psychophysiological consequence of any event challenging an individual's capacity to cope. Stressful life events are situations likely to *objectively* require some degree of coping in ongoing life adjustment, while perceived stress is defined as the degree to which situations in one's life are *subjectively* appraised as stressful. Anxiety is a related concept measuring individual psychological and physical manifestation of exposure to perceived stress. Anxiety is traditionally separated into state anxiety (an emotional response to stimuli perceived as dangerous, threatening, or stressful, typically experienced as tension, worry, or nervousness – or how one feels at a given moment, for example, because of an upcoming interview or test) and trait anxiety (the predisposition to react to a wider range of stimuli by experiencing anxiety – or the anxiety one feels generally).

Research on PSP has examined the roles of both objective stress constructs (i.e., exposures measured independently of the individual's perception of them such as a death in the family, becoming unemployed, natural disasters or war-related violence) and subjective measures of stress levels. Studies have also explored the role of pregnancy-related stress and anxiety, that is, stress and anxiety stemming from the physical, psychological, and social experience of pregnancy. Measures of pregnancy-related anxiety capture this concept by asking about fears and concerns specifically related to the pregnancy. Pregnancy-related stressors include physical changes naturally associated with pregnancy, concerns about the experience of childbirth and parenting, and relationship strains due to pregnancy. Examining the role played by pregnancy-related versus non-pregnancy-related stressors and anxiety is crucial to understanding how psychosocial stress and anxiety differ in pregnant women compared to other populations, and to clarifying what kinds of stressors and fears are most strongly associated with birth outcomes.

Stressful Life Events, Their Timing, and Perceived Impact

Stressful life events during pregnancy have been associated with PTB or shortened gestation in some [10, 11] but not all [12, 13] studies. Effects of stressful life events during pregnancy on PTB have been found in studies conducted in several different countries, with sample sizes ranging from less than 200 to more than 8,000 and using both prospective and retrospective cohort and case-control designs. As the techniques used in measuring stressful life events have been refined, timing within the pregnancy and subjective perception of stress have usually been found to be more relevant to the risk of PTB than objective event counts across pregnancy [9]. The maternal hypothalamic-pituitary-adrenal (HPA) axis has been shown to be progressively downregulated over the course of pregnancy [14], suggesting that biological and emotional stress responses are likely to be attenuated toward the end of pregnancy. In light of this evidence, it is not surprising that life events experienced at the beginning of pregnancy were perceived as more stressful than similar events occurring in the third trimester [15]. Specifically, the z-score for mean stress appraisal across all life events was 0.14 in the first trimester and 0.03 in the second trimester, compared to -0.34 in the third trimester ($F(2,196) = 4.77$, $p < .01$). Fourteen of the 18 life events analyzed were reported as less upsetting when occurring in the third trimester compared to the first trimester (binomial test, $p < .05$) [15]. Recent studies have also found that earlier exposure to stressful life events or acute traumatic events was most likely to be associated with PTB [10]. In sum, observational research supports a stronger role for subjectively perceived stress in the prediction of PTB compared to objectively defined stressful events, as well as a stronger role for stressors experienced early compared to later in the pregnancy [9].

General Perceived Stress and Maternal Anxiety

An important limitation of the "life event" approach to stress in PTB research is that it often fails to capture relevant chronic stressors such as racism, domestic violence and less severe 'daily hassles.' In contrast, the assessment of perceived stress is not necessarily tied to specific events and is thus likely to capture individuals' actual stress levels more precisely than objective scales of stressful life events [9]. Measures of anxiety also share this feature in that they are not bound to specific events experienced by an individual.

Both anxiety and general perceptions of stress (independent of its source) have been associated with shortened gestation in many [11, 16] but not all [12, 13] studies. Studies with null findings have tended to be characterized by study populations of higher socio-economic status and exposure measurement scales not specific to pregnancy. Trait anxiety measures have generally not shown strong direct relationships with birth outcomes, likely because they are not sensitive to the presence of stressful stimuli that may trigger state anxiety. In contrast to trait anxiety, several studies have found positive associations between pregnancy-related anxiety and PTB or shortened gestation [11, 16], though these effects were weak in one study [12]. Overall, the literature suggests that pregnancy-related anxiety may be more strongly associated with adverse birth outcomes than non-pregnancy-related stressors.

Other Psychosocial Factors

Evidence suggests that the prevalence of some clinical anxiety disorders may be higher in samples of pregnant women compared to the general population [17]. In addition to the impact of anxiety disorders on quality of life, clinical anxiety may be related to pregnancy outcomes as well. As with subclinical anxiety, severe mental illnesses can lead to pregnancy-related medical disorders and obstetric complications, operating through neuroendocrine, immune-related and inflammatory mechanisms [18]. Depressive symptoms and clinical depression may also be related to preterm labor and birth [6]. While some psychotropic medications may cross the placental barrier and harm the fetus, untreated psychiatric disorders also pose risks to the mother and eventually to the child. Accordingly, care must be taken to balance the risks and benefits of symptoms and treatments. The role of non-pharmacological treatment of depression and anxiety disorders in pregnancy must not be discounted either. For example, omega-3 fatty acids are an emerging alternative therapy that may be effective for the prevention and treatment of antenatal depression and psychiatric disorders [19].

Methodological Concerns

In addition to challenges relating to exposure definition, other methodological issues may contribute to mixed findings on PSP and PTB. For example,

pregnancy-related anxiety and other subjective stress measures could plausibly stem from threatened preterm labor, other pregnancy complications or previous adverse pregnancy outcomes [12]. Existing studies have not always been able to adequately address this potential reverse causality. Secondly, the role of social support in mitigating the severity or effects of stress as it relates to PTB is not well understood [5, 20]. Some suggest that greater levels of family social support and/or lower stress levels among Latino immigrants in the United States may in part explain the "Hispanic paradox" (in which immigrants have better health outcomes, including perinatal outcomes, than expected based on their socioeconomic profile) as it relates to PTB [21]. Several other studies have explored social support interventions as a strategy for PTB prevention, though randomized trials have shown limited success [5]. Systematic measurement of social support in epidemiologic studies could help clarify whether it may partially account for inconsistent associations found between PSP with PTB.

Summary

The epidemiologic literature on PSP and PTB presents mixed results that stem in part from a multitude of exposure definitions and other methodological limitations. If psychosocial factors influence biological perinatal outcomes, the intervening mechanisms must have a biological signature. Examining the biological mechanisms connecting PSP to PTB is thus crucial, as the correspondence between psychosocial stress, its subjective perception, and biological stress measures is not straightforward. By anchoring subjective perceptions of stress with biological mechanisms more proximal to PTB, such work can help identify the most relevant psychosocial measures of stress in pregnancy and the conditions under which the mechanisms operate. The following sections outline existing knowledge and potential directions for future research in this area.

Mechanisms Linking Psychosocial Stress during Pregnancy with Preterm Birth

Potential biological mediators of the relationship between PSP and PTB include neuroinflammatory, immune and neuroendocrine pathways [6, 9, 22]. In addition, stress-related behaviors, including smoking, substance abuse and poor nutritional intake have been implicated in the etiology of PTB [6]. Finally, pregnancy-related anxiety could sometimes stem from medical risk that itself leads to PTB.

Hormonal and Neurological Correlates of Psychosocial Stress

The biological manifestations of stress have been assessed by the measurement of hormone levels in plasma or saliva samples, as well as through measurement of prefrontal functional connectivity using positron emission tomography and functional magnetic resonance imaging [23]. Importantly, chronic stress was associated with reduced attention control and functional connectivity in the prefrontal cortex in a manner that persisted in the absence of any acute stressor, but that was reversible in response to reduced chronic stress [23].

Cortisol is known to be a mediator of the physiologic stress response [24], and psychosocial stress also activates hypothalamic release of corticotropin-releasing hormone (CRH) [25]. However, these mechanisms are altered during pregnancy [24] and may in fact influence pregnancy outcomes, as described in the following sections.

Neuroendocrine Pathways Linking Psychosocial Stress during Pregnancy and Preterm Birth

The maternal HPA axis constitutes the principal neuroendocrine mechanism hypothesized to mediate the link between PSP with PTB [6]. In pregnancy, maternal cortisol stimulates placental gene expression that increases placental CRH production. While cortisol inhibits maternal hypothalamic CRH production, placental CRH production increases maternal CRH and stimulates maternal adrenal cortisol secretion, creating a positive feedback loop. Ultimately, maternal CRH concentrations increase up to a thousand fold across the course of pregnancy [24]. However, it has not been conclusively shown that CRH mediates the relationship between PSP and PTB [26], and epidemiologic studies measuring all three factors have yielded conflicting results, as we will see next.

Psychosocial Stress during Pregnancy, Corticotropin-Releasing Hormone and Preterm Birth

CRH is one mechanism hypothesized to function as a 'placental clock' controlling parturition, and CRH

trajectories across pregnancy have predicted timing of delivery [27]. In one study, CRH as measured at 28–30 weeks' gestation was found to mediate the relationship between anxiety and gestational age at delivery [28]. However, other studies have failed to find associations between stress or anxiety and maternal CRH. For example, one study of women in mid-pregnancy found job stress and stressful life events were unrelated to serum CRH at 28 weeks' gestation [29]. An additional study found an association between perceived stress and PTB; however, that association was not mediated by maternal CRH as measured in the second trimester [30].

In addition to these varied findings on the mediating role of CRH in a link between PSP and PTB, moderating effects have also been observed between stress and CRH on PTB in two studies. In one study, Guendelman et al. [31] found that the association between CRH and preterm delivery was stronger in women exposed to chronic stressors during pregnancy than in unexposed women. In a second study, Hobel et al. [32] compared preterm with matched term deliveries, finding a positive association between perceived stress and maternal plasma CRH for the PTB cases but a negative association for controls. Interestingly, stress was also inversely associated with CRH in the study by Guendelman et al. [31], who hypothesized that reduced CRH may be a protective placental response to *prolonged* gestation in cases of stress. Taken together, these results suggest that CRH does not consistently mediate or modify the association between PSP and PTB.

Effects of Chronic Stress on Physiologic Stress Response and Infection

Results from both animal and human studies using general population samples show associations between psychosocial stressors and altered response in the amygdala and hippocampus to novel stressors, as well as with elevated serum CRH levels and CRH gene expression in the amygdala [25]. This suggests that chronic stress may prime an individual to an adaptive state of hypervigilance and, by a process of sensitization, increase the physiological responses to future acute stressors [33]. Conversely, chronic stress is also hypothesized to blunt HPA function and has been shown to desensitize the stress response in the entorhinal cortex and striatum of adult rats exposed to chronic prenatal stress [34]. Finally, chronic stress increases susceptibility to infection and is associated with maternal infection during pregnancy [35]. Further research is needed to clarify the relative contribution of chronic versus acute stress to PTB.

Neuroinflammatory Pathways

Inflammation is the basic process by which tissues of the body respond to injury through the effects of cytokines and other inflammatory mediators. Cytokines are small soluble peptides or glycoproteins including interleukins, chemokines and tumor necrosis factor (TNF), among others. Cytokines' primary function is intercellular communication, and their role in the inflammatory response functions largely through regulation of the immune response [36]. PSP is hypothesized to bring about parturition in part through pro-inflammatory mechanisms, specifically pro-inflammatory cytokines [22].

While conclusive links connecting psychosocial stress, inflammation, and PTB have not been demonstrated, there is some evidence suggesting that the process of inflammation mediates a link between PSP and PTB. For example, psychosocial stress leads to increased production of pro-inflammatory cytokines in the general population [8], and altered levels of inflammatory cytokines have been observed in pregnant women with increased psychosocial stress [7, 8]. While cytokine levels have also been linked with PTB, their role as a mediator of the relationship between stress and PTB is still unclear. It has been shown that an inflammatory response in the form of overexpression of toll-like receptors in the chorioamniotic membranes is part of normal term labor [37]. Further supporting the role of inflammation in parturition, inflammatory cytokines increase the production of prostaglandins, which are implicated in term and preterm labor [38]. Through induction of matrix metalloproteinases, inflammatory cytokines can also weaken fetal membranes and ripen the cervix [39]. A recent meta-analysis found that the inflammatory cytokine interleukin-6 (IL-6) and C-reactive protein were strongly associated with spontaneous PTB [40], and biologic evidence also supports the role of tumor necrosis factor alpha (TNFα) in preterm parturition [36].

Recent work has begun to describe a cholinergic anti-inflammatory pathway (CAP) in which the release of inflammatory cytokines is controlled through the vagus nerve. Specifically, action potentials transmitted through the vagus nerve result in the release of acetylcholine, which inhibits cytokine production by innate immune cells in tissues innervated by the vagus nerve. Evidence in support of this pathway comes from suppression of inflammation (decreased production of pro-inflammatory cytokines with no change in production of anti-inflammatory cytokines) in response to stimulation of the vagus nerve in adult animal models [41]. Specifically, vagus nerve stimulation inhibits inflammatory cytokine production in an adult rat model of sepsis [42], in a mouse model of pancreatitis [43] and in postoperative ileus [44]. In addition, clinical-pathological studies in adult human subjects with chronic inflammatory conditions show that increased spontaneous CAP activity is correlated to decreased levels of pro-inflammatory cytokines such as IL-1β.

The relevance of this line of research to the link between PSP and PTB is suggested by results showing a strengthening of the association between depression (i.e., mouse model studied through monoamine depletion and maternal separation) and inflammation in response to decreased vagal nerve activity [45]. This line of investigation is beginning to map out connections between the brain and the inflammatory response that could provide a crucial link connecting neural responses to stress during pregnancy with inflammation-mediated adverse birth outcomes. Of note, CAP activity can be monitored non-invasively via heart rate variability (HRV) derived from maternal or fetal ECG. This opens a new, very cost-effective venue for exploring the relationship between PSP, maternal CAP and inflammation as well as PTB in prospective clinical studies. A recent intervention study of HRV biofeedback in patients with preterm labor showed reductions in reported stress levels in the intervention group [46].

Infectious Pathways and Maternal Microbiome

Infection is a well-documented risk factor for PTB and is likely to partially mediate the relationship between PSP and PTB [4, 7]. Advances in diagnostic techniques may eventually improve the predictive value of this risk factor for PTB. Bacterial vaginosis, the most common lower genital tract infection in women of reproductive age, is associated with stress in pregnant women and with a two- to fourfold increase in risk for spontaneous PTB [47]. However, the current characterization of intrauterine infection is imprecise. Numerous different bacteria are known to comprise the vaginal flora, yet clinical tests for infection rely on measures that are relatively crude and sometimes inconsistent, and intrauterine infections during pregnancy are frequently subclinical and escape diagnosis. Furthermore, many intrauterine infections are caused by bacteria that resist cultivation, thus limiting the utility of culture-based detection [48].

Understanding of the mediating role played by infection in the relationship between PSP and PTB is limited. However, culture-independent detection methods are becoming more common and are enabling a more advanced understanding of the genetic content of the vaginal microbial community, known as the vaginal microbiome [49]. Recent improvements in DNA sequencing allow detailed characterization of the microbiome of both the vagina and the colon and elucidation of the relationship between microbiota patterns and the central nervous system. For example, prenatal stress has been associated with altered patterns of microbial colonization and reduced dominance of lactobacilli (the bacteria that dominate the vaginal flora of healthy women) in the intestinal microbiota of infants [50]. Should this pattern translate to the maternal vaginal microbiome as well, it would provide important insights into the biological pathways mediating infectious causes of PTB and their relationships with the maternal nervous system's response to psychosocial stress.

Summary and Future Directions

Epidemiologic and physiologic evidence suggests a possible role of psychosocial stress as an etiologic risk factor for PTB. Set against a context of poor prediction coupled with increasing incidence of PTB, the importance of psychosocial stress is further highlighted by its potential amenability to intervention. Psychometric research has made significant advances in identifying the most sensitive tools to measure PSP, while clinical research has begun elucidating the intersecting biologic pathways through which PSP could be linked to PTB. Nevertheless, epidemiologic findings remain mixed and do not consistently support an effect of psychosocial stress on PTB risk in the overall population.

At the physiological level, biomarkers, including cortisol and CRH, help clarify the role of the neuroendocrine system in the stress response and the initiation of parturition. Inflammation and infection are other important biological factors that are likely to be involved in the relationship between PSP and PTB.

While these physiologic pathways have not conclusively explained the connection between psychosocial exposures and PTB, several novel advances show considerable promise in this area. The ability to monitor CAP activity via HRV presents an exciting possibility for the safe and inexpensive exploration of the link between stress and inflammation, and of the role of inflammation in term and preterm parturition. Characterization of the structure and function of the maternal microbiome will enable a clearer and richer understanding than currently available of the role played by infection in the relationship between stress and length of gestation. Research joining the fields of psychometrics, epidemiology and physiology suggests promising possibilities for a deeper understanding of PTB, which in turn can point the way toward future preventive strategies.

Key Points

- Preterm birth (PTB) is the leading cause of infant mortality in industrialized countries, accounting for 60% of perinatal mortality and about half of long-term neurologic morbidity.
- While understanding of biological risk factors for PTB is more advanced than for psychosocial risk factors, a growing literature supports the role of psychosocial stress during pregnancy (PSP) in the etiology of preterm labor and birth.
- The epidemiologic literature on PSP and PTB presents mixed results that stem in part from a multitude of exposure definitions and other methodological limitations.
- Observational research shows that life events experienced at the beginning of pregnancy tend to be perceived as more stressful than similar events occurring in the third trimester.
- The literature suggests that pregnancy-related anxiety may be more strongly associated with adverse birth outcomes than non-pregnancy-related stressors.
- Potential biological mediators of the relationship between PSP and PTB include neuroinflammatory, immune and neuroendocrine pathways.
- The maternal hypothalamic-pituitary-adrenal (HPA) axis constitutes the principal neuroendocrine mechanism hypothesized to mediate the link between PSP and PTB.

- Chronic stress increases susceptibility to infection and is associated with maternal infection during pregnancy.
- Culture-independent methods of detecting genital tract infection are now broadly available and are enabling a better characterization of the vaginal microbiome. This will promote the understanding of the mediating role played by bacterial colonization in the relationship between PSP and PTB.

References

1. Goldenberg, R.L., The management of preterm labor. *Obstet Gynecol*, 2002. **100**(5 Pt 1): 1020–37.

2. Frey, H.A., Klebanoff, M.A., The epidemiology, etiology, and costs of preterm birth. *Semin Fetal Neonatal Med*, 2016. **21**(2): 68–73.

3. Institute of Medicine (US) Committee on Understanding Premature Birth and Assuring Healthy Outcomes, *Preterm Birth: Causes, Consequences, and Prevention*, ed. R.E. Behrman and A.S. Butler. 2007, Washington DC: National Academy of Sciences.

4. Harrison, M.S., Goldenberg, R.L., Global burden of prematurity. *Semin Fetal Neonatal Med*, 2016. **21**(2): 74–9.

5. Shapiro, G.D., Fraser, W.D., Frasch, M.G., et al., Psychosocial stress in pregnancy and preterm birth: Associations and mechanisms. *J Perinat Med*, 2013. **41**(6): 631–45.

6. Dunkel Schetter, C., Psychological science on pregnancy: Stress processes, biopsychosocial models, and emerging research issues. *Annu Rev Psychol*, 2011. **62**: 531–58.

7. Wadhwa, P.D., Entringer, S., Buss, C., et al., The contribution of maternal stress to preterm birth: Issues and considerations. *Clin Perinatol*, 2011. **38**(3): 351–84.

8. Christian, L.M., Psychoneuroimmunology in pregnancy: Immune pathways linking stress with maternal health, adverse birth outcomes, and fetal development. *Neurosci Biobehav Rev*, 2012. **36**(1): 350–61.

9. Hobel, C.J., Goldstein, A., Barrett, E.S., Psychosocial stress and pregnancy outcome. *Clin Obstet Gynecol*, 2008. **51**(2): 333–48.

10. Zhu, P., Tao, F., Hao, J., et al., Prenatal life events stress: Implications for preterm birth and infant birthweight. *Am J Obstet Gynecol*, 2010. 203(1): 34 e1–8.

11. Dole, N., Savitz, D.A., Hertz-Picciotto, I., et al., Maternal stress and preterm birth. *Am J Epidemiol*, 2003. **157**(1): 14–24.

12. Shapiro, G.D., *Links between obstetric history, nutritional and genetic risk factors, perinatal mental health and length of gestation*. Doctoral thesis, 2015, Université de Montréal: Montreal.

13. Abeysena, C., Jayawardana, P., Seneviratne Rde, A., Effect of psychosocial stress and physical activity on preterm birth: A cohort study. *J Obstet Gynaecol Res*, 2010. **36**(2): 260–7.

14. Sarkar, P., Bergman, K., Fisk, N.M., et al., Maternal anxiety at amniocentesis and plasma cortisol. *Prenat Diagn*, 2006. **26**(6): 505–9.

15. Glynn, L.M., Schetter, C.D., Wadhwa, P.D., et al., Pregnancy affects appraisal of negative life events. *J Psychosom Res*, 2004. **56**(1): 47–52.

16. Orr, S.T., Reiter, J.P., Blazer, D.G., et al., Maternal prenatal pregnancy-related anxiety and spontaneous preterm birth in Baltimore, Maryland. *Psychosom Med*, 2007. **69**(6): 566–70.

17. Goodman, J.H., Chenausky, K.L., Freeman, M.P., Anxiety disorders during pregnancy: A systematic review. *J Clin Psychiatry*, 2014. **75**(10): e1153–84.

18. Paschetta, E., Berrisford, G., Coccia, F., et al., Perinatal psychiatric disorders: An overview. *Am J Obstet Gynecol*, 2014. **210**(6): 501–9 e6.

19. Dennis, C.L., Dowswell, T., Interventions (other than pharmacological, psychosocial or psychological) for treating antenatal depression. *Cochrane Database Syst Rev*, 2013. 7: CD006795.

20. Hetherington, E., Doktorchik, C., Premji, S.S., et al., Preterm birth and social support during pregnancy: A systematic review and meta-analysis. *Paediatr Perinat Epidemiol*, 2015. **29**(6): 523–35.

21. Dunkel Schetter, C., Schafer, P., Lanzi, R.G., et al., Shedding light on the mechanisms underlying health disparities through community participatory methods: The stress pathway. *Perspect Psychol Sci*, 2013. **8**(6): 613–33.

22. Voltolini, C., Torricelli, M., Conti, N., et al., Understanding spontaneous preterm birth: From underlying mechanisms to predictive and preventive interventions. *Reprod Sci*, 2013. **20**(11): 1274–92.

23. Liston, C., McEwen, B.S., Casey, B.J., Psychosocial stress reversibly disrupts prefrontal processing and attentional control. *Proc Natl Acad Sci U S A*, 2009. **106**(3): 912–17.

24. Murphy, S.E., Braithwaite, E.C., Hubbard, I., et al., Salivary cortisol response to infant distress in pregnant women with depressive symptoms. *Arch Women's Ment Health*, 2015. **18**(2): 247–53.

25. Fuchs, E., Flugge, G., Modulation of binding sites for corticotropin-releasing hormone by chronic psychosocial stress. *Psychoneuroendocrinology*, 1995. **20**(1): 33–51.

26. Thomson, M., The physiological roles of placental corticotropin releasing hormone in pregnancy and childbirth. *J Physiol Biochem*, 2013. **69**(3): 559–73.

27. McLean, M., Bisits, A., Davies, J., et al., A placental clock controlling the length of human pregnancy. *Nat Med*, 1995. **1**(5): 460–3.

28. Mancuso, R.A., Dunkel Schetter, C., Rini, C.M., et al., Maternal prenatal anxiety and corticotropin-releasing hormone associated with timing of delivery. *Psychosom Med*, 2004. **66**(5): 762–9.

29. Petraglia, F., Hatch, M.C., Lapinski, R., et al., Lack of effect of psychosocial stress on maternal corticotropin-releasing factor and catecholamine levels at 28 weeks' gestation. *J Soc Gynecol Investig*, 2001. **8**(2): 83–8.

30. Himes, K.P., Simhan, H.N., Plasma corticotropin-releasing hormone and cortisol concentrations and perceived stress among pregnant women with preterm and term birth. *Am J Perinatol*, 2011. **28**(6): 443–8.

31. Guendelman, S., Kosa, J.L., Pearl, M., et al., Exploring the relationship of second-trimester corticotropin releasing hormone, chronic stress and preterm delivery. *J Matern Fetal Neonatal Med*, 2008. **21**(11): 788–95.

32. Hobel, C.J., Dunkel-Schetter, C., Roesch, S.C., et al., Maternal plasma corticotropin-releasing hormone associated with stress at 20 weeks' gestation in pregnancies ending in preterm delivery. *Am J Obstet Gynecol*, 1999. **180**(1 Pt 3): S257–63.

33. Lupien, S.J., Parent, S., Evans, A.C., et al., Larger amygdala but no change in hippocampal volume in 10-year-old children exposed to maternal depressive symptomatology since birth. *Proc Natl Acad Sci U S A*, 2011. **108**(34): 14324–9.

34. Fumagalli, F., Bedogni, F., Slotkin, T.A., et al., Prenatal stress elicits regionally selective changes in basal FGF-2 gene expression in adulthood and alters the adult response to acute or chronic stress. *Neurobiol Dis*, 2005. **20**(3): 731–7.

35. Nansel, T.R., Riggs, M.A., Yu, K.F., et al., The association of psychosocial stress and bacterial vaginosis in a longitudinal cohort. *Am J Obstet Gynecol*, 2006. **194**(2): 381–6.

36. Gotsch, F., Romero, R., Kusanovic, J.P., et al., The fetal inflammatory response syndrome. *Clin Obstet Gynecol*, 2007. **50**(3): 652–83.

37. Blank, V., Hirsch, E., Challis, J.R., et al., Cytokine signaling, inflammation, innate immunity and preterm labour – a workshop report. *Placenta*, 2008. **29**(Suppl A): S102–4.

38. Challis, J.R., Lockwood, C.J., Myatt, L., et al., Inflammation and pregnancy. *Reprod Sci*, 2009. **16**(2): 206–15.

39. Snegovskikh, V., Park, J.S., Norwitz, E.R., Endocrinology of parturition. *Endocrinol Metab Clin North Am*, 2006. **35**(1): 173–91, viii.

40. Wei, S.Q., Fraser, W., Luo, Z.C., Inflammatory cytokines and spontaneous preterm birth in asymptomatic women: A systematic review. *Obstet Gynecol*, 2010. **116**(2 Pt 1): 393–401.

41. Tracey, K.J., Reflex control of immunity. *Nat Rev Immunol*, 2009. **9**(6): 418–28.

42. Borovikova, L.V., Ivanova, S., Zhang, M., et al., Vagus nerve stimulation attenuates the systemic inflammatory response to endotoxin. *Nature*, 2000. **405**(6785): 458–62.

43. van Westerloo, D.J., Giebelen, I.A., Florquin, S., et al., The vagus nerve and nicotinic receptors modulate experimental pancreatitis severity in mice. *Gastroenterology*, 2006. **130**(6): 1822–30.

44. de Jonge, W.J., van der Zanden, E.P., The, F.O., et al., Stimulation of the vagus nerve attenuates macrophage activation by activating the Jak2-STAT3 signaling pathway. *Nat Immunol*, 2005. **6**(8): 844–51.

45. Ghia, J.E., Blennerhassett, P., Collins, S.M., Impaired parasympathetic function increases susceptibility to inflammatory bowel disease in a mouse model of depression. *J Clin Invest*, 2008. **118**(6): 2209–18.

46. Siepmann, M., Hennig, U.D., Siepmann, T., et al., The effects of heart rate variability biofeedback in patients with preterm labour. *Appl Psychophysiol Biofeedback*, 2014. **39**(1): 27–35.

47. Nadeau, H.C., Subramaniam, A., Andrews, W.W., Infection and preterm birth. *Semin Fetal Neonatal Med*, 2016. **21**(2): 100–5.

48. Gregory, K.E., Microbiome aspects of perinatal and neonatal health. *J Perinat Neonatal Nurs*, 2011. **25**(2): 158–62; quiz 163–4.

49. Witkin, S.S., The vaginal microbiome, vaginal anti-microbial defence mechanisms and the clinical challenge of reducing infection-related preterm birth. *BJOG*, 2015. **122**(2): 213–18.

50. Zijlmans, M.A., Korpela, K., Riksen-Walraven, J.M., et al., Maternal prenatal stress is associated with the infant intestinal microbiota. *Psychoneuroendocrinology*, 2015. **53**: 233–45.

Tokophobia

Kristina Hofberg and Yana Richens

Introduction

The gravid state and parturition are normal and often desired by women from early adulthood and beyond. Nevertheless, pregnancy can be a time of anxiety with emotional lability, especially for the primigravida entering her third trimester. The conception, pregnancy and postnatal period will be influenced by the woman's expectations, personality, previous life and health experiences, as well as her sexuality. Conflicting feelings are common. Women have access to stories of childbirth through literature, social settings and media. These may be reassuring or anxiety-inducing. Fear of pregnancy and childbirth are also features of mental health disorders, including eating disorder, anxiety and mood disorder. Fear of birth (FOB) can be consequent to female genital mutilation (FGM), childhood sexual abuse (CSA) or rape. A woman may request a caesarean section (CS) due to fear of childbirth (FOC). Some women experience significant anxiety, dread and fear of death or mutilation of herself or her fetus during childbirth. This pathological dread and avoidance of childbirth is tokophobia.

FOB was described in 1858, by the French psychiatrist Marcé [1]. He stated of women, '*If they are primiparous, the expectation of unknown pain preoccupies them beyond all measure, and throws them into a state of inexpressible anxiety. If they are already mothers, they are terrified of the memory of the past and the prospect of the future*' [1].

Although FOB is recognized internationally as a distressing state affecting women in relation to childbirth, there remains a lack of consensus regarding its definition. Consequently, the terms 'fear of birth', 'fear of childbirth' and 'tokophobia/tocophobia' have been used in research and the literature. Diagnostic tests have been developed and some validated for FOB/FOC. The term 'tokophobia' is now included in the National Institute for Health and Care Excellence (NICE) guidelines [CG192], 'Antenatal and postnatal mental health: clinical management and service guidance' [2]. The addition of tokophobia in 2014 highlights the pathological nature of this condition. However, as ambiguity remains regarding its definition and many women with FOB do not experience tokophobia, there remains work to be done within obstetrics, midwifery, perinatal psychiatry and with these women who can suffer significant distress. The authors address caution over the use of the term 'tokophobia' when a woman may be suffering from FOB or appropriate anxiety regarding impending parturition.

The Spectrum Disorder and Classification

Although the state of pregnancy is both normal and often desired, anxiety is not uncommon with the physical and emotional consequences of the gravid state. It is not the purpose of this chapter to comment on the 'normal' pregnancy or 'normal' anxiety. However, when anxiety is the primary symptom of a pathological mental state, this is fear of birth or tokophobia.

Tokophobia was described and classified by Hofberg and Brockington in 2000. They stated, 'When this specific anxiety (fear of parturition) or fear of death during parturition precedes pregnancy and is so intense that *tokos* ("childbirth") is avoided whenever possible, this is a phobic state called "tokophobia"' [1].

Hofberg and Brockington (2000) classified primary and secondary tokophobia, with a third category, 'tokophobia as a symptom of depression'. The reported cases had been referred to a specialist perinatal psychiatry service. Hence, tokophobia is the morbid psychological state of fearful women at the severe end of the FOB spectrum [1].

Primary Tokophobia

Primary tokophobia affects nulliparous women. FOB is common and more intense in pregnant, nulliparous women than in pregnant parous women. Nulliparous women report fear of the unknown and of pain as well as psychological factors, including parenthood [3].

Secondary Tokophobia

Secondary tokophobia affects women with previous experience of pregnancy. It is characterized either by a woman's previous traumatic birth experience or a poor perinatal outcome. Traumatic birth includes deliveries, whether preterm or full term, which are physically traumatic (for example, instrumental or assisted deliveries or emergency CSs, severe perineal tears, postpartum haemorrhage), as well as births that are experienced as traumatic, even when the delivery is obstetrically straightforward [4]. Women who have a negative experience or previous traumatic birth are five times more likely to report FOB in subsequent pregnancies. Between 7 and 26% of women in Western countries fear childbirth [5], with 6% of women reporting the fear as disabling [6]. Studies suggest that secondary FOB is associated with prolonged second stage of delivery [7]. Women who experience secondary tokophobia as a phobic state may avoid further pregnancies.

Tokophobia as a Symptom of Depression

Rarely, women with major depressive disorder present with FOB as a symptom of illness. This reported fear is in stark contrast to previously held beliefs on pregnancy and childbirth. This presentation has been reported in women suffering from antepartum depression [1] as well as non-pregnant women suffering from major depressive disorder [8]. This 'symptom' may be ameliorated by pharmacological treatment of the depressive disorder.

FOB and Tokophobia

FOB is internationally recognized as a cause for increasing concern, and this is in spite of a lack of consensus on a definition. An agreed definition is required to ensure the term is used consistently in literature and research. The most reliable tool for assessing FOB is the Wijma Delivery Expectancy/Experience Questionnaire W-DEQ [9]. Version A of the questionnaire (W-DEQ-A) measures prenatal FOC while version B (W-DEQ-B) measures fearful childbirth experience. However, W-DEQ has been used as a research tool only due to the length and complexity of the questionnaire. The Fear of

Childbirth Visual Analogue Scale [10] correlates well with W-DEQ and is a simple method for screening FOC. In clinical practice FOB is mainly self-reported. With no clear guidelines on assessing or treating FOB, women regularly request CS as a way of alleviating or bypassing their anxieties, and hence are referred to obstetricians.

The perinatal psychiatric formulation of Hofberg and Brockington [1] does not capture the range of fears as well as the degree of resilience seen in women with FOB. It is this FOB spectrum disorder that needs clarifying and defining, for treatment, research and mothering.

FOB Spectrum and Co-morbidity

PTSD and FOB

What is PTSD?

The International Classification of Diseases (ICD10) states that post-traumatic stress disorder (PTSD) arises as a delayed or protracted response to a stressful event or situation (of either brief or long duration) of an exceptionally threatening or catastrophic nature, which is likely to cause pervasive distress in almost anyone.

Although predisposing factors such as personality traits (e.g. compulsive, asthenic) or previous neurotic illness may lower the threshold or aggravate the course of PTSD, they are neither necessary nor sufficient to explain its occurrence.

Typical features include episodes of repeated reliving of the trauma in intrusive memories ('flashbacks'), dreams or nightmares, occurring against the persisting background of a sense of 'numbness' and emotional blunting, detachment from other people, unresponsiveness to surroundings, anhedonia, and avoidance of activities and situations reminiscent of the trauma. There is usually a state of autonomic hyperarousal with hypervigilance, an enhanced startle reaction and insomnia.

Anxiety and depression are commonly associated with the above symptoms and signs, and suicidal ideation is not infrequent. The onset follows the trauma with a latency period that may range from a few weeks to months. The course is fluctuating but recovery can be expected in the majority of cases. In a small proportion of cases the condition may follow a chronic course over many years, with eventual transition to an enduring personality change.

The *Diagnostic and Statistical Manual of Mental Disorders, Fifth Edition* (American Psychiatric Association, 2013), describes the 'trauma' as 'exposure to actual or threatened death, serious injury, or sexual violence' and includes, but is not limited to, exposure to war, threatened or actual physical assault, threatened or actual sexual violence, kidnap and torture. The trauma can include being witness to such events. PTSD is more prevalent among females across the life span and has a longer duration in females than males. Some of this increased morbidity for females is their greater likelihood of exposure to traumatic events such as rape, domestic and other violence. Tedstone and Tarrier [11] estimate lifetime prevalence for PTSD in the general population as 5–6% for men and 10–11% for women.

PTSD following Childbirth

For some women, their experience of childbirth is sufficiently distressing to be described as a trauma in the context of PTSD (see Chapter 39). With this in mind, researchers have looked for predictors as well as treatments of PTSD associated with childbirth [12]. A systematic review [13] reported risk factors for developing PTSD, such as poor coping strategies, poor response to stress and certain personality factors.

PTSD and FOB

There is lack of clarity regarding the link between PTSD and FOB. They are actually distinct conditions. It is postulated that PTSD is a retrospective phenomenon following birth trauma. It is also possible that PTSD may co-exist with a fear of subsequent pregnancy/birth [14]. Although PTSD and secondary FOB can occur as a consequence of a traumatic birth, some women have reported symptoms of PTSD but did not perceive their birth as traumatic. Consequently, PTSD and FOB can co-exist in multiparous women. Hence, accurate diagnosis is crucial.

Increased rates of postpartum PTSD are noted in women denied their choice of delivery [1], women who delivered preterm or stillborn infants or experienced complications during pregnancy and labour [15]. Garthus-Niegel et al. [16] reported that it is the overall birth experience which is a central factor in the development of PTSD symptoms.

Of particular relevance, approximately 6% of women experience PTSD following obstetric or gynaecological procedures; this is associated specifically with traumatic experiences. It can be challenging to differentiate between postnatal depression and PTSD following childbirth.

It is noted that women may experience FOB before conception but are not necessarily susceptible to PTSD. For example, not all women who develop PTSD have FOB and vice versa. Although predisposing factors are similar to those for FOB, PTSD is more strongly associated with negative birth experiences [17], pain during labour, concerns over well-being of baby [14], assisted birth or emergency sections as well as prior non-obstetric events such as sexual abuse or domestic violence.

A meta-synthesis of qualitative evidence on the impact of traumatic birth by Fenech et al. highlights the negative effects of PTSD [18] for women and includes powerful narratives. It is essential that obstetricians, midwives and mental health services recognize and understand both FOB and PTSD.

CSA and FOB

Significant numbers of women describe being sexually abused before the age of 16. It is known that the psychological morbidity secondary to CSA is both immense and diverse. As adults these women suffer increased rates of sexual dysfunction, anorexia and PTSD. A history of CSA is sometimes associated with an aversion to gynaecological examinations, including routine smears and obstetric care. The trauma of vaginal delivery or even the contemplation of it may cause a resurgence of distressing memories. This can lead to anxiety, dread and avoidance of childbirth, even when a woman wants a baby. Women who have been the victims of CSA or rape may experience flashbacks during certain procedures that mimic abuse. Women may approach pregnancy with their own clear birth plan. This may include CS in the absence of an obstetric indication. Research suggests that women with abuse histories more frequently experience FOB and request CS [19].

FGM and FOB

FGM has been practised for centuries and, in specific communities, was seen as a part of a girl's rite of passage into womanhood. FGM is a procedure that intentionally alters or causes injury to the female genital organs for non-medical reasons [20]. This practice is illegal in the UK. It is also illegal for a child to be taken from the UK for FGM (Female

Genital Mutilation Act 2003). FGM is prevalent in Africa, the Middle East and Asia. In the UK, FGM is seen in areas with larger populations of communities who practise FGM, such as first-generation immigrants, refugees and asylum seekers. It is estimated that over 20,000 girls under the age of 15 are at risk of FGM in the UK each year, and that 66,000 women in the UK are living with the consequences of FGM. The true extent is unknown.

Of all aspects of FGM, the psychological and emotional consequences are least reported. Toubia [21] cites three psychological cases: 'anxiety state' originating from lack of sleep and hallucinations, 'reaction depression' from delayed healing and 'psychotic excitement' from childlessness and divorce. FGM is traumatic and young women have reported feeling betrayed by family and elders.

FOB is a significant feature in women who have undergone FGM. Lundberg and Gerezgiher [22] interviewed 15 Eritrean immigrant women in Sweden during pregnancy and the postnatal period. Each had experienced FGM. Themes were identified, and these included fear and anxiety about childbirth as well as reports of extreme pain in childbirth and long-term gynaecological complications of FGM. FOB may be associated with this trauma of FGM, concerns about health professionals' knowledge of FGM and concerns about de-infibulation. The women were obliged to maintain the safety of their own daughters against cultural pressures to perform FGM and the legal status of FGM in Sweden. The women reported flashbacks to the FGM trauma during pregnancy and childbirth. There are real and increased risks for the labouring mother and fetus following FGM. It is not the intention of the authors to describe FGM further. FGM is discussed elsewhere in this book (Chapter 9) but has been included in this chapter to note this vulnerable group of women, experiencing FOB in the wake of the trauma of FGM procedure. FOB occurs in the context of mutilated or abnormal anatomy, vaginismus and virgo intacta, and this is broadening the field for FOB studies.

FOB and Treatment Studies

Women with FOB are vulnerable to increased surgical intervention and subsequent psychological complications. Historical studies investigating alleviation of FOB are few. However, psychoprophylaxis was investigated in the 1950s and the use of hypnosis in the 1990s. Swedish clinicians and researchers have been at the forefront of research in the field of FOB over the last 25 years.

A psychoprophylactic preparation course offered to pregnant women afraid of childbirth made no significant difference to obstetric outcome [23]. Ryding [24], an obstetrician and psychotherapist, offered either counselling or short-term psychotherapy to pregnant women demanding a CS that the obstetrician thought unnecessary. At term, half these women chose vaginal delivery. Similar results were found when Sjögren [25] investigated 72 women with severe anxiety about childbirth. They were offered psychotherapy or extra obstetric support. Subsequently, some women chose vaginal delivery. These women experienced the delivery positively as a reference group. Tokophobic women who strongly desired a surgical delivery and were refused, suffered greater psychological morbidity than those granted their chosen delivery method [1].

Patel and Hollins [26] highlight the benefits of joint obstetric and psychiatric management of phobic anxiety disorders in pregnancy. They advocate early identification so treatment may be offered to manage fears and improve coping strategies. A positive birth experience may facilitate more successful mother–infant bonding.

Rouhe [10], an obstetrician, submitted an academic dissertation describing a randomized controlled trial offering group psychoeducation with relaxation to nulliparous women suffering from severe FOB in Finland. In total, 131 women were randomized to a psychoeducation group with relaxation and 240 to standard care by community nurses. Psycho-emotional and psychosocial evaluations, Edinburgh Postnatal Depression Scale (EPDS), social support, Maternal Adjustment and Attitudes (MAMA), Traumatic Events Scale (TES) and the Wijma Delivery Experience Questionnaire (W-DEQ-B) were completed twice during pregnancy and/or three months postpartum. Results showed that postnatal maternal adjustment and childbirth experience were better in the intervention group. In hierarchical regression, social support, participating in intervention and less fearful childbirth experience predicted better maternal adjustment. The level of postnatal depressive symptoms was significantly lower in the intervention group. There were no differences in the frequency of PTSD between the groups. The researchers concluded that for nulliparous women with severe FOB, participation in a targeted psychoeducative group resulted in better maternal adjustment, a less fearful childbirth experience and fewer post-natal depressive symptoms, compared with conventional care.

'Tokophobia', Elective CS and NICE Guidelines

It is known that CS rates are increasing internationally. In the United Kingdom, between 20 and 25% of births are by CS [4]. In the United States, the rate is higher at 32.2% [27]. These increasing rates majorly concern other high-resource countries such as Italy, Norway and Sweden. CS is associated with increased maternal mortality and morbidity compared to vaginal birth [28]. Consequently, national and international guidance has been published and research continues to attempt to identify the reasons behind a woman's choice for operative delivery in the context of FOB [29].

Women in the UK today are more likely to request or demand a delivery of their choice than a generation ago. Indeed, the NICE guidelines [4], 'Caesarean section. Guidance and Guidelines', state clearly that 'when a woman requests a CS because she has anxiety about childbirth, [the clinician should] offer referral to a healthcare professional with expertise in providing perinatal mental health support to help her address her anxiety in a supportive manner'. The guidelines continue,

> For a woman requesting a CS, if after discussion and offer of support (including perinatal mental health support for women with anxiety about childbirth), a vaginal birth is still not an acceptable option, [the clinician should] offer a planned CS. An obstetrician unwilling to perform a CS should refer the woman to an obstetrician who will carry out the CS. (NICE 2011)

This guidance allows any woman in the UK to request an operative delivery. Clinical work and research must continue to understand and manage both the aetiology leading to the request for CS psychopathology and further choice regarding vaginal delivery.

In 2004, the Department of Health in UK advocated the need for health professionals to attend to the psychological needs of mothers in the Choosing Health Report [30]. Previously, the focus on midwifery and obstetric research was predominated by physiological aspects of care. Now clinicians have the opportunity to examine more closely FOB and PTSD.

Whose Responsibility Is It to Recognize Mental Health Needs in Pregnancy?

It is known that the range and prevalence of anxiety disorders as well as depression are under-recognized throughout pregnancy and the postnatal period. Women may be unwilling to disclose or discuss these difficulties, dreading stigma, negative perceptions of them as mother or fearing their baby may be removed. CEMACH [31] reported in line with earlier research [32] that many women who developed mental illness in pregnancy had identifiable risk factors, including a previous history of mental illness or a first-degree relative affected. Although midwives were already asking women about personal and family history of mental illness in line with NICE guidance [33], it was unclear exactly how questions were asked. The Whooley questions [34] or 'depression identification questions' were incorporated in NICE guidance to help identify women with mental disorder [33]. These are as follows:

> *During the past month, have you often been bothered by feeling down, depressed or hopeless?*
> *During the past month, have you often been bothered by having little interest or pleasure in doing things?*

If the woman answers in the affirmative to either question or to the third enquiry, '*Is this something you feel you need or want help with?*' (NICE, 2007), a referral is made.

NICE guidance (CG192) 2014 [2] added recommendations to try and identify women with anxiety disorders using the two-item Generalized Anxiety Disorder scale (GAD-2):

> *During the past month, have you been feeling nervous, anxious or on edge?*
> *During the past month have you not been able to stop or control worrying?*

Hence, there is now an expectation from primary care, midwifery and obstetric services to identify mental health needs of pregnant women. NICE [2] goes on to suggest the use of the EPDS, the PHQ-9 and the GAD-7 scale for further assessment of the woman's mental well-being. Women should thus be referred either to her GP or, if a severe mental health problem is suspected, to a mental health professional.

Whilst this advice was written more in relation to pre-existing and new anxiety and depression, it is probably as relevant to patients who have primary and secondary tokophobia.

NICE Recommendations for Tokophobia (CG192 2014)

In 2014, NICE made recommendations for anxiety disorders and included the term 'tokophobia' [2].

> For a woman with tokophobia (an extreme fear of childbirth), offer an opportunity to discuss her fears with a healthcare professional with expertise in providing perinatal mental health support in line with NICE guidance on caesarean section. (NICE guideline CG132)

Thus, in 2014, this statement on tokophobia marries NICE guidelines for antenatal and postnatal mental health (CG192 2014) [2] to section 1.2.9 of the guideline on CS [4] in relation to maternal request for CS. The text on CS does not refer directly to tokophobia but instead to 'anxiety about childbirth'.

Recommended Treatment Times for Psychological Morbidity in Pregnancy

When a woman with a known or suspected mental health problem is referred in pregnancy or the postnatal period, she must be assessed for treatment within two weeks of referral and offered psychological interventions within one month of this assessment [2]. If there is failure to improve within two weeks of treatment, high-intensity psychological intervention should be offered.

The woman with tokophobia is offered the opportunity for perinatal mental health support to help her address her anxiety. NICE does not appear to recommend high-intensity psychological intervention for tokophobia as a treatment method as it does for PTSD or other anxiety disorders. Instead, the referral suggests clarity is sought for the intensity of the fear, thus validating the maternal request for CS.

Mother–Infant Attachment and FOB

FOB may inhibit mother–baby attachment. Nationally, the importance of the mother–infant relationship is recognized [2]. It is reported that new mothers who have experienced a traumatic birth may suffer serious and enduring morbidities which can impact on the infant and the family well-being [18]. It is important that the nature of the mother–baby relationship is assessed, noting verbal interaction, emotional sensitivity and physical care of the baby at all postnatal contacts. A mother expressing concern about her attachment to the newborn must be endorsed and treatment for any postnatal mental illness considered a priority. If the relationship with the baby does not ameliorate, intervention for the mother and baby should be offered.

Early identification and support for women who have FOB is required as, in the UK, women are not currently screened or assessed for FOB using any screening tool as highlighted in a survey of UK maternity units [35]. There are several reasons for this. A national online survey highlighted that in the UK there are few NHS Trusts with a care/referral pathway in place for women suffering from FOB. Only 35 out of 203 maternity units surveyed responded as having services for women with FOB in place [35].

Discussion

Failure to identify women who have FOB along with the sparse provision of services could potentially lead to women feeling isolated and unsupported. Thus, more needs to be done to raise awareness of FOB and improve the care available for women in order to improve their physical and psychological outcomes. Integral to providing good-quality maternity care is having efficient strategies for its identification. However, this is not always so simple, as a variance in diagnostic testing has led to a lack of consensus on a universal definition. Criteria used for FOB risk inclusion in the diagnosis of conditions ranging from anxiety to a pathological fear. Also there is currently no consensus on which is the most effective tool to use with women to measure FOB in clinical practice.

Key Points

- There is no consensus on the definition and measurement of tokophobia. FOB manifests as a spectrum of anxiety states, and the term 'tokophobia' applies to the severe end of the spectrum, where there is a pathological level of anxiety, or phobia. This pathological state may apply to nulliparous women (primary tokophobia) or result from a previous negative birth experience (secondary tokophobia).

- Rarely, women may present with FOB as a symptom of depression.
- The most reliable tool for assessing FOB is the W-DEQ. The simpler Fear of Childbirth Visual Analogue Scale correlates well with W-DEQ.
- There are some shared risk factors between FOB and PTSD, but the two are distinct conditions.
- Women with a history of sexual abuse frequently experience FOB and request caesarean delivery.
- With no clear guidelines on assessing or treating FOB, women regularly request caesarean delivery as a way of alleviating or bypassing their anxieties.
- There is some evidence that psychotherapy and psychoeducation are beneficial in the management of FOB.

References

1. Hofberg K, Brockington I. Tokophobia: An unreasoning dread of childbirth. *A series of 26 cases. Br J Psychiatry* 2000;**176**:83–5.

2. National Institute for Health and Care Excellence (NICE) guidelines [CG192], 'Antenatal and postnatal mental health: Clinical management and service guidance' 2014.

3. Saisto T, Halmesmäki E. Fear of childbirth: A neglected dilemma. *Acta Obstet Gynecol Scand* 2003;**82**:201–8.

4. National Institute for Health and Care Excellence (NICE) guidelines [CG132] Caesarean section. 2011.

5. Fenwick J, Gamble J, Nathan E, et al. Pre- and postpartum levels of childbirth fear and the relationship to birth outcomes in a cohort of Australian women. *J Clin Nurs* 2009 **18**(5):667–77.

6. Searle J. Fearing the worst – why do pregnant women feel 'at risk'? *ANZ J Obstet Gynaecol* 1996;**36**(3):279–86.

7. Sydsjö G, Angerbjörn L, Palmquist S, et al. Secondary fear of childbirth prolongs the time to subsequent delivery. *Acta Obstet Gynecol Scand* 2013;**92**(2):210–14.

8. Bhatia SB, Jhanjee A. Tokophobia: A dread of pregnancy. *Case report. Industrial Psychiatry Journal* 2012;**21**(2):158–9.

9. Wijma K, Wijma B, Zar M. Psychometric aspects of the W-DEQ: A new questionnaire for the measurement of fear of childbirth. *J Psychosom Obstet Gynecol* 1998;**19**(2):84–97.

10. Rouhe H, Salmela-Aro K, Toivanen R, et al. Group psychoeducation with relaxation for severe fear of childbirth improves maternal adjustment and childbirth experience – a randomised controlled trial. *J Psychosom Obstet Gynecol* 2015;**36**(1):1–9.

11. Tedstone JE, Tarrier N. Posttraumatic stress disorder following medical illness and treatment. *Clin Pychol Rev* 2003May;**23**(3):409–48.

12. Alder J, Breitinger G, Granado C, et al. Antenatal psychobiological predictors of psychological response to childbirth. *J Am Psych Nurses Association* November/December 2011;**17**(6):417–25.

13. DiGangi J, Guffanti G, McLaughlin KA, et al. Considering trauma exposure in the context of genetics studies of posttraumatic stress disorder: A systematic review. *Biology of Mood & Anxiety Disorders* 2013;**3**:2.

14. Ballard CG, Stanley AK, Brockington IF. Post-traumatic stress disorder (PTSD) after childbirth. *B J Psych* 1995;**166**(4):525–8.

15. Ghorbani M, Dolatian M, Shams J, et al. Anxiety, post-traumatic stress disorder and social supports among parents of premature and full-term infants. *Iran res Crescent Med J* 2014 March;**16**(3).

16. Garthus-Niegel S, von Soest T, Vollrath M, et al. The impact of subjective birth experiences on post-traumatic stress symptoms: A longitudinal study. *Arch Women's Mental Health* 2013;**16**(1):1–10.

17. Ayers S. Thoughts and emotions during traumatic birth: A qualitative study. *Birth* 2007;**34**(3):253–63.

18. Fenech G, Thomson G. 'Tormented by ghosts from their past': A meta-synthesis to explore the psychosocial implications of a traumatic birth on maternal well-being. *Midwifery* 2014;**30**(2):185–93.

19. Lukasse M, Vangen S, Øian P, et al. Fear of childbirth, women's preference for caesarean section and childhood abuse: A longitudinal study. *Acta Obstet Gynecol Scand* 2011;**90**:33–40.

20. Royal College of Midwives, Royal College of Nursing, Royal College of Obstetricians and Gynaecologist. *Tackling FGM in the UK: Intercollegiate recommendations for identifying and recording and reporting.* Royal College of Midwives, 2013.

21. Toubia N. *Female Genital Mutilation: A Call for Global Action.* 1993. New York: Women Ink; p19.

22. Lundberg PC, Gerezgiher A. Experiences from pregnancy and childbirth related to female mutilation among Eritrean immigrant women in Sweden. *Midwifery* 2008;**24**(2):214–25.

23. Di Renzo GC, Polito PM, Volpe A, et al. Multicentric study on fear of childbirth in pregnant women at term. *J Psychosomatic Obstet Gynecol* 1984;**3**:155–63.

24. Ryding EL. Investigation of 33 women who demanded a caesarean section for personal reasons. *Acta Obstet Gynecol Scand* 1993;**72**:280–5.

25. Sjögren B. Fear of childbirth and psychosomatic support: A follow up of 72 women *Act Obstet Gynecol Scand* 1998;**77**:819–25.

26. Patel R, Hollins K. Clinical report: The joint obstetric and psychiatric management of phobic anxiety disorders in pregnancy *J Psychosom Obstet Gynecol* 2015;**36**(1):10–14.

27. MacDorman M, Declercq E, Menacker F, et al. Recent trends and patterns in cesarean and vaginal birth after cesarean (VBAC) deliveries in the United States. *Clinics in Perinatology* 2011;**38**(2):179–92.

28. van Dillen J, Zwart J, Schutte J, et al. Severe acute maternal morbidity and mode of delivery in the Netherlands. *Acta Obstet Gynecol Scand* 2010;**889**(11): 1460–5.

29. Hildingsson, I. Swedish couples' attitudes towards birth, childbirth fear and birth preferences and relation to mode of birth – A longitudinal cohort study. *Sexual and Reproductive Healthcare* 2014;**5**(2):75–80.

30. Choosing Health: Making healthy choices easier, Department of Health, 16 November 2004, Public Health White Paper.

31. Saving Mothers' Lives: Reviewing maternal deaths to make motherhood safer – 2003–2005. The Seventh Report of the Confidential Enquiries into Maternal Deaths in the United Kingdom.

32. Jones I, Craddock N. Familiality of the puerperal trigger in bipolar disorder: Results of a family study. *Am J Psychiatry* 2001;**158**(6):913–7.

33. National Institute for Health and Care Excellence (NICE) guidelines [CG45] Antenatal and postnatal mental health: Clinical management and service guidance 2007.

34. Whooley MA, Avins AL, Miranda J, Browner WS. Case-finding instruments for depression: Two questions are as good as many. *J Gen Intern Med* 1997 July;**12**(7):439–45.

35. Richens Y. A national online survey of UK maternity unit service provision for women with fear of birth. *British Journal of Midwifery* 2015;**23**(8): 472–475.

Chapter 35

Psychiatric Disorders in Pregnancy and Lactation

Angelika Wieck

Introduction

Mental disorder is the most common complication of childbearing with one in five women being affected. There are complex interactions between the two conditions. Childbearing can alter the course of mental illness and mental illness can affect pregnancy and child outcome. Perinatal mental illness can also lead to long-term disadvantages in the physical and neurobehavioural development of the offspring. The resulting enormous costs to families and society are now beginning to be realized. In the UK, appropriate services are as yet available only to a minority of pregnant women suffering from mental illness, but plans are underfoot to extend them across the population.

Maternity services have a crucial role in identifying, assessing and managing women with pre-existing or new disorders in pregnancy and those who develop acute psychiatric episodes in the immediate postnatal period. In this chapter, the presentation and management of the main psychiatric disorders presenting in childbearing women are discussed.

Non-Psychotic Mental Disorders in the Perinatal Period

Postpartum Blues

More than half of recently delivered mothers experience mild mood changes such as anxiety, irritability, low mood and tearfulness in the first 10 days after childbirth, with a peak incidence around day 3–5 postnatal. These changes usually resolve spontaneously after a few hours or days and do not require any intervention.

Depressive Illness

In high-income countries, the point prevalence of major and minor depression ranges between 8.5 and 11.0% in the different stages of pregnancy and from 6.5 to 12.9% in the 12 months after childbirth [1]. In low-

and middle-income countries, rates are usually reported to be higher. Epidemiological data have usually not found significant differences in comparison with non-pregnant women. There are also no major qualitative differences in the psychopathology except that the content of the depressive thoughts are frequently coloured by themes of motherhood. Women might think, for example, that they have failed as mothers and wives or that their children should be looked after by someone else. Often, depressed women have comorbid anxious or intrusive obsessional thoughts that they might harm their children. Because of their depression women may be unable to bond with their unborn or newborn child. This is particularly distressing to sufferers and they often feel that they are to blame for what they regard as an unnatural state.

In more than half of women with postnatal depression, symptoms commence in pregnancy or pre-conception [2]. In fact, findings from one recent large study suggest that postnatal depression is heterogeneous and that conditions with an onset in pregnancy represent more severe states [3].

The risk of perinatal depression is increased by psychiatric factors, including a past history of depression, anxiety, post-traumatic stress disorder (PTSD), substance misuse and neurotic personality traits, and psychosocial adversities such as low socio-economic status, particularly in low- and middle-income countries, exposure to trauma, childhood sexual abuse, chronic and acute negative life stress, domestic violence, migration, relationship problems and low levels of social support [4, 5].

Women with postnatal depression have an approximately 40% risk of a recurrence after a subsequent birth [6] and an increased risk of having non-perinatal episodes [7].

Anxiety Disorders

The period prevalence of common anxiety disorders, including panic disorder, social phobia, specific phobias and generalized anxiety disorder, has been estimated as 13.0% in pregnant and 12.3% in postnatal women and as no different from women who have not recently been childbearing [8]. Although anxiety disorders can exist in isolation they more commonly occur with other psychiatric disorders, particularly other anxiety states, depression and bipolar disorder. In a childbearing woman, anxious thinking or ruminations often relate to serious harm coming to either herself or the child or that the mother may not be a good parent or be viewed by others as such.

Post-traumatic Stress Disorder

PTSD develops in response to traumatic events such as severe accidents, interpersonal violence or military action. Traumatic or perceived traumatic delivery can be a significant cause of PTSD (see Chapter 39). Symptoms of most types of PTSD usually emerge within a month of the trauma, although there may be a delay of several months or even years. People with PTSD have repetitive, involuntary and distressing memories or nightmares of the event, or experience flashbacks in which they feel or act as if the event is recurring. In severe cases, this can lead sufferers to lose awareness of their surroundings. When exposed to cues that resemble or symbolize aspects of the trauma, the person may become intensely distressed or show marked physical reactions. The presentation is accompanied by avoidance of trauma reminders, hypervigilance for threat, insomnia, amnesia for parts of the trauma and emotional changes, such as feeling detached from other people, losing interest in activities and being unable to feel positive emotions.

PTSD in childbearing women may have been pre-existing or related to childbearing. In the postnatal period, the prevalence is about 1–2% [9], and the most important risk factors are subjective distress in labour and obstetric emergencies [9]. However, infant complications, low support during labour and delivery, psychological difficulties in pregnancy and previous traumatic experiences are also factors that are related to the development of postnatal PTSD [9].

Obsessive Compulsive Disorder

Obsessive compulsive disorder (OCD) is characterized by the presence of repetitive and unwanted thoughts (obsessions) or repetitive and unproductive behaviours (compulsions). Often the two types of symptoms occur together.

The prevalence of OCD in the perinatal period has been estimated as approximately 2%, which is about twice higher than in the general female population [10]. In fact, about one-third of female sufferers report that they first became ill in pregnancy or after childbirth. Symptoms are highly distressing to the sufferer and can significantly impair day-to-day functioning and parenting.

A common theme for obsessional thoughts is being responsible for harm to others. As the attention of pregnant and postnatal women is focused on the baby, obsessive thoughts often concern accidental or deliberate harm coming to the child. The mother may worry about exposing her unborn or newborn to toxic substances or germs through the food she eats, the air she breathes or the things she touches. She may also worry that she might turn into someone who is abusing children. She may develop compulsive behaviour in the form of excessive cleaning and washing of baby clothes, checking, repeating, ordering, counting and sometimes praying. Some mothers may avoid changing soiled nappies due to fears of being a paedophile, isolate their children to prevent contamination and remove knives or sharp objects from the home so that they cannot stab their infant. There is as yet little known how perinatal OCD may affect maternal bonding and parenting. In one controlled study [11] mothers with OCD were less likely to breastfeed, less confident, reported more marital distress and were rated as less sensitive in their interaction with their infant. With appropriate treatment the disorder usually improves significantly or resolves altogether.

Tokophobia

Tokophobia (see Chapter 34) is a severe fear of parturition that can be caused by a previous traumatic delivery, although it can also develop in nulliparous pregnant women. Women who have poor mental health, a history of sexual abuse and poor social support are more vulnerable. Women are often highly distressed and request deliveries by caesarean section.

Eating Disorders

Anorexia nervosa, bulimia nervosa and binge eating disorders have been reported to occur in about 2% of pregnant women [12]. Pregnancy can exacerbate symptoms or trigger new onsets, but more often symptoms reduce in intensity [13]. After childbirth they usually become more severe again [13]. Anorexia nervosa and bulimia nervosa have been found to affect pregnancy outcomes adversely with a consistent finding of low birthweight [13]. About 30% of women with current or past eating disorders have comorbid depression if they are assessed postnatally [7].

Personality Disorders

In a Swedish study the prevalence of personality disorders in pregnancy was reported as 4.5% [14]. In clinical samples borderline personality disorder (BPD) is the most common type in females. Its main features are pervasive instability in regulation of emotion, self-image, interpersonal relationships and impulse control. Comorbidity is high with increased rates of other psychiatric disorders, such as substance misuse, anxiety, mood disorders and other personality disorders. In severe cases, BPD can lead to severe functional impairment, substantial use of health services and high rates of mortality by suicide.

Symptoms typically worsen with stress and women are therefore more likely to function less well in pregnancy and after childbirth. Little is known about the effects of BPD itself on pregnancy and infant outcomes but more about the effects of the frequent comorbidities. The long-term course of the disorder is varied. The initial peak in adolescence and early adulthood may be followed by rapid improvement within a few months or a more gradual amelioration across the life span.

Psychotic Disorders in the Peripartum Period

This section refers to bipolar disorder, psychotic depression and schizophrenia and schizophrenia-related disorders. New onsets or recurrences of such illnesses are not more common in pregnancy. In contrast, childbirth is followed by a large increase in severe psychiatric morbidity. This is illustrated by a dramatic rise in first and recurrent hospital admissions after childbirth, with a peak in the first postnatal month. The incidence of psychiatric hospital admissions within three months is usually reported as 1–2/1000 deliveries.

The majority of severe mental illnesses after childbirth are affective in nature [15]. They usually commence abruptly and very early – within the first few days after delivery – progress rapidly, are severe and pose serious risks to the safety of mother and child [15]. These illnesses need to be identified early, regarded as psychiatric emergencies, managed decisively and monitored closely.

Bipolar Disorder

Patients with bipolar disorder suffer from depressive or manic mood episodes or mixed states, where both kinds of symptoms co-exist. The condition commences on average in the early twenties, although patients often report a degree of mood instability from teenage years or even childhood onwards.

Bipolar disorder is associated with a high level of psychiatric comorbidity, with the majority of sufferers having other conditions such as anxiety disorders, behaviour disorders and substance use disorders. As many as 4–5 patients report a suicide attempt in the last 12 months [16], and the rate of completed suicide in the 15 years from first psychiatric contact is reported to be as high as 4.8% in women [17]. Cognitive and psychosocial functioning can be significantly impaired, although individuals vary greatly in the course and nature of their illness. The prognosis can be markedly improved by a comprehensive treatment plan and close collaboration between the patient, family or carers, primary care and mental health professionals.

Although pregnancy does not seem to alter the course of bipolar disorder, studies that have followed patients who discontinued mood stabilizers around preconception have found that women who discontinue medication are at a much higher risk of relapsing in pregnancy than women who continue. This risk increases after childbirth, which is a very potent trigger for bipolar recurrences. One in two women will have another episode and one in five women will become severely ill.

Postpartum Psychosis

The term 'puerperal psychosis' or 'postnatal psychosis' refers to severe mood disorders which commence after childbirth and include manic states, mixed affective states and psychotic depression but not non-psychotic depression [15]. Psychotic depression is included in this term because it shares with manic states the close temporal relationship with childbirth and stormy course in the postnatal period. The manic and severe depressive episodes of bipolar disorder can therefore be regarded as subtypes of postpartum psychosis, and some research refers to this group of disorders together.

As many as 54.4% of women with a past history of puerperal psychosis (including puerperal mania or psychotic depression) have been reported to experience another severe episode after the next delivery

[18]. It is important to note that as many as half or more women developing a puerperal psychosis have no antecedent psychiatric history [18]. This means that, in the early postpartum period, clinicians need to be particularly vigilant when affective symptoms develop even in women with no prior history of an affective psychosis.

A family history of postpartum psychosis (mania or psychosis) significantly increases the risk of major affective episodes in the postpartum [19]. The other consistent risk factor for affective psychoses in the postpartum is primiparity [15].

Schizophrenia

The annual prevalence of schizophrenia in women is approximately 7/1000 [20]. The prevalence in pregnant women has not been investigated but is likely to be a little lower because of a reduced fertility rate. The core symptoms of schizophrenia are abnormal beliefs, thought disorder, abnormal perceptions, thought alienation, feelings of one's actions being made by an outside agency, reduced social engagement, blunted affect, lack of drive and altered social behaviour. The disease is often accompanied by other mental health problems such as anxiety disorders, major depressive illness or substance use disorder. Symptoms typically develop gradually, begin in young adulthood, and can be long-lasting.

Men and women with severe mental illness have high rates of childhood abuse and domestic violence in adulthood. In addition, women suffering from schizophrenia have been reported to have high rates of coerced sex and high-risk sexual behaviour and tend to use less contraception. They are therefore particularly vulnerable to unintended pregnancies [21]. These factors can sometimes result in complex presentations in childbearing women that require careful assessment and management by a multi-disciplinary and multi-agency team.

Suicide

In the UK, the latest confidential enquiry [22] found a continuing decline in the overall maternal mortality rate. However, maternal deaths due to indirect causes, including those due to mental illness, remain high and have not changed since 2003. In almost a quarter of women who died between six weeks and one year after childbirth the cause was mental illness and 1 in 7 died from suicide. Within the perinatal period, 12% of suicides occurred in pregnancy, 9% in the first six weeks postnatal and the remainder later in the postnatal year [22]. Most mothers had a pre-existing mental disorder and the most common diagnosis was recurrent depressive disorder. Fortunately, extended suicides, where the mother also killed her baby, were a very rare occurrence. They related to a diagnosis of depressive illness and safeguarding issues.

'Red flag' clinical features for maternal death due to psychiatric causes were a recent significant change in mental state or emergence of new symptoms, new thoughts or acts of violent self-harm, new or recurrent feelings of incompetence as a mother and feeling estranged from the child.

The MBRRACE-UK report [22] revealed a number of failings in the management of these women. The key recommendations for achieving a reduction in mental illness related maternal deaths were to improve the effectiveness of communication between health professionals and other agencies, to raise awareness of mental illnesses in the perinatal period and to provide additional training to all involved health professionals. In addition, it was recommended that regional clinical networks for perinatal mental health should be set up. In all of these, improvements the participation of maternity services is essential.

Identification of Mental Illness in the Perinatal Period

Since mental illnesses can have serious consequences for mother and child, it is important that they are identified early in pregnancy and the postnatal period and managed effectively. Initial identification should be followed by a comprehensive assessment of mental health and social needs.

In the UK, the NICE guidelines for antenatal and postnatal mental health [23] recommend to ask brief screening questions for common mental illnesses at a woman's first contact with primary care or her booking visit and during the early postnatal period. If a woman responds positively to the depression or anxiety screening questions, it is recommended that she either completes self-rating scales for a fuller assessment (such as the Edinburgh Postnatal Depression Scale, the Generalized Anxiety Scale, or the Patient Health Questionnaire) or is referred to either her GP or secondary health services, according to the severity of her condition.

At all further contacts, the health visitor and other healthcare professionals who have regular contact with the woman in pregnancy and in the first postnatal year should consider asking the depression and anxiety screening questions as part of a general discussion about her mental health well-being and use self-rating scales as part of monitoring.

NICE guidance also specifies brief questions about past or present severe mental illness at the first contact with services [23]. Because there is a genetic contribution to developing severe mood disorders in the postnatal period, a question about perinatal illnesses in female first-degree relatives is included. If the response to any of these questions is positive, the woman should be referred to secondary mental health services and, preferably, perinatal mental health services. It is important to note that, if a woman has a sudden onset of symptoms suggesting postpartum psychosis, this should be regarded as an emergency. She should be referred to a general adult mental health service, and preferably a perinatal mental health team, for urgent assessment within 4 hours [23].

The Organiziation of General and Specialist Perinatal Mental Health Services in the UK

Stepped Care

At present much of the UK mental healthcare system is organized around the principles of stepped care [24]. This provides a framework for best-practice clinical pathways to care. Patients step through progressive levels of treatments with increasing intensity of their disorder. The vast majority of common mental disorders are treated in primary care, but patients who are unresponsive to treatment can be referred to mental health services. Patients who present with severe or particularly complex forms of either anxiety, depression or OCD, and impaired social functioning, or patients with high suicide risk are usually directly referred to specialized mental health services. Patients with suspected psychosis or severe depression are also usually directly referred to secondary care services.

Perinatal Mental Health Services

Perinatal psychiatry is a sub-specialty within general adult psychiatry and provides specialist care at secondary and tertiary care levels. NICE [23] recommends that each locality should have a perinatal mental health clinical network that includes healthcare professionals as well as commissioners, managers, service users and carers. Its responsibilities are to provide a specialist multi-disciplinary perinatal mental health service for direct clinical care and advice to maternity services, other mental health and community services. The network should also provide access to specialist expert advice on the benefits and risks of psychotropic medication in the perinatal period, write referral and management protocols for services across the stepped care framework, ensure effective transfer of information and continuity of care and design pathways of care [23]. A specialized service should consist of perinatal mental health community team and a specialized psychiatric mother and baby unit. In the UK, current availability of specialized care is patchy with around half of affected women having no access [25]. However, NHS England is currently planning an expansion of perinatal mental health clinical networks and specialized services.

In several maternity departments in the UK, specialist mental health midwives provide a service for pregnant women with mental illness. The aim is to improve early identification of mental illness in pregnancy, facilitate access to the appropriate level of care, provide support to women with severe mental illness and monitor their mental health. Often this is combined with a safeguarding children role. Because of the wide remit of this role, it is important that a robust identification system is in place and that women with the greatest need and risk are selected for specialized input.

Individual consultant obstetricians around the country have also developed a specialist interest in recent years. A recent survey [26] has shown that clinical practice in this area varies widely and that there is a need for a greater definition of the role and training in perinatal mental health.

In some maternity departments a perinatal psychiatrist or liaison psychiatrist sees patients in the antenatal clinics alongside specialist mental health midwives and consultant obstetricians.

Assessment and Care-Planning in the Perinatal Period

The following recommendations on the assessment of women with mental illness in pregnancy and the postnatal period are a summary of the respective sections in the NICE guidelines on antenatal and postnatal mental health [23].

If a mental illness is suspected in a woman during pregnancy or postnatal period, further assessment should include the history of the mental health problem, any previous perinatal episodes, her physical well-being and medical history, past and current substance misuse, the woman's attitude and experience towards the pregnancy and her unborn or newborn child, and any past or present treatments and her response to them. Her social networks and quality of key relationships, her living conditions, any past or current experience of domestic violence, sexual abuse, trauma or childhood maltreatment should be included in the assessment. Her current housing, employment, economic and immigration status as well as her responsibilities as carer for other children and younger adults and other adults should be enquired about. It is also important to take account of any learning disabilities or other cognitive disabilities and to assess whether there is a need to consult with a specialist.

The clinician should make a diagnosis and an assessment whether there is a risk of self-neglect, self-harm, suicidal thoughts and intent and risks to others, including the baby. If there is a risk of suspected child maltreatment, local safeguarding protocols should be followed. Should the woman be at risk of self-harm or suicide, her level of support should be assessed, help appropriate to the level of risk should be arranged and all relevant health professionals should be informed. The woman and those close to her should be advised to seek further help if the situation deteriorates.

Professionals in secondary mental health services, including specialist perinatal mental health services, should develop a written care plan in collaboration with the woman, and as appropriate her partner, a family member or carer. The plan should be comprehensive, cover pregnancy, childbirth and the postnatal period and should be distributed to all relevant health professionals.

Management of Non-Psychotic Mental Disorders in the Perinatal Period

Psychotropic Medication for Non-Psychotic Disorders

The threshold for the use of psychotropic medication is higher in the perinatal period than at other times of a woman's life and it should only be considered if a condition is at least of moderate severity, or if talking therapy is not accepted by the patient or has not been effective. Antidepressants, and in particular selective serotonin inhibitors, are the most commonly used medications in perinatal patients and are effective not only for the treatment of depression but also for the treatment of anxiety disorders, including OCD and PTSD and bulimia. There are as yet few studies that specifically have tested the efficacy in perinatal patients.

Psychosocial and Social Interventions for Non-Psychotic Disorders

The NICE guidelines [23] state that psychological interventions should be provided within 1 month of initial assessment. A wide range of effective psychological and social interventions are available which vary with the condition. The intensity of intervention is dependent on the degree of functional impairment and patient preference [24]. If the functional impairment is mild, low-intensity treatments should be offered at primary care level, such as self-help materials or brief individual therapy by telephone. If the functional impairment is greater, more intensive 1:1 interventions may be offered. Psychological therapy should be adapted to the perinatal situation, take account of the mother's anxieties concerning how her illness may affect the development of the child and aim to improve her bond and interaction with the child.

Where the patient suffers severe functional impairment, combined psychological, social and pharmacological therapy can be offered and a referral to the community mental health team made. In the following sections psychological and psychosocial interventions are discussed for individual non-psychotic disorders.

Depression

Little is also yet known how to prevent depression in pregnancy, but a number of psychosocial and psychological interventions for the prevention of depression after childbirth have been tested. Several interventions have been found to be effective, including intensive, individualized postpartum home visits provided by public health nurses or midwives, peer-based telephone support and interpersonal psychotherapy, particularly if the intervention is delivered after childbirth and targeted at women with risk factors [27]. Whether CBT may also be effective is not clear. For the treatment of postnatal depression, psychosocial interventions, such as peer or partner support, non-directive or cognitive behavioural counselling, cognitive therapy and interpersonal psychotherapy are effective [4].

Treatment of Anxiety Disorders

A range of interventions are effective in the management of anxiety disorders, including behavioural, cognitive-behavioural and cognitive therapy. In moderate to severe cases psychological approaches often have to be combined with medications enhancing serotonergic neurotransmission. Since there are no randomized controlled trials specifically for the perinatal period, evidence needs to be extrapolated from general guidelines.

Despite the high personal and health costs, the treatment of tokophobia has received little attention. Promising preliminary results have been reported for midwife-led psycho-education but further research is needed.

Eating Disorders

In addition to usual interventions, pregnant women with current eating disorders require careful monitoring throughout pregnancy and the postpartum period and more intensive prenatal care, consisting of support to achieve adequate prenatal nutrition and fetal development [23]. However, this advice has not yet been subjected to randomized controlled trials [4].

Borderline Personality Disorder

Support by a community mental health team and talking therapy, such as dialectic-behavioural therapy, mentalization-based therapy or therapeutic communities are recommended as the primary approaches to the management of BPD in general. Although the transition to motherhood poses particular challenges to women with BPD and despite some evidence that their care practices and involvement with their infants are negatively affected, no specific interventions have yet been adequately tested for this patient group. Medication has a place in ameliorating specific symptoms and treating comorbid conditions.

Management of Severe Mental Illness in the Perinatal Period

When her pregnancy becomes known, a woman with a past or current severe mental illness should be referred within two weeks to secondary mental health services and seen by a psychiatrist, and if possible by a perinatal psychiatrist or other experienced perinatal mental health professional.

In severe perinatal mental illness, the management should include psychological and social support of the mother and her partner from a community mental health team, preferably a service specialized in perinatal mental health and specific talking therapies. In addition to behavioural and cognitive therapies, formal education about the illness and interventions aimed at relapse prevention or coping with psychotic symptoms may be part of the treatment programme. Depending on the complexities of the presentation a large number of professionals may be involved that include specialists in housing, substance misuse, domestic violence, immigration specialists and others.

Pharmacological treatment is usually an important part of the management of a severe mental illness and enables the patient to participate in other forms of therapy. Severe depression is responsive to antidepressants, sometimes in combination with antipsychotic drugs. Drugs that are effective in the treatment of bipolar disorder include mainly mood stabilizers, antipsychotic medication and antidepressant medication, and they are often used in combination. Antipsychotic medications are also effective in the acute and maintenance therapy of paranoid schizophrenia. In the most severe depressive states, when either drug therapy has failed to bring about sufficient relief from suffering or where the risks are so high that urgent improvement is required, electro-convulsive therapy can be a life-saving intervention.

A comprehensive treatment plan is formulated by the community mental health team under the leadership of the psychiatrist. It should cover the needs of the patient, actions to be taken to ameliorate for social problems, psychological therapies, medication, a description of early symptoms of a recurrence, an emergency plan, contact details of all involved professionals and other aspects. Because of the complexity of the presentations in the perinatal period and the high risks involved, it is important that care planning is started early in pregnancy, that a clear strategy is established for the antenatal, intra-partum and postnatal period, and that the management plan is available at the latest around 32 weeks of gestation. Copies should be given to the patient and all involved healthcare professionals and be part of the handheld and hospital notes. The implementation of the care plan is directed and monitored by a named care coordinator who is a member of the community mental health team. If a woman requires inpatient treatment in late pregnancy or in the first postnatal year, she should be admitted jointly with her child to a specialized mother-and-baby unit.

Many women with severe or complex mental illness are judged to parent their children successfully, particularly if they have access to social support. However, if there are any concerns that a pregnant woman may have significant difficulties in parenting, clinicians should discuss this with the patient and make a referral to Children and Families Social Services. Clear safeguarding children procedures are available in most maternity services.

Psychotropic Medication: Reproductive Safety and Prescribing in the Perinatal Period

The reproductive safety of pharmacological treatments is difficult to assess in childbearing women with mental illness because there are a host of other parameters that can determine pregnancy and child outcomes. These include confounding by indication, psychiatric comorbidities, physical illnesses, concomitant medication, smoking, maternal age, high BMI and low socioeconomic status. In women with mental illness, several of these characteristics are often present. In addition, randomized controlled trials cannot be conducted in perinatal women and existing research often suffers from small sample sizes, poor design, little adjustment for confounding factors and frequently no adjustment for the psychiatric indication.

A detailed discussion of the current literature on the reproductive safety of psychotropic drugs is beyond the scope of this chapter and the reader is referred to recent reviews [4, 28, 29, 30]. In the following sections the main findings from current evidence on commonly used psychotropic drugs is summarized.

When discussing the use of psychotropic medication with the patient, it is important that she and her partner or a significant other person know the risks of different options. This includes continuing medication, or stopping and restarting it in the second trimester, before delivery or in the early postnatal period. Drugs with higher teratogenic risk and with the least safety data should be avoided. However, it is important to recognize that the woman's past response to treatment is in many cases the decisive factor in the choice of agent. Abrupt discontinuation of medication when the pregnancy is discovered should be avoided unless the drug is

valproate. Polypharmacy should be avoided as much as possible. Although it is important to avoid higher doses, it is equally important not to undertreat. Weighing up the risks and benefits of psychotropic medication in pregnancy is often complex and the patient may need time until the next appointment to make a decision.

Selective Serotonin Reuptake Inhibitors

Selective Serotonin Reuptake Inhibitors (SSRIs) have in most recent studies not shown to be associated with an increased teratogenic potential, although a few studies suggest a small increase of major congenital malformations accounted for mostly by cardiac septal defects. Paroxetine is an SSRI that has been most frequently associated with cardiac defects. Current evidence suggests that there may be a maximally 2.5-fold increase of pulmonary hypertension of the newborn in children exposed in the second half of pregnancy to SSRIs whilst the base rate is extremely low (about 0.5–1.0/1000). There is consistent evidence that late pregnancy exposure is associated with an increase of poor neonatal adaptation from a base rate of about 1:10 to 1:3 babies, but symptoms are mild and usually resolve spontaneously within 10 days of birth. There is currently a debate whether an about 2-fold increase in the rate of autism spectrum disorders in exposed offspring is related to a medication effect or confounding factors.

There seem to be few differences between individual serotonin reuptake inhibitors and the choice of agent should be primarily determined by the patient's previous response. Paroxetine should be avoided.

Antipsychotic Medications

Current evidence does not suggest that antipsychotic drugs are major teratogens. It has not yet been clarified whether the small observed increase of major congenital anomalies (mostly cardiovascular and especially septal defects) is due to the medication or the large number of potential confounding factors. There is also a lack of clarity about the aetiology of a small increase in stillbirths and whether the medication can lead to a maximally 2-fold increase in the rate of gestational diabetes. An oral glucose tolerance test at 24–28 weeks of pregnancy is recommended by the NICE guidelines [23]. The body of evidence does not allow us to determine whether there are differences in the reproductive safety of individual antipsychotic agents, although recently introduced agents with particularly few data, such as paliperidone and lurasidone, should be avoided in perinatal patients.

Anti-Epileptic Mood Stabilizers

Because of its widespread teratogenic and adverse effects on children's neurodevelopment, the mood stabilizer valproate should not be prescribed to pregnant or breastfeeding women. The mood stabilizer carbamazepine has an uncertain place in the treatment of bipolar disorder and causes congenital spina bifida and should therefore also not be prescribed to perinatal patients. It is important to note that recent studies have failed to show that peri-conceptual intake of folic acid prevents anti-epileptic teratogenicity. The more recently introduced lamotrigine, which has efficacy in the treatment and prevention of bipolar depression, has significantly less teratogenic effects than valproate, but there are as yet insufficient data to judge whether it has any teratogenic potential. Current evidence does not suggest that it causes neurodevelopmental impairment and it can be used cautiously in bipolar disorder if other treatment is not effective.

Lithium

Initial findings about lithium causing a high rate of cardiovascular anomalies in children exposed in the first trimester have been shown to be incorrect. Recent studies have conflicted whether there is either a much smaller increase or no increase in major congenital malformations. No systematic studies are available for other fetal or neonatal effects. Because of these uncertainties, lithium should only be prescribed in the first trimester of pregnancy if it is considered that a switch to a safer drug would mean a high risk of a recurrence. If a woman has taken it in the first trimester, she should be offered not only structural ultrasounds but also fetal echocardiograms. Lithium can be replaced by an antipsychotic agent that has proven efficacy in bipolar disorder in the first trimester or for the entire pregnancy. Because lithium has to be dosed so that its blood level is within the therapeutic window and because of its changing pharmacokinetics in pregnancy, it is essential that dosing is undertaken by a psychiatrist. Detailed prescribing recommendations can be found in the NICE guidelines [23].

Sleep-Inducers and Anxiolytics

Benzodiazepines are probably not teratogenic but may cause floppiness and respiratory depression in newborn babies. These drugs should, in adults, only be used for severe anxiety or agitation in pregnancy on a short-term basis and short-acting agents should be preferred

in late pregnancy. Hypnotic benzodiazepine receptor agonists are also not thought to be teratogenic, but zolpidem possibly causes a small increase in the rates of preterm birth and delivery of small for gestational age babies (birthweights below the 10th percentile for babies of the same gestational age). These drugs should also only be used in the short term for severe insomnia and zolpidem should be avoided. There is either very little or poor quality data on the reproductive safety of trazodone, promazine, promethazine or pregabalin, and they should be avoided in perinatal patients if possible. Low doses of the antipsychotic quetiapine, which has strong sedative effects, can be used as an alternative to other anxiolytics or sleep inducers.

Breastfeeding

All psychotropic drugs are transferred into breast milk. The relative infant dose, which is the weight-adjusted dose that a fully breastfed infant ingests compared to the maternal dose, has been calculated for many psychotropic medications, although the numbers of cases on which these calculations are based are often still small. For most psychotropic drugs, the relative infant dose is below 10% which is regarded by paediatric pharmacologists as a relatively safe range. There are no systematic clinical studies of the effects on breastfed children, but existing case reports do not suggest that most psychotropic drugs lead to significant adverse effects. However, there are some drugs that should be avoided during breastfeeding: lithium because of a high relative infant dose and potential toxic effects in the infant, and the antipsychotic clozapine because of the risk of agranulocytosis. The advice given under 'Sleep inducers and Anxiolytics' also applies to breastfeeding women. For further reference, the electronic Drugs and Lactation Database [31] provides an excellent up to date resource for prescribing clinicians.

Key Points

- The main non-psychotic mental disorders in the perinatal period include postpartum blues, anxiety disorders, depressive illness, post-traumatic stress disorder, personality disorders, eating disorders, tokophobia and obsessive compulsive disorder.
- Psychotic disorders in the perinatal period include bipolar disorder, psychotic depression and schizophrenia and schizophrenia-related disorders.

- Childbirth is a strong trigger for bipolar recurrence. One in two women will suffer a recurrence and, in one in five women, this is a severe episode.
- Postnatal mania and psychotic depression are combined in the term 'postpartum psychosis'. These states start abruptly, usually within a few days of childbirth and escalate rapidly. They need to be regarded as psychiatric emergencies, requiring urgent assessment and assertive management.
- Studies of women who discontinued mood stabilizers around conception have found increased recurrence rates in pregnancy compared to women who continued medication.
- 'Red flag' clinical features for maternal death due to psychiatric causes include a recent significant change in mental state or emergence of new symptoms, new thoughts or acts of violent self-harm, new or recurrent feelings of incompetence as a mother or feeling estranged from the child.
- The threshold for the use of psychotropic medication for non-psychotic disorders is higher in the perinatal period than at other times of a woman's life and it should only be considered if a condition is at least of moderate severity, if talking therapy is not accepted by the patient or has not been effective. Antidepressants, and in particular selective serotonin inhibitors, are effective not only for the treatment of depression but also for the treatment of anxiety disorders, including OCD and PTSD, and bulimia.
- Psychosocial interventions for non-psychotic disorders include guided self-help, brief individual therapy by telephone and psychological therapy. Where the patient suffers severe functional impairment, combined psychological, social and pharmacological therapy can be offered and a referral to the community mental health team made.
- Pharmacological treatment is usually an important part of the management of a severe mental illness. Drugs that are effective in the treatment of bipolar disorder include mood stabilizers, antipsychotic medication and antidepressant medication, and they are often used in combination.
- If there are any concerns that a pregnant woman may have significant difficulties in parenting, clinicians should discuss this with the patient and make a referral to Children and Families Social Services.
- Abrupt discontinuation of medication when the pregnancy is discovered should be avoided unless the drug is valproate. Polypharmacy should be avoided as much as possible.
- All psychotropic drugs are transferred into breastmilk. In most cases the relative infant dose is below 10%. The antipsychotic clozapine and the mood stabilizers lithium, valproate and carbamazepine should not be prescribed to breastfeeding women.

References

1. Gavin NI, Gaynes BN, Lohr KN, et al. Perinatal depression: A systematic review of prevalence and incidence. *Obstet Gynecol* 2005; **106**:1071–83.

2. Wisner KL, Sit DK, McShea MC, et al. Onset timing, thoughts of self-harm, and diagnoses in postpartum women with screen-positive depression findings. *JAMA Psychiatry* 2013; **70**:490–8.

3. Postpartum Depression: Action Towards Causes and Treatment (PACT) Consortium. Heterogeneity of postpartum depression: A latent class analysis. *Lancet Psychiatry* 2015; January **2**(1):59–67.

4. Howard LM, Molyneaux E, Dennis CL, et al. Non-psychotic mental disorders in the perinatal period. *Lancet* 2014; November **15**(384):1775–88.

5. Wosu AC, Gelaye B, Williams MA. History of childhood sexual abuse and risk of prenatal and postpartum depression or depressive symptoms: An epidemiologic review. *Arch Women's Ment Health* 2015; **18**:659–71.

6. Wisner KL, Perel JM, Peindl KS, et al. Timing of depression recurrence in the first year after birth. *J Affect Disord* 2004; **78**:249–52.

7. Cooper PJ, Murray L. Course and recurrence of postnatal depression: Evidence for the specificity of the diagnostic concept. *Br J Psychiatry* 1995; **166**:191–5.

8. Vesga-López O, Blanco C, Keyes K, et al. Psychiatric disorders in pregnant and postpartum women in the United States. *Arch Gen Psychiatry* 2008; **65**:805–15.

9. Andersen LB, Melvaer LB, Videbech P, et al. Risk factors for developing post-traumatic stress disorder following childbirth: A systematic review. *Acta Obstet Gynecol Scand* 2012; **91**:1261–72.

10. Russell EJ, Fawcett JM, Mazmanian D. Risk of obsessive-compulsive disorder in pregnant and postpartum women: A meta-analysis. *J Clin Psychiatry* 2013; **74**:377–85.

11. Challacombe FL, Salkovskis PM, Woolgar M, et al. Parenting and mother-infant interactions in the context of maternal postpartum obsessive-compulsive disorder: Effects of obsessional symptoms and mood. *Infant Behav Dev* 2016; **44**:11–20.

12. Easter A, Bye A, Taborelli E, et al. Recognising the symptoms: How common are eating disorders in pregnancy? *Eur Eat Disord Rev* 2013; **21**:340–4.

13. Micali N. Management of eating disorders during pregnancy. *Progress in Neurology and Psychiatry* 2010; **14**:24–26.

14. Börjesson K, Ruppert S, Wager J, et al. Personality disorder, psychiatric symptoms and experience of childbirth among childbearing women in Sweden. *Midwifery* 2007; **23**:260–8.

15. Jones I, Chandra PS, Dazzan P, et al. Bipolar disorder, affective psychosis, and schizophrenia in pregnancy and the post-partum period. *Lancet* 2014; **384**:1789–99.

16. Merikangas KR, Jin R, He JP, et al. Prevalence and correlates of bipolar spectrum disorder in the world mental health survey initiative. *Arch Gen Psychiatry* 2011; **68**:241–51.

17. Nordentoft M, Mortensen PB, Pedersen CB. Absolute risk of suicide after first hospital contact in mental disorder. *Arch Gen Psychiatry* 2011; **68**:1058–64.

18. Blackmore ER, Rubinow DR, O'Connor TG, et al. Reproductive outcomes and risk of subsequent illness in women diagnosed with postpartum psychosis. *Bipolar Disord* 2013; **15**:394–404.

19. Jones I, Craddock N. Familiality of the puerperal trigger in bipolar disorder: Results of a family study. *Am J Psychiatry* 2001; **158**:913–17.

20. Bamrah JS, Freeman HL, Goldberg DP. Epidemiology of schizophrenia in Salford, 1974–84: Changes in an urban community over ten years. *Br J Psychiatry* 1991; **159**:802–10.

21. Seeman MV. Clinical interventions for women with schizophrenia: Pregnancy. *Acta Psychiatr Scand* 2013; **127**:12–22.

22. MBRRACE-UK. Saving Lives, Improving Mothers' Care. National Perinatal Epidemiology Unit, University of Oxford. 2015.

23. NICE – National Institute for Care and Health Excellence. Antenatal and postnatal mental health – Clinical management and service guidance. Updated edition. (2015). NICE clinical guideline 192.

24. NICE – National Institute for Care and Health Excellence. Common Mental Health Disorders – Identification and Pathways to Care. 2011. National Clinical Guideline 123.

25. Bauer A, Parsonage M, Knapp M, et al. The costs of perinatal mental health problems. *Centre for Mental Health and London School of Economics*. 2014. Available at www.centreformentalhealth.org.uk/costs-of-perinatal-mh-problems. Accessed 26 March 2017.

26. Wieck A, Mountain E, Edozien L. A survey of consultant obstetricians with a special interest in perinatal mental health. Abstract. International Conference of the Royal College of Psychiatrists, London, June 2016.

27. Dennis CL, Dowswell T. Psychosocial and psychological interventions for preventing postpartum depression. *Cochrane Database Syst Rev* 2013; **28**(2): CD001134.

28. NICE – National Institute for Care and Health Excellence. Antenatal and postnatal mental health: Clinical management and service guidance. Full guideline. Clinical Guideline 192. December 2014. Updated June 2015.

29. Wieck A, Reis M. Pharmacological treatment of mental health problems in pregnancy and lactation. In: Castle DJ, Abel KM eds : *Comprehensive Women's Mental Health*. Cambridge, Cambridge University Press. 2016; 122–36.

30. Wieck A, Abel KM. Sexual, reproductive and antenatal care of women with mental illness. In: Castle DJ, Abel KM eds : *Comprehensive Women's Mental Health*. Cambridge, Cambridge University Press. 2016; 90–100.

31. Drugs and Lactation Database (LactMed) (2017). http://toxnet.nlm.nih.gov/newtoxnet/lactmed.htm. Accessed 26 March 2017.

Chapter 36

Psychotherapy in Pregnancy and Following Birth

Basic Principles and Transcultural Aspects

Mary Steen and Tahereh Ziaian

Introduction

This chapter introduces and discusses maternal mental health and includes a review of what psychotherapy is and the different approaches are described and discussed. Stigma and shame are strongly associated with mental health problems; this is particularly true for pregnant and new mothers from culturally and linguistically diverse (CALD) backgrounds. Pregnant and new mothers from CALD backgrounds are at increased risk of mental health problems and more likely not to access psychotherapy. This is mainly due to modern psychotherapy not always meeting the needs of a diverse population. Consequently, people from CALD backgrounds are either reluctant to access psychotherapy, withdraw from therapy or less likely to show positive outcomes.

Therefore, cultural and ethnic issues concerning pregnant and new mothers are considered in this chapter to assist the reader to gain knowledge of the complexities surrounding mental health and the difficulties accessing psychotherapy. Two disguised case studies are included; firstly, a pregnant woman demonstrating increasing levels of anxiety and stress and, secondly, a new mother from a CALD background with post-traumatic stress symptoms are illustrated to aid the reader's understanding of the benefits of psychotherapy when mental health problems have been identified.

Maternal Mental Health

Being pregnant, then giving birth and the transition to motherhood can be an emotional time for many women. It is, therefore, not too surprising that many women will experience some level of anxiety and stress during this time period. Anxiety and stress can present alone as a mental health problem but can occur as a comorbidity with other mental health problems such as depression. It appears that many women manage their anxiety and stress without the need for referral to receive psychotherapy. However, many women go undetected and stigma and shame are linked to mental health; this can be a reason why pregnant women and new mothers do not seek help or support [1]. Mental health problems that are not identified and treated can lead to lifelong illness and are a significant public health issue [2]. It is, therefore, important for health professionals to be aware of this potential risk and consider women's emotional status and the need for referral to receive psychotherapy if there appears to be an indication.

Mental health problems often occur during the childbirth continuum and this can have adverse effects on women's physical health and well-being. Approximately one in seven women will experience a mental health problem at some point during pregnancy and the postnatal period [2]. Women who suffer from an existing mental illness are at an increased risk of relapse during pregnancy. It is recognized that pregnant women and mothers from culturally and linguistically diverse (CALD) backgrounds are at increased risk of mental health problems. Social isolation, language barriers, lack of opportunities to integrate with local communities and different cultural and traditional aspects associated with pregnancy and motherhood can be predisposing factors [3]. Other socioeconomic influences and life circumstances can also have an effect on a pregnant woman's mental health status, such as financial problems, domestic violence and sexual abuse [4]. There is also a strong link between mental health and physical health [5]. Birth trauma can be a trigger for post-traumatic stress disorder (PTSD). It is estimated that up to 16% of women may require a mental health intervention during the antenatal and postnatal period [6].

It is also recognized that maternal mental health problems can have a negative impact upon the health and well-being of infants which can contribute to

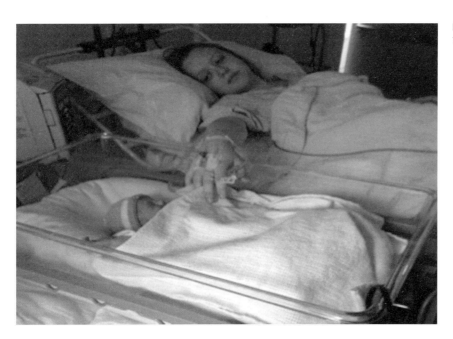

Figure 36.1 A mother's first touch

bonding and attachment issues [7]. A systematic literature review of prenatal depression and adverse birth outcomes reported an association between depression and low birth weight but not pre-term birth [8]. A recent review investigating the long-term economic and social costs associated with maternal mental health problems has estimated that £8.1 billion for each one-year cohort of births in the UK is spent; a higher percentage of these costs relates to the adverse impacts on the infant rather than the mother [9]. This evidence strengthens the reason why it is vital that the needs of expectant and newly birthed mothers who are at risk of developing a mental health problem or are at risk of relapse of an existing one during the childbirth continuum are met. However, mental health is not as well understood as other areas of health and the improving access to psychological therapies (IAPT) strategy indicates a lower threshold for access to women in pregnancy [10]. Nevertheless, there is some evidence of benefits of psychotherapies during the childbirth continuum. Psychological therapies have been demonstrated to be effective in the treatment of mild to moderate mental health problems [2].

What Is Psychotherapy?

Psychotherapy (talking therapies) involves talking about feelings and life problems with a psychotherapist in a safe and calming environment. There are several types of psychotherapy and a psychotherapist may use different approaches to meet individual pregnant or new mother needs. Depending on individual circumstances a psychotherapist may arrange one-to-one sessions or invite a woman's partner and/or other family members along or encourage participation in a psychotherapy group session.

Psychotherapy, in whatever format, can help pregnant and new mothers to feel better about themselves and enable them to develop coping strategies to deal with life problems and traumatic events more effectively [7]. Some approaches to psychotherapy make use of art, drama, poetry, stories, music and increasingly digital computer aids.

Different Types of Psychotherapy

According to the American Psychological Association [11] there are five broad approaches to psychotherapy: (i) Psychoanalysis/psychodynamic, (ii) behaviour, (iii) cognitive, (iv) humanistic, (v) integrative or holistic therapies.

These approaches guide psychotherapists to understanding a person's problems and developing appropriate solutions.

Psychoanalysis/psychodynamic therapies focus on changing problematic behaviours, feelings and thoughts by discovering their unconscious meanings and motivations. Psychoanalytic theory viewed mental life and overt behaviour as representing intrapsychic conflict between opposing aims and wishes of different aspects of personality (id, ego and superego); an inability to resolve conflict resulted in psychopathology. A close working relationship is established between the therapist and client, and clients learn about themselves by exploring their interactions in this therapeutic relationship.

Behavioural therapy utilizes principles of learning theory (classical and operant conditioning) to change pathological or maladaptive behaviour patterns [12]. The focus is on the consequences of behaviour, not intrapsychic conflicts or processes. In classical conditioning, new behaviours are learned by association; in Pavlov's famous experiments, dogs learned to salivate upon hearing the bell because they associated the bell sound with food. The technique of *desensitization*, for example, utilizes classical conditioning principles to assist clients with phobias by repeatedly exposing them to their anxiety (e.g. heights, confined spaces). In operant conditioning, positive reinforcement of adaptive behaviours and negatively reinforcing maladaptive behaviours are used to facilitate behavioural change. Several variations of behavioural therapy have been developed, including cognitive-behavioural therapy (CBT) and the third-wave behavioural therapies (see below).

Cognitive therapies focus on changing dysfunctional thinking patterns, thereby positively impacting on mood and behaviour. Prominent proponents of the cognitive approach are Albert Ellis and Aaron Beck [13, 14, 15, 16], who influenced the development of CBT. Their psychotherapy was based on the idea that emotional problems such as depression emerged from illogical, irrational or incorrect thinking; cognitive restructuring to be more accepting of reality could improve mood and normalize behaviour. Therapy also included directive techniques and actively engaged clients to change their thinking.

CBT is probably the most researched and frequently practiced psychotherapy today [17]. CBT incorporates a mix of *cognitive therapy* and *behavioural therapy* depending on individual needs. Cognitive elements focus on pattern of thinking; behavioural elements focus on associated actions. CBT not only helps people overcome their current symptoms but also teaches them new skills and strategies which they can apply to future problems.

CBT is continually evolving; and third-wave CBT therapies such as mindfulness-based cognitive therapy (MBCT), acceptance and commitment therapy (ACT) and dialectical behavioural therapy (DBT) are increasingly being used for a variety of emotional, behavioural and psychiatric problems.

MBCT is designed to help people suffering from repeated bouts of depression and chronic unhappiness. It combines traditional CBT with mindfulness/meditative practices. Cognitive methods can include educating a person about depression while mindfulness focuses on becoming aware of incoming thoughts and feelings and then accepting them [18].

ACT also includes mindfulness and behaviour change techniques to traditional CBT. ACT breaks mindfulness skills down into 3 categories: (i) diffusion – distancing from and letting go of unhelpful thoughts, beliefs and memories; (ii) acceptance – making room for painful feelings, urges and sensations and allowing them to come and go without a struggle; and (iii) contact and connect with the present moment – engaging fully with the here-and-now experience, with an attitude of openness and curiosity [19].

DBT is a specific type of CBT developed to treat borderline personality disorder which, since its development, has been successful with other types of mental health disorders. DBT helps a person to identify their strengths and build on them; to identify thoughts, beliefs and assumptions that make life harder; to work out problems in their relationships with the therapists; and to practise new skills individually [20].

Humanistic therapy: This approach emphasizes people's capacity to make rational choices and develop to their maximum potential. Concern and respect for others are important aspects. Significant humanistic therapies include *person-centred therapy* that rejects the idea of therapists as authorities on their clients' inner experiences and instead helps a person change by emphasizing their concern, care and interest. *Gestalt therapy* emphasizes 'organismic holism', the importance of being aware of the present moment and accepting responsibility for oneself; *existential therapy* focuses on free will, self-determination and the search for meaning [21].

Integrative or holistic therapy: Increasingly, there has been recognition that psychotherapy can be most effective when elements of different approaches are integrated to meet each client's need for maximum benefit. The growing interest in integrative theories, also referred to as multimodal or eclectic approaches, includes the proliferation of therapies and the need to reduce fragmentation; recognition that change in human behaviour is far too complex to be explained by a single theoretical approach.

Four types of psychotherapy integration have been proposed [22].

(i) Assimilative integration: consisting of a main therapy combined with techniques from other systems of psychotherapy, for example, MBCT [23].

(ii) Sequential and parallel concurrent integration: separate forms of therapy are used in sequential order or during the same phase of treatment in separate sessions, for example, traditional CBT.

(iii) Theoretical integration: clear theory guides intervention that includes techniques from one or more psychotherapies, for example, ACT [24].

(iv) Technical eclecticism: the use of psychotherapy without regard to their theoretical origins; when clients are matched to treatments in order to maximize therapy outcome, for example, multimodal therapy [25].

Case Study (1) Anxiety and Stress in Pregnancy

Julie and her partner Tom had been trying to conceive for several months, and after what seemed like an eternity, Julie conceived, and this was confirmed by a pregnancy test. They decided not to tell any family members or friends until Julie had had a dating scan. Julie, accompanied by Tom, went to have a first antenatal contact visit with a midwife at the local health centre. From her last menstruation, her expected date for birth was calculated and her pregnancy gestation was estimated to be nearly 8 weeks. The dating scan was arranged to take place in a month's time and Julie was also made a further appointment for a booking appointment for the week before the scan appointment. Julie and Tom were given a contact number if any problems should happen in the mean time.

Unknown to Tom and the midwife, Julie had had a termination of pregnancy, five years earlier. Julie chose not to disclose this information. However, she began to worry about this and steadily over the next few weeks of her pregnancy became more and more anxious. She developed several symptoms associated with anxiety and stress. She became increasingly nervous and had problems sleeping. Julie had difficulty concentrating at work, had a dry mouth and felt palpations. She was feeling nauseated and felt physically sick. She made an appointment to see her General Practitioner (GP) and was advised to take some sick leave until she felt better. Tom was concerned about Julie's health and increasing anxiety but reassured himself that it was due to the pregnancy and would subside.

Whilst Julie was on sick leave, her mother (Ann) became concerned and suspected that her daughter maybe pregnant and decided to visit her at home. On the morning her mother decided to visit, Julie had had a small vaginal bleed and was displaying panic symptoms; becoming increasingly distressed she started to hyperventilate and became very frightened and felt like she was going to die. Her mother held her in her arms and was able to calm her down. Julie began to cry and confirmed her mother's suspicion that she was pregnant. She informed her mother that she had had a vaginal bleed that morning and she felt it was all her fault. Her mother telephoned the contact number that was given to Julie and a viability scan was arranged for later that day. Julie became increasingly anxious again and kept repeating that it was all her fault as she had had a termination. Her mother reassured her that it was not her fault and made her a cup of tea. Julie's mother was aware of Julie's termination and advised her to disclose this information to the ultrasonographer during the viability scan and seek advice as to whether this vaginal bleed was linked to the termination. Julie felt too ashamed to disclose this information and declined to ask the ultrasonographer. The scan confirmed a viable pregnancy and this temporarily reassured her. Julie's mother was still concerned about her state of mind and encouraged her to seek help. She made an appointment to see her GP and an appointment with a psychotherapist was arranged. Julie was taught some coping techniques to help her when she was feeling panicky and anxious. She learnt about the biological basis of her symptoms and how to develop some helpful ways to reduce her anxiety and induce a calm state. Some mindfulness, deep relaxation and self-hypnosis techniques were taught and practised during a series of sessions. During this time Julie utilized mindfulness techniques that she was taught which enabled her to become aware of the incoming thoughts and her shame and guilt feelings, accepting them, without attaching, judging or reacting to them. This new free feeling of detachment from her strong emotions allowed her to disclose her termination to her midwife and coped fairly well with the remainder of her pregnancy. She continued to use some mindfulness, deep relaxation techniques and self-hypnosis following the birth of a live baby girl and joined a local support group for mums where she gained some peer support.

Pregnant and New Mothers from CALD Backgrounds

There is good evidence that high levels of anxiety and stress, and/or depression during pregnancy, whether diagnosed or not, predict various adverse physical and psychological health outcomes for mother and infant from all ethnic backgrounds [26, 27]. Christian [28] has highlighted that environmental stressors such as, low socioeconomic status, stressful life events, daily hassles, past traumatic experiences, racial discrimination, disconnection from cultural and ethnic roots and domestic violence can lead to subjective distress; but coping resources, such as social support, reconnecting to religion and spirituality and self-efficacy are helpful.

It is, therefore, not too surprising that a meta-analysis reported a higher risk of adverse birth outcomes for pregnant women from developing countries who had a lower socioeconomic status and now residing in the US and were suffering from depression [29]. In addition, when a pregnant woman experiences traumatic events, both natural (hurricanes, earthquakes, floods) and man-made (terrorist attacks, bomb blasts), these are also associated with poor pregnancy outcomes [27]. Therefore, when considering susceptibility to mental health problems and the need for psychotherapy, special considerations are required for migrant and refugee pregnant and new mothers.

Special Considerations of Migrant and Refugee Women

Research exploring pregnancy and postnatal experiences of recent immigrants and refugees has focused on pregnancy outcomes, mental health and access/utilization of health services [30]. According to the literature, women from recent immigrant and refugee communities are particularly at risk of poor pregnancy outcomes and suffer higher rates of maternal complications and interventions such as gestational diabetes, caesarean section, postpartum haemorrhage, perineal trauma, all leading to a greater risk of postnatal depression [31, 32, 33].

Migration and pregnancy are both major life events; hence, it can be reasonably hypothesized that pregnant women who are also recent migrants experience environmental stressors and adverse life events over and above mainstream women. Pregnant women from CALD backgrounds may encounter discrimination, unemployment, underemployment, acculturation stress and social isolation. In addition, women with refugee backgrounds may have experienced severe trauma (torture, rape, serious injury), loss or separation from family members and may continue to worry about the safety of their family left behind. Pregnant women seeking asylum often find themselves in limbo, have heightened stress about their asylum applications being rejected and being returned to the countries they fled. Not surprisingly, they are prone to anxiety and stress and/or depression. These vulnerable pregnant women will be very anxious about giving birth in an unfamiliar environment, with lack of support from family or friends, unable to engage in culturally familiar behaviours and rituals relating to childbirth.

Social isolation during and after pregnancy has been identified as a major cause of mental distress among immigrant mothers. Being socially isolated and separated from their families was a contributing factor to their poor mental health status [30]. These mothers reported not having time to connect to their own community groups or join multicultural groups. Their inadequate English-language skills prevented greater engagement with community workers and health services.

An Australian report that reviewed pregnancy and post-birth experiences of women from refugee backgrounds identified communication as the most significant challenge to address [35]; language difficulties, lack of translated information and issues surrounding cultural responsiveness were highlighted. In addition, accredited interpreters were not always available at antenatal appointments, during the birthing experience, when completing consent forms or during postnatal home visits.

It has been shown that professional accredited interpreters can improve clinical outcomes for immigrant women with limited English proficiency [35]. Offering this service enables this vulnerable cohort of women to feel less anxious and have a better understanding of maternity care. Correa-Velez and Ryan [36] have identified an urgent need for adequate education programmes for immigrant women regarding antenatal and postnatal care to reduce anxiety and stress and also increase awareness of services.

Alongside this identified need, it is also important for health professionals to have education and an understanding of different cultural practices; to enable them to respond to individual needs of pregnant and new mothers from CALD backgrounds and support them in either practising their cultural norms or adopting the ways of their second culture [30]. Culture and ethnicity can influence the concepts of health and well-being during the childbirth continuum and therefore these attributes need to be considered when mental health problems have been identified and a referral for psychotherapy is being recommended.

Psychotherapy: Cultural and Ethnic Considerations

Psychotherapy, as a product of western civilization, often reflects the western cultural context [37]. Many psychotherapists have received training developed for western communities and therefore are limited in their approaches to provide culturally appropriate forms of therapy. As a result, psychotherapy may not always meet the needs of pregnant and new mothers from CALD backgrounds. Alongside the issue of stigma and shame associated with mental health, the lack of cultural and ethnic appropriate therapies can lead to CALD pregnant

Case Study (2) –PTSD Following an Emergency Caesarean Section

Mairo, a recent immigrant from Abuja, Nigeria, had an emergency caesarean section (CS) for fetal distress. Everything seemed to happen so fast; one minute everything seemed to be fine and then all of a sudden her baby's heart was erratic, beating very fast then a lot slower than what is within the normal fetal heart range (100–160 bpm). All she remembers is being wheeled on a trolley to the operating theatre and the anaesthetist inserting a tube down her throat; she could hear voices and could not move. Her last thoughts were I'm going to die and my baby too. When Mairo awoke from the general anaesthetic she did not know where she was or where her baby was. She then saw her partner Dapu, who smiled and reassured her that everything was fine and that their baby boy was healthy. Their baby had been admitted to the neonatal intensive care unit for some observations and the next day was transferred to the postnatal ward to be with Mairo. Two days later, both Mairo and her baby were transferred home to receive postnatal care in the community.

Everything seemed to be progressing normally and Mairo was recovering from her CS; baby was breastfeeding and fixing on well and settling. However, Mairo was having some problems sleeping. When she closed her eyes she could see herself being wheeled on the trolley to theatre and the anaesthetist trying to intubate her. She could not breathe, felt like she was suffocating, started to feel panicky and her heart was pounding. She also had begun to have flashbacks of being assaulted and robbed in her home city Abuja, where she had also struggled to breathe when a stranger had grabbed her from behind and put his hand over her mouth. Mairo did not tell anyone how she was feeling. During the week that followed she became increasingly tired and weepy due to lack of sleep and the flashbacks she was having. She started to feel more and more anxious, having palpitations, sweaty hands and a dry mouth. Her mother and partner became increasingly worried about her. The following week Mairo was becoming increasingly stressed, showing signs of exhaustion and could not breastfeed her baby. A midwife visited and was concerned about Mairo's well-being; she arranged for Mairo to see her GP. Her GP suspected PTSD and possibly postnatal depression as a comorbidity. Mairo was prescribed some antidepressants and referred to see a psychotherapist. PSTD was confirmed by the psychotherapist following an initial assessment being undertaken and upon Mairo disclosing her symptoms and later her traumatic experiences. A combination of narrative therapy, some mindfulness and CBT techniques were used to manage Mairo's symptoms and help to reduce her anxiety and stress. She developed some coping strategies to counteract her anxiety and fears. After a few sessions she began to feel better and was able to sleep. A few weeks later, the flashbacks became less frequent and she started to relax more. She had stopped breastfeeding but was bonding with her baby well. She was able to go out and started to feel less anxious and fearful; she stopped taking antidepressants. Three months later she stopped seeing the psychotherapist and was adjusting to motherhood well.

and new mothers being less likely to access and utilize psychotherapy, withdraw from therapy or fail to indicate improvement. However, researchers and practitioners have been advocating for changes in the mental health system to better match or fit with the cultural lifestyle and experiences of CALD people.

This led to the concept of cultural competence being developed. Cultural competence is the ability of systems, agencies and practitioners to provide care and deliver services to effectively meet the needs of a culturally, socially and linguistically diverse population [37].

Cultural competency regarding psychotherapy can be achieved by modifying or adapting existing psychotherapies or developing new treatments for specific cultural groups [38]. There is some evidence of traditional psychotherapies, such as CBT, being successfully modified to meet the needs of culturally and ethnically diverse populations. Some therapies have been specifically developed for a particular ethno-cultural group, for example: folk healing, network therapy, ethnic narratives and liberation psychology-psychotherapy [39]. Therefore, psychotherapy that is specifically adapted to meet the needs of CALD pregnant and new mothers will promote better engagement in therapy, with a resulting improvement in mental health status.

Building Resilience for Better Maternal Mental Health

Building resilience to promote better health and well-being is an important aspect for maternal healthcare. Mind and Mental Health Foundation in the UK recently developed a model for building resilience to promote better mental health [40]. This model involves learning about mood and mind to develop coping strategies, based on principles of mindfulness and CBT, undertaking physical activities such as pram walks, needlework, arts and crafts and social capital aspects, such as befriending and peer support to build self-esteem and confidence [41]. A mixed methods evaluation of this building resilience model piloted with pregnant mothers and new mothers from a diverse population residing in both urban and rural regions of England has demonstrated that this combined approach to promote well-being is effective [42]. This approach has been designed to fill a gap in maternity services and focuses on preventative ways to maintain and manage maternal mental health.

Conclusions

Maternal health and well-being is an important aspect of women's healthcare. Pregnant and new mothers can be at increased risk of developing mental health problems. Socioeconomic and life events can take their toll and increase levels of anxiety and stress during pregnancy and the transition to motherhood. Pregnant and new mothers from CALD backgrounds are at increased risks of developing or exacerbating mental health problems. Previous experiences of trauma and birth trauma can also put mothers at further risk.

Psychotherapy can help pregnant and new mothers to feel better about themselves and enable them to develop coping strategies to deal with life problems and traumatic events more effectively. Psychotherapy can be adapted to meet the needs of pregnant and new mothers from CALD backgrounds. Cultural competence is an important aspect of health professionals' education and practice. It is essential to provide care and deliver maternity services to effectively meet the needs of a culturally, socially and linguistically diverse population.

Supporting pregnant women and new mothers who are particularly at risk of mental health problems to build resilience and stay well is an important preventative measure that has been identified. A combined approach to promote well-being appears to be effective. Physical activities, developing coping strategies based on the principles of psychotherapy and strong social networks all contribute to the promotion of better maternal mental health.

Key Points

- There are five broad approaches to psychotherapy: Psychoanalysis/ Psychodynamic, behaviour, cognitive, humanistic and integrative/holistic.
- psychotherapy can be most effective when elements of these different approaches are integrated to meet each client's need.
- Culture and ethnicity can influence the concepts of health and well-being during the childbirth continuum and therefore these attributes need to be considered when mental health problems have been identified and a referral for psychotherapy is being recommended. Cultural competence is the ability of systems, agencies and practitioners to provide care and deliver services to

effectively meet the needs of a culturally, socially and linguistically diverse population.

- A model for building resilience to promote better mental health in pregnant mothers and new mothers has been shown to be effective. This model involves learning about mood and mind to develop coping strategies, based on principles of mindfulness and CBT, undertaking physical activities such as pram walks, needlework, arts and crafts and social capital aspects, such as befriending and peer support to build self-esteem and confidence.

References

1. Steen M & Jones A. Maternal mental health: Stigma and shame. *The Practising Midwife*, 2013; **16**:6, 5.

2. National Institute for Health and Care Excellence (NICE). *Antenatal and postnatal mental health.* Clinical Guideline 45. London: NICE, 2007.

3. Steen M & Green B. Mental health in pregnancy and early parenthood. In: Steen M, Thomas M. (eds.). *Mental health across the life span.* Routledge: Taylor Francis, 2016. 60–87.

4. World Health Organisation (WHO). *Maternal mental health and child health and development,* Geneva: WHO, 2013.

5. Drake M. The physical health needs of individuals with mental health problems – setting the scene. In: Collins E, Drake M, & Deacon M (eds.). *The physical care of people with mental health problems: A guide for best practice,* London: Sage Publications Ltd, 2013. 1–15.

6. NICE. Antenatal care: Routine care for the healthy pregnant woman. CG 62, London, NICE, 2008.

7. Steen M, Jones A, & Woodsworth B. Anxiety, bonding and attachment during pregnancy, the transition to parenthood and psychotherapy. *British Journal of Midwifery*, 2013; **21**:12, 768–774.

8. Accortt EE, Cheadle A, & Dunkel-Schetter C. Prenatal depression and adverse birth outcomes: An updated systematic review. *Maternal and Child Health Journal,* 2014; **19**:6, 1306–1337.

9. Bauer A, Parsonage M, Knapp M, Lemmi V, & Adelaja B. *The costs of perinatal mental health problems.* London: Centre for Mental Health and London School of Economics, 2014.

10. Department of Health. Improving Access to Psychological Therapies (IAPT). *Perinatal: Positive practice guide.* London: Department of Health, 2009. Available at www.uea.ac.uk/documents/246046/11919343/perinatal-positive-practice-guide-2013.pdf/aa054

d07-2e0d-4942-a21f-38fba2cbcceb (Accessed 26 March 2017).

11. American Psychological Association (APA) Different approaches to psychotherapy. www.apa.org/topics/therapy/psychotherapy-approaches.aspx (Accessed 26 March 2017).

12. Skinner BF. *The behavior of organisms: An experimental analysis.* Englewood Cliffs, NJ: Prentice-Hall, 1938.

13. Ellis A. *Reason and emotion in psychotherapy.* New York, NY: Lyle Stuart, 1962.

14. Ellis A. *Reason and emotion in psychotherapy: A comprehensive method of treating human disturbances:* New York NY: Carol Publishing Group, 1994.

15. Beck AT. Cognitive therapy: Nature and relation to behavior therapy. *Behavior Therapy*, 1970; **1**: 184–200. doi: 10.1016/S0005-7894(70)80030–2.

16. Beck AT. *Cognitive therapy and the emotional disorders.* New York, NY: Meridian, 1976.

17. Hollon SD & DiGiuseppe R. Cognitive theories of psychotherapy. In Norcross JC, VandenBos GR, & Freedheim DK (eds.). *History of psychotherapy: Continuity and change.* 2nd ed, Washington, DC: American Psychological Association, 2011. 203–241.

18. Segal Z, Williams J, & Teasdale J. Your guide to Mindfulness-Based Cognitive Therapy.2017. www.mbct.com/ (Accessed 26 March 2017).

19. Harris R & Hayes SC. *ACT made simple: An easy-to-read primer on acceptance and commitment therapy:* Oakland, CA; New Harbinger Publications, 2009. ISBN-10: 1572247053.

20. Psych Central. An Overview of Dialectical Behavior Therapy. *Psych Central*, 2016. http://psychcentral.com/lib/an-overview-of-dialectical-behavior-therapy/ (Accessed 26 March 2017).

21. Watson JC, Goldman RN, & Greenberg LS. Humanistic and experiential theories of psychotherapy, In JC. Norcross, GR. VandenBos, & DK. Freedheim (eds.). *History of Psychotherapy: Continuity and Change*, 2nd ed., Washington, DC: American Psychological Association Books, 2011. 141–172.

22. Goldfried MR, Glass CR, & Arnkoff DB. Integrative approaches to psychotherapy, In JC. Norcross, GR. VandenBos, DK. Freedheim (eds.). *History of Psychotherapy: Continuity and Change*, 2nd ed., Washington, DC: American Psychological Association Books, 2011. 269–296.

23. Segal Z, Williams J, & Teasdale J. *Mindfulness-based cognitive therapy for depression: A new approach to relapse prevention.* New York: Guilford Press, 2002.

24. Hayes SC, Strosahl KD, & Wilson KG. *Acceptance and commitment therapy: An experiential approach to behavior change*: New York: Guilford Press, 1999.

25. Lazarus AA. Multimodal therapy: Technical eclecticism with minimal integration. In: Norcross JC & Goldfried MR (eds.). *Handbook of psychotherapy integration*, 1992.

26. Dunkel-Schetter C. Psychological science on pregnancy: Stress processes, biopsychosocial models, and emerging research issues. *Annual Review of Psychology*, 2011; **62**: 531–558.

27. Guardino CM & Dunkel-Schetter C. Coping during pregnancy: A systematic review and recommendations. *Health Psychology Review*, 2014; **8**:1, 70–94.

28. Christian LM. Stress and immune function during pregnancy an emerging focus in mind-body medicine. *Current Directions in Psychological Science*, 2015; **24**:1, 3–9.

29. Grote NK, Bridge JA, Gavin AR, Melville JL, Iyengar S, & Katon WJ. A meta-analysis of depression during pregnancy and the risk of preterm birth, low birth weight, and intrauterine growth restriction. *Archives of General Psychiatry*, 2010; **67**:10, 1012–1024.

30. Renzaho A & Oldroyd JC. Closing the gap in maternal and child health: A qualitative study examining health needs of migrant mothers in Dandenong, Victoria, Australia. *Maternal and Child Health Journal*, 2014; **18**:6, 1391–1402.

31. Carolan M. Pregnancy health status of sub-Saharan refugee women who have resettled in developed countries: A review of the literature. *Midwifery*, 2010; **26**:4, 407–414.

32. Gibson-Helm ME, Teede HJ, Block AA, Knight M, East CE, Wallace EM, & Boyle JA. Maternal health and pregnancy outcomes among women of refugee background from African countries: A retrospective, observational study. *BMC Pregnancy and Childbirth*, 2014; **14**:1, 392.

33. Murray L, Windsor C, Parker E, & Tewfik O. The experiences of African women giving birth in Brisbane, Australia. *Health Care for Women International*, 2010; **31**:5, 458–472.

34. Each Social & Community Health Report (EACH Report). The pregnancy and post birth experience of women from refugee backgrounds living in the Outer East of Melbourne, 2011.

35. Karliner LS, Jacobs EA, Chen AH, & Mutha S. Do professional interpreters improve clinical care for patients with limited English proficiency? A systematic review of the literature. *Health Services Research*, 2007; **42**:2, 727–754.

36. Correa-Velez I & Ryan J. Developing a best practice model of refugee maternity care. *Women and Birth*, 2012; **25**:1, 13–22.

37. Betancourt JR, Green AR, Carrillo JE, & Ananeh-Firempong O. Defining cultural competence: A practical framework for addressing racial/ethnic disparities in health and health care. *Public Health Reports*, 2003; **118**:4, 293.

38. Kirmayer LJ. Rethinking cultural competence. *Transcultural Psychiatry*, 2012; **49**:2, 149–164. doi: 10.1177/1363461512444673.

39. Comas-Diaz L. Multicultural approaches to psychotherapy. In: Norcross JC, VandenBos GR, & Freedheim DK (eds.), *History of Psychotherapy: Continuity and Change*, 2nd ed. Washington DC: American Psychological Association, 2011.

40. Mind and MHF. Building resilient communities. Making every contact count for public mental health. London: Mind and MHF, 2013.

41. Steen M, Robinson M, Robertson S, & Raine G. Pre and post survey findings from the Mind 'Building resilience programme for better mental health: Pregnant women and new mothers'. *Evidence Based Midwifery*, 2015; 13:3, 92–99.

42. Robinson M, Steen M, Robertson S, & Raine G. *Evaluation of the local Mind resilience programme: Final report*. 2014 www.mithn.org.uk/uploaded_files/c kfinder/files/Final%20Mind%20resilience%20report% 20unemployed%20men%20and%20perinatal%20wom en%202014(1).pdf (Accessed 26 March 2017).

Chapter 37

Biopsychosocial Factors in Intrapartum Care

Leroy C. Edozien

Women's Experiences of Childbirth

Is childbirth simply a matter of the mechanical progress of the baby through the birth canal, or the final exhilarating experience of bringing forth the life which has been nurtured unseen, but felt within, for so many weeks? [1]

Obstetricians and midwives have often concentrated on clinical outcomes and been oblivious of negative psychological experiences of women under their care. After a 'straightforward' instrumental delivery, an obstetrician's perception may be that all is well with the woman. The woman's subjective experience of her care may, however, be that of a psychologically traumatic birth. By adopting a biopsychosocial model of intrapartum care, doctors and midwives can enhance the birth experience of women under their care and achieve optimal clinical outcomes while also securing psychological well-being.

Research conducted in Australia in the 1980s showed that access to information during labour, relationships to care-givers, the extent of women's involvement in decisions about their care and exposure to intervention were critical to women's satisfaction with care [2]. Despite advances in technology, little has changed in the subsequent three decades: recent studies in Western Australia found that pregnant women valued a sensitive, respectful, shared relationship with competent clinicians who aimed to provide woman-focused care [3, 4].

Factor analysis of responses in a survey of mothers in Montreal, Canada [5], identified five dimensions to women's satisfaction: (a) the delivery itself, (b) medical care, (c) nursing care, (d) information received and participation in the decision-making process, and (e) physical aspects of the labour and delivery rooms. Two decades later, the first national survey of women's experience of maternity services in Canada [6] showed that 3 in 4 women were 'very satisfied' with the respect shown to them, the perceived competence of the healthcare providers, the concern shown for their privacy and dignity, and with their personal involvement in decision-making.

In the United Kingdom, 3 in 4 women responding to the 2015 national maternity survey felt that they were always involved enough in decisions about their care during labour and birth, a significant increase since the 2007 national survey, but there were substantial variations between hospitals [7].

A review of studies reporting from developing countries showed that the process of care dominated the determinants of maternal satisfaction [8]. These process determinants included provider behaviour, communication, provision of adequate information, privacy, perceived provider competency and emotional support.

A positive birth experience enhances maternal well-being and mother–child bonding; it reinforces the woman's confidence in herself and lays a good foundation for family health and future childbearing. A negative birth experience is associated with inhibition of breastfeeding, post-traumatic stress disorder (see Chapter 39), fear of birth, delay in having another baby, stress in the next pregnancy and maternal request for a planned caesarean delivery in the absence of medical indications.

A number of instruments are available for assessing women's satisfaction with intrapartum care [9]. These vary in scope and psychometric properties and include the Labour and Delivery Satisfaction Index (LADSI), the Perceptions of Care Adjective Checklist (PCACL-R), the Intrapartal care in relation to WHO recommendations (IC-WHO), Patient Perception Score (PPS, designed for operative births), the Questionnaire to assess clients' satisfaction (CliSQ), the Intrapartal-Specific QPP-questionnaire (QPP-I), the Six Simple Questions (SSQ), Maternal Satisfaction for Caesarean Section (MSCS) and the Consumer Satisfaction Questionnaire (CSQ).

BOX 37.1 Components of a biopsychosocial model of intrapartum care

BOX 37.1 Components of a biopsychosocial model of intrapartum care

P – Person-centred care; culturally sensitive care

R – Relief of pain: optimal, holistic

E – Environment: home or 'home-away-from-home'

C – Continuous midwifery support

E – Education: pre-labour and intrapartum

D – Dysfunctional labour optimally managed

E – Engagement of partner

N – Information giving, during and after labour

C – Consent; informed choice; involvement in decision-making

E – Empathy; compassionate care

The findings of a systematic scoping review of what women want, need and value in pregnancy suggest that current maternity care across the globe might provide only a small proportion of what matters to women and their families [10]. On the basis of their findings, the authors propose a model of care comprising three domains: clinical care/therapeutic practices; relevant and timely information (physiological, biomedical, as well as behavioural and sociocultural); and support (social, cultural, emotional and psychological).

Women's experiences of childbirth, combined with evidence-supported maternity care, provide the framework for a biopsychosocial model of intrapartum care in which the needs of the individual woman are accorded precedence (Box 37.1). The components of this model include pre-labour and intrapartum education of the woman; a salutary environment; continuous support in labour; person-centred and culturally sensitive care; empathic, compassionate care; provision of adequate and tailored information; engagement of the woman in decision-making; a holistic approach to pain relief; engagement of the partner; optimal management of dysfunctional labour and evidence-based management of the first, second and third stages of labour. Each component is discussed in the following sections.

Person-Centred Care

Person-centred care takes into consideration the person's personal preferences, cultural traditions, values and beliefs. Care of the pregnant woman during labour and delivery needs to be tailored to the individual woman and what they would find acceptable within their social values and beliefs.

Doctors and midwives should proactively seek the opinion of the woman in labour, and respect that opinion. The woman should be constructively engaged in decision-making about her care, and decisions about choices such as what to eat and when should be made not solely on the basis of medical opinion but also on the woman's preferences and her culture. Women allowed freedom to adopt the position of their choice – like standing, walking, sitting, kneeling or squatting in the first stage of labour – cope with pain better and show reduced requirements for pain relief. They also feel more in control of their labour and have less anxiety. Similarly, women should be involved in decisions about medical interventions (see section titled 'Consent' below).

The adoption of a person-centred approach helps to build trust and transparency in the relationship between the woman and her midwife and doctor. When a woman in labour receives support from a person she trusts, she enjoys a more conducive environment and has a more positive birth experience.

Environment: Home or 'Home-Away-from-Home'

In the UK – and other countries such as Canada and the USA – most women give birth in hospital, a change from what was the norm about 50 years ago. The change in the birth setting from a familiar home environment to a room on the delivery unit induced a biomedicalization of labour and delivery, with less attention being paid to the psychological and social correlates of childbirth.

Childbirth does not need to be in the obstetric environment for it to be safe. The assurance of a timely referral to specialist services when indicated would allow a woman to labour in a setting away from the obstetric environment but have access to emergency care when needed, and thus be able to avoid or minimize morbidities which could follow from complications of labour and childbirth. As an alternative to the home and obstetric environments, there is the option of birth in a midwifery-led unit. The midwifery-led unit could be freestanding or co-located with an obstetric unit. The rate of intervention in freestanding or alongside midwifery-led units is lower and neonatal outcome is no different compared to an obstetric unit [11].

BOX 37.2 List of NICE intrapartum care quality statements [25]

Statement 1. Women at low risk of complications during labour are given the choice of all birth settings and information about local birth outcomes.

Statement 2. Women in established labour have one-to-one care and support from an assigned midwife.

Statement 3. Women at low risk of complications do not have cardiotocography as part of the initial assessment of labour.

Statement 4. Women at low risk of complications who have cardiotocography because of concern arising from intermittent auscultation have the cardiotocograph removed if the trace is normal for 20 minutes.

Statement 5. Women at low risk of complications are not offered amniotomy or oxytocin if labour is progressing normally.

Statement 6. Women do not have the cord clamped earlier than 1 minute after the birth unless there is concern about cord integrity or the baby's heartbeat.

Statement 7. Women have skin-to-skin contact with their babies after the birth.

Source: National Institute of Health and Care Excellence (NICE). Intrapartum care: NICE quality standard [QS105]. London; NICE, December 2015.

Having a baby is an intense life experience for the woman, so she should be empowered to make decisions regarding her own care and all healthcare persons should respect the woman's choice regarding place of birth and other birth options. National policy and service guidelines seek to minimize medical intervention in uncomplicated labour and the UK National Institute for Health and Care Excellence (NICE) guidance for intrapartum care recommends that low-risk women should be supported in their decision to give birth in a setting of their choice [12]. The NICE guidance also encourages low-risk nulliparous women to consider birth in freestanding or alongside midwifery-led units. For the same reasons, low-risk multiparous women are encouraged to consider birth at home or in a midwifery-led unit (freestanding or alongside). The corresponding NICE Quality Statement stipulates that 'women at low risk of complications during labour are given the choice of all birth settings and information about local birth outcomes' (see Box 37.2).

The 2015 survey of women's experiences of UK maternity care showed that more women (41%) were offered a choice of delivery in a midwife-led unit or birth centre (35% in 2013) [13].

Where possible, women should be granted the choice of labouring and/or delivering in water. For women who take up this option, it is a helpful way of minimizing the anxiety and pain associated with labour and, ultimately, of enhancing the birth experience.

Regardless of where birth takes place, healthcare personnel attending a labour or delivery should possess the appropriate skills for a biopsychosocial model of care.

Education

Doctors and midwives may enhance a woman's birth experience through education. Education provides a basis for informed decision-making and helps to shape expectations. Regrettably, doctors are not usually involved in formal antenatal education sessions.

Childbirth education sessions should cover positioning for labour and delivery, monitoring in labour, pain relief, relaxation techniques, coping skills, nutrition and potential interventions in labour. NICE recommends that nulliparous women should be educated on issues such as how to differentiate between Braxton Hicks contractions and active labour contractions, recognition of amniotic fluid and pain relief. Women should also be provided with information on how to access the midwifery care team in an emergency or when help is needed.

Prenatal education helps to build the woman's confidence in her body's ability to give birth. In technical language, prenatal education strengthens the woman's 'sense of coherence' (SoC). The concept of 'sense of coherence' was derived from the salutogenic approach, which advocates a focus on factors that support human health and well-being, rather than on factors that cause disease. It is the extent to which one is able to use one's personal attributes and social support to maintain and improve health. Higher SoC scores have been found to be an independent protective factor for the prediction of uncomplicated delivery [14].

Continuous Support

The most important intervention proven to be beneficial in labour is for the woman to have continuous presence of a supportive companion. It is hypothesized that psychological support during labour reduces stress and prevents the release of catecholamines, thus improving uterine contractility. Meta-analysis of random allocation trials assessing the effects of continuous, one-to-one intrapartum support compared with usual care shows that women allocated to continuous support had shorter labours [15]. They were more likely to have a spontaneous vaginal birth and less likely to have intrapartum analgesia or to report dissatisfaction. They were less likely to have regional analgesia or a baby with a low five-minute Apgar score.

The companion may be a midwife or, ideally, someone chosen by the woman to support her in labour. A NICE Quality Statement stipulates that 'women in established labour have one-to-one care and support from an assigned midwife' (see Box 37.2).

It is best if continued support was provided by a single midwife, but often it is a team of midwives which provides the 'one-to-one' support in labour. Staff should be introduced when a handover of care takes place, and the woman should be kept informed when her attending midwife takes a break or is deployed elsewhere.

Companionship should be maintained if the woman is transferred from one birth setting to another. NICE recommends that the arrangements for transfer should be explained to the woman and her birth companion(s), and that a midwife who has been involved in her care up to that point should travel with her and carry out a handover of care that involves the woman.

Empathy

Whatever birth setting is chosen, healthcare personnel should ensure that there is a culture of respect for a woman undergoing an intense life experience. The woman should be listened to and cared for with compassion. Women who feel cared for during labour are likely to report their birth experience as a positive one.

The initial assessment of a woman in labour, and her subsequent care, should address her preferences and her emotional and psychological needs. Indicators of actual or impending emotional exhaustion include the woman expressing fear, asking an excessive number of questions, being overly demanding, displaying an antipathy to doctor or midwife or being hypersensitive to touch or suggestions. Particular attention should be paid to the needs of a woman with a history of sexual abuse, neglect, domestic violence, mental health disorder, previous traumatic birth or other sources of chronic stress.

The woman's dignity and privacy should be protected at all times and a private environment to give birth should be provided, with limited access to third parties according to need. Staff and visitors should knock and wait to be invited before entering a woman's room.

Recommended good practice [12] should be followed when conducting a vaginal examination. The recommendations include the following:

- Be sure that the examination is necessary and will add important information to the decision-making process
- Recognize that a vaginal examination can be very distressing for a woman, especially if she is already in pain, highly anxious and in an unfamiliar environment
- Explain the reason for the examination and what will be involved
- Ensure the woman's informed consent, privacy, dignity and comfort
- Explain sensitively the findings of the examination and any impact on the birth plan to the woman and her birth companion(s)

Information Giving

The labouring woman should be given adequate information regarding every intervention and every procedure offered or carried out. She should be given as much information as she desires, and in a language she understands. The information should also be provided to the partner who is providing emotional support to the woman.

The amount of information provided by the doctor or midwife does not have to be overwhelming in order to be adequate. What is more important is that the information is intelligible to the woman and tailored to her needs. Concise and clear explanations of *what* is being proposed (or what is happening), *why* this is necessary, *how* it will be done and *when* it will be done are generally adequate – but often not provided.

Information giving is a critical element in the women's sense of empowerment and control. Women who feel in control of decisions about their care and of unfolding events are more likely to report having a positive birth experience.

Consent

The pregnant woman, like any other recipient of medical treatment, has the right to determine what treatment to accept or to decline. In exercising the right to self-determination in pregnancy care, the woman relies on the information provided by the doctor or midwife, and the right cannot be said to have been upheld if the woman is not in a position to make an informed choice. Unfortunately, interventions are frequently (in some cases, routinely) delivered in the absence of informed choice.

It is not good practice to shove a consent form in front of a woman in the throes of labour when she is *en route* to the operating theatre or after arrival in the theatre [16]. It is likely that the court will deem this woman, who is in severe pain and may even have had a narcotic analgesic, not to be in a position to make a well-considered choice. The way to protect the woman's right to self-determination in such cases is to ensure that all women are provided with pertinent information throughout the care pathway from antenatal care through intrapartum care, so that she is aware of unfolding events and what potential developments and options are in the horizon. That is to say, consent should be viewed not just as an event (the signing of a form) but as a process. Also, a legitimately obtained verbal consent is just as valid as a written one.

If a woman who has capacity declines an intervention after full discussion and explanation, her wish should be respected even if this means that her life or that of the unborn baby would be at risk.

If a doctor performs an illegal operation, he or she cannot use the patient's consent to the operation as an acceptable defence. This is particularly pertinent to female genital cutting/mutilation (FGC/FGM), which is illegal in the Republic of Ireland under the Criminal Justice (Female Genital Mutilation) Act 2012 and in the UK under corresponding legislation (in England, Wales and Northern Ireland the Female Genital Mutilation Act 2003, and in Scotland the Prohibition of Female Genital Mutilation (Scotland) Act 2005). Reversal of a defibulation after childbirth is an offence under this legislation, so a doctor who attempts this at the request or 'consent' of the woman or her husband faces criminal prosecution (see Chapter 9).

Pain Relief

The degree of pain felt or perceived by a woman in labour is influenced by the cultural expectations and emotional state of mind in labour. The continuous presence of a supportive birth attendant reassures and relaxes the woman and she feels less pain and can cope better with labour.

If and when a woman does require pain relief then non-pharmacological forms of pain relief may be preferable to pharmacological forms as first-line analgesia, and the woman should be encouraged to use them as much as possible. Examples of coping mechanisms for labour pain include being as ambulant as possible and trying different positions to achieve more comfort. The woman and her birthing partner should be informed that relaxation techniques like breathing exercises, immersion in water, distraction or visual imagery 'which takes the mother away for a few moments' are known to be effective in reducing pain in the latent phase of labour. Massage techniques have also been known to help with reducing pain in labour. NICE recommends that aromatherapy, acupressure or yoga should not be offered for pain relief in the acute stage of labour but that if the woman wishes to use them then she should be supported with her wishes [12]. Transcutaneous electrical nerve stimulation is of little beneficial effect in established labour.

Encouraging the woman to say how well she is coping with the pain of labour also helps her in dealing with it. Psychologically expressing pain provides a way of coping with it.

Pain associated with interventions should be minimized. All necessary examinations should be done in a sensitive manner and in between contractions to reduce pain.

Entonox (a mixture of 50:50 oxygen and nitrous oxide) should be made available in birth settings, but women should be informed that it could make them feel dizzy or lightheaded.

Opioid analgesia is commonly used. Opioids help in reducing pain of labour but could make the woman sleepy and could potentially slow down the birth process. They also potentially make the baby sleepy after birth, especially if the injection is administered within an hour of delivery, and thus could interfere with the establishment of breastfeeding.

Epidural analgesia provides the most effective pain relief but is associated with an increase in prolonged labour and the need for instrumental deliveries. The woman is not able to feel contractions and not able to push in response to her contractions. Maternal mobility in labour is severely hampered by a regional anaesthetic and the woman may experience backache and headaches after the epidural, which hamper with mother–baby bonding in the postnatal period. For some women these may detract from the birth experience.

Further research is needed before categorical statements can be made regarding the value of aromatherapy and hypnosis in the management of labour pain [17, 18]. Massage, acupuncture or acupressure, relaxation and yoga may have a role in reducing childbirth pain and/or improving the birth experience, but further research is needed [19–21].

Notwithstanding the pros and cons of the different forms of pain relief, the woman should be given adequate informational and instrumental support in her choice of pain relief.

Engagement of Partner

The woman's partner is usually (but not invariably) in a good position to support her during labour and, as discussed above, such support is associated with good clinical and psychological outcomes. Engagement of the partner during pregnancy and delivery enhances the prospects of his continuing involvement in the care of the offspring during childhood and this in turn has an impact on the child's cognitive and behavioural development.

Separate from their role in supporting the woman in labour, men have their own anxieties and needs as they play out this role. Some men may feel that they are under pressure to attend the birth, to comply with societal expectations. Enforced attendance at women's labour puts partners at risk of psychological disturbances if staff do not pay sufficient attention to partners' expectations, fears and needs. Witnessing a birth that is traumatic, or perceived as traumatic, can leave the partner with long-term psychological problems. Post-traumatic stress, depression and negative effect on the relationship and on sex life have been reported in the aftermath of traumatic deliveries.

A meta-synthesis of the pertinent literature showed that men expressed a strong desire to support their partners and to be fully engaged but their experience of maternity care was often as 'not-patient and not-visitor' [22]. Fathers see themselves as much more than just passive supporters for their partners; they want to be authentically engaged. Fathers struggle to balance their own unknown and uncertain journey to fatherhood with the desire to provide some certainty and support for the mother. Their expectation of active engagement leads to profound trauma where events do not go well (clinical events or dehumanizing behaviour from staff). A study in Canada showed differences in mothers' and fathers' birth satisfaction, highlighting the need to take into account the birth experience of each parent [23].

Health professionals' beliefs about the father's role and the way they treat men affect both how engaged the partner feels and how comfortable he is giving support to the mother. Doctors and midwives who adopt a family-centred approach are more likely to engage partners than those who only see a pregnant woman as their concern. The engagement of partners could also be inhibited, if not forestalled, by safeguarding concerns. Sometimes, the midwife or doctor may find it difficult to distinguish the intentions of a man who is simply being keen or concerned about his partner's well-being and their baby's safety from those of a man who is manifesting a controlling streak. Good communication skills will help to resolve the dilemma.

Dysfunctional Labour

The term 'dysfunctional labour' refers to the stalling of cervical dilatation in the active phase of labour or arrest of fetal descent in the second stage of labour. The rate of cervical dilatation is stalled if it is slower than one centimetre per hour, in association with irregular or weak uterine contractions. Arrest of descent is diagnosed if there is no change in the station of the bony presenting part or if the baby is not delivered after one hour of active pushing.

This is not just a mechanical issue. It may be caused or prevented by biopsychosocial factors, and may cause psychological problems. Women can feel more negative about a birth if they perceive labour as being prolonged [24]. As dysfunctional labour is more common in nulliparous women, this means that a substantial proportion of first-time mothers are potentially at risk of negative birth experience, so doctors and midwives should be mindful of this risk.

The progress of labour should be plotted on a partogram and discussed with the woman. She should be reassured by the midwife or doctor if labour is progressing normally. This keeps up the morale and confidence of the woman. Where progress of labour is slow, appropriate and timely intervention should be offered. Malposition, feto-pelvic disproportion and asynclitism should be excluded.

The first step in preventing dysfunctional labour is to create a calm, friendly environment, make the women feel psychologically secure and enhance her SoC (see discussion under 'Education' above). The use of a bath, ball or other means of promoting comfort should be encouraged.

The woman should be encouraged to be mobile in early labour and to change positions regularly during labour. The dorsal position is associated with weaker contractions, compared to other positions, and may cause supine hypotension. In cases of occipito-posterior position, it may inhibit rotation to occipito-anterior position. The range of alternative positions available to the woman include lateral, knee-chest, hands and knees, standing, semi-prone and leaning (on a chair, ball or partner) positions.

Dehydration inhibits uterine contraction. A full bladder not only predisposes to dysfunctional labour but also may cause long-term urinary incontinence (detrusor instability). The woman should drink appropriate fluids (isotonic fluids) during labour to maintain hydration, and the bladder should be emptied hourly.

Traditionally, women were not allowed to eat in labour, for fear of the risk of gastric aspiration syndrome were they to require a general anaesthetic during delivery. It is now believed that stomach contents would be less acidic if women were to have a light diet in labour, and women are now given a choice whether (and what) they would like to eat and drink in labour. This helps women feel more in control of their labour. The risk of maternal ketoacidosis secondary to starvation is also reduced. Women with high-risk labour are offered histamine H2-receptor antagonist (ranitidine) to reduce the stomach acid formation in labour.

While early recognition and management of dysfunctional labour are important, unnecessary augmentation with oxytocin should be avoided. In one study, some women progressing well in labour received treatment for prolonged labour while some women with prolonged labour were not treated [24]. Unnecessary use of oxytocin puts the woman at risk of needing additional pain relief (in particular, epidural analgesia) and at risk of interventions for fetal distress.

Conclusion

Childbirth is a unique event in the life of the mother and her partner. It has effects on marital relationships, mother–child bonding and the psychological health of the mother. In severe situations, a bad experience during labour may bring about a revulsion to childbirth and affect the woman's perceptions of self as a woman and mother. Women want good clinical outcomes for themselves and their babies but they also want to be treated humanely, with dignity and with respect for their right to self-determination. A biopsychosocial approach to intrapartum care combines the best available evidence with person-centred care to achieve the best clinical and psychological outcomes for the woman, her partner and their baby.

Key Points

- By adopting a biopsychosocial model of intrapartum care, doctors and midwives can enhance the birth experience of women under their care and achieve optimal clinical outcomes while also securing psychological well-being.
- Birth experience has implications for maternal well-being, mother–child bonding, family health and future childbearing.
- Women's experiences of childbirth, combined with evidence-supported maternity care, provides the framework for a biopsychosocial model of intrapartum care in which the needs of the individual woman are accorded precedence.
- Regardless of where birth takes place, healthcare personnel attending a labour or delivery should possess the appropriate skills for a biopsychosocial model of care.
- Doctors and midwives should proactively seek the opinion of the woman in labour, and respect that opinion. Women who feel cared for during labour are likely to report their birth experience as a positive one.

- Information giving is a critical element in the woman's sense of empowerment and control, and her satisfaction with care in labour.
- Dysfunctional labour may cause or be caused by biopsychosocial factors. The first step in its prevention is enhancement of the woman's 'sense of competence'.

References

1. Prince J, Adams ME. *The Psychology of Childbirth.* An introduction for Mothers and Midwives. Second edition. Edinburgh; Churchill Livingstone 1987, p59.

2. Brown S, Lumley J, Small R, Astbury J. *Missing Voices, The Experience of Motherhood.* Melbourne; Oxford University Press 1994, p78.

3. Lewis L, Hauck YL, Ronchi F, Crichton C, Waller L. Gaining insight into how women conceptualize satisfaction: Western Australian women's perception of their maternity care experiences. *BMC Pregnancy Childbirth* 2016;**16**:29. doi: 10.1186/s12884-015-0759-x.

4. Jenkins MG, Ford JB, Morris JM, Roberts CL. Women's expectations and experiences of maternity care in NSW–what women highlight as most important. *Women Birth* 2014;**27**(3):214–9. doi: 10.1016/j.wombi.2014.03.002.

5. Seguin L, Therrien R, Champagne F, Larouche D. The components of women's satisfaction with maternity care. *Birth* 1989;**16**:109–13. doi: 10.1111/j.1523-536X.1989.tb00878.x.

6. Public Health Agency of Canada. What Mothers Say: The Canadian Maternity Experiences Survey. Ottawa, 2014. Available at www.phac-aspc.gc.ca/rhs-ssg/survey-eng.php. Accessed 27 March 2017.

7. Care Quality Commission. Survey of women's experiences of maternity care. CQC. December 2015.

8. Srivastava A, Avan BI, Rajbangshi P, Bhattacharyya S. Determinants of women's satisfaction with maternal health care: A review of literature from developing countries. *BMC Pregnancy Childbirth* 2015;**15**:97. doi: 10.1186/s12884-015-0525-0.

9. Sawyer A, Ayers S, Abbott J, Gyte G, Rabe H, Duley L. Measures of satisfaction with care during labour and birth: A comparative review. *BMC Pregnancy Childbirth* 2013;**13**:108. doi: 10.1186/1471-2393-13-108.

10. Downe S, Finlayson K, Tunçalp Ö, Metin Gülmezoglu A. What matters to women: A systematic scoping review to identify the processes and outcomes of antenatal care provision that are important to

11. Sandall J, Soltani H, Gates S, Shennan A, Devane D. Midwife-led continuity models versus other models of care for childbearing women. *Cochrane Database Syst Rev* 2015;**9**:CD004667. doi: 10.1002/14651858.CD004667.pub4.

12. National Institute of Health and Care Excellence (NICE). Intrapartum care for healthy women and babies. NICE guidelines [CG190]. London; NICE, December 2014.

13. Care Quality Commission. NHS patient survey programme. 2015 survey of women's experiences of maternity care. Newcastle; Care Quality Commission, December 2015.

14. Oz Y, Sarid O, Peleg R, Sheiner E. Sense of coherence predicts uncomplicated delivery: A prospective observational study. *J Psychosom Obstet Gynecol* 2009;**30**:29–33.

15. Hodnett ED, Gates S, Hofmeyr GJ, Sakala C. Continuous support for women during childbirth. *Cochrane Database Syst Rev* 2013;7:CD003766. doi: 10.1002/14651858.CD003766.pub5.

16. Edozien LC. Self-determination in childbirth: The law of consent. In O'Mahony D, (Ed,). *Medical Negligence and Childbirth.* Dublin; Bloomsbury Professional, 2015.

17. Smith CA, Collins CT, Crowther CA. Aromatherapy for pain management in labour. *Cochrane Database Syst Rev* 2011;(7):CD009215. doi: 10.1002/14651858.CD009215.

18. Madden K, Middleton P, Cyna AM, Matthewson M, Jones L. Hypnosis for pain management during labour and childbirth. *Cochrane Database Syst Rev* 2012;**11**:CD009356. doi: 10.1002/14651858.CD009356.pub2.

19. Smith CA, Collins CT, Crowther CA, Levett KM. Acupuncture or acupressure for pain management in labour. *Cochrane Database Syst Rev* 2011;(7):CD009232. doi: 10.1002/14651858.CD009232.

20. Smith CA, Levett KM, Collins CT, Jones L. Massage, reflexology and other manual methods for pain management in labour. *Cochrane Database Syst Rev* 2012;2:CD009290. doi: 10.1002/14651858.CD009290.

21. Smith CA, Levett KM, Collins CT, Crowther CA. Relaxation techniques for pain management in labour. *Cochrane Database Syst Rev* 2011;(**12**):CD009514. doi: 10.1002/14651858.CD009514.

22. Steen M, Downe S, Bamford N, Edozien L. Not-patient and not-visitor: A metasynthesis fathers' encounters with pregnancy, birth and maternity care. *Midwifery* 2012;**28**(4):362–71. doi: 10.1016/j.midw.2011.06.009.

healthy pregnant women. *BJOG* 2016;**123**(4):529–39. doi: 10.1111/1471-0528.13819.

23. Bélanger-Lévesque MN, Pasquier M, Roy-Matton N, Blouin S, Pasquier JC. Maternal and paternal satisfaction in the delivery room: A cross-sectional comparative study. *BMJ Open* 2014;**4**(2):e004013. doi: 10.1136/bmjopen-2013–004013.

24. Nystedt A, Hildingsson I. Diverse definitions of prolonged labour and its consequences with sometimes subsequent inappropriate treatment. *BMC Pregnancy Childbirth* 2014;**14**:233. doi: 10.1186/1471–2393-14–233.

Chapter 38

Biopsychosocial Factors in Postnatal Care

Caroline Hunter and Hannah Rayment-Jones

The birth of a baby is usually a time to celebrate for most women and their families. However, it is also a period of significant transition and adaptation that may trigger a variety of challenges to the physical and psychological health, well-being and social status of women. For some women and families, it can also be a time of loss and grief. Provision and planning of effective, high-quality care for women and babies in the postnatal period could be improved by the application of a model which acknowledges the influence of psychological, sociological, environmental and biological factors in women's well-being and seeks to understand the associations between these elements. Whilst provision of postnatal care may vary widely in terms of where it takes place, who provides it and for how long, similarities with respect to the impact of childbirth on maternal postnatal health have been reported in a range of high-income country settings regardless of the health system in which women have given birth. Therefore, the biopsychosocial challenges women and their families might face in the first year of their child's life will be explored here with a focus on how healthcare professionals can offer support throughout this transition to positively influence women's mental and physical health and well-being, bonding and infant development.

Birth in high-income countries is increasingly safe in terms of obstetric outcomes. However, indicators of postnatal maternal morbidity are also high [1–3]. Whilst for most women health problems will be non-life-threatening, they may still cause pain, distress or anxiety, impact negatively on their daily lives and persist well beyond the 6–8 week postnatal period [4]. For others, the consequences of physical and psychological ill-health after the birth of a baby may be more serious and could inform decisions about future pregnancies and mode of birth. As more women become pregnant with co-existing chronic health issues such as diabetes, cardiac disease or obesity, the complexity of their healthcare needs in the postnatal period and beyond increases. Data from the UK triennial confidential enquiries into maternal deaths demonstrate the reality that the postnatal period is the time when women face increased risk of morbidity and mortality, with over 51% of maternal deaths in the UK occurring within the first six weeks post-birth [3]. Despite this, the content, timing and provision of postnatal care have been neglected, with limited change to provision of care other than reductions in the duration of in-patient stay [5].

Women are not only at risk from medical or obstetric complications after giving birth. Increasingly, evidence demonstrates associations between physical and psychological health, emotional well-being and social support, suggesting that poor mental health, isolation, poor-quality relationships or low socio-economic status are as likely to impact on the well-being of women as physical morbidity. Furthermore, the evidence illustrates that these factors do not stand alone but rather are intertwined with, promote and influence each other [1, 6, 7]. Maternal health and well-being must therefore be understood within the context of all these influences in order to plan and provide the most effective care for women and babies. Postnatal care that ignores or marginalizes the role of emotional and/or social aspects may severely impact on a woman's experiences of early motherhood and influence her future reproductive and longer-term health.

The importance of timely, effective and appropriate postnatal care to support the well-being of women and their families is a key tenet of current UK maternity policy [8], with effective care viewed as essential to improve the life-course health of women and their infants [9]. The last decade has seen government policy in England reflect concerns that this well-being should not be limited merely to physical recovery but should also encompass psychological and social factors [8, 10, 11]. However, despite policy recommendations and the changing health profile of women giving birth in the UK, the only changes in the timing, content and structure of UK postnatal care over the last 20–30 years include much earlier discharge from hospital (within 48 hours or less) [12] and fewer community-based contacts from a midwife or other healthcare provider when emotional health and support could be evaluated and promoted [13]. A Cochrane systematic review reported maternity care in UK settings as highly fragmented, with social isolation prevalent for significant numbers of women [3, 14]. The review found that little evidence exists to suggest that current service provision is adequate for meeting health needs or indeed that guidelines and recommendations are being routinely implemented [15].

In many areas, limited resources directed to postnatal services have resulted in a task-oriented 'tickbox' schedule of care, mainly focused on markers of physical recovery, with little attention paid to psychological well-being or the availability of supportive social structures around postnatal women [16]. Women can be left feeling isolated, ignored, unsatisfied with their care and unprepared for the challenges of motherhood [14, 17]. In some cases where physical, mental or social issues are not identified, the consequences for women can be serious, long-lasting and even fatal [3].

The Structure of Postnatal Care

NICE guidelines for routine postnatal care [8] define the postnatal period as the 6–8 weeks following the birth of the baby, although there is no evidence base to inform this definition of 'postnatal'. The end of maternity care is usually signified by the '6-week check' of mother and baby which is offered to all women who give birth in the UK and is usually carried out by the family doctor. The implication is that most women will have physically recovered from the birth by this time and will be adapting to their new role. Indeed, midwifery care – in the form of home visits from the midwife, a clinic appointment or follow-up telephone call – will have ceased much earlier (around 10–14 days post-birth) for the majority of new mothers. However, the assumption inherent in this routine provision of care, that the postnatal period of recovery and adjustment is similar for all women, has been challenged by several authors [2, 18, 19] who suggest that the postnatal period should be revised to last beyond 6 weeks and up to a year post-birth if women's health needs are to be better met. It seems likely that

the prescriptive definition of the postnatal period as lasting less than 2 months is insufficient to capture the variety of maternal experience even for those mothers with an apparently straightforward physical recovery from birth and who have not experienced any problems with adaptation to motherhood.

The majority of women who have had a vaginal birth in a UK hospital will be discharged home with their baby within 6–24 hours, whilst those who have undergone a planned or emergency caesarean section will usually be discharged by day two or three after delivery [12]. This represents a significant decrease in the length of postnatal stay since the 1970s and 1980s, when women could expect to spend several days in hospital after birth. Despite its almost universal adoption within UK postnatal services, the subject of 'early discharge' has been a controversial one. It has been suggested that decreased length of hospital stay promotes a more family-centred approach to postnatal care, moving its focus from the inflexible routines of the medical model back towards the domestic, social sphere and allowing closer involvement with the woman's social and psychological support networks from an early point. Women may find it easier to sleep, eat and maintain necessary standards of personal hygiene in their own, familiar environment. Continuity of contact from a community midwife, as opposed to various members of staff covering differing shifts, may reduce the amount of conflicting advice a woman receives in the early days and increase her confidence and self-efficacy, particularly around issues such as breastfeeding [20, 21].

Negative aspects have been identified in the literature as possible consequences of early hospital discharge, namely a reduction in maternal confidence, a lower initiation and continuation of breastfeeding, increasing incidence of postnatal depression and reduced detection of morbidity leading to an increase in readmissions from the community [22, 23]. These are significant issues that may affect a woman's functioning beyond the initial postnatal period and should be regarded as potential public health concerns. It must also be acknowledged that widespread implementation of reduced postnatal hospital stays are more likely to reflect resourcing issues than evidence-based practice focused on the women's needs; a return to longer postnatal stays is unlikely due to current demographic and policy drivers [17]. Of interest, the Cochrane review of clinical trials by Brown et al (2002) found that early postnatal discharge did not appear to have a negative impact on markers such as continuation of breastfeeding or on rates of postnatal depression [13].

With this in mind, it is essential to consider the efficacy of postnatal care offered to women and babies at home following hospital discharge. A Cochrane review by Yonemoto et al (2014) found no evidence that home visits from a midwife were associated with improvements in maternal and neonatal morbidity, and no strong evidence that more postnatal visits at home were associated with improvements in maternal health [24]. However, the findings of the 2002 UK trial by MacArthur et al were reported incorrectly in this review; rather than reporting that a new model of community-based midwifery care was associated with *more positive* mental health outcomes as assessed using the EPDS and SF-36 at 4 months postnatally [18], the reviewers reported a *negative* association (see comment on published review by MacArthur and Bick in 2015). The review did find some evidence that postnatal contacts at home may reduce infant health service utilization in the weeks following the birth, and that more home visits may encourage more women to exclusively breastfeed their babies. There was some evidence that home visits were associated with increased maternal satisfaction with postnatal care. Further analyses from the large community-based trial of a new model of midwifery-led postnatal care published by MacArthur et al (2003) found that the positive impact on maternal mental health outcomes in the intervention arm persisted at 12 months postnatally [25].

Women have reported practical help received from their partners and other family members (particularly their mothers), for example with household chores and infant care, to be of great importance although conversely breastfeeding duration may be affected if a woman's own mother is a main source of advice and support [26]. Providing support for women in caring for their infants in the postnatal period is an important concern with previous research showing that social support can facilitate women's transition to motherhood [21, 27–29], especially among women who find the transition psychologically stressful [30].

Physical Symptoms

Postnatal care traditionally revolves around the surveillance and monitoring of the woman's physiological recovery to a pre-pregnancy state, with women being discharged from maternity care at around 6–8 weeks once involution of the uterus has occurred and heavy lochia has ceased. Women are encouraged to report any concerns they may have about their physical symptoms during postnatal contacts [8]; however, in practice these often remain limited to questions from healthcare providers regarding, for example, perineal discomfort or 'abnormal' bleeding. Whilst often transient, these symptoms should not be viewed in isolation by the healthcare provider. In a 2008 study, Webb et al found a significant and consistent correlation between 'minor' postnatal health problems and measures of emotional well-being, including depressive symptomatology. Over 1,300 women were interviewed at 9 and 12 months postpartum and the study concluded that careful assessment of the physical, functional and emotional health status of women in the year after childbirth may improve the quality of postpartum care [7]. These findings were echoed in an Australian study by Woolhouse et al (2014) who found that women in their study reporting five or more health problems had a six-fold increase in their likelihood of reporting concurrent depressive symptoms at 3 months postpartum than those who reported only one or two symptoms [19]. Over 1,500 women who completed questionnaires at 3, 6 and 12 months postpartum reported being unprepared for the cumulative effects of supposedly minor health issues such as fatigue, backache, sore nipples, headaches or constipation, suggesting that the prevalence of these issues is either not discussed in the antenatal period or, perhaps more likely, is dismissed as 'normal' when reported postpartum.

Physical symptoms apparently unrelated to pregnancy or birth (e.g. colds, pain perception) have also been seen to increase in the postnatal period when women report higher levels of depressive symptomatology or lower levels of satisfaction with social support [1]. Healthcare professionals have a clear role to play in ensuring that the vicious circle of ill-health and emotional distress is arrested by preparing women more effectively for the physical consequences of childbirth and taking their concerns seriously when reported postpartum.

Women have long reported the challenges associated with the first few months postpartum, including the need to respond to their infant's needs whilst recovering physically and emotionally from the pregnancy and birth [31, 32]. It is generally considered that during the first 6 months post-birth, muscle tone and connective tissue restore to the pre-pregnant state. However, the genitourinary system can take much longer to heal, and sometimes may never be restored to its pre-pregnant state; there is a growing evidence base associating childbirth with conditions, including stress urinary incontinence, incontinence of flatus or faeces, uterine prolapse, cystocele and rectocele [33], although it is important that analysis undertaken is able to adjust for potential confounding factors, such as age and parity of a woman. Around a third of women suffer from urinary incontinence after giving birth and around 10% of women experience either frank faecal incontinence or flatus [34]. Researchers have recommended that healthcare professionals discuss birth options during the antenatal period in order to minimize a woman's risk of instrumental birth, and encourage women to practise pelvic floor exercises to reduce the risk of urinary and faecal incontinence [35]. However, Hay-Smith et al's (2008) systematic review concluded that there was not enough evidence to suggest pelvic floor exercises have any long-term effects on incontinence. Worryingly, several studies have reported that women who suffer urinary and/or faecal incontinence are reluctant to report it to a healthcare professional, despite significant disruption to their daily lives and relationships [36, 37]. Reasons behind this non-disclosure include a belief that nothing can be done to improve the incontinence, not knowing who to approach, feelings of embarrassment and shame, and perceiving that healthcare professionals will not be interested [38]. In addition, a large cohort study by Brown et al (2015) found robust evidence that many women experiencing severe symptoms of postpartum incontinence do not receive adequate primary care follow up in the first 12 months postpartum [39].

It can therefore be assumed that other commonly experienced morbidities remain unreported and unidentified due to a postnatal care structure that does not enable women to access ongoing support and treatment or ensure healthcare providers specifically ask women about their health. From a societal perspective, normal physical adjustments and slow healing processes are often overlooked as focus shifts to the infant and the expectation that women should be 'back to normal' within 6 to 8 weeks of giving birth persists. Women in Wray's ethnographic study reported up to a year to physically recover from birth, and that their

own expectations and the societal pressures on them added to feelings of failure and disappointment [40].

Breastfeeding

While the health benefits of breastfeeding for both a woman and her baby are well known [41], the number of UK babies who are still exclusively breastfed at 6 months old remains extremely low at around 1% [12]. The decision whether or not to breastfeed may be a complex one for many women and research suggests that there are myriad influencing factors that affect the initiation and continuation of breastfeeding [42, 43]. Women who choose to breastfeed may face discrimination in an environment that still positions bottle-feeding as the socio-cultural 'norm', and those who choose to feed formula milk to their babies may encounter difficulties negotiating a health service culture wherein 'alternatives to breastfeeding are routinely portrayed as inferior' [44]. The myth of 'the good mother' is intimately connected to infant feeding practices, with women who either choose not to breastfeed or who are unable to maintain breastfeeding beyond a few days or weeks, reporting feelings of inadequacy, shame and guilt [44, 45]. In light of this, some commentators have called for a shift in education around breastfeeding towards a more realistic, family-centred conceptualization of infant feeding choices [44, 46].

In 2013, a systematic review of the literature found that several psychosocial factors were strongly predictive of breastfeeding outcomes [47]. Maternal intention and self-efficacy, social support and mental health status all affect breastfeeding duration. Maternal self-efficacy was examined in five out of the eight studies included in the review, and was found to be the major pre-disposing factor to mothers breastfeeding for the recommended 6 months or more. The review also found that these influencing psychosocial factors could be changed through intervention, suggesting that midwives and other health professionals may have a role to play in enhancing maternal self-efficacy and increasing rates of longer-term breastfeeding. Paying more attention to the diverse values, meanings and emotions around infant feeding within families could help to reconcile health ideals with reality.

Postnatal Mental Health

The transition to parenthood has long been described as a major life crisis and time of significant psychological adjustment [48], with the weeks and months after birth being exciting, tiring and stressful. Although a certain amount of anxiety is expected during significant life changes such as parenthood, for some women these issues are significant risk factors for postnatal depression [30]. It is important that healthcare professionals are able to recognize differences in normal psychological change during this transition, such as 'the baby blues' – a common mood lability, weepiness and irritability lasting a few days in the early postpartum period, and more acute and severe mental illness. As well as anxiety and postnatal depression, women can experience a number of mental health issues during the postpartum period, such as puerperal psychosis, the onset or recurrence of personality disorders, self-harm and eating disorders (NICE, 2014).

Postnatal depression (PND) is known to be the most significant and commonly occurring severe mental health morbidity in the ongoing postnatal period, affecting 7–12% of women over the first year postpartum [49]. The detrimental and sometimes fatal consequences to both maternal well-being and longer-term infant development are significant and have been well documented [50]. PND can compromise maternal functioning and the developing mother–infant relationship in early motherhood at this crucial time [51]. Despite its relatively high incidence, postnatal depression can be difficult to detect, in part because new mothers are often reluctant to report depressive symptoms to healthcare professionals and in part because healthcare professionals do not ask about symptoms. A report from the Royal College of General Practitioners [52] stated that only around half of mothers with perinatal depression and anxiety are identified despite frequent routine contact with a range of primary care services at this time; and even fewer receive adequate treatment'. The most significant factor in the duration of postnatal depression has been found to be the length of delay to early recognition and adequate treatment [53]. Effective interventions for postnatal depression need to be initiated as soon as possible; therefore, early detection is imperative for this to be realized. Evidence reviewed by Khan's 2015 report of perinatal mental health services identified common barriers to identification such as insufficient training, time pressures, a lack of contact and communication between healthcare professionals and women, lack of focus on well-being of mother and baby after 6 weeks

postpartum and women's feelings of dismissal. It was subsequently recommended that equal attention was paid to the well-being and physical health of the entire family, improvement in GP's responses to women who are concerned about their mental health through further training, and support for partners to identify symptoms and raise concerns.

Lifestyle and Expectations

Unrealistic expectations placed on new parents either by society or themselves are a growing concern, with overly optimistic views of parenthood having a detrimental effect on a couple's adjustment to parenthood [54]. These expectations may include the 'perfect pregnancy and birth', self-as-woman (the 'yummy mummy'), infant feeding, sleep patterns and routines, relationships with partner, support from friends and family, physical changes and the child's developmental milestones. The disappointment and frustration felt when these expectations are not met can often be intensified by conflicting advice between healthcare professionals, family members and content of online websites or other social-media sources. Beck's meta-synthesis found that a common theme reported by women suffering from postnatal depression was an incongruity between expectations and the reality of motherhood [51]. The paper concluded that these myths operating amongst health professionals set expectations that are impossible for women to attain and placed their mental health at risk, particularly for development of postnatal depression. Because these harmful myths are so common in our society, women believed that no others shared the same negative experiences and thoughts. They viewed themselves as bad or abnormal mothers who were unable to cope with their new infants, although the likely reality was that they would have benefited from additional support and reassurance. Equally, Harwood's 2007 study of first-time mothers' expectations of parenthood also found that where women's postnatal experiences were negative, compared to their expectations, there was greater depression symptomatology and poorer relationship adjustment.

Parenthood is no longer as central to adulthood as it traditionally was, with more women viewing motherhood as a choice rather than inevitability. Evidence suggests that the more that women see motherhood as just one of a variety of life-course choices they could have taken, the more they seem to blame themselves for the negative feelings they have as they adjust [55]. This coincides with the 'yummy mummy' phenomenon – an unrealistic media representation of celebrity mothers – and intensifies the gap between expectation and reality. The National Childbirth Trust champions the idea of discussion groups with parents-to-be and experienced parents to challenge these ideals, ease pressures and enable new parents to embrace the changes parenthood brings in a more realistic context [14]. Healthcare professionals can also help ease this transition by discussing the expectations and concerns new parents may have, ensuring they are not offering conflicting advice through effective inter-professional communication, and providing new parents with contact details of local support networks. Continuity of carer, for example a named midwife, is invaluable in achieving these recommendations as they are not only known and trusted by families but also able to follow up concerns and refer to specific support in the community [56, 57].

Relationships

Couples' relationships during the postnatal period have been explored and debated in a number of previous studies over recent decades, with limited agreement among researchers about the impact of the transition to parenthood on relationship functioning. Earlier researchers agreed that the stress experienced throughout this transition impacted negatively on the quality of a couple's relationship [48, 58]. However, later research suggested that data are limited to support the view that parenthood negatively affects marital satisfaction [59]. It is generally considered, however, that there are numerous factors – some of which are detailed throughout this chapter – that could influence a couple's relationship in the postnatal period and beyond. High-quality qualitative research studies are providing much more information on those factors that affect this complex transition [60] The importance of this understanding does not only concern parents' relationships and emotional well-being but also infant bonding, attachment and development, with some research suggesting that a child's psychological, social and educational functioning is related to the status and quality of their parent's relationship during their early years [61]. Healthcare professionals

can support couples to maintain healthy relationships by addressing their expectations and promoting constructive communication between parents. These discussions might include issues such as parental roles, finances, childcare, returning to work, support networks, infant temperament and generally how they expect their lives will change. Depending on individual need, some couples may benefit from counselling, although this is not routinely offered in the UK [62].

Learning to Become a Parent

In order for new parents to feel confident in their parenting role and tackle the realities of caring for their new baby, they often need to acquire new knowledge and skills. In 2013, a systematic review of 27 trials focused on the effects of postnatal education on infant general health or care and the parent–infant relationships [63]. Although many of the papers linked positive parenting to healthy child development, the review concluded that the benefits of postnatal education remained unclear, and that larger and better-designed studies are required to confirm or refute this link. It is recognized that for many new parents in western society, the immediate postnatal period is the first opportunity they have had to hold, soothe, teach children and learn from them, whereas in low-income societies that live more simply there is a constant psychological preparation for parenting through social learning and observation [64]. In addition to this, as it is now more common for extended families to live further apart, so many new parents do not have the social support around them to teach them these positive parenting behaviours.

Parent education delivered by health and social care professionals is consequently often the first point of learning for new parents, and it has the potential to play a key role in easing some of the difficulties associated with the transition to parenting as well as affect child development. Although the effectiveness of antenatal parent education remains largely unclear [65], a number of studies of postnatal parent education interventions have been effective in improving parenting and infant outcomes such as maternal-infant interaction, infant language development, parental attitudes and knowledge [66], paternal competence in parenting – including fostering infant cognitive growth and awareness of cues [67] – and use of infant health clinics [68].

Bonding and Attachment

As well as positive parenting, a growing number of studies have linked levels of bonding between parent and infant, with later secure attachment and mental well-being of the child. It is important to remember the difference between the two terms when reviewing literature as they are often confused; attachment refers to an ongoing relationship and the infant's emotional connection to the parent, whereas bonding refers solely to the parents' feelings and connection to the child. The large 'Copenhagen child cohort study' [69] found that disturbances to this relationship, for example postnatal depression, a breakdown in parent's relationship or physical illness, played a major role in infant emotional, behavioral, eating and sleeping disorders. A recent Cochrane review was undertaken to assess the effectiveness of parent–infant psychotherapy as an intervention to improve bonding, attachment and optimal infant development [70]. It concluded that although there seemed to be some promising results associated with the psychotherapy and infant attachment, there were no further benefits related to other outcomes and therefore it was not recommended as a routine treatment for parents and infants. Clinicians nevertheless require an awareness of how parents and infants are bonding due to these disturbances in the postnatal period, playing a significant role in infant development, healthy relationships and family well-being. If detected early, families and clinicians can work together to establish effective care plans and interventions to minimize long-lasting effects. These plans could be as simple as extra support with household chores and childcare to more structured interventions such as counselling and therapy.

Conclusion

Postnatal care remains an overlooked and under-resourced aspect of maternity care, yet its centrality to the health and well-being of women, infants and families in the short- and long-term should not be underestimated. The current model of postnatal care in many countries is unsupported by the evidence around best outcomes for women and their infants, and despite national and international policy drivers which emphasize the need for holistic, flexible care encompassing the physical, emotional and social needs of individual women, they are often still poorly served by routine maternity service provision. Furthermore, despite an understanding from policy-makers that the postnatal period can be a time in which to initiate and support behaviour change to promote health and well-being, the early discharge of women and babies from hospital, a reduction in home-visiting schedules and overstretched community services equally mean that the longer-term care provision required to embed these changes is frequently unavailable.

It can be seen from the issues presented in this chapter that the care of women and infants in the weeks and months after birth is situated within a complex system of social, political and culturally-mediated assumptions around motherhood and the transition to the parental role. Presented with an image of new motherhood as a self-actualizing, fulfilling experience, many women in fact frequently experienced feelings of self-doubt, isolation and inadequacy during the postnatal period. Physical morbidities often go unreported and/or untreated as women feel ill-equipped and unsupported to seek out essential treatment, and a tendency on the part of health professionals to regard such issues as minor and inevitable discomforts. Inadequate or inappropriate care therefore has significant implications across the biopsychosocial model, affecting not just physical health but long-term psychological and social outcomes.

The potential for better outcomes and more holistic, socially relevant care is offered – particularly in the earliest postnatal period – by a continuity-based approach which allows women, families and midwives the chance to develop an effective partnership that can mitigate against some of the most damaging elements of fragmented care delivery. However, postnatal care does not end when the midwife discharges the woman and the transition to parenthood requires the input of professionals across the healthcare spectrum for an extended period. What is required for truly effective postnatal care is a multi-disciplinary approach which gives equal consideration to women's social and psychological needs as well as physical recovery, and acknowledges that the biopsychosocial transition that takes place during this time can have significant repercussions for women and their families for years to come.

Key Points

- Postnatal care, as currently delivered, is often a task-oriented 'tickbox' schedule of care, mainly focused on markers of physical recovery, with little attention paid to psychological well-being or the availability of supportive social structures around postnatal women. With the current model of postnatal care, the opportunity to initiate behaviour change to promote health and well-being is not fully utilized.

- High-quality care for women and babies in the postnatal period calls for the application of a model which acknowledges the influence of psychological, sociological, environmental and biological factors in women's well-being and seeks to understand the associations between these elements.

- Early discharge from hospital after childbirth has advantages and disadvantages. It can promote a more family-centred approach to postnatal care, moving its focus from the rigid routines of the medical model back to the domestic, social sphere and allowing closer involvement of the woman's social and psychological support networks from an early point. The potential disadvantages include reduction in maternal confidence, lower initiation and continuation of breastfeeding, increased incidence of postnatal depression and reduced detection of morbidity leading to an increase in readmissions from the community. A Cochrane review found, however, that early postnatal discharge did not appear to have a negative impact on continuation of breastfeeding or on rates of postnatal depression.

- One in every 3 women suffers from urinary incontinence after giving birth and 1 in 10 women experiences anal incontinence. These morbidities often go underreported and/or untreated.

- Supposedly minor health issues such as fatigue, backache, sore nipples, headaches or constipation can have a significant impact on postnatal psychological health. They should be discussed in the antenatal period and should not be dismissed as 'normal' when reported postpartum.

- Only around half of mothers with perinatal depression and anxiety are identified despite frequent routine contact with healthcare services, and even fewer receive adequate treatment.

- Positive parenting is linked to subsequent healthy child development. Healthcare professionals should help ease the transition to parenthood by discussing the expectations and concerns that new parents may have, and by offering consistent rather than conflicting advice.

References

1. Buultjens, M., et al., The perinatal period: a literature review from the biopsychosocial perspective. *Clinical Nursing Studies*, 2013. **1**(3): 19.

2. Furuta, M., et al., The relationship between severe maternal morbidity and psychological health symptoms at 6–8 weeks postpartum: A prospective cohort study in one English maternity unit. *BMC Pregnancy and Childbirth*, 2014. **14**(1): 133.

3. Knight, M., et al., *Saving Lives, Improving Mothers' Care Lessons learned to inform future maternity care from the UK and Ireland Confidential Enquiries into Maternal Deaths and Morbidity 2009–2012*. London; MBRRACE-UK 2014. Available at www.npeu.ox.ac.uk/mbrrace-uk/reports. Accessed 27 March 2017.

4. MacArthur, C., et al., Effects of redesigned community postnatal care on womens' health 4 months after birth: A cluster randomised controlled trial. *Lancet*, 2002. **359**(9304): 378–385.

5. Bick, D.E., et al., Improving inpatient postnatal services: Midwives' views and perspectives of engagement in a quality improvement initiative. *BMC Health Serv Res*, 2011. **11**: 293.

6. Fahey, J.O. and E. Shenassa, Understanding and meeting the needs of women in the postpartum period: The perinatal maternal health promotion model. *Journal of Midwifery & Women's Health*, 2013. **58**(6): 613–621.

7. Webb, D.A., et al., Postpartum physical symptoms in new mothers: Their relationship to functional limitations and emotional well-being. *Birth*, 2008. **35**(3): 179–187.

8. National Institute for Health and Care Excellence (NICE), Routine Postnatal Care of Women and their Babies, in *Clinical Guideline 37*, NICE 2006.

9. Lewis, I. and C. Lenehan. *Report of the children and young people's health outcomes forum*. London: Children and Young People's Health Outcomes Forum. 2012.

10. DH, *National service framework for children, young people and maternity services*. Department of Health London, 2004.

11. DH, *Maternity matters: Choice, access and continuity of care in a safe service*, Department of Health London, 2007.

12. HSCIC, *Hospital Episode Statistics: NHSMaternity Statistics, England 2013–2014*. Health and Social Care Information Centre, 2015.

13. Brown, S., et al., *Early postnatal discharge from hospital for healthy mothers and term infants*. The Cochrane Library, 2002.

14. Bhavnani, V. and M. Newburn, *Left to your own devices: The postnatal care experiences of 1260 first-time mothers*. London: NCT, 2010.

15. Beake, S., D. Bick, and A. Weavers, Revising care to meet maternal needs post birth: An overview of the hospital to home postnatal study. *The Practising Midwife*, 2012. **15**(6): 10–13.

16. Bick, D., et al., Improving postnatal outcomes using continuous quality improvement: A pre and post intervention study in one English maternity unit. *BMC Pregnancy and Childbirth*, 2012. **12**(1): 41.

17. Schmied, V. and D. Bick, Postnatal care–Current issues and future challenges. *Midwifery*, 2014. **30**(6): 571–574.

18. MacArthur, C., et al., Effects of redesigned community postnatal care on womens' health 4 months after birth: A cluster randomised controlled trial. *The Lancet*, 2002. **359**(9304): 378–385.

19. Woolhouse, H., et al., Physical health after childbirth and maternal depression in the first 12 months post partum: Results of an Australian nulliparous pregnancy cohort study. *Midwifery*, 2014. **30**(3): 378–384.

20. Darvill, R., H. Skirton, and P. Farrand, Psychological factors that impact on women's experiences of first-time motherhood: A qualitative study of the transition. *Midwifery*, 2010. **26**(3): 357–366.

21. Emmanuel, E.N., et al., Maternal role development: The impact of maternal distress and social support following childbirth. *Midwifery*, 2011. **27**(2): 265–272.

22. Cargill, Y., et al., Postpartum maternal and newborn discharge. *Journal of obstetrics and gynaecology Canada : JOGC = Journal d'obstetrique et gynecologie du Canada : JOGC*, 2007. **29**(4): 357–363.

23. Malkin, J.D., et al., Infant Mortality and Early Postpartum Discharge. *Obstetrics & Gynecology*, 2000. **96**(2): 183–188.

24. Yonemoto, N., et al., Schedules for home visits in the early postpartum period. *Evidence-Based Child Health: A Cochrane Review Journal*, 2014. **9**(1): 5–99.

25. MacArthur, C., et al., *Redesigning postnatal care: A randomised controlled trial of protocol-based midwifery-led care focused on individual women's physical and psychological health needs*. National Co-ordinating Centre for Health Technology Assessment, 2003.

26. Bick, D.E., C. MacArthur, and R.J. Lancashire, What influences the uptake and early cessation of breast feeding? *Midwifery*, 1998. **14**(4): 242–247.

27. Logsdon, M.C. and D.W. Davis, Social and professional support for pregnant and parenting women. *MCN: The American Journal of Maternal/Child Nursing*, 2003. **28**(6): 371–376.

28. Razurel, C. and B. Kaiser, The Role of Satisfaction with Social Support on the Psychological Health of Primiparous Mothers in the Perinatal Period. *Women & Health*, 2015. **55**(2): 167–186.

29. Wilkins, C., A qualitative study exploring the support needs of first-time mothers on their journey towards intuitive parenting. *Midwifery*, 2006. **22**(2): 169–180.

30. Leahy-Warren, P., G. McCarthy, and P. Corcoran, First-time mothers: Social support, maternal parental self-efficacy and postnatal depression. *Journal of Clinical Nursing*, 2012. **21**(3-4): 388–397.

31. Harwood, K., N. McLean, and K. Durkin, First-time mothers' expectations of parenthood: What happens when optimistic expectations are not matched by later experiences? *Developmental Psychology*, 2007. **43**(1): 1.

32. Tulman, L. and J. Fawcett, Functional status during pregnancy and the postpartum: A framework for research. *Image: The Journal of Nursing Scholarship*, 1990. **22**(3): 191–194.

33. Romano, M., et al., Postpartum period: Three distinct but continuous phases. *Journal of Prenatal Medicine*, 2010. **4**(2): 22.

34. Hay-Smith, J., et al., Pelvic floor muscle training for prevention and treatment of urinary and faecal incontinence in antenatal and postnatal women. *Cochrane Database Syst Rev*, 2008. 4. doi: 10.1002/14651858.CD007471.

35. Boyle, R., et al., Pelvic floor muscle training for prevention and treatment of urinary and faecal incontinence in antenatal and postnatal women. *The Cochrane Library*, 2012;10:CD007471. doi: 10.1002/14651858.CD007471.pub2.

36. Hannestad, Y.S., G. Rortveit, and S. Hunskaar, Help-seeking and associated factors in female urinary incontinence. The Norwegian EPINCONT Study. *Scandinavian Journal of Primary Health Care*, 2002. **20**(2): 102–107.

37. Solans-Domènech, M., et al., Urinary and anal incontinence during pregnancy and postpartum: Incidence, severity, and risk factors. *Obstetrics & Gynecology*, 2010. **115**(3): 618–628.

38. Koch, L.H., Help-Seeking behaviors of women with urinary incontinence: An integrative literature review. *Journal of Midwifery & Women's Health*, 2006. **51**(6): e39–e44.

39. Brown, S., et al., Consultation about urinary and faecal incontinence in the year after childbirth: A cohort study. *BJOG: An International Journal of Obstetrics & Gynaecology*, 2015. **122**(7): 954–962.

40. Wray, J., *Bouncing back?: An ethnographic study exploring the context of care and recovery after birth through the experiences and voices of mothers*, 2011, University of Salford.

41. WHO, *Exclusive breastfeeding for six months best for babies everywhere*, 2011, World Health Organisation: Geneva.

42. Brown, A., P. Raynor, and M. Lee, Healthcare professionals' and mothers' perceptions of factors that influence decisions to breastfeed or formula feed infants: A comparative study. *Journal of Advanced Nursing*, 2011. **67**(9): 1993–2003.

43. Renfrew, M.J., et al., Support for healthy breastfeeding mothers with healthy term babies. *Cochrane Database Syst Rev*, 2012. 5: CD001141.

44. Lee, E., *Feeding babies and the problems of policy*. Centre for Parenting Culture Studies, University of Kent. 2011. Available at https://blogs.kent.ac.uk/parentingculture studies/files/2011/02/CPCS-Briefing-on-feeding-babies -FINAL-revised1.pdf. Accessed 27 March 2017.

45. Knaak, S.J., Contextualising risk, constructing choice: Breastfeeding and good mothering in risk society. *Health, risk & society*, 2010. **12**(4): 345–355.

46. Hoddinott, P., et al., A serial qualitative interview study of infant feeding experiences: Idealism meets realism. *BMJ Open*, 2012. **2**(2): e000504.

47. de Jager, E., et al., Psychosocial correlates of exclusive breastfeeding: A systematic review. *Midwifery*, 2013. **29**(5): 506–518.

48. LeMasters, E.E., Parenthood as crisis. *Marriage and family living*, 1957;**19**: 352–355.

49. Gavin, N.I., et al., Perinatal depression: A systematic review of prevalence and incidence. *Obstet Gynecol*, 2005. **106**(5 Pt 1): 1071–1083.

50. Goodman, S.H., et al., Maternal depression and child psychopathology: A meta-analytic review. *Clin Child Fam Psychol Rev*, 2011. **14**(1): 1–27.

51. Beck, C.T., Postpartum depression: A metasynthesis. *Qual Health Res*, 2002. **12**(4): 453–472.

52. Khan, L., *Falling through the gaps: Perinatal mental health and general practice*, 2015, Royal College of General Practitioners and Centre for Mental Health: London.

53. Stewart, D.E., et al., *Postpartum depression: Literature review of risk factors and interventions*. Toronto: University Health Network Women's Health Program for Toronto Public Health, 2003.

54. Harwood, K., N. McLean, and K. Durkin, First-time mothers' expectations of parenthood: What happens when optimistic expectations are not matched by later experiences? *Dev Psychol*, 2007. **43**(1): 1–12.

55. Newburn, M., Becoming a mother–regaining the balance. *The practising midwife*, 2006. **9**(7): 13.

56. Sandall, J., et al., Midwife-led continuity models versus other models of care for childbearing women. *Cochrane Database Syst Rev*. 2016. 4: CD004667. doi: 10.1002/14651858.CD004667.pub5.

57. Rayment-Jones, H., T. Murrells, and J. Sandall, An investigation of the relationship between the caseload model of midwifery for socially disadvantaged women and childbirth outcomes using routine data–a retrospective, observational study. *Midwifery*, 2015. **31**(4): 409–417.

58. Cowan, C.P. and P.A. Cowan, Interventions to ease the transition to parenthood: Why they are needed and what they can do. *Family Relations*, 1995; **44**:412–423.

59. Huston, T. and E.K. Holmes, Becoming parents. *Family Communication*. 2003. 105.

60. Coleman, L. and F. Glenn, The varied impact of couple relationship breakdown on children: Implications for practice and policy. *Children & Society*, 2010. **24**(3): 238–249.

61. Amato, P.R., Children of divorce in the 1990s: An update of the Amato and Keith (1991) meta-analysis. *J Fam Psychol*, 2001. **15**(3): 355–370.

62. Doss, B.D., et al., The effect of the transition to parenthood on relationship quality: An 8-year prospective study. *J Pers Soc Psychol*, 2009. **96**(3): 601–619.

63. Bryanton, J., C.T. Beck, and W. Montelpare, *Postnatal parental education for optimizing infant general health and parent-infant relationships*. The Cochrane Library, 2013.

64. Gerhardt, S., Why love matters: How affection shapes a baby's brain. *Infant Observation*, 2006. **9**(3): 305–309.

65. Gagnon, A.J. and J. Sandall, Individual or group antenatal education for childbirth or parenthood, or both. *Cochrane Database Syst Rev*, 2007(3): CD002869.

66. Mercer, R.T. and L.O. Walker, A review of nursing interventions to foster becoming a mother. *J Obstet Gynecol Neonatal Nurs*, 2006. **35**(5): 568–582.

67. Magill-Evans, J., et al., Interventions with fathers of young children: Systematic literature review. *J Adv Nurs*, 2006. **55**(2): 248–264.

68. El-Mohandes, A.A., et al., The effect of a parenting education program on the use of preventive pediatric health care services among low-income, minority mothers: A randomized, controlled study. *Pediatrics*, 2003. **111**(6 Pt 1): 1324–1332.

69. Skovgaard, A.M., et al., Predictors (0–10 months) of psychopathology at age 1½ years–a general population study in the Copenhagen child cohort CCC 2000*. *Journal of Child Psychology and Psychiatry*, 2008. **49**(5): 553–562.

70. Barlow, J., et al., Parent-infant psychotherapy for improving parental and infant mental health. *Cochrane Database of Systematic Reviews*, 2015; 8;1:CD010534. doi: 10.1002/14651858.CD010534.pub2.

Chapter 39

Birth Trauma and Post-Traumatic Stress

Pauline Slade and Elinor Milby

Post-Traumatic Stress following Childbirth: An Overview

Definition

Post-traumatic stress disorder (PTSD) is a psychological response following exposure to an event that involves actual or threatened death, serious injury or sexual violation to self or others [1]. There are four distinct symptom clusters. Firstly, there are re-experiencing symptoms which include spontaneous and intrusive thoughts and images, typically occurring involuntarily. These are often in the form of flashbacks (when the person feels as if they are back in the traumatic situation) and nightmares. Secondly, there is avoidance of reminders of the traumatic event, such as people, places or situations that may trigger re-experiencing. Thirdly, the person experiences negative cognitions and mood, which can range from a persistent sense of blame to diminished interest in activities and an impaired memory of the event. Fourthly, there are arousal symptoms, which include hypervigilance for threat so that the person is wary and on edge. These can include heightened irritability, sleep disturbance and problems of concentration. These symptoms must cause clinically significant distress and impairment to the individual's level of functioning and have a minimum duration of four weeks to fulfil diagnostic criteria [1]. However, it is now recognized that high levels of distress can accompany experiences which do not meet diagnostic thresholds and it may be more helpful to think about responses to traumatic events as representing a continuum of distress.

PTSD after Childbirth

PTSD was first identified in relation to adverse psychological responses following exposure to experiences of war and initially diagnostic criteria stipulated that the traumatic event must be 'outside the range of normal human experience'. However, clinicians have long been aware that precipitants of PTSD are not confined to external triggers such as military combat, assault or traffic collisions but may also include health-related events.

Increasing recognition that post-traumatic stress symptoms can occur after events that, whilst societally normal, are outside the range of usual daily experience for an individual led to childbirth being formally recognized as a potential precipitant of PTSD [2]. Growing public recognition of PTSD following childbirth has also been evidenced by the emergence of the Birth Trauma Association (www.birthtraumaassociation.org.uk), a self-help information site for people who have been affected by traumatic childbirth experiences, which receives 150,000 hits per year.

While there are clear similarities between PTSD following childbirth and PTSD following other events, there are also important differences which require consideration. Unlike other potentially traumatic events, childbirth is often a planned event entered into voluntarily, and although the exact timing may be uncertain, it is anticipated that it will occur. Again, unlike other events, childbirth is generally viewed as a positive experience at a societal level and women are expected to respond positively. There are also key differences during the event itself. For example, a traumatic childbirth will always involve at least two people (mother and baby); usually occurs while under the care of health professionals; and often whilst the woman is receiving pain-relieving drugs which may alter perception. Childbirth happens during a period of major life transition whilst other traumatic events may occur at any time. These context-specific factors inevitably influence how PTSD is experienced following childbirth and also have theoretical and clinical implications which will be further considered in the following.

Current Theoretical Understanding

How context influences theoretical understandings also merits consideration. Extensive literature exists in this area on other traumatic events but research specific to PTSD following childbirth is limited [3].

The Cognitive Model and PTSD following Childbirth

One of the models that has received support in the general literature is the cognitive model of PTSD [4]. This model argues that PTSD symptoms are perpetuated by negative appraisals of the traumatic event and/or its sequelae and that recovery is hindered by the use of maladaptive coping strategies such as rumination and thought suppression.

Recently, researchers have looked at the predictive value of this model in the childbirth context. Ford, Ayers and Bradley [5] found that the model accounted for 23% of the variance in acute stress symptoms three weeks after birth and 9% of PTS symptoms at 3 months. This increased to 16% when social support was added to the model.

Vossbeck-Elsebusch et al. [6] assessed the predictive value of cognitive variables in the development of PTSD following childbirth whilst controlling for other established predictors of PTSD (discussed later in the chapter). Established pre- and perinatal variables explained 33% of variance in trauma symptoms in the 1–6 month postnatal period. The inclusion of cognitive variables (negative appraisals of the traumatic event and its sequelae and maladaptive cognitive strategies) increased the amount of explained variance to 68%. These preliminary findings show the potential utility of applying the cognitive model in the childbirth context; however, there remains a significant proportion of unexplained variance in symptoms which requires further investigation.

Recent research has begun to explore this gap. Iles and Pote [7] used a grounded theory approach to develop a theoretical model of PTSD following childbirth. A strength of their model is its recognition of childbirth-specific variables that influence women's experience of trauma. For example, childbirth as an expected event is accompanied by a variety of anticipatory beliefs and coping strategies that impact on women's emotional states. Factors implicated in the development of PTSD symptoms included prenatal anxiety about childbirth, rigid expectations about labour and delivery and how women assimilated their birth experience into their role as a new mother.

Attachment Theory and PTSD following Childbirth

Another area that has recently begun to receive attention in relation to PTSD following childbirth is attachment theory. Attachment patterns develop in infancy and can be characterized as secure, anxious or avoidant. It is thought that attachment patterns established in childhood continue into adulthood affecting our relationships and interactions. Having a secure attachment pattern has been shown to protect individuals against stressful situations [8] and may be particularly relevant during the transition to parenthood given the adjustment required within relationships between mothers, their partners and newly born infants. Furthermore, in the non-childbirth literature, a relationship has been found between attachment style and perceptions of pain [9]. It is therefore possible that certain adult attachment patterns increase vulnerability to PTSD following childbirth by influencing: how women experience childbirth (i.e. levels of pain and perceptions of care received); and postnatal coping strategies and perceived social support. Recent work has identified a link between insecure attachment patterns, perceptions of partner support and PTS symptoms in the postpartum period [10].

Impact of PTSD following Childbirth

The impact of post-traumatic stress symptoms can be severe and far reaching and is associated with major functional impairment. In the postnatal context this burden is compounded by the impact on maternal and infant health, future reproductive plans and mothers' relationships with their infants and partners. Box 39.1 provides a case illustration of PTSD following childbirth.

Women's relationships with their partners may be adversely affected. Women may avoid sex and intimacy following a traumatic birth for fear of becoming pregnant again and triggering further PTSD symptoms [11]. PTSD following childbirth may also be comorbid between couples and trauma responses in men can exacerbate mental health difficulties in their partners [10]. PTSD following childbirth has also been found to be associated with higher levels of parenting stress two years later [12] and may interfere with maternal bonding and attachment to the infant, although comorbid postnatal depression may also contribute to this [13].

Future family plans may also be affected with women with PTSD up to four times more likely than non-sufferers to have no further children [14]. Where

BOX 39.1 Marie's Story – A Subjectively Traumatic Birth

Marie's pregnancy went over term and she was admitted to hospital for an induction. Nothing happened for 12 hours and her husband went home and she was told by staff to get some sleep. Around the time of shift changeover she began to experience very intense pain. She felt she was no longer coping and that she did not know what was happening. Staff tried to reassure her that nothing was happening and she was told to just relax. Marie's pain intensified and she asked for an epidural. When she was finally examined she was found to be 4.5 cm dilated and labour had progressed very rapidly. By the time staff were available she was too late to have an epidural. She experienced very intense pain and there were then concerns about fetal distress. She was told she needed to 'try harder' when she felt she was already giving all she had. Eventually, her baby was delivered by ventouse and two episiotomies. At the birth Marie felt so exhausted and frightened she felt nothing but relief when her baby was given to her.

Two years after the birth of her daughter Marie was referred to a clinical psychologist who specialized in trauma-related responses. At this time she was reporting that most days she would experience the feeling of being back in labour. Images would run through her head like a film and she would feel very frightened. She would try to block this and distract herself but this didn't usually work. Whilst this usually happened at home alone or with her daughter, she had actually missed getting off at her bus stop on several occasions when reliving had been triggered by the sight of a pregnant woman getting on the bus. Marie did her best to avoid talking about the birth as she knew this would trigger reliving, so she avoided other women with babies and young children. This led her to become socially isolated postnatally. She had been unable to go to mother and baby groups and avoided work colleagues. Factors associated with the birth acted as triggers. If she heard the mention of or saw an advert for 'a cocktail' this could trigger reliving of the birth as at the height of her distress her midwife suggested she 'imagine lying on a beach with a daquiri'.

Marie was not experiencing birth-related dreams and she was not depressed. She had no previous mental health difficulties. She did however feel more irritable and on edge than usual which led to some tensions at home, but she had a supportive partner. She felt angry towards staff. Marie had a good relationship with her child, although she felt guilty that she had not had a feeling of overwhelming warmth to her baby at the birth that she had expected of herself. She had always wanted two children but was adamant she would never become pregnant again. Whilst she was using contraception, this fear adversely affected her sexual relationship with her partner.

women do go on to have further children, a previous traumatic birth experience can contribute to fear of childbirth in subsequent pregnancies [15] and secondary tokophobia in some cases [16]. It has been reported that women who experience fear of childbirth are two to six times more likely to request caesarean sections [17, 18]. While opting for a caesarean may enable some women with PTSD following childbirth to have further children, this is also associated with higher incidence of some postnatal complications and increased costs to the NHS [19]. Where there is high fear, in accordance with NICE guidelines [19], then early maternity care should make it clear that if a woman does want a caesearan section because of fear then she can have this. However, consultation with a psychologist whose aim is to enable a woman to have the most positive birth experience *whatever* mode is advised. There is then scope to provide psychological help to alleviate anxieties and/or post-traumatic stress symptoms whilst still allowing a woman to retain her all-important control.

Experiencing Childbirth as Traumatic and Subsequent Experience of PTSD: Prevalence

How Many Women Experience Childbirth as Traumatic?

Research to date in this area has largely been based on DSM-IV criteria [2] which specified that a person must experience actual or threatened death or serious injury (criterion A1) and respond with intense fear, helplessness or horror (criterion A2). An early Canadian study reported that approximately one-third of women experience childbirth as traumatic [20], while a more recent Australian study found that 46% of the sample reported a traumatic birth when asked at 4–6 weeks postpartum [21]. Another Australian study found that 14% of women met criteria for a traumatic birth, which doubled to 29% when criterion A2 was removed [22]. A recent pilot study undertaken in Liverpool, UK (the findings of which are currently being prepared for publication), found that a third of women self-identified as having a traumatic birth experience.

How Many Women Develop PTSD at Full and Sub-diagnostic Levels Following Childbirth?

The first comprehensive review of studies investigating the prevalence of PTSD following childbirth reported a rate of women fitting a PTSD profile of between 2.8–5.6% at 6 weeks postpartum and approximately 1.5% at 6 months postpartum [23]. A systematic review of studies carried out in Western Europe identified a prevalence rate of 1.3%–2.4% between 1 and 2 months postpartum and 0.9%–4.6% between 3 and 12 months postpartum [24].

However, two key methodological flaws have been identified relating to the above reviews. Firstly, they did not distinguish between studies that clearly identified childbirth as the traumatic stressor meaning prevalence rates may have included women with PTSD resulting from events other than childbirth. Secondly, they did not distinguish between studies focusing on community and at-risk study samples which is likely to affect prevalence estimates. Heterogeneity among the studies reviewed in relation to the measures used to assess PTSD and definitions of what constitutes a traumatic birth are also problematic.

A recent systematic review which addressed these issues estimated a prevalence rate of 3.1% in community samples and 15.7% in at-risk samples [25]. The most methodologically sound study of prevalence carried out to date found that, after controlling for PTSD due to previous trauma and anxiety and depression during pregnancy, rates of full PTSD following childbirth were 1.2% at 4–6 weeks and 3.1% at 3 months and 6 months postpartum [21].

As noted before, it is helpful to view responses to trauma as existing on a continuum. It is therefore important to consider women who experience trauma symptoms following childbirth, but who do not meet full diagnostic criteria as they are still likely to experience significant distress at a key time for transitions in roles and relationships. Recent studies have reported a prevalence rate of 5.6% at 4–6 weeks [21] and 8.6% at 8 weeks postnatally [26] when also taking into account clinically significant symptoms at sub-diagnostic levels. Based on the number of women giving birth in England and Wales [27] this equates to between 39,000 and 60,000 women who experience clinically significant symptoms of post-traumatic stress following childbirth each year.

What Is the Longitudinal Course of PTSD following Childbirth?

Current evidence relating to the natural course of PTSD following childbirth is limited. A recent review of the literature on the longitudinal course of PTSD following other events found that only half of people recover naturally from PTSD after an average of 3 years [28]. However, again the postnatal context may influence the course of PTSD as women are simultaneously caring for their babies. This could potentially exacerbate symptoms by triggering more re-experiencing or conversely decrease symptoms by reducing avoidance [29]. Alcorn et al. [21] found that rates of PTSD increased over the first three months postpartum but then stabilized by six months. Although the longitudinal course of PTSD following childbirth is still to be firmly established, its long-term impact has been documented with evidence from clinical case studies highlighting the persistence of adverse responses for up to 9 years [30].

Risk Factors

Various risk factors have been implicated in the development of PTSD following childbirth. Slade [31] provides a useful conceptual framework for understanding risk factors. Essentially, this follows a formulation approach which considers why a person may experience psychological distress at this point in their life. This involves taking account of not just what happens during labour and delivery (precipitating factors) but also what a person brings into that situation (predisposing factors that are present before or during pregnancy), which may influence how events are experienced, and what happens postnatally (perpetuating/maintaining factors) which may influence resolution of responses.

The second dimension in Slade's model relates to the source of the risk factor and whether at each time frame this is internal (relating to aspects of the individual), external (relating to aspects of the environment) or a result of an interaction between the two. Table 39.1 shows an updated summary of risk factors that have been established in the literature in the context of Slade's model.

Table 39.1 Evidence-based predictors of PTSD following childbirth in the context of Slade's (2006) conceptual framework

	Internal	External	Interactional
Predisposing Factors	Depression during pregnancy PTSD/anxiety during pregnancy History of mental health difficulties Trait anxiety High fear of labour *Younger age*	History of sexual abuse *Previous traumatic life experiences*	Unplanned pregnancy Perceptions of low social support *Insecure attachment*
Precipitating Factors	Perceived loss of control Severe pain High fear for self and/or baby Negative gap between expectation and experience *Peritraumatic dissociation* *Negative emotions*	Emergency caesarean section Instrumental delivery Partner not present *Maternal complications* *Elective caesarean section*	Perceived low support from partner Perceived low support from staff Feeling poorly informed
Perpetuating/ Maintaining Factors	*Negative appraisals of childbirth* *Dysfunctional cognitive coping strategies*		*Low social support*

Note: Items in italics represent updates to the literature since the model was first published.

Antenatal (Predisposing) Factors

A history of mental health difficulties, trait anxiety, a history of sexual or other types of trauma and mental health difficulties during pregnancy (particularly depression) have all been found to be strong predictors of PTSD following childbirth [6, 24, 25]. There is some evidence that younger age and having an unplanned pregnancy also increase risk, although this is not universally supported [24].

Perinatal (Precipitating) Factors

In a recent review, women's subjective distress during labour and delivery (including negative emotions, perception of loss of control, dissociation, pain, fear for self or baby, and fear of labour) emerged as the key determinant for developing subsequent PTS symptoms [24]. A recent study provides further support for this with negative subjective appraisal of childbirth (intensity of fear, helplessness and horror) and feelings of fear, anger and shame found to predict later PTS symptoms [32]. Although obstetric interventions such as having an emergency caesarean or instrumental delivery also increase risk, women who have an objectively normal birth in terms of duration and mode of delivery may still be highly traumatized. Other perinatal factors linked to the development of symptoms are other obstetric complications, low levels of perceived support from partner and staff [24, 25] and perinatal dissociation [6].

A recent meta-ethnography provides further support for the importance of women's perceptions of a traumatic birth, with key findings highlighting their experiences of feeling out of control and degraded or dehumanized by healthcare professionals during labour and delivery, feeling trapped by the recurring nightmare of childbirth, going through a rollercoaster of emotions and needing to atone for failure in the postnatal period [33].

Postnatal (Maintaining) Factors

When Slade's model [31] was first developed there was not enough evidence regarding the hypothesized factors that maintain PTSD following childbirth and they were therefore omitted from the framework. In the non-childbirth literature negative appraisals

---

BOX 39.2 Marie's Story: Risk Factors

Predisposing Factors

Marie sets herself high standards in everything she does. She seeks information, plans and puts in maximum effort. She must always do her best or feels guilty. These attributes have served her well through her life and she is highly educated and successful. She had adopted the same strategies for planning her childbirth.

Precipitating Factors

During labour Marie felt she wasn't coping and that she did not know what was happening (*perceived loss of control/feeling poorly informed*). She felt alone, vulnerable and unlistened to as new staff tried to reassure her that nothing was happening and she should just relax (*perceived low support*). As her pain intensified Marie experienced very high levels of fear and panic (*severe pain/negative emotions*). Her labour and delivery were nothing like what she had planned for (*negative gap between expectation and experience*).

Perpetuating/Maintaining Factors

Marie returned home and her family and partner were supportive. After about a week she began to experience intrusive images and thoughts. She tried hard to put these out of her mind and avoid anything that would trigger intrusions (*dysfunctional cognitive coping strategies*). She tried to just carry on and take the advice of her family that she had a happy healthy baby and needed to put the birth behind her and look forward. After the first month it was rarely discussed as she would get upset and everyone thought it was for the best (*avoidance*). In a year she went back to work part time and although friends had noticed a reclusiveness and change (*low social support*) she outwardly managed to get by.

Marie's story highlights how it is not the objective complexity or threat that is important but the subjective experience of the individual.

---

of the event and its sequelae and a lack of social support are key processes that have been identified [34]. Recent research has shown that cognitive processing factors, specifically negative appraisals of childbirth, viewing intrusions as a sign of abnormality and maladaptive coping strategies (ruminating about childbirth and trying to block intrusive memories), are also implicated in the maintenance of PTSD symptoms in a postnatal context [6].

These factors have the adverse effects of preventing the cognitive processing required to achieve successful adjustment after childbirth and reducing conversation about the traumatic experience with others. This may be an attempt to avoid further distress for self or others but also reduces the woman's level of perceived social support. This is highly relevant as high perceived social support has been found to be a key protective factor against PTSD postnatally [10]. Box 39.2 provides a case illustration of risk factors for PTSD following childbirth.

The Role of Attachment

Recent research has highlighted the role of adult attachment patterns in the development and maintenance of PTS symptoms following childbirth. Both anxious and avoidant attachment styles have been found to predict trauma symptoms in the postpartum period [10]. Attachment may also influence precipitating risk factors. For example, a recent study found that higher levels of anxious adult attachment were associated with pain severity during childbirth, whilst higher avoidant attachment scores were associated with feeling less respected by staff during labour and delivery [35]. As noted above, perceived social support is important after childbirth. In order to benefit from social support, individuals need the capacity to form and maintain social bonds with others. Insecure attachment patterns may lower women's perceptions of support or their ability to make use of the support available [10].

The literature on predictors of PTSD following childbirth is highly relevant from a clinical perspective as it offers insight into potential preventative measures. Antenatal and postnatal mental health guidance advises that midwives should routinely ask women about their birth experience in order to identify women who have had a traumatic experience and are therefore at risk of developing PTSD [36]. The guidance also states that services should provide timely treatment from specialist staff for women with partial and full PTSD. However, there is currently no specific guidance on screening procedures, prevention or treatment as the evidence for effective interventions for PTSD following childbirth is sparse. The following sections consider the potential for and evidence concerning antenatal and postnatal prevention and then intervention.

Prevention and Early Intervention

Antenatal Prevention

Low perceived support has consistently been shown to be a predictor of PTSD following childbirth, highlighting the importance of good communication from staff during labour and delivery. A recent targeted prevention study aimed to improve effective clinical communication by implementing and evaluating a pink sticker communication system to alert staff to vulnerable women who may require extra support [37]. Preliminary findings were encouraging with no women going on to develop PTSD as a result of perceived poor care. A reduction in the number of psychology service referrals relating to birth trauma was also observed whilst the sticker system was in place.

Postnatal Prevention

Most of the research to date in this area has focused on postnatal 'debriefing', which is commonly offered in the UK [38] despite ambiguity over its definition and effectiveness. A review of the non-childbirth-related literature concluded that debriefing as an early intervention for PTSD was ineffective and may even increase the risk of developing PTSD [39]. As a result debriefing is not recommended in national guidelines on the management of PTSD [40].

As recognized earlier, differences in both the nature of childbirth as a potentially traumatic event and the social context of childbirth may also influence the salience and consequences of interventions. Findings from the postnatal context report mixed results in terms of outcomes of debriefing interventions [41]. Inconsistencies may be due to heterogeneity between studies including variations in terminology, content, timing of delivery and whether interventions are offered universally or targeted to women at risk.

A recent systematic review of the debriefing literature specifically related to childbirth identified that there is some utility in targeting provision of debriefing to women who perceive their childbirth as traumatic and when this is offered shortly after

childbirth or at the woman's specific request [42]. Furthermore, there is evidence that women view the opportunity to discuss their childbirth experience positively and achieve a sense of validation through talking and being heard [43]. Given that a key finding of a recent review of qualitative studies is that women who have had a traumatic childbirth may feel dehumanized, the subsequent experience of being heard is likely to be highly valued. However, due to the differences between what is commonly employed postnatally (which is not critical incident debriefing), the adoption of the term 'childbirth review' to describe this type of early intervention has been recommended [42].

Screening Issues

A key change in the diagnostic criteria for PTSD in DSM-V [1] is the removal of criterion A2, which required that a person experienced intense fear, helplessness or horror in response to the traumatic event [2]. The subjective appraisal element was removed following a review which found evidence of the lack of effect of this criterion on PTSD prevalence and the presence of PTSD symptomology [44]. However, none of the evidence reviewed originated in a postnatal context and as noted earlier, childbirth presents a unique set of circumstances in which a women's subjective experience is the key determinant of subsequent distress.

Although related, criterion A1 (perceived threat) and A2 (responding with intense fear, helplessness and horror) do occur independently of each other. Boorman et al. [22] found that slightly over half of women who perceived threat to themselves or their baby during childbirth did not experience an intense fear response. Furthermore, subjective appraisal of threat has also been found to have predictive value over and above the experience of a traumatic childbirth in postnatal levels of distress [32].

These findings have clinical implications for screening women for PTSD postnatally and targeting interventions. The elimination of the emotional response to childbirth has the potential to double the number of women who are identified as requiring further assessment. Disadvantages associated with erroneously categorizing birth as traumatic include pathologizing normal responses to the risk and uncertainty associated with birth; increasing demand on postnatal health services; and diluting the care available for women in actual need of help [22].

Intervention

The lack of information on effective treatments for PTSD following childbirth once established is a significant gap in the current literature, with research to date limited to case studies. It is widely recognized in the non-childbirth literature that cognitive behavioural therapy (CBT) and eye movement desensitization and reprocessing (EMDR) are effective treatments for PTSD [40], but these treatment approaches have yet to be rigorously tested in a postnatal context.

Cognitive Behavioural Therapy

Ayers et al. [45] describe two cases in which CBT was tailored to the women's traumatic childbirth experience with positive results. This study also highlighted the need to incorporate prior trauma and core beliefs into formulations and treatment plans. A recent study also found that trauma-focused CBT was effective in reducing PTSD symptoms in mothers of pre-term infants [46].

Eye Movement Desensitization and Reprocessing

Two further studies have reported encouraging results using EMDR [47, 48]. In the first EMDR was used to treat four pregnant women who presented with PTSD as a result of a previous childbirth experience [47]. The authors concluded that EMDR is a promising avenue for addressing fear of childbirth following birth trauma with the potential to enable women to continue with plans for future pregnancies. The second study [48] also reported on three cases where EMDR was successfully used to reduce PTSD symptoms in pregnant women who went on to reflect positively on their second childbirth experience despite complications during delivery.

In Summary

Childbirth has the potential to be a traumatic event that can involve actual or threatened harm to mothers and their babies. Childbirth presents a unique set of cultural and contextual circumstances which influence women's psychological responses to the event. Approximately one-third of women experience childbirth as traumatic, with a significant minority going on to develop clinically significant symptoms of post-traumatic stress. Trauma symptoms may be detrimental to the well-being of women and adversely impact their relationships. It is women's subjective experience rather than objectively traumatic events that is the key determinant in subsequent trauma responses. Several risk factors have been established in the development of symptoms which may relate to what women bring to childbirth (predisposing factors) and what occurs during labour and delivery (precipitating factors). Recently, research has also identified factors which maintain distress postnatally (perpetuating factors). Evidence for effective prevention is limited, though recent innovations show promising results and there is a case for targeted input in the form of a childbirth review. The criteria used for screening women for targeted interventions should be carefully considered as this has the potential to confound prevalence rates. Although CBT and EMDR are recognized as effective treatments for PTSD, this has yet to be firmly established in the childbirth context.

Key Points

- In England and Wales, between 39,000 and 60,000 women experience clinically significant symptoms of PTSD following childbirth each year.
- In PTSD there are four distinct symptom clusters: re-experiencing symptoms (often in the form of flashbacks and nightmares); avoidance of reminders of the traumatic event; negative cognitions and mood; and arousal symptoms (which include hypervigilance, heightened irritability, sleep disturbance and problems of concentration). High levels of distress can accompany experiences which do not meet diagnostic thresholds.
- There are clear similarities, but also important differences, between PTSD following childbirth and PTSD following other events.
- The cognitive model argues that PTSD symptoms are perpetuated by negative appraisals of the traumatic event and/or its sequelae and that recovery is hindered by the use of maladaptive coping strategies. Attachment theory posits attachment patterns (secure, anxious or avoidant) established in childhood continue into adulthood, affecting our relationships and interactions, and certain adult attachment patterns increase vulnerability to PTSD following childbirth.

- PTSD affects the mother's future reproductive plans and her relationships with her infant and partner. Women with PTSD are up to four times more likely than non-sufferers to have no further children and tend to have higher levels of parenting stress.
- PTSD following childbirth may be comorbid between couples
- The longitudinal course of PTSD following childbirth is still to be firmly established but adverse responses could persist for up to nine years
- In Slade's conceptual model, risk factors for PTSD after childbirth could be precipitating, predisposing or perpetuating/maintaining factors; they could be internal (relating to aspects of the individual), external (relating to aspects of the environment) or a result of an interaction between the two.
- There is currently no specific guidance on screening procedures, prevention or treatment as, currently, the evidence for effective interventions for PTSD following childbirth is sparse.
- Good communication from staff during labour and postnatally could reduce the number of women who develop PTSD as a result of perceived poor care.
- In the childbirth context CBT and EMDR have shown some promise but are yet to be firmly established.

References

1. American Psychiatric Association. *Diagnostic and Statistical Manual of Mental Disorders.* 5th ed. Washington, DC: Author; 2013.

2. American Psychiatric Association. *Diagnostic and Statistical Manual of Mental Disorders.* 4th ed. Washington, DC: Author; 1994.

3. McKenzie-McHarg K, Ayers S, Ford E, Horsch A, Jomeen J, Sawyer A, et al. Post-traumatic stress disorder following childbirth: An update of current issues and recommendations for future research. *Journal of Reproductive and Infant Psychology.* 2015; 33(3): 219–237.

4. Ehlers A, Clark D. A cognitive model of posttraumatic stress disorder. *Behaviour Research and Therapy.* 2000; 38(4): 319–345.

5. Ford E, Ayers S, Bradley R. Exploration of a cognitive model to predict post-traumatic stress symptoms following childbirth. *Journal of Anxiety Disorders.* 2010; 24: 353–359.

6. Vossbech-Elsebusch A, Freisfeld C, Ehring, T. Predictors of posttraumatic stress symptoms following childbirth. *BMC Psychiatry.* 2014; 14: 200.

7. Iles J, Pote H. Postnatal posttraumatic stress: A grounded theory model of first-time mothers' experiences. *Journal of Reproductive and Infant Psychology.* 2015; 33(3): 238–255.

8. Ditzen B, Schmidt S, Strauss B, Nater UM, Ehlert U, Heinrichs U. Adult attachment and social support interact to reduce psychological but not cortisol responses to stress. *Journal of Psychosomatic Research.* 2008; 64: 479–486.

9. Meredith P, Strong J, Feeney J. Adult attachment, anxiety and pain self-efficacy as predictors of pain intensity and disability. *Pain.* 2006; 123: 146–154.

10. Iles J, Slade P, Spiby H. Posttraumatic stress and postnatal depression in couples after childbirth: The role of partner support and attachment. *Journal of Anxiety Disorders.* 2011; 25: 520–530.

11. Ayers S, Wright DB, Wells N. Post-traumatic stress in couples after birth: Association with the couple's relationship and parent-baby bond. *Journal of Reproductive and Infant Psychology.* 2007; 25(1): 40–50.

12. McDonald S, Slade P, Spiby H, Iles J. Post-traumatic stress symptoms, parenting stress and mother-child relationships following childbirth and at 2 years postpartum. *Journal of Psychosomatic Obstetrics and Gynecology.* 2011; 32: 141–146.

13. Davies J, Slade P, Wright I, Stewart P. Post traumatic stress symptoms following childbirth and mothers' perceptions of their infants. *Infant Mental Health Journal.* 2008; 29: 537–554.

14. Czarnocka J, Slade P. Prevalence and predictors of post traumatic stress symptoms following childbirth. *British Journal of Clinical Psychology.* 2000; 39: 35–52.

15. Hildingsson I. Swedish couples' attitudes towards birth, childbirth fear and birth preferences and relation to mode of birth – A longitudinal cohort study. *Sexual and Reproductive Healthcare.* 2014; 5: 75–80.

16. Hofberg K, Brockington I. Tokophobia: An unreasoning dread of childbirth. *British Journal of Psychiatry.* 2000; 176: 83–85.

17. Waldenström U, Hildingsson I, Ryding EL. Antenatal fear of childbirth and its association with subsequent caesarean section and experience of childbirth. *BJOG: An International Journal of Obstetrics and Gynaecology.* 2006; 113: 638–646.

18. Ryding EL, Lukasse M, Van Parys A-S, Wangel A-M, Karro H, Kristjansdottir H, et al. Fear of childbirth and risk of cesarean delivery: A cohort study in six European countries. *Birth.* 2015; 42: 48–55.

19. National Institute for Health and Care Excellence. *Caesarean section. NICE clinical guideline 132*. London: Author; 2011.

20. Soet JE, Brack GA, Dilorio C. Prevalence and predictors of women's experience of psychological trauma during childbirth. *Birth*. 2003; **30**: 36–46.

21. Alcorn KL, O'Donovan A, Patrick JC, Creedy D, Devilly GJ. A prospective longitudinal study of the prevalence of post-traumatic stress disorder resulting from childbirth events. *Psychological Medicine*. 2010; **40**(11): 1849–1859.

22. Boorman RJ, Devilly GJ, Gamble J, Creedy DK, Fenwick J. Childbirth and criteria for traumatic events. *Midwifery*. 2014; **30**: 255–261.

23. Olde E, van der Hart O, Kleber R, van Son M. Posttraumatic stress following childbirth: A review. *Clinical Psychology Review*. 2006; **26**: 1–16.

24. Andersen LB, Melvaer LB, Videbech P, Lamont RF. Risk factors for developing post traumatic stress disorder following childbirth: A systematic review. *Acta Obstetrica and Gynaecologica Scandinavica*. 2012; **91**: 1261–1272.

25. Grekin R, O'Hara MW. Prevalence and risk factors of postpartum posttraumatic stress disorder: A meta-analysis. *Clinical Psychology Review*. 2014; **34** (5): 389–401.

26. Garthus-Niegel S, Ayers S, van Soest T, Torgersen L, Eberhard-Gran M. Maintaining factors of posttraumatic stress symptoms following childbirth: A population-based, two-year follow-up study. *Journal of Affective Disorders*. 2015; **172**: 146–152.

27. Office for National Statistics. *Births in England and Wales 2013*. Hampshire: Author; 2014.

28. Morina N, Wicherts JM, Lobbrecht J, Priebe S. Remission from post-traumatic stress disorder in adults: A systematic review and meta-analysis of long term outcome studies. *Clinical Psychology Review*. 2014; **34**: 249–255.

29. Ayers S, Joseph S, McKenzie-McHarg K, Slade P, Wijma K. Post-traumatic stress disorder following childbirth: Current issues and recommendations for research. *Journal of Psychosomatic Obstetrics and Gynecology*. 2008; **29**(4): 240–250.

30. Fones C. Posttraumatic stress disorder occurring after painful childbirth. *Journal of Nervous Mental Disorders*. 1996; **184**: 195–196.

31. Slade P. Towards a conceptual framework for understanding post-traumatic stress symptoms following childbirth and implications for further research. *Journal of Psychosomatic Obstetrics and Gynecology*. 2006; **27**(2): 99–105.

32. Devilly GJ, Gullo MJ, Alcorn KL, O'Donovan A. Subjective appraisal of threat (Criterion A2) as a predictor of distress in childbearing women. *Journal of Nervous and Mental Disease*. 2014; **202**(12): 877–882.

33. Elmir R, Schmied V, Wilkes L, Jackson D. Women's perceptions and experiences of a traumatic birth: A meta-ethnography. *Journal of Advanced Nursing*. 2010; **66**(10): 2142–2153.

34. Holeva V, Tarrier NT, Wells A. Prevalence and predictors of acute stress disorder and PTSD following road traffic accidents: Thought control strategies and social support. *Behaviour Therapy*. 2001; **32**: 65–83.

35. Quinn K, Spiby H, Slade P. A longitudinal study exploring the role of adult attachment in relation to perceptions of pain in labour, childbirth memory and acute traumatic stress responses. *Journal of Reproductive and Infant Psychology*. 2015; **33**(3): 256–267.

36. National Institute for Health and Care Excellence. *Antenatal and postnatal mental health: Clinical management and service guidance. NICE clinical guideline 192*. London: Author; 2014.

37. Olander EK, McKenzie-McHarg K, Crockett M, Ayers S. Think pink! A pink sticker alert system for women with psychological distress or vulnerability during pregnancy. *British Journal of Midwifery*. 2014; **22**(8): 590–595.

38. Ayers S, Claypool J, Eagle A. What happens after a difficult birth? Postnatal debriefing services. *British Journal of Midwifery*. 2006; **14**: 157–161.

39. Rose S, Bisson J, Churchill R, Wesley S. Psychological debriefing for preventing post-traumatic stress disorder (PTSD). *Cochrane Database Systematic Reviews*. 2002; **2**(2): CD000560.

40. National Institute for Health and Care Excellence. *Post-traumatic Stress Disorder (PTSD): The management of PTSD in adults and children in primary and secondary care. NICE clinical guideline 26*. London: NICE; 2005.

41. Lapp LK, Agbokou C, Peretti CS, Ferreri F. Management of post-traumatic stress disorder after childbirth: A review. *Journal of Psychosomatic Obstetrics and Gynecology*. 2010; **31**(3): 113–122.

42. Sheen K, Slade P. The efficacy of 'debriefing' after childbirth: Is there a case for targeted intervention? *Journal of Reproductive and Infant Psychology*. 2015; **33** (3): 308–320.

43. Baxter J, McCourt C, Jarrett PM. What is current practice in offering debriefing services to post partum women and what are the perceptions of women in accessing these services: A critical review of the literature. *Midwifery*. 2014; **30**: 194–219.

44. Friedman MJ, Resick PA, Bryant RA, Brewin CR. Considering PTSD for DSM-5. *Depression and Anxiety*. 2011;**28**(9):750–69. doi: 10.1002/da.20767

45. Ayers S, McKenzie-McHarg K, Eagle A. Cognitive behaviour therapy for postnatal post-traumatic stress disorder: Case studies. *Journal of Psychosomatic Obstetrics and Gynecology*. 2007; **28**: 177–184.

46. Shaw RJ, St John N, Lilo E, Jo B, Benitz W, Stevenson DK, et al. Prevention of traumatic stress in mothers of preterms: 6-month outcomes. *Pediatrics*. 2014; **134**(2): e481–488.

47. Sandstrom M, Wiberg B, Wikman M, Willman AK, Hoberg U. A pilot study of eye movement desensitisation and reprocessing treatment (EMDR) for post-traumatic stress after childbirth. *Midwifery*. 2008; **24**: 62–73.

48. Stramrood CA, van der Velde J, Doornbos B, Paarlberg KM, Weijmar Schultz WC, van Pampus MG. The patient observer: Eye-movement desensitization and reprocessing for the treatment of posttraumatic stress following childbirth. *Birth*. 2012; **39**: 70–76.

Chapter

40

Vicarious Traumatization in Maternity Care Providers

Pauline Slade, Kayleigh Sheen and Helen Spiby

Maternity professionals, through providing care during childbirth, may sometimes encounter adverse events that fulfil criteria for trauma. Exposure to events that caregivers experience as traumatic (whether or not the same events are actually experienced as traumatic by the woman giving birth) can elicit the same psychological response in those present as can occur in those directly affected by the event, with adverse implications for staff personal well-being [1]. Staff well-being is important not just for themselves but because it has the potential to impact upon quality of care they can provide.

Most of the existing literature on the impact of vicarious exposure to trauma focuses on events such as natural disasters, road traffic accidents and accidents resulting in emergency care. However, healthcare professionals engaged in the provision of care during childbirth may experience trauma that is qualitatively different to this. Childbirth in the developed world generally occurs in a positive social context. When birthing events involve threat to the life of the mother or child, there is juxtaposition between anticipation and reality that is absent in other types of trauma exposure. Therefore, specific consideration of the impact of indirect exposure to traumatic perinatal events (events occurring during labour, delivery or in the early postpartum) is important.

This chapter provides an overview of current evidence pertaining to the experience and impact of traumatic perinatal events in maternity care providers. The first section will describe the nature of psychological responses to vicarious trauma. The second section will discuss current understandings about the nature of events perceived as traumatic by care providers and consider the prevalence of work-related traumatic stress responses, aspects associated with increased risk and supportive strategies. The final section will highlight key areas for further research, and present recommendations that require further testing in clinical settings.

Theoretical Issues

Responding to Indirect Trauma

Vicarious or indirect exposure to trauma can include witnessing or listening to an account of an event, recalled by the individual directly affected. Indirect exposure has the potential to elicit the same adverse psychological responses as identified in individuals who are directly affected by trauma. The most commonly considered response in this context is post-traumatic stress disorder (PTSD). Additional frameworks have been developed (secondary traumatic stress, compassion fatigue, vicarious traumatization) to specifically conceptualize responses to indirect trauma. However, due to a high degree of overlap between criteria for onset and resulting symptomatology, their utility is uncertain. PTSD and the additional frameworks are considered in the following sections.

Post-traumatic Stress Disorder

PTSD is a trauma and stressor-related disorder that can occur following direct or indirect exposure to a traumatic event involving threat to physical integrity or life (to the self or someone else) [1]. Symptoms of PTSD include four dimensions: (1) intrusions (involuntary, distressing recollections of the event), (2) avoidance of reminders, (3) heightened arousal (e.g., feeling 'on edge', difficulty concentrating or sleeping and (4) negative alterations to beliefs or mood (e.g., anger, guilt). The latter dimension was recently introduced following amendments to the DSM-IV-TR [2] criteria in 2013 [1] and acknowledges the potential for PTSD to include cognitive as well as emotional or behavioural responses. PTSD is diagnosed when symptoms remain for a minimum of 1 month after experiencing a traumatic event, and when they are accompanied by severe levels of perceived impairment to daily functioning [1].

The development of PTSD following exposure to trauma is not inevitable. Initial stress responses are indicative of normal cognitive processing, required for the assimilation of trauma event information into autobiographical memory [3]. However, for a proportion of people exposed to trauma, the event is processed in a way that results in strong feelings of current threat [4]. In these instances, when symptoms remain for several months, responses are no longer indicative of normal cognitive processing and intervention may be required. It is also recognized that symptoms not fulfilling diagnostic levels can be highly distressing and require input.

Secondary Traumatic Stress

Secondary traumatic stress (STS) is defined as the stress arising from 'helping or wanting to help a traumatised or suffering person' [5; p. 7]. Symptoms occur soon after exposure to details of a traumatic event, or in response to exposure to multiple accounts of trauma from several recipients of care, and are essentially the same as the intrusive, avoidant and heightened arousal symptoms of PTSD [5].

Compassion Fatigue

The term compassion fatigue (CF) was originally developed by Beck and colleagues [6], to describe the general, negative impact of providing care. The term 'compassion fatigue' has since been incorporated into a wider concept – professional quality of life (ProQOL), which relates to the quality felt by an individual in relation to their work as a care provider [7].

Professional quality of life consists of two components: compassion satisfaction and compassion fatigue. Compassion satisfaction is the positive attribute held by an individual in relation to their work as a care provider. Compassion fatigue relates to the negative impact of care-giving, and consists of two further elements: burnout and STS symptoms. Burnout relates to an enduring, gradual negative impact of work-related stress. STS symptoms are conceptualized as the development of fear following exposure to primary or secondary trauma experienced as part of the professional role. Within this, primary exposure refers to witnessing a traumatic event occurring and secondary exposure relates to listening to an account of a traumatic event from a recipient of care. Compassion satisfaction and compassion fatigue operate on two ends of a spectrum; higher compassion satisfaction is associated with lower compassion

fatigue and vice versa. According to this theory, STS symptoms can occur soon after trauma exposure and are acute in their nature.

Vicarious Traumatization

Vicarious traumatization (VT) is conceptualized as a response to repeated exposure to details of multiple traumatic accounts. It is not event-specific, and instead represents a gradual cumulative response to traumatic material [8].

VT manifests as negative and enduring alterations to cognitive schema or worldview. Schema (or beliefs) about the self or other people are vulnerable to disruption. These include beliefs about safety (safe when alone, other people are safe), trust (in own judgement of feelings, other people), intimacy (disengagement from others, uncomfortable when alone), esteem (not deserving of praise, viewing others with disrespect) and control (uncomfortable with others in charge, need to control self) [9]. When schemas are disrupted they become more negative and general in their application to the world [10].

Burnout

Burnout occurs in response to chronic strain experienced through emotional and interpersonal stressors that are encountered in the workplace [11]. It is characterized by symptoms of emotional exhaustion, depersonalization of (i.e., attempts to distance oneself from) recipients of care and perceptions of reduced accomplishment in one's professional role. Symptoms of burnout are highly convergent with, yet distinct from, those associated with traumatic stress [12]. Consequences of burnout include increased staff turnover and absenteeism, and reduced productivity and quality of work [11]. Although burnout is not a response to trauma, the association of burnout with traumatic stress symptoms highlights this as a potential component to trauma exposure in care providers [13].

Summary

The recent reconceptualization of PTSD in the *DSM-V* has strengthened the case to primarily consider a PTSD framework when investigating responses to vicarious traumatization. Since the DSM-IV, the stressor criterion for PTSD has acknowledged vicarious exposure to trauma (witnessing, being 'confronted with' details of an event) to elicit the same symptomatic profile as associated with direct trauma exposure [2]. This was strengthened for the DSM-V to include work-related exposure to trauma [1]. The intrusive, avoidant and arousal symptoms of STS are identical in nature to those of PTSD. Whilst VT was previously unique in its acknowledgement of enduring cognitive changes in response to trauma exposure, the symptom criterion for PTSD now includes a dimension for cognitive belief and mood-related disruption.

It is clear that there is considerable overlap between terms used to describe responses to indirect trauma. Prior arguments for utility of STS, CF and VT included the specific focus on vicarious exposure to trauma [7]. However, when considering the stressor criterion and revised symptom profile of PTSD, the concepts of STS, CF or VT are redundant. Instead, individualized responses to vicarious trauma in care providers should be investigated and conceptualized using the PTSD framework. In the context of care providers, it is also recommended that a separate dimension of burnout is incorporated into investigations, to acknowledge within-role disruption relating specifically to the workplace.

The Experience and Impact of Traumatic Perinatal Events on Care Providers

The limited research investigating the impact of vicarious exposure to traumatic perinatal events in healthcare providers was reviewed by Sheen, Slade and Spiby [14]. Of 42 papers retrieved, only four included health professionals who had indirectly experienced trauma within a childbirth context. Whilst research with midwives, nurse-midwives and nurses engaged in the provision of labour and delivery care has since increased, the experiences of medical staff are largely unexplored.

Type of Events

The types of maternity events most frequently perceived as traumatic by staff include demise or neonatal death, shoulder dystocia, infant resuscitation and maternal death [15, 16, 17]. However, perception of trauma is subjective. Although it is useful to identify the type of maternity events that may be perceived as traumatic, understanding why some events are perceived as traumatic may enable more effective identification of those at risk for traumatic stress.

Aspects influencing the perception of trauma during traumatic perinatal events have been identified through qualitative methodology. Feeling helpless during a birthing event due to disagreement with decisions made by other clinicians, perceiving physicians to be using overly forceful approaches, feeling unable to access resources or additional personnel when required and having an existing bond with a mother have been cited as contributing to trauma perception [15, 17, 18, 19, 20].

Prevalence of Traumatic Stress

Wallbank and Robertson [21] conducted a survey investigating the impact of experiencing loss (miscarriage, neonatal death and stillbirth) among UK doctors (n= 38), nurses (n= 42) and midwives (n= 104). Over half (55%) of the total sample exceeded the clinical cut off for 'severe' symptoms of intrusion and avoidance. Symptoms of intrusion and avoidance in doctors and midwives following similar experiences of loss were also identified in an earlier survey [22]. However, for both of these studies [21, 22], levels of response were not disaggregated by professional role and therefore conclusions regarding the experiences of each professional group are limited.

Sheen, Spiby and Slade [13] conducted the first large-scale UK investigation of midwives' experiences of traumatic perinatal events. Midwives (n= 421, 16% response rate) were recruited using the national membership database of the UK Royal College of Midwives. Findings confirmed that a proportion, representative of approximately one in six, of UK midwives had experienced trauma corresponding to the DSM-IV Criterion A for PTSD (APA, 2000). Approximately one in 20 midwives reported clinically significant symptoms of PTSD. These figures are highly likely to underestimate the true proportion of midwives with traumatic stress responses, as it makes the assumption that all midwives who did not return their survey were entirely non-symptomatic [13]. As a key feature of PTSD is avoidance, it is possible that a proportion of midwives contacted will not have returned their questionnaire due to the distress elicited by recounting their traumatic experience.

A similar prevalence for traumatic stress responses was identified by Beck and Gable [16] in a survey of US labour and delivery ward nurses (n= 464). The authors measured symptoms of intrusion, avoidance and arousal (conceptualized as STS) and identified that 35% were experiencing moderate to severe levels of traumatic stress. Beck et al. [17] also conducted an electronic survey of US-certified nurse-midwives' responses to traumatic birthing events. Clinically relevant levels of PTS symptomatology were reported by 36% (n= 170) of the sample. The large sample sizes and national recruitment strategies used by Sheen et al. [13], Beck and Gable [16] and Beck et al. [17] strengthen the generalizability of findings. However, response rates between all three studies are similarly low (16%, 15% and 5% respectively), which introduces the potential for selection bias.

Further research specifically considering experiences of obstetricians is required. One small qualitative study with Irish consultants identified the emotional impact of encountering stillbirth through the provision of care. Although responses were not conceptualized within a PTSD framework, responses reported by consultants reflected this symptom pattern [23].

Aspects Increasing Vulnerability to Traumatic Stress

Empathy

Empathy is a primary feature of maternity care, cited by both care providers and women in receipt of care as integral to a positive birthing experience [24]. The sensitivity of maternity care provided is an important determinant of women's experiences of giving birth and postpartum mental health [25]. Whilst empathy can facilitate sensitive care, it may also increase risk for the care provider to experience traumatic stress as empathic engagement can increase the extent to which an adverse event is internalized [5].

Rice and Warland [19] conducted qualitative interviews with 10 midwives in Australia. Midwives identified that having a bond with the mother increased their own levels of distress during an adverse event. Such bonds may come from having developed relationships with the woman in maternity care systems that involve continuity of care provider or from providing support through the process of labour care. Sheen et al. [13] reported that midwives scoring high on a measure of empathic concern reported significantly higher levels of PTS symptomatology. Further research, especially with obstetricians, is required in order to explore the extent to which

empathy may increase vulnerability to traumatic stress responses.

Organizational Stress

Symptoms of traumatic stress are often highly associated with elevated levels of burnout in care providers exposed to trauma [13, 14]. Sheen et al. [13] reported that higher levels of PTS symptomatology significantly predicted elevated levels of emotional exhaustion and depersonalization. Burnout is associated with increased absenteeism, increased staff turnover and a poorer quality of work [26], with implications for organizational efficiency. It is not clear whether PTS predisposes individuals to increased burnout, whether elevated burnout increases vulnerability to traumatic stress responses, or whether this relationship is bi-directional. However, evidence to date indicates that organizational climate is an intrinsic factor in the perception of trauma and subsequent psychological response.

Prior Trauma Exposure

Prior trauma exposure has been identified as a risk factor for PTSD [27]. In Sheen et al.'s [13] study, midwives who had experienced a previous traumatic event in their personal lives (unrelated to childbirth) reported higher levels of PTS symptomatology. In addition, midwives who had experienced a larger number of traumatic perinatal events whilst providing care for women reported higher levels of PTSD symptoms. This latter finding indicates a potential for repeated exposure to traumatic perinatal events in the workplace to be associated with higher levels of PTSD symptoms. Both findings highlight the potential for personal and workplace-related traumatic events to increase vulnerability to PTS responses.

Extent of Professional Experience

The extent of professional experience at the time of vicarious trauma exposure may influence the development of PTSD responses. Fewer years in the profession was associated with more frequent symptoms of intrusion, avoidance and arousal (conceptualized as STS) in labour and delivery nurses [16]. However, the duration of professional experience was not associated with symptoms of PTSD in UK midwives [13]. It is highly likely that professional experience is not linearly related to traumatic stress responses. It is also possible that care providers with longer professional experience represent those more 'resilient' to trauma exposure. Studies to date have included maternity care professionals who were registered in their profession at the time of completion; therefore, further investigations with those who choose to leave their profession altogether is required. In addition, there is only limited understanding about maternity care professionals' experiences prior to qualification. Research with midwives, nurse-midwives and obstetricians during training would further understanding about the association between the duration of experience as a care provider, trauma experience and the development of PTSD responses.

Implications

Experiencing trauma and traumatic stress responses can adversely impact upon personal and professional well-being. Traumatic stress responses are by their nature highly distressing for the individual. Literature highlighting the impact of trauma exposure with medical professionals is limited; however, Gold et al. [28] conducted a large survey with US physicians (n= 804) to investigate the impact of stillbirth or neonatal death on care providers. Over a fifth (22%) of respondents strongly agreed that the experience of stillbirth had an 'emotional toll' on them and over a third (34%) felt guilty and blamed themselves. Feelings of self-blame and guilt reflect findings from studies with midwives, nurse-midwives and labour and delivery ward nurses after experiencing a traumatic perinatal event [16, 17]. Sadness and fear have also been reported by studies with midwives, nurse-midwives and labour and delivery ward nurses [15, 17, 19, 18]. The impact of experiencing trauma is reported as enduring, with distinct memories easily recalled for several years afterwards [15, 17, 18].

The experience of trauma has also been associated with considerations to leave midwifery or nurse-midwifery practice altogether, change the location of clinical work, take sick leave or move to a non-clinical role [13, 16, 17, 28]. In a sample of UK midwives who had experienced a traumatic perinatal event whilst providing care, Sheen et al. [13] reported that 35% of respondents had seriously considered leaving midwifery altogether following a traumatic perinatal experience. Midwives with symptoms meeting criteria for clinical PTSD were significantly more likely to report that they had considered leaving the profession. Avoidance of clinical areas associated with the event or increased anxiety at subsequent similar births has also been reported [15]. Additional impacts include

practising in an increasingly defensive manner (e.g., intervening sooner to avoid a similar result) [13] or 'distancing' oneself in order to cope [18]. Findings indicate that if PTSD develops following indirect exposure to trauma, then implications can involve either desensitization and avoidant behaviour, or burnout and loss from the clinical workforce. In either case, there is a loss of highly skilled staff, and a loss of original investment in pre-registration education, appointment and continuing professional development.

Furthermore, the experience of PTS responses and high emotional exhaustion is likely to impact upon caregivers' ability to engage in compassionate care. A care provider who is emotionally exhausted, or who is experiencing symptoms of PTSD, may unconsciously avoid engagement with recipients of care. This holds implications for the experiences of mothers, for whom the experiencing of birthing and subsequent postpartum health can be influenced by the nature of care provided [25].

The potential for increased organizational stress in response to investigative procedures taking place after an adverse maternity event has also been identified [15, 18]. A qualitative study with labour and delivery ward nurses who were present during a shoulder dystocia reported feeling 're-traumatized' by subsequent investigations and litigation procedures that took place [15]. Investigations following an adverse maternity event are important for maintaining safe and effective maternity care. However, there is the additional potential for these to exacerbate care providers' responses to the event.

Supportive Strategies

The impact of adverse perinatal events on staff is largely unacknowledged [19]. Working within a supportive working environment has been identified as beneficial [17]. Peer support and reflection on practice are reported as helpful for maintaining midwives' well-being and resilience [29].

Talking about the event and debriefing with colleagues without fear of repercussion have been reported as beneficial for overcoming the impact of traumatic perinatal event exposure [17, 19]. The term 'debriefing' is often used in an ambiguous and unspecific way. Traditionally, the term 'debriefing' included a structured and formal approach to investigating cognitive, emotional and affective responses to a traumatic event, for example, Critical Incident

Stress Debriefing (CISD) [30]. However, it has also been used to refer to a conversation about an event that has been difficult [31]. The provision of structured CISD is controversial and is contraindicated for the prevention of PTSD [32]. However, there is emerging evidence with postpartum women to suggest that the provision of an opportunity to discuss a childbirth experience with a care provider reduces symptoms of PTSD and depression [33]. In the current context of care providers, the term 'debriefing' was used to refer to an informal discussion with colleagues about a maternity event [19], and not the provision of a structured debriefing programme. It is possible that the provision of an opportunity to discuss a maternity event that has been perceived as difficult may beneficially impact upon care providers.

Interventions

A limited number of studies have investigated the utility of interventions aimed at reducing the development of PTS responses in care providers who are exposed to a traumatic perinatal event.

A pilot study with midwives, obstetricians and gynaecologists (n= 30) indicated that supervision from a clinical psychologist reduced PTSD symptoms following neonatal death, stillbirth or miscarriage [22]. Staff members received six sessions with a clinical psychologist, lasting up to one hour. The supervision adopted a 'restorative' approach, aimed at supporting individual emotional and psychological needs and included strategies for processing anxiety and emotions, in addition to a focus on interpersonal relationships with women in receipt of care. Foureur et al. [34] piloted a mindfulness-based stress reduction intervention with midwives (n= 20) and nurses (n= 20) in Australia. Although trauma exposure and response were not measured, there was a significant reduction in depression and stress, and an increased perceived ability to cope with stress 8 weeks later.

Recommendations

Recommendations for Research

Whilst current evidence indicates that medical staff encounter events they perceive as traumatic [21, 22, 28], this needs to be further explored. It is likely that there will be similarities between the clinical events perceived as traumatic by medical and midwifery or nursing staff. However, differences between professional roles may also introduce different predisposing factors.

Therefore, specific consideration of obstetricians' experiences is required.

Greater understanding of factors predisposing, precipitating and maintaining PTSD responses in care providers is also required, taking into account personal and workplace variables (e.g., organizational climate, support). From this, a framework for predicting vulnerability to traumatic stress responses can be developed to aid early identification of individuals who may be vulnerable to traumatic stress.

There is also a need to systematically develop and evaluate methods of preparing care providers for the potential to experience trauma, and to prevent the development of PTSD symptoms. Increased understanding about the nature of traumatic experiences and potential responses can reduce the likelihood that PTSD occurs [35]. Care providers need to be provided with information about the potential to experience trauma, nature of initial symptoms and when responses may indicate a need to seek further input. Increased understanding of this nature can aid the 'normalization' of responses should they occur following a difficult event, which can reduce the likelihood that PTSD develops [35].

Consideration of the experiences of trainee care providers is also required. One qualitative study investigating the experience of traumatic events with student midwives, who were two-thirds of the way through their training, identified responses synonymous with PTSD [36]. The student midwives reported reliving events and fearing entering the same clinical area on their own. Some reported that they felt unprepared for experiencing some of the maternity events that had occurred and doubted their ability to work as a midwife. A potential implication of not preparing student care providers prior to trauma exposure is attrition from training programmes; therefore, understanding ways to prepare and support trainees is essential.

Clinical Recommendations

The importance of staff well-being is paramount to the provision of effective, safe maternity care and to maintaining a healthy and efficient workforce. Vicarious exposure to trauma holds adverse impacts at both the individual and organizational level. It is important that managers are aware that some maternity events may be perceived as traumatic by care providers, and that timely identification of those experiencing difficulty is essential. In addition, awareness of impacts to the organization through staff retention and absenteeism is required.

There is currently no specific guidance for care providers to be aware of the potential for traumatic perinatal events to impact upon them. The development and evaluation of interventions to prepare care providers for trauma exposure, as described in the previous section, will inform the potential utility of providing additional information for care providers at both the pre- and post-registration stages.

Finally, it is essential that care providers who are experiencing PTSD are provided with appropriate assessment and psychological input. Current recommendations advocate the provision of trauma-focused cognitive behavioural therapy (TF-CBT) or eye movement desensitization and reprocessing (EMDR) [37]. The provision of non-directive counselling for individuals with PTSD is contraindicated [37].

Conclusion

Vicarious exposure to traumatic perinatal events has the potential to adversely influence care providers' well-being, their professional practice and the experiences of women in receipt of care. Vicarious exposure to trauma can result in PTSD, is associated with elevated burnout syndrome and may influence decisions to leave the profession. Despite emerging interest in the impact of vicarious trauma on care providers, the available evidence for maternity professionals is small and there is a paucity of research specifically considering the experiences of obstetric staff. Further research identifying factors that predispose care givers to PTSD, or indeed what may prevent this, is required. It is also essential that methods of preparing staff for trauma exposure, increasing support and facilitating access to effective interventions for those with PTSD are developed. Through this, the health and well-being of staff, quality of care and efficiency of the maternity services will be enhanced.

Key Points

- Vicarious exposure to trauma has the potential to elicit the same adverse psychological responses as identified in individuals who are directly affected by trauma. The potential consequences include PTSD, secondary traumatic stress, compassion fatigue and vicarious traumatization.
- The types of maternity events most frequently perceived as traumatic by staff include demise or neonatal death, shoulder dystocia, infant resuscitation and maternal death. However, perception of trauma is subjective.
- At least 1 in 6 of UK midwives have experienced trauma corresponding to the DSM-IV Criterion A for PTSD and at least one in 20 midwives report clinically significant symptoms of PTSD.
- Empathy can facilitate sensitive care, but may also increase risk for the care provider to experience traumatic stress.
- Organizational climate is an intrinsic factor in health professionals' perception of trauma and their subsequent psychological response.
- Repeated exposure to traumatic events in the personal lives of health professionals or in their workplace is associated with higher levels of PTSD symptoms. If PTSD develops following indirect exposure to trauma, then the potential implications include inability to engage in compassionate care, desensitization and avoidant behaviour, burnout and loss from the clinical workforce.

References

1. American Psychological Association. *Diagnostic and Statistical Manual of Mental Disorders (V)*. Washington DC, American Psychiatric Association, 2013.

2. American Psychological Association. *Diagnostic and Statistical Manual of Mental Disorders (IV-TR)*. Washington DC, American Psychiatric Association, 2010.

3. Brewin CR, Dalgleish T, Joseph S. A dual representation theory of posttraumatic stress disorder. *Psychological Review* 1996; **103**(4): 670–686. doi: 10.1037//0033-295x.103.4.670.

4. Ehlers A, Clark, DM. A cognitive model of posttraumatic stress disorder. *Behaviour Research and Therapy* 2000; **38**(4): 319–345. doi: 10.1016/s0005-7967(99)00123-0.

5. Figley CR. Compassion fatigue as secondary traumatic stress disorder: An overview. In: Figley CR, ed. *Compassion fatigue: Coping with secondary traumatic stress disorder in those who treat the traumatized*. New York, Routledge, 1995; 1–20.

6. Joinson C. Coping with compassion fatigue. *Nursing* 1992; **22**(4): 118–120.

7.   Stamm BH. The Concise ProQOL Manual. 2nd ed. Pocatello (ID). 2010. www.proqol.org/ProQOl_Test_Manuals.html. (Accessed 26 March 2017).

8.   Pearlman L, Mac Ian PS. Vicarious traumatization: An empirical study of effects of trauma work on trauma therapists. *Professional Psychology-Research and Practice* 1995; **26**(6): 558–565. doi: 10.1037/0735–7028.26.6.558.

9.   Pearlman LA. *Trauma and attachment belief scale.* Los Angeles, Western Psychological Services, 2003.

10. Pearlman L, Saakvitne KW. *Trauma and the therapist: Countertransference and vicarious traumatization in psychotherapy with incest survivors.* New York, Norton and Company, 1995.

11. Maslach C, Shaufeli WB, Leiter MP. Job burnout. *Annual Review of Psychology* 2001; **52**: 397–422.

12. Jenkins S, Baird S. Secondary traumatic stress and vicarious trauma: A validational study. *Journal of Traumatic Stress* 2002; **15**(5): 423–432.

13. Sheen K, Spiby H, Slade P. Exposure to traumatic perinatal experiences and posttraumatic stress symptoms in midwives: Prevalence and association with burnout. *International Journal of Nursing Studies* 2015; **52**(2): 578–587. doi: 10.1016/j.ijnurstu.2014.11.006.

14. Sheen K, Slade P, Spiby H. An integrative review of the impact of indirect trauma exposure in health professionals and potential issues of salience for midwives. *Journal of Advanced Nursing* 2014; **70**(4): 729–743. doi: 10.1111/jan.12274.

15. Beck CT. The obstetric nightmare of shoulder dystocia: A tale from two perspectives. *Mcn-the American Journal of Maternal-Child Nursing* 2013; **38**(1): 34–40. doi: 10.1097/NMC.0b013e3182623e71.

16. Beck CT, Gable RK. A Mixed Methods Study of Secondary Traumatic Stress in Labor and Delivery Nurses. *Journal of Obstetric Gynecologic and Neonatal Nursing* 2012; **41**(6): 747–760. doi: 10.1111/j.1552–6909.2012.01386.x.

17. Beck CT, LoGiudice J, Gable RK. A mixed-methods study of secondary traumatic stress in certified nurse-midwives: Shaken belief in the birth process. *Journal of Midwifery & Women's Health* 2015; **60**(1): 16–23. doi: 10.1111/jmwh.12221.

18. Puia DM, Lewis L, Beck CT. Experiences of obstetric nurses who are present for a perinatal loss. *Journal of Obstetric Gynecologic and Neonatal Nursing* 2013; **42**(3): 321–331. doi: 10.1111/1552–6909.12040.

19. Rice H, Warland J. Bearing witness: Midwives experiences of witnessing traumatic birth. *Midwifery* 2013; **29**(9): 1056–1063. doi: 10.1016/j.midw.2012.12.003.

20. Sheen K, Spiby H, Slade P. The experience and impact of traumatic perinatal event experiences in midwives: A qualitative investigation. *International Journal of Nursing Studies* 2016; **53**: 61–72. doi: 10.1016/j.ijnurstu.2015.10.003.

21. Wallbank S, Robertson N. Predictors of staff distress in response to professionally experienced miscarriage, stillbirth and neonatal loss: A questionnaire survey. *International Journal of Nursing Studies* 2013; **50**(8): 1090–1097. doi: 10.1016/j.ijnurstu.2012.11.022.

22. Wallbank S. Effectiveness of individual clinical supervision for midwives and doctors in stress reduction: Findings from a pilot study. *Evidence Based Midwifery* 2010; **8**(2): 65–70.

23. Nuzum D, Meaney S, O'Donoghue K. The impact of stillbirth on consultant obstetrician gynaecologists: A qualitative study. *BJOG: An International Journal of Obstetrics & Gynaecology* 2014; **121**(8): 1020–1028. doi: 10.1111/1471–0528.12695.

24. Hunter B. The importance of reciprocity in relationships between community-based midwives and mothers. *Midwifery* 2006; **22**(4): 308–322. doi: 10.1016/j.midw.2005.11.002.

25. Elmir R, Schmied V, Wilkes L, Jackson D. Women's perceptions and experiences of a traumatic birth: A meta-ethnography. *Journal of Advanced Nursing* 2010; **66**(10): 2142–2153. doi: 10.1111/j.1365–2648.2010.05391.x.

26. Maslach C, Jackson SE, Leiter MP, Schaufeli WB, Schwab RL. *MBI: The maslach burnout inventory: Manual.* Palo Alto, Consulting Psychologists Press, 1996.

27. Ozer EJ, Best SR, Lipsey TL, Weiss DS. Predictors of posttraumatic stress disorder and symptoms in adults: A meta-analysis. *Psychological Bulletin* 2003; **129**(1): 52–73. doi: 10.1037//0033–2909.129.1.52.

28. Gold KJ, Kuznia AL, Hayward RA. How physicians cope with stillbirth or neonatal death: A national survey of obstetricians. *Obstetrics and Gynecology* 2008; **112**(1): 29–34. doi: 10.1097/AOG.0b013e31817d0582.

29. Hunter B, Warren L. *Investigating resilience in midwifery: Final report.* Cardiff, Cardiff University, 2013.

30. Mitchell JT. When disaster strikes . . . the critical incident stress debriefing process. *Journal of Emergency Medical Services* 1997; **8**: 36–39.

31. Alexander J. Confusing debriefing and defusing postnatally: The need for clarity of terms. *purpose and value. Midwifery* 1998; **14**(2): 122–124.

32. Rose S, Bisson J, Churchill R, Wessel S. Psychological debriefing for preventing post traumatic stress disorder (PTSD). *Cochrane Database Systematic Reviews* 2002; **2**(2): CD000560.

33. Sheen K, Slade P. The efficacy of 'debriefing' after childbirth: Is there a case for targeted intervention? *Journal of Reproductive and Infant Psychology* 2015; **33**(3): 308–320. doi: 10.1080/02646838.2015.1009881.

34. Foureur M, Besley K, Burton G, Yu N, Crisp J. Enhancing the resilience of nurses and midwives: Pilot of a mindfulness-based program for increased health, sense of coherence and decreased depression, anxiety and stress. *Contemporary Nurse* 2013; **45**(1): 114–125.

35. Wessley S, Bryant R, Greenberg N, Earnshaw M, Sharpley J, Hughes J. Does psychoeducation help prevent posttraumatic psychological stress? *Psychiatry* 2008; **71**: 287–307.

36. Davies S, Coldridge L. 'No Man's Land': An exploration of the traumatic experiences of student midwives in practice. *Midwifery* 2015; **31**(9): 858-64. doi: 10.1016/j.midw.2015.05.001.

37. National Institute for Health and Care Excellence. Post-traumatic stress disorder (PTSD): The management of PTSD in adults and children in primary and secondary care. 2005. https://www.nice.org.uk/Guidance/cg26 (Accessed 27 March 2017).

Biopsychosocial Care after the Loss of a Baby

Chapter 41

Leroy C. Edozien

Introduction

Parents who lose their baby through miscarriage, ectopic gestation, stillbirth or termination for genetic or structural anomalies face a difficult time; historically, the care they receive following this traumatic event has not always taken cognizance of the emotional element of their care. Universally the care of women and partners after the loss of a baby falls below their expectations: studies of parents' experiences in both westernized [1, 2] and low-income countries [3, 4] show gross inadequacies in the provision of biopsychosocial care. Studies also show that the behaviours and actions of staff have a memorable impact on parents. There are unmet educational needs for doctors, midwives and nurses. The deficiencies in education and clinical practice are accompanied by a paucity of clinical research in what is clearly a major concern in maternity care [5].

The Psychological Impact of Losing a Baby

Emotional Impact

The loss of a baby is a deeply saddening event that occurs at a time when joy and fulfilment are anticipated. The emotional impact may include feelings of disbelief, anger, blame, guilt or helplessness as well as crying openly or privately. There may be a loss of self-esteem and loss of confidence in the prospect of becoming a parent. It is important for doctors, midwives and nurses to appreciate that each parent may respond in their own way. The ability to maintain steady psychological and physical functioning (i.e. resilience) in the aftermath of a bereavement varies from person to person. After the initial shock, the parent(s) may suffer continued emotional distress as they mentally revisit the events surrounding the loss or when they see parents with healthy babies.

In addition to and associated with the emotional dimension, there may be behavioural, physical and cognitive dimensions to the parent(s) reaction. The grief reaction may lead them to isolate themselves from family and friends, to sleep a lot or to have disordered eating patterns. Cognitive elements include intrusive and anxious thoughts. Physically, the parent may feel tired all the time or have other symptoms such as palpitations.

Prolonged Grief and Risk of Persisting Mental Health Disorder

The grief reaction is a natural response to bereavement. Various coping mechanisms are employed by the parent and substantial psychological recovery occurs after a few months. In some cases, however, there is continued inability to resume normal psychological and physical functioning. This state has variously been termed 'prolonged grief disorder', 'complicated grief' or 'pathological grief'. Predictors of the development of complicated grief after the loss of a baby include pre-existing relationship difficulties, inadequate social support, presence of other life crises, absence of surviving children and physical or psychological traumatic health care [6]. Parents may be at risk of developing post-traumatic stress disorder (PTSD) as a consequence of perinatal loss [7] (see Chapter 39). Prolonged grief could persist even after the subsequent birth of a healthy child. The quality of care given by doctors, midwives and nurses can help reduce the chances that the parent(s) will progress from a physiological to a pathological grief process, so it is of critical importance that staff should be competent in delivering care that addresses biopsychosocial factors.

Sometimes, perinatal loss occurs in a woman who has a background history of mental health disorder and this combination, as well as the synergistic effect, goes unrecognized by health-care providers.

Impact on the Father

Compared to mothers, much less is known about the impact of perinatal loss on fathers [8]. Generally, fathers' grief responses appear to be similar to mothers'. They suffer the same feelings of shock, anger, emptiness, helplessness and loneliness, but some quantitative studies have shown these to be less intense than mothers' grief responses. It is hypothesized that the social requirement for the father to support his spouse through a difficult time explains the less intense grief reaction. The mother rather than father being treated as a 'patient' in hospital may also be a factor. Given the heterogeneity and methodological limitations of existing studies, no robust conclusions can be drawn and so each couple should be treated according to their own circumstances and wishes. What is important is for health professionals to appreciate that the father has his own need for support while also supporting the mother. Renaissance man was expected to be stoic but in modern times it has become acceptable for men to cry, as was the case in biblical times.

Impact on the Couple's Relationship

Parental relationships have a higher risk of dissolving after miscarriage or stillbirth, compared with live birth [9]. Differing patterns of grief could potentially lead to a decline in the couple's relationship. If, for example, the father wishes to move on but the mother is still grieving (or progressing to prolonged grief disorder) this could introduce conflict. Anxieties about the prospects of another pregnancy may induce tension in the relationship. One partner may blame the other for the unfortunate outcome of the pregnancy. While a live birth could enhance the security of a relationship, the stress of losing an unborn or stillborn baby could overwhelm the relationship, especially if there was pre-existing strain. The loss could, on the other hand, bind a couple more strongly. As with other aspects of bereavement care, doctors, midwives and nurses should sensitively and non-judgmentally ascertain the needs of the particular couple and tailor their professional support accordingly.

Implications for Other Children

The impact on the couple's relationships with their other children also varies [10]. While some may neglect the siblings, albeit temporarily, others may become more attached to the siblings. Bereavement midwives should support parents in recognizing the potential impact of their grief reaction on other children (where this applies) and in particular the potential impact of prolonged grief reaction on the child or children.

Peri-partum Care Following Stillbirth

The care received during and after stillbirth may have lasting impact on parents' future well-being. There is a lack of high-quality randomized trials of support interventions for mothers, fathers and families after perinatal death [11]. There is enough evidence, however, concerning what parents want [12–16], and authoritative clinical practice guidance is available [17–19].

The key elements in the management of a woman and her partner after a perinatal loss are communication; emotional support; support in decision-making, particularly (for stillbirths/neonatal deaths) in relation to holding the baby and post-mortem examination. Additionally, there is the importance of the investigations to determine the cause of perinatal loss.

Communication

Doctors, midwives and nurses should communicate with bereaved parents in an empathic and sensitive manner. Informing the woman and her partner in an appropriate manner that their baby has died requires communication skills (see Chapter 4). Information provided to the parent(s) about what has happened, what will be done, what support is available and their options regarding delivery and disposal of the baby or fetal tissue should be clear. This includes not only information on clinical issues such as induction of labour but also information on administrative issues such as how to register their baby's birth and how to arrange for a funeral.

The parent(s) should be given a contact telephone number on which they can contact the unit at any time, day or night.

Emotional Support

The parent(s) should be cared for in a physical and psychological environment that is conducive to their emotional well-being. In most contemporary maternity units there is a dedicated room or suite for bereaved mothers and their partner. This insulates them, to some extent, from the noise and the crying babies in the delivery unit. The wishes of the parent(s) should be continually ascertained and respected. This helps reduce psychological distress. For example, some parents may want the midwife or doctor to remain in the room and support them for a while after the demise of their baby while others will want a period of privacy, to be alone. If their preference is not elicited, the midwife or doctor leaving or remaining in the room may be seen as abandoning the couple or intruding on their privacy.

As much as possible continuity of carer should be maintained, so that a relationship of empathy and trust is sustained and the parent is protected from distress associated with repetition of the same questions and answers.

Parents should be reassured that their feelings (see section on 'Emotional Impact' above) are normal and that recovery may take a few months. Those particularly at risk of prolonged grief or post-traumatic stress disorder should be identified. Counselling should be offered as appropriate.

When a woman has experienced a stillbirth, some mothers wish to proceed immediately with delivery of the baby. Others wish to go back home, take some time for emotional recovery in a familiar environment and then return to hospital for delivery of the baby. If there are no compelling medical reasons (sepsis, haemorrhage, severe pre-eclampsia or ruptured membranes), there should be no rush to effect immediate delivery. Stillborn babies will usually be delivered spontaneously within three weeks of their demise, but many parents will find it more emotionally traumatic to carry a dead baby for more than a few days. Retaining the baby *in utero* for up to 4 weeks increases the risk of maternal coagulopathy. Also, if the baby is not delivered within 2–3 days the body becomes macerated and this poses difficulties when the baby is seen and held by the parents after birth and when post-mortem examination is performed.

The parent(s) should be offered contact with local and national support groups which offer informational, instrumental and emotional support to bereaved parents. Sands, originally known as the Stillbirths and Neonatal Death Society (SANDS), is well known for its work in this regard [20]. Referrals for professional support should also be made as appropriate.

Mementos such as photographs, locks of hair and hand and foot prints are also emotional supports for some, and the staff should guide the parents in choosing which mementos they wish to keep.

Clinical Management

Following a miscarriage, the method of disposal of the products of conception should be discussed with the woman and her partner, and local protocols should be followed. In cases of stillbirth, mode of delivery and decisions regarding burial or cremation of the baby should be discussed. Following a stillbirth diagnosed antenatally, induction of labour and vaginal birth is the usual course but a caesarean delivery may be indicated for medical reasons or occasionally for maternal preference. Caesarean delivery of a dead baby in the absence of a medical indication may rightly be considered to be a drastic intervention, and the implications should be explained to the woman and her partner. If it remains her preference to have a caesarean birth, then this should be respected. Persistent attempts to persuade her to have vaginal birth would cause more distress at a time when the objective of care is to provide optimal emotional support.

For induction of labour, a single dose 200 mg oral mifepristone is given to ripen the cervix and the woman is admitted 24–48 hours later for administration of prostaglandin (usually misoprostol). Pain relief should be administered as required.

After delivery, an external examination of the baby should be performed and the baby's weight should be plotted on a customized growth chart (where this is in use) to exclude fetal growth restriction and to explore the possibility of placental insufficiency. Lactation is suppressed with cabergoline 1 mg, single oral dose (contraindicated in women with hypertensive disease or psychosis). Before discharge, advice is given on contraception.

The parents should be advised that there is no specific time interval that must elapse before they try for another pregnancy; they can start once they feel physically and psychologically ready for this.

Investigations

The investigations performed after a miscarriage or stillbirth will depend on the circumstances of the particular case. It is important for the parent(s) to know that, often, the cause of fetal death may remain unknown despite extensive investigation. The following investigations are usually performed after a stillbirth:

Kleihauer test – to exclude fetomaternal haemorrhage

Serology –Toxoplasma, Rubella, Cytomegalovirus, Herpes simplex and Parvovirus B19

Bile salts

HbA1 c

Thyroid function tests

Fetal chromosome analysis

Swab taken from the baby's axilla and sent for microscopy and culture

Swabs of the maternal and fetal surfaces of the placenta taken for microscopy and culture

Histopathological examination of the placenta

Sepsis screen, if indicated – maternal blood culture, urine microscopy and culture, culture of vaginal and endocervical swabs

Thrombophilia screen (indications: recurrent perinatal loss, pre-eclampsia, coagulopathy, fetal growth restriction)

Maternal urine for toxicology, if indicated (e.g. cocaine use)

Administrative Matters

The mother's GP is formally informed of the stillbirth.

All pending antenatal and scan appointments are cancelled. A clinic appointment letter or reminder sent routinely because the appointment has not been cancelled could cause substantial emotional distress to the family.

The birth is registered. Arrangements for a funeral or cremation are agreed with the mother and partner.

A postnatal follow up appointment is arranged. This would be the time to review events and results and discuss the management of the next pregnancy. The woman's psychological well-being is assessed and features of post-traumatic stress disorder are sought.

To Hold the Baby or Not to Hold?

It is common practice to encourage parents to have contact with their dead baby. There are advantages and disadvantages to this and the subject should be carefully discussed with the parent(s) as soon as is possible. Seeing the baby, holding the baby and spending time with the baby could be beneficial to the grieving and recovery processes and provide succour

and memories that are cherished for a lifetime. Being with the baby also affords the opportunity for the family to grieve together. On the other hand, a parent may be psychologically traumatized by seeing a dead baby and particularly one with gross abnormality, and may be put at risk of post-traumatic stress disorder [21]. As with other aspects of the management of perinatal loss, there is only limited research on this topic and the existing work gives variable results. A narrative synthesis of studies comparing outcomes for parents who held their baby or engaged in other memory-making activities and those who did not showed mixed results regarding the impact of holding the stillborn baby on mental health and well-being [22]. An Australian study showed that mothers who saw and held their baby had higher levels of grief (measured by the Perinatal Grief Scale) than mothers who chose not to see their baby [23]. This may be a reflection of mother–baby bonding (see Chapter 28). One study found an overall beneficial effect of having held a stillborn baby born after 37 gestational weeks, whereas findings for having held a stillborn baby born at gestational weeks 28–37 were uncertain [24].

For some parents, not seeing the baby facilitates detachment and closure and prevents unwanted imprinting of the baby in their memory, but other parents prefer to have this imprinting [25].

In some instances, even where mothers experienced intense distress during the contact with their stillborn baby, they reported that this contact was still important to them and they felt in retrospect that they had made the right decision [26].

It appears that women who had a multiple birth and those whose pregnancy resulted from fertility treatment are less likely to hold their baby [27, 28].

Further research could inform clinical practice but it is likely that personal, cultural and spiritual factors and the role of the care provider will remain influential. Each parent is different and the care provided should be in tune with her/his informed preferences. The way in which maternity staff present the subject of seeing the baby and explore the confidence of the parent(s) in coping with this will influence the long-term impact of their seeing the baby [29, 30]. It is a very difficult time for the parent(s) and they need support in their decision-making. Some parents would subsequently regret their decision not to see the baby and care providers should endeavour, in a gentle and respectful way, to give the parents every opportunity to reconsider their decision while it is still possible to do so.

Parents wishing to spend time with the baby should be offered the use of the cooling cot (if available) to maintain baby's skin condition, making it possible for the parents to spend more time with the baby.

Perinatal Loss of a Co-twin

Parents who have lost one baby of a twin or higher-order multiple birth face a different set of challenges from parents of deceased singletons [31, 32]. They face the challenge of grieving for one baby while welcoming, bonding with, and looking after the other(s). In many cases, the surviving baby is in the neonatal intensive or special care unit, which poses further challenges.

The parent may grieve for the lost baby and not bond with the surviving baby/babies. At the other end, the parent may focus on the survivor(s) and defer the grief process, only to suffer psychological distress downstream. Between these extremes is the parent that is torn between grief and parenthood, and is confused. Doctors and midwives should avoid the tendency to ask the parent to 'focus on the positive'. The bereavement support should be no less than the parent would receive had their baby been a singleton. Casual, insensitive comments should be avoided.

Post-mortem Examination

There are some cases of perinatal loss where the cause of death is obvious and a post-mortem examination would add little or no additional information. In other cases, however, a post-mortem examination has the potential to provide new information that explains or confirms the cause of death. When post-mortem examination yields this information, it helps the parents understand the cause of death and, importantly, facilitates closure. Further, it informs the management of the next pregnancy. In many cases, however, post-mortem examination fails to explain the cause of death. It is important that bereaved parents should be made aware of this possibility (or probability) at the time of discussing the advisability of the examination, otherwise the failure of post-mortem examination to provide answers to their question could result in frustration, anger and further emotional turmoil. It is important also to provide balanced information on the value and limitations of post-mortem examination as parents could be distraught at the thought that their baby could be cut up for no benefit and they may

for this reason decline consent for the examination. Post-mortem examinations should be performed by appropriately trained perinatal pathologists, as this reduces the number of cases where a plausible explanation for fetal demise is not found. Other reasons for declining post-mortem examination of the baby are religious and cultural (in particular, the belief in, and practice of, burying the dead as soon as possible). In the United Kingdom, the scandal of unauthorized paediatric organ retention by pathologists appears to account for a significant fall in the number of parents consenting to post-mortem examination of their babies. This has been addressed through an improvement in consent and governance procedures.

About 1 in 3 of parents who decline post-mortem examination would subsequently regret their decision. The quality of explanation or counselling about this examination may influence not only the decision of the parents but also the prospect that they will subsequently regret their decision. For this and other reasons, obstetricians and midwives should have the appropriate training [33, 34].

The consent discussion should be held at a time that suits the parents and should not be rushed. They should be given every opportunity to ask questions and given time to consider their options.

The doctor or midwife obtaining consent should understand the autopsy process and be able to explain to the parents that the examination will entail the preparation of tissue blocks and slides, and also to explain the option of a less invasive autopsy – see Judge-Kronis et al for outline descriptions [35]. Less invasive autopsy usually entails post-mortem imaging (MR scan, CT scan or X-ray) and/or selective tissue sampling. The doctor or midwife should be familiar with the legal framework that applies in their country. In England, Wales and Northern Ireland, the handling of babies' bodies is regulated by the Human Tissue Act 2004. In Scotland, the Human Tissue (Scotland) Act 2006 applies. These laws require that specific consent should be obtained for each of the following: post-mortem examination, genetic testing, retention of organs, retention of DNA, imaging and use of materials for education or research.

Pregnancy after a Perinatal Loss

When a woman becomes pregnant after a perinatal loss the predominant emotions are not, as in most wanted pregnancies, those of joy and relief but those of fear and anxiety [36, 37]. The psychological distress and anxiety increase the risk of adverse short-term and long-term outcomes (see Chapter 30 'Maternal Psychosocial Distress'). The anxiety tends to increase as the pregnancy approaches the gestational age at which the preceding stillbirth occurred. Heightened anxiety also occurs when critical tests such as fetal anatomy scan are to be performed. Pregnancies that follow a stillbirth are associated with an increased risk of intrauterine growth restriction (IUGR), premature birth and another stillbirth. Compared with women who had a live birth in their first pregnancy, those who had already experienced a stillbirth were almost five times more likely to experience a stillbirth in their second pregnancy [38].

Not surprisingly, the emphasis of medical staff in the subsequent pregnancy is on more monitoring and more technology. While this is valued by the parents, they also need biopsychosocial support, but this is often neglected by care providers. Doctors and midwives should assist the parents in devising strategies for coping with their feelings of uncertainty and bonding with the unborn baby.

Of course, this facilitator role cannot be played if the doctor or midwife does not recognize the parent's emotional status and needs in the first place. The key elements in the management of a woman and her partner during the subsequent pregnancy are similar to those outlined above for perinatal loss: communication; emotional support; support in decision-making. Empathy, listening skills and sensitive communication are critical to ensuring positive experience for the parents in a pregnancy after stillbirth [39].

Tailored care extends to the provision of antenatal education. Parents with a history of previous stillbirth feel uncomfortable attending classes with first-time parents and other parents who have not had the experience of a stillbirth. They feel more comfortable in the company of parents with similar experience from whom they can derive peer support, and this is an advantage provided by dedicated clinics held for women with a previous stillbirth. Even in such company, however, peers could drift apart and lose that support if one couple has a smooth-sailing pregnancy while another has obstetric complications in the index pregnancy.

Training of Doctors and Midwives

While the quality of care provided to parents at the time of perinatal loss and in their subsequent pregnancy strongly influences their grieving process

and their longer-term psychological well-being, many obstetricians and midwives do not feel sufficiently equipped and confident to provide the support that the parents require. This is partly due to the absence or inadequacy of specific training on the management of perinatal loss in undergraduate and post-qualification training, but also on the absence of a biopsychosocial approach across the board in obstetrics, gynaecology and maternity care. A qualitative study of UK senior obstetricians identified a training gap that needs to be bridged [40]. While some training needs are generic (e.g. communication skills), others are specific. For example, specific training should be provided on the obtaining of consent under the provisions of the United Kingdom legislation on consent, and perinatal pathologists have a role to play in this [41]. Training should also recognize the emotional toll of bereavement care on doctors, midwives and nurses and equip them to deal with this as best as they can.

Conclusion

Parents who lose a baby face severe psychological trauma, regardless of the gestational age at which the loss happens. They need tailored support and optimal care during this challenging time. Often, however, the quality of care delivered does not meet their expectations or has not been adapted to meet the particular needs and circumstances of the parents. Communication failures or inadequacies add to their grief. Recognition of the biopsychosocial factors described in this chapter and delivery of care that is underpinned by the biopsychosocial approach could provide psychological safety for the parents and potentially enhance their long-term well-being. Delivery of this quality of care calls for inclusion of these factors in undergraduate and postgraduate training.

Key Points

- The ability to maintain steady psychological and physical functioning (i.e. resilience) in the aftermath of a bereavement varies from person to person. Each bereaved parent will respond in their own way, and care should be tailored to their needs.
- Some bereaved parents remain unable to resume normal psychological and physical functioning ('prolonged grief disorder').

- The quality of care given by doctors, midwives and nurses can help reduce the chances that the parent(s) will progress from a physiological to a pathological grief process.
- Doctors, midwives and nurses should be aware of the potential impact of perinatal loss on the father, on the couple's relationship and on other children of the family.
- The key elements in the management of a woman and her partner after a perinatal loss are communication; emotional support; support in decision-making, particularly (for stillbirths) in relation to holding the baby and post-mortem examination; and investigations to determine the cause of perinatal loss.
- The wishes of the couple regarding aspects of care after birth, such as holding the baby, should be ascertained and respected. Appropriate information should be provided. This will help reduce the likelihood of later regret by the parents.
- Doctors and midwives should be aware of the legal framework and communication requirements for obtaining consent to post-mortem examination after perinatal loss.
- Parents need the same level of empathy and sensitive communication in the subsequent pregnancy.

References

1. Redshaw M, Rowe R, Henderson J. *Listening to parents after stillbirth or the death of their baby after birth.* Oxford; National Perinatal Epidemiology Unit, April 2014.

2. Kelley MC, Trinidad SB. Silent loss and the clinical encounter: Parents' and physicians' experiences of stillbirth-a qualitative analysis. *BMC Pregnancy Childbirth* 2012;**12**:137. doi: 10.1186/1471–2393-12-137.

3. Sereshti M, Nahidi F, Simbar M, Ahmadi F, Bakhtiari M, Zayeri F. Mothers' perception of quality of services from health centers after perinatal loss. *Electron Physician* 2016;**8**(2):2006–17. doi: 10.19082/2006.

4. Simwaka AN, de Kok B, Chilemba W. Women's perceptions of Nurse-Midwives' caring behaviours during perinatal loss in Lilongwe, Malawi: An exploratory study. *Malawi Med J* 2014;**26**(1):8.

5. Koopmans L, Wilson T, Cacciatore J, Flenady V. Support for mothers, fathers and families after perinatal death. *Cochrane Database Syst Rev* 2013;(**6**):CD000452. doi: 10.1002/14651858.CD000452.pub3.

6. Kersting A, Wagner B. Complicated grief after perinatal loss. *Dialogues Clin Neurosci* 2012;**14**(2):187–94.

7. Christiansen DM, Elklit A, Olff M. Parents bereaved by infant death: PTSD symptoms up to 18 years after the loss. *Gen Hosp Psychiatry* 2013;**35**(6):605–11. doi: 10.1016/j.genhosppsych.2013.06.006.

8. Badenhorst W, Riches S, Turton P, Hughes P. The psychological effects of stillbirth and neonatal death on fathers: Systematic review. *J Psychosom Obstet Gynecol* 2006;**27**(4):245–56.

9. Gold KJ, Sen A, Hayward RA. Marriage and cohabitation outcomes after pregnancy loss. *Pediatrics* 2010;**125**(5):e1202–7. doi: 10.1542/peds.2009–3081.

10. Human M, Green S, Groenewald C, Goldstein RD, Kinney HC, Odendaal HJ. Psychosocial implications of stillbirth for the mother and her family: A crisis-support approach. *Social Work (Stellenbosch)* 2014;**50**(4).pii:392.

11. Koopmans L, Wilson T, Cacciatore J, Flenady V. Support for mothers, fathers and families after perinatal death. *Cochrane Database Syst Rev* 2013;(**6**):CD000452. doi: 10.1002/14651858.CD000452.pub3.

12. Peters MD, Lisy K, Riitano D, Jordan Z, Aromataris E. Caring for families experiencing stillbirth: Evidence-based guidance for maternity care providers. *Women Birth* 2015;**28**(4):272–8. doi: 10.1016/j.wombi.2015.07.003.

13. Lisy K, Peters MD, Riitano D, Jordan Z, Aromataris E. Provision of meaningful care at diagnosis, birth, and after stillbirth: A qualitative synthesis of parents' experiences. *Birth* 2016;**43**(1):6–19. doi: 10.1111/birt.12217.

14. Gausia K, Moran AC, Ali M, Ryder D, Fisher C, Koblinsky M. Psychological and social consequences among mothers suffering from perinatal loss: Perspective from a low income country. *BMC Public Health* 2011;**11**:451. doi: 10.1186/1471–2458-11–451.

15. Ellis A, Chebsey C, Storey C, Bradley S, Jackson S, Flenady V, Heazell A, Siassakos D. Systematic review to understand and improve care after stillbirth: A review of parents' and healthcare professionals' experiences. *BMC Pregnancy Childbirth* 2016;**16**:16. doi: 10.1186/s12884-016-0806-2.

16. Sutan R, Miskam HM. Psychosocial impact of perinatal loss among Muslim women. *BMC Women's Health* 2012;**12**:15. doi: 10.1186/1472–6874-12–15.

17. Peters MD, Lisy K, Riitano D, Jordan Z, Aromataris E. Caring for families experiencing stillbirth: Evidence-based guidance for maternity care providers. *Women Birth* 2015;**28**(4):272–8. doi: 10.1016/j.wombi.2015.07.003.

18. Heazell AE, Leisher S, Cregan M, Flenady V, Frøen JF, Gravensteen IK, de Groot-Noordenbos M, de Groot P, Hale S, Jennings B, McNamara K, Millard C, Erwich JJ. Sharing experiences to improve bereavement support and clinical care after stillbirth: Report of the 7th annual meeting of the International Stillbirth Alliance. *Acta Obstet Gynecol Scand* 2013;**92**(3):352–61. doi: 10.1111/aogs.12042.

19. Royal College of Obstetricians and Gynaecologists. Intrauterine fetal death and stillbirth. Green-top guideline 55. London: RCOG; 2010.

20. Sands, the stillbirth and neonatal death charity. www .sands.org.uk/. Accessed 27 March 2017.

21. Cacciatore J, Rådestad I, Frederik Frøen J. Effects of contact with stillborn babies on maternal anxiety and depression. *Birth* 2008;**35**(4):313–20. doi: 10.1111/j.1523-536X.2008.00258.x.

22. Hennegan JM, Henderson J, Redshaw M. Contact with the baby following stillbirth and parental mental health and well-being: A systematic review. *BMJ Open* 2015;**5**(11):e008616. doi: 10.1136/bmjopen-2015–008616.

23. Wilson PA, Boyle FM, Ware RS. Holding a stillborn baby: The view from a specialist perinatal bereavement service. *Aust N Z J Obstet Gynaecol* 2015;**55**(4):337–43. doi: 10.1111/ajo.12327.

24. Rådestad I, Surkan PJ, Steineck G, Cnattingius S, Onelöv E, Dickman PW. Long-term outcomes for mothers who have or have not held their stillborn baby. *Midwifery* 2009;**25**(4):422–9.

25. Sun JC, Rei W, Sheu SJ. Seeing or not seeing: Taiwan's parents' experiences during stillbirth. *Int J Nurs Stud* 2014;**51**(8):1153–9. doi: 10.1016/j.ijnurstu.2013.11.009.

26. Ryninks K, Roberts-Collins C, McKenzie-McHarg K, Horsch A. Mothers' experience of their contact with their stillborn infant: An interpretative phenomenological analysis. *BMC Pregnancy Childbirth* 2014;**14**:203. doi: 10.1186/1471–2393-14–203.

27. Redshaw M, Hennegan JM, Henderson J. Impact of holding the baby following stillbirth on maternal mental health and well-being: Findings from a national survey. *BMJ Open* 2016;**6**(8):e010996. doi: 10.1136/bmjopen-2015–010996.

28. Swanson PB, Kane RT, Pearsall-Jones JG, Swanson CF, Croft ML. How couples cope with the death of a twin or higher order multiple. *Twin Res Hum Genet* 2009;**12**(4):392–402. doi: 10.1375/twin.12.4.392.

29. Erlandsson K, Warland J, Cacciatore J, Rådestad I. Seeing and holding a stillborn baby: Mothers' feelings in relation to how their babies were presented to them after birth–findings from an online

30. questionnaire. *Midwifery* 2013;**29**(3):246–50. doi: 10.1016/j.midw.2012.01.007.

30. Kingdon C, O'Donnell E, Givens J, Turner M. The role of healthcare professionals in encouraging parents to see and hold their stillborn baby: A meta-synthesis of qualitative studies. *PLoS One* 2015;**10**(7):e0130059. doi: 10.1371/journal.pone.0130059.

31. Richards J, Graham R, Embleton ND, Campbell C, Rankin J. Mothers' perspectives on the perinatal loss of a co-twin: A qualitative study. *BMC Pregnancy Childbirth* 2015;**15**:143. doi: 10.1186/s12884-015–0579-z.

32. Swanson PB, Kane RT, Pearsall-Jones JG, Swanson CF, Croft ML. How couples cope with the death of a twin or higher order multiple. *Twin Res Hum Genet* 2009;**12**(4):392–402. doi: 10.1375/twin.12.4.392.

33. Downe S, Kingdon C, Kennedy R, Norwell H, McLaughlin MJ, Heazell AE. Post-mortem examination after stillbirth: Views of UK-based practitioners. *Eur J Obstet Gynecol Reprod Biol* 2012;**162**(1):33–7. doi: 10.1016/j.ejogrb.2012.02.002.

34. Heazell AE, McLaughlin MJ, Schmidt EB, Cox P, Flenady V, Khong TY, Downe S. A difficult conversation? the views and experiences of parents and professionals on the consent process for perinatal postmortem after stillbirth. *BJOG* 2012;**119**(8):987–97. doi: 10.1111/j.1471–0528.2012.03357.x.

35. Judge-Kronis L, Hutchinson JC, Sebire NJ, Arthurs OJ. Consent for paediatric and perinatal postmortem investigations: Implications of less invasive autopsy. *Journal of Forensic Radiology and Imaging* 2016;(4):7–11.

36. Mills TA, Ricklesford C, Cooke A, Heazell AE, Whitworth M, Lavender T. Parents' experiences and expectations of care in pregnancy after stillbirth or neonatal death: A metasynthesis. *BJOG* 2014;**121**(8):943–50. doi: 10.1111/14 71–0528.12656.

37. Campbell-Jackson L, Bezance J, Horsch A. 'A renewed sense of purpose': Mothers' and fathers' experience of having a child following a recent stillbirth. *BMC Pregnancy Childbirth* 2014;**14**:423. doi: 10.1186/s12884-014–0423-x.

38. Lamont K, Scott NW, Jones GT, Bhattacharya S. Risk of recurrent stillbirth: Systematic review and meta-analysis. *BMJ* 2015;**350**:h3080. doi: 10.1136/bmj.h3080.

39. Mills TA, Ricklesford C, Heazell AE, Cooke A, Lavender T. Marvellous to mediocre: Findings of national survey of UK practice and provision of care in pregnancies after stillbirth or neonatal death. *BMC*

Pregnancy Childbirth 2016;**16**:101. doi: 10.1186/s12884-016-0891-2.

40. Nuzum D, Meaney S, O'Donoghue K. The impact of stillbirth on consultant obstetrician gynaecologists: A qualitative study. *BJOG* 2014;**121**(8):1020–8. doi: 10.1111/1471-0528.12695.

41. Heazell AE, McLaughlin MJ, Schmidt EB, Cox P, Flenady V, Khong TY, Downe S. A difficult conversation? the views and experiences of parents and professionals on the consent process for perinatal postmortem after stillbirth. *BJOG* 2012;**119**(8):987–97. doi: 10.1111/j.1471-0528.2012.03357.x.

Appendix: RCOG Checklist of Hints and Tips to Support Clinical Practice in the Management of Gender-Based Violence

1. **Get knowledgeable**

   Find out how domestic and sexual violence affects women and girls.

   Broaden your understanding of domestic and sexual violence.

   Find your local and domestic abuse professional support services and ask their advice.

   Encourage colleagues and reception staff to do the same.

   What is the situation in your local community?

2. **Be open-minded and ready for the unknown**

   Think about missed opportunities.

   Learn to recognize behaviours.

   Make sure you're not stereotyping – you can't tell by looking at people.

   Be prepared for hidden stories – don't make assumptions.

3. **Create a safe and welcoming environment**

   Display information and helplines for patients in waiting rooms.

   Remember what your options are – e.g. chaperone, translator, panic button, inviting a female colleague.

   Avoid escalating the situation.

4. **Build rapport and trust**

   Think about your body language – is it encouraging your patient to trust you?

   Show you care, understand and believe your patient.

   Give your patient your full attention and explain you can and will help.

   Recognize that your patient has strength and courage.

5. **Keep an eye out for red flags**

   Multiple attendances for different problems (or non-attendance).

   'Inexplicable' or 'vague' symptoms invite deeper enquiry – other vulnerabilities, repeat terminations or losses, no contraception, a 'controlling' partner.

   Review a patient's notes – the red flags may appear.

   Think about the danger your patient might be in.

   Use the word 'harm' rather than 'violence'.

   Note down potential patterns of abuse.

6. **Trust your instincts**

   Listen to your gut feelings or hunches about a situation.

   Pay attention to that 'uneasy' feeling when you think something is wrong.

   BUT don't leap to a diagnosis – it's better to say 'I don't know' than get it wrong.

   Alert the next person about your concerns and feelings.

7. **Your responses – what do you do when a patient discloses?**

   Listen, validate and don't judge.

   Avoid clumsy responses, e.g. looking shocked.

   Protect confidentiality but check with your patients what they consent to being disclosed to other agencies – e.g. police, social services.

   Have telephone numbers to hand for help, especially if the patient is in immediate danger and needs a refuge.

   Tell the patient what you are going to do next.

   Remember – doing a little is better than nothing but doing nothing is better than harm.

8. **Safe reporting and safe referral**

   Is this an emergency? Is there immediate danger?

Think about referrals and ongoing care.

Are there any children involved?

Document everything and share with colleagues if given consent to do so.

Document potential patterns to avoid missed opportunities in future.

9. **Follow up**

Involve a wider sphere of professionals, including domestic violence experts.

Try to arrange another appointment with the patient at a suitable time and follow up.

Don't act alone, discuss cases in confidence with supervisors/trusted experts.

Remember – social service referral is available at any stage.

10. **Strengthening systems**

Seek training for you and your team from experts in domestic violence.

Be especially aware and informed of vulnerability of younger girls.

Work together as a team with colleagues (medical and admin) to provide a safe, informative environment.

Demonstrate and encourage professional curiosity among your colleagues.

Look to institutionalize the practice of reflective learning.

Index